Advances in Autism Research

Editor
Antonio Narzisi
IRCCS Stella Maris of Calambrone (Pisa)
Adjunct Professor at University of Pisa
Italy

Editorial Office
MDPI
St. Alban-Anlage 66
4052 Basel, Switzerland

This is a reprint of articles from the Special Issue published online in the open access journal *Actuators* (ISSN 2076-0825) (available at: https://www.mdpi.com/journal/brainsci/special_issues/Advance_Autism_Research).

For citation purposes, cite each article independently as indicated on the article page online and as indicated below:

LastName, A.A.; LastName, B.B.; LastName, C.C. Article Title. *Journal Name* **Year**, *Volume Number*, Page Range.

Volume 1
ISBN 978-3-0365-0162-8 (Hbk)
ISBN 978-3-0365-0163-5 (PDF)

Volume 1-2
ISBN 978-3-0365-0204-5 (Hbk)
ISBN 978-3-0365-0205-2 (PDF)

Cover image courtesy of pixabay.com user John Silver.

© 2021 by the authors. Articles in this book are Open Access and distributed under the Creative Commons Attribution (CC BY) license, which allows users to download, copy and build upon published articles, as long as the author and publisher are properly credited, which ensures maximum dissemination and a wider impact of our publications.

The book as a whole is distributed by MDPI under the terms and conditions of the Creative Commons license CC BY-NC-ND.

Advances in Autism Research

Volume 1

Editor

Antonio Narzisi

MDPI • Basel • Beijing • Wuhan • Barcelona • Belgrade • Manchester • Tokyo • Cluj • Tianjin

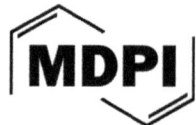

Contents

About the Editor ix

Antonio Narzisi
The Challenging Heterogeneity of Autism: Editorial for Brain Sciences Special Issue
"Advances in Autism Research"
Reprinted from: *Brain Sci.* **2020**, *10*, 948, doi:10.3390/brainsci10120948 1

Antonio Narzisi
Handle the Autism Spectrum Condition during Coronavirus (COVID-19) *Stay at Home* Period:
Ten Tips for Helping Parents and Caregivers of Young Children
Reprinted from: *Brain Sci.* **2020**, *10*, 207, doi:10.3390/brainsci10040207 17

Gabriele Masi, Silvia Scullin, Antonio Narzisi, Pietro Muratori, Marinella Paciello, Deborah Fabiani, Francesca Lenzi, Maria Mucci and Giulia D'Acunto
Suicidal Ideation and Suicidal Attempts in Referred Adolescents with High Functioning Autism Spectrum Disorder and Comorbid Bipolar Disorder: A Pilot Study
Reprinted from: *Brain Sci.* **2020**, *10*, 750, doi:10.3390/brainsci10100750 21

Jacopo Troisi, Reija Autio, Thanos Beopoulos, Carmela Bravaccio, Federica Carraturo, Giulio Corrivetti, Stephen Cunningham, Samantha Devane, Daniele Fallin, Serguei Fetissov, Manuel Gea, Antonio Giorgi, François Iris, Lokesh Joshi, Sarah Kadzielski, Aletta Kraneveld, Himanshu Kumar, Christine Ladd-Acosta, Geraldine Leader, Arlene Mannion, Elise Maximin, Alessandra Mezzelani, Luciano Milanesi, Laurent Naudon, Lucia N. Peralta Marzal, Paula Perez Pardo, Naika Z. Prince, Sylvie Rabot, Guus Roeselers, Christophe Roos, Lea Roussin, Giovanni Scala, Francesco Paolo Tuccinardi and Alessio Fasano
Genome, Environment, Microbiome and Metabolome in Autism (GEMMA) Study Design: Biomarkers Identification for Precision Treatment and Primary Prevention of Autism Spectrum Disorders by an Integrated Multi-Omics Systems Biology Approach
Reprinted from: *Brain Sci.* **2020**, *10*, 743, doi:10.3390/brainsci10100743 33

Jinhee Lee, Min Ji Son, Chei Yun Son, Gwang Hun Jeong, Keum Hwa Lee, Kwang Seob Lee, Younhee Ko, Jong Yeob Kim, Jun Young Lee, Joaquim Radua, Michael Eisenhut, Florence Gressier, Ai Koyanagi, Brendon Stubbs, Marco Solmi, Theodor B. Rais, Andreas Kronbichler, Elena Dragioti, Daniel Fernando Pereira Vasconcelos, Felipe Rodolfo Pereira da Silva, Kalthoum Tizaoui, André Russowsky Brunoni, Andre F. Carvalho, Sarah Cargnin, Salvatore Terrazzino, Andrew Stickley, Lee Smith, Trevor Thompson, Jae Il Shin and Paolo Fusar-Poli
Genetic Variation and Autism: A Field Synopsis and Systematic Meta-Analysis
Reprinted from: *Brain Sci.* **2020**, *10*, 692, doi:10.3390/brainsci10100692 49

Cecilia Perin, Giulio Valagussa, Miryam Mazzucchelli, Valentina Gariboldi, Cesare Giuseppe Cerri, Roberto Meroni, Enzo Grossi, Cesare Maria Cornaggia, Jasmine Menant and Daniele Piscitelli
Physiological Profile Assessment of Posture in Children and Adolescents with Autism Spectrum Disorder and Typically Developing Peers
Reprinted from: *Brain Sci.* **2020**, *10*, 681, doi:10.3390/brainsci10100681 75

Sanae Tanaka, Aiko Komagome, Aya Iguchi-Sherry, Akiko Nagasaka, Teruko Yuhi,
Haruhiro Higashida, Maki Rooksby, Mitsuru Kikuchi, Oko Arai, Kana Minami,
Takahiro Tsuji and Chiharu Tsuji
Participatory Art Activities Increase Salivary Oxytocin Secretion of ASD Children
Reprinted from: *Brain Sci.* 2020, *10*, 680, doi:10.3390/brainsci10100680 93

Flavia Marino, Paola Chilà, Chiara Failla, Ilaria Crimi, Roberta Minutoli, Alfio Puglisi,
Antonino Andrea Arnao, Gennaro Tartarisco, Liliana Ruta, David Vagni
and Giovanni Pioggia
Tele-Assisted Behavioral Intervention for Families with Children with Autism Spectrum
Disorders: A Randomized Control Trial
Reprinted from: *Brain Sci.* 2020, *10*, 649, doi:10.3390/brainsci10090649 103

Amy Jane Griffiths, Amy Hurley Hanson, Cristina M. Giannantonio, Sneha Kohli Mathur,
Kayleigh Hyde and Erik Linstead
Developing Employment Environments Where Individuals with ASD Thrive:Using Machine
Learning to Explore Employer Policies and Practices
Reprinted from: *Brain Sci.* 2019, *10*, 632, doi:10.3390/brainsci10090632 115

Rehab H. Alsaedi
An Assessment of the Motor Performance Skills of Children with Autism Spectrum Disorder in
the Gulf Region
Reprinted from: *Brain Sci.* 2020, *10*, 607, doi:10.3390/brainsci10090607 137

Jessica Barsotti, Gloria Mangani, Roberta Nencioli, Lucia Pfanner, Raffaella Tancredi,
Angela Cosenza, Gianluca Sesso, Antonio Narzisi, Filippo Muratori, Paola Cipriani and
Anna Maria Chilosi
Grammatical Comprehension in Italian Children with Autism Spectrum Disorder
Reprinted from: *Brain Sci.* 2020, *10*, 510, doi:10.3390/brainsci10080510 157

Elisa Leonardi, Antonio Cerasa, Francesca Isabella Famà, Cristina Carrozza, Letteria Spadaro,
Renato Scifo, Sabrina Baieli, Flavia Marino, Gennaro Tartarisco, David Vagni,
Giovanni Pioggia and Liliana Ruta
Alexithymia Profile in Relation to Negative Affect in Parents of Autistic and Typically
Developing Young Children
Reprinted from: *Brain Sci.* 2020, *10*, 496, doi:10.3390/brainsci10080496 169

Chiara Cristofani, Gianluca Sesso, Paola Cristofani, Pamela Fantozzi, Emanuela Inguaggiato,
Pietro Muratori, Antonio Narzisi, Chiara Pfanner, Simone Pisano, Lisa Polidori,
Laura Ruglioni, Elena Valente, Gabriele Masi and Annarita Milone
The Role of Executive Functions in the Development of Empathy and Its Association
with Externalizing Behaviors in Children with Neurodevelopmental Disorders and Other
Psychiatric Comorbidities
Reprinted from: *Brain Sci.* 2020, *10*, 489, doi:10.3390/brainsci10080489 183

Stefano Damiani, Pietro Leali, Guido Nosari, Monica Caviglia, Mariangela V. Puci,
Maria Cristina Monti, Natascia Brondino and Pierluigi Politi
Association of Autism Onset, Epilepsy, and Behavior in a Community of Adults with Autism
and Severe Intellectual Disability
Reprinted from: *Brain Sci.* 2020, *10*, 486, doi:10.3390/brainsci10080486 199

Patricia Garcia Primo, Christoph Weber, Manuel Posada de la Paz, Johannes Fellinger,
Anna Dirmhirn and Daniel Holzinger
Explaining Age at Autism Spectrum Diagnosis in Children with Migrant and Non-Migrant
Background in Austria
Reprinted from: *Brain Sci.* 2020, *10*, 448, doi:10.3390/brainsci10070448 207

Antonio Narzisi, Mariasole Bondioli, Francesca Pardossi, Lucia Billeci, Maria Claudia Buzzi,
Marina Buzzi, Martina Pinzino, Caterina Senette, Valentina Semucci, Alessandro Tonacci,
Fabio Uscidda, Benedetta Vagelli, Maria Rita Giuca and Susanna Pelagatti
"Mom Let's Go to the Dentist!" Preliminary Feasibility of a Tailored Dental Intervention for
Children with Autism Spectrum Disorder in the Italian Public Health Service
Reprinted from: *Brain Sci.* 2020, *10*, 444, doi:10.3390/brainsci10070444 225

Natascia Brondino, Stefano Damiani and Pierluigi Politi
Effective Strategies for Managing COVID-19 Emergency Restrictions for Adults with Severe
ASD in a Daycare Center in Italy
Reprinted from: *Brain Sci.* 2020, *10*, 436, doi:10.3390/brainsci10070436 245

Valentina Bianco, Alessandra Finisguerra, Sonia Betti, Giulia D'Argenio and Cosimo Urgesi
Autistic Traits Differently Account for Context-Based Predictions of Physical and Social Events
Reprinted from: *Brain Sci.* 2020, *10*, 418, doi:10.3390/brainsci10070418 251

Roberto Keller, Silvia Chieregato, Stefania Bari, Romina Castaldo, Filippo Rutto,
Annalisa Chiocchetti and Umberto Dianzani
Autism in Adulthood: Clinical and Demographic Characteristics of a Cohort of Five Hundred
Persons with Autism Analyzed by a Novel Multistep Network Model
Reprinted from: *Brain Sci.* 2020, *10*, 416, doi:10.3390/brainsci10070416 271

Pamela Papangelo, Martina Pinzino, Susanna Pelagatti, Maddalena Fabbri-Destro and
Antonio Narzisi
Human Figure Drawings in Children with Autism Spectrum Disorders: A Possible Window on
the Inner or the Outer World
Reprinted from: *Brain Sci.* 2020, *10*, 398, doi:10.3390/brainsci10060398 285

Lucia Billeci, Ettore Caterino, Alessandro Tonacci and Maria Luisa Gava
Behavioral and Autonomic Responses in Treating Children with High-Functioning Autism
Spectrum Disorder: Clinical and Phenomenological Insights from Two Case Reports
Reprinted from: *Brain Sci.* 2020, *10*, 382, doi:10.3390/brainsci10060382 297

Angela Caruso, Letizia Gila, Francesca Fulceri, Tommaso Salvitti, Martina Micai,
Walter Baccinelli, Maria Bulgheroni and Maria Luisa Scattoni
Early Motor Development Predicts Clinical Outcomes of Siblings at High-Risk for Autism:
Insight from an Innovative Motion-Tracking Technology
Reprinted from: *Brain Sci.* 2020, *10*, 379, doi:10.3390/brainsci10060379 311

Kimon Runge, Ludger Tebartz van Elst, Simon Maier, Kathrin Nickel, Dominik Denzel,
Miriam Matysik, Hanna Kuzior, Tilman Robinson, Thomas Blank, Rick Dersch,
Katharina Domschke and Dominique Endres
Cerebrospinal Fluid Findings of 36 Adult Patients with Autism Spectrum Disorder
Reprinted from: *Brain Sci.* 2020, *10*, 355, doi:10.3390/brainsci10060355 327

Marco Colizzi, Elena Sironi, Federico Antonini, Marco Luigi Ciceri, Chiara Bovo and Leonardo Zoccante
Psychosocial and Behavioral Impact of COVID-19 in Autism Spectrum Disorder: An Online Parent Survey
Reprinted from: *Brain Sci.* **2020**, *10*, 341, doi:10.3390/brainsci10060341 343

Simonetta Panerai, Raffaele Ferri, Valentina Catania, Marinella Zingale, Daniela Ruccella, Donatella Gelardi, Daniela Fasciana and Maurizio Elia
Sensory Profiles of Children with Autism Spectrum Disorder with and without Feeding Problems: A Comparative Study in Sicilian Subjects
Reprinted from: *Brain Sci.* **2020**, *10*, 336, doi:10.3390/brainsci10060336 357

Mariangela Gulisano, Rita Barone, Salvatore Alaimo, Alfredo Ferro, Alfredo Pulvirenti, Lara Cirnigliaro, Selena Di Silvestre, Serena Martellino, Nicoletta Maugeri, Maria Chiara Milana, Miriam Scerbo and Renata Rizzo
Disentangling Restrictive and Repetitive Behaviors and Social Impairments in Children and Adolescents with Gilles de la Tourette Syndrome and Autism Spectrum Disorder
Reprinted from: *Brain Sci.* **2020**, *10*, 308, doi:10.3390/brainsci10050308 373

About the Editor

Antonio Narzisi is Lead Psychologist at the Department of Child Psychiatry and Psychopharmacology (Head: Gabriele Masi) at the IRCCS Stella Maris Foundation sited in Calambrone (Pisa) and Adjunct Professor at University of Pisa. He was born in Avola in the province of Siracusa (Sicily). Narzisi studied in Rome where he graduated in Psychology at La Sapienza University (Advisor: Massimo Ammaniti). He then moved to Tuscany, where he obtained his PhD in Developmental Neurosciences at the University of Pisa (Advisor: Filippo Muratori). He was certified as Psychotherapist at the Gestalt Institute HCC-Italy, Milan (Advisor: Margherita Spagnuolo Lobb). Narzisi is a recognized expert in the field of Autism Spectrum Disorder (ASD) and is specialized in evidence-based treatment models and gold standard diagnostic protocols. His clinical and research activity is focused on the diagnosis of Autism Spectrum Disorder, treatment outcomes, and the application of new technologies in the clinical and daily living settings. During the years, Narzisi was an active participant in the COST Action BM1004 (Enhancing the scientific study of early autism: A network to improve research, services, and outcomes) and has Full Membership at INSAR – International Society for Autism Research. In 2012, he was a visiting scientist at the Institute of Brain, Behavior and Mental Health, University of Manchester (UK) (Head: Jonathan Green). He has served as co-investigator in several research projects funded by the European Commission and Italian Ministry of Health. Narzisi is the author of numerous publications in recognized international journals. Narzisi has presented the results of his research in international conferences (USA, Canada, UK, France, Malta, Belgium, Morocco, and Italy). He teaches "Autism Best Practices" in several Italian universities, Masters and Clinical Institute that are accredited by the Italian National Health Service. He was recently nominated Local Coordinator (for IRCCS Stella Maris Foundation) of the bio-behavioral bank of ITAN (Italian Autism Network).

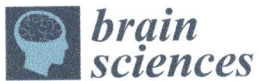
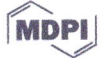

Editorial

The Challenging Heterogeneity of Autism: Editorial for Brain Sciences Special Issue "Advances in Autism Research"

Antonio Narzisi

Department of Child Psychiatry and Psychopharmacology, IRCCS Stella Maris Foundation, 56018 Pisa, Italy; antonio.narzisi@fsm.unipi.it

Received: 23 November 2020; Accepted: 30 November 2020; Published: 7 December 2020

1. Introduction

My personal experience as Guest Editor of the Special Issue (SI) entitled "Advances in Autism Research" began with a nice correspondence with Andrew Meltzoff, from the University of Washington, Seattle (WA, USA), which, in hindsight, I consider as a good omen for the success of this Special Issue: "*Dear Antonio . . . .I am happy you are editing a special issue on this important topic. It will be useful for society, as well as for psychology, neuroscience, and of course the children and families . . . . . . .Best, Andy.*"

Advances in Autism Research was a unique experience from a scientific and human point of view; 50 contributions took part in this SI from five Continents (see Appendix A). Globally, all the articles involved 356 authors and 156 reviewers between researchers and clinicians actively engaged in the field of autism spectrum disorder (ASD).

The SI saw, alongside a significant representation of the major Italian institutions that deal with ASD, the contribution of worldwide recognized experts in ASD such as Professor Sally Rogers from MIND Institute, CA, USA.

The SI took place during a very important historical period for the world community; the COVID-19 pandemic has profoundly changed our way of living every day as human beings and the way in which we are carrying out our work as researchers and clinicians.

The SI addressed many topics including: (1) COVID-19 pandemic; (2) Epidemiology and prevalence; (3) Screening and early behavioural markers; (4) Diagnostic and phenotypic profile; (5) Treatment and intervention; (6) Etiopathogenesis (Biomarkers, Biology, Genetic, Epigenetic and Risk Factor); (7) Autism and comorbidity; (8) Autism and adulthood; and (9) Broader Autism Phenotype (BAP).

2. COVID-19 Pandemic

The SI hosted three papers that described the COVID pandemic. First, Narzisi's editorial [1] whose goal was to help clinicians and parents manage the difficult moment of the lockdown that people with autism and their families have had to endure. Second, the research paper of Colizzi and colleagues [2] aimed to investigate the impact of the COVID-19 pandemic on ASD individuals. COVID-19 emergency resulted in a challenging period for 93.9% of families, increased difficulties in managing daily activities, especially free time and structured activities and children presenting with more intense and more frequent behavior problems. Third, the retrospective study of Brondino and colleagues [3] evaluated the impact of COVID-19 restrictions on challenging behaviors in a cohort of people with severe ASD attending a daycare center at the beginning of the pandemic. Authors showed that during the first two weeks of the pandemic, there were no observed variations in challenging behaviors. This suggested that adaptations used to support individuals with ASD in adapting to the COVID-19 emergency restrictions were effective for managing their behavior.

3. Epidemiology and Prevalence

In the field of epidemiology, Chiarotti and Venerosi [4], from the Italian National Institute of Health, presented an interesting review of the ASD prevalence estimates published since 2014. Data confirmed a high variability in prevalence across the world, likely due to methodological differences in case detection, and the consistent increase of prevalence estimates within each geographical area.

4. Screening and Early Behavioural Markers

The SI included six papers about the screening of ASD. Petrocchi and colleagues' study [5] provided a systematic review of level 1 and level 2 screening tools for the early detection of ASD under 24 months of age. Levante and colleagues [6] examined the cross-cultural generalisability of the First Year Inventory (FYI) on an Italian sample, testing its construct validity, consistency, and structural validity. Their findings supported the generalisability of the Italian version of the FYI and its validity. Devescovi and colleagues [7] aimed to identify early signs of atypical development consistent with ASD or other developmental disorders in a population of 224 low-risk toddlers through a two-stage screening approach applied at 12 and 18 months of age using the Communication and Symbolic Behavior Scales Developmental Profile (CSBS DP) Infant–Toddler Checklist (I-TC) and the Quantitative Checklist for Autism in Toddlers (Q-CHAT). Their results showed that autistic signs can be detected as early as the first year even though a few questions extrapolated from both screeners with potential benefit in terms of the screening procedure. Taresh and his group [8] presented a conceptual framework aimed to utilize the current literature to present a discussion on preschool teachers' knowledge, belief, identification skills, and self-efficacy (KBISSE) in identifying children with ASD and making decisions to refer children suspected with ASD to specialists. The conceptual framework emphasized the need for preschool teachers to be educated in ASD via an educational module that could increase teachers' self-efficacy in identifying children with ASD. Finally, the studies of Baccinelli [9] and Caruso [10], coordinated by Maria Luisa Scattoni from the Italian National Institute of Health, were aimed to investigate the early motor trajectories of infants at high-risk (HR) of ASD through MOVIDEA, a semi-automatic software developed to analyze 2D and 3D videos and provide objective kinematic features of their movements. Results revealed that early developmental trajectories of specific motor parameters were different in HR infants later diagnosed with Neuro-Developmental Disorders from those of infants developing typically.

5. Diagnostic and Phenotypic Profile

5.1. Motor Profile

Alsaedi's study [11] aimed to determine the prevalence, severity, and nature of the motor abnormalities in children with ASD as well as to elucidate the associated developmental profiles. The short-form of the Bruininks–Oseretsky Test of Motor Proficiency, Second Edition (BOT-2) was used to assess various aspects of the motor performance of children with ASD and typically developing from three Gulf states. The results revealed the high prevalence of motor abnormalities among the ASD group when compared with the normative data derived from the BOT-2 manual as well as with the data concerning the typically developing group.

5.2. Language Profile

Barsotti and colleagues [12] aimed to study the grammatical comprehension of children with ASD. The presence of receptive difficulties in school-age ASD children with relatively preserved non-verbal cognitive abilities could provide important hints to establish rehabilitative treatments. The main finding of the study showed that language comprehension is the most impaired language domain in ASD. The Gladfelter and Barron's study [13] explored whether global–local processing differences influence the type of semantic features children with ASD, developmental language disorder (DLD), and their neurotypical peers learn to produce when learning new words. Results indicated that the children with ASD and DLD produced more global, rather than local, semantic features in their definitions than the children with typical language. Shield [14] presented a longitudinal case study of a single child with ASD, a hearing, signing child of Deaf parents. Lexical signs and fingerspelled letters were coded for the four parameters of sign articulation (handshape, location, movement, and palm orientation). Longitudinal data suggested that palm orientation errors could be rooted in both imitation differences and motoric difficulties.

5.3. Neuropsychological Profile

Cristofani and colleagues [15] aimed to examine the role of empathic dimensions and executive skills in regulating externalizing behaviors. This study further corroborated developmental models of empathy and their clinical implications, for which externalizing behaviors could be attenuated by enhancing executive functioning skills.

The aim of the Andreou and Skrimpa's review [16] was to present the most recent available studies with respect to the connection between the function of mirror neurons in individuals with ASD and ToM-reflecting sensorimotor, social and attentional stimuli. The majority of these studies approach the theory of broken mirror neurons critically. Findings from electroencephalography (EEG) studies so far indicate that further research is necessary to shed more light on the mechanisms underlying the connection(s) between ToM and neurophysiological operations.

The study of Papangelo and the group of Maddalena Fabbri-Destro [17], from the Institute of Neurology of National Council of Research of Parma, was aimed to evaluate the performance of human figure drawings (HFD) of children with ASD relative to typically developing (TD) controls. Findings suggested that the use of HFD tests with individuals with ASD may not be used in clinical practices. However, in basic research, HFDs could be used to highlight dependencies between drawing performance and neuropsychological features, thus possibly providing hints on the functioning of autism.

5.4. Sensory Profile

The study of Panerai and colleagues [18] was aimed to better understand the relationship between sensory and feeding problems in ASD by comparing the sensory responsiveness of ASD children with (ASD-W) and without (ASD-WO) feeding problems. Both groups showed strengths in Visual/Auditory sensitivity, Low-Energy/Weak, and Movement sensitivity, again more marked in ASD-WO. The work of Perin and his group [19] was aimed to investigate the Physiological Profile Assessment (PPA) in children and adolescents with ASD compared with age-matched typically developing (TD) individuals and examine the relationship between the PPA subset within the ASD and TD participants according to different age groups. Performance in most of the PPA tests significantly improved with older age in the TD group but not in the ASD group. Molinaro and colleagues [20] conducted a review of visual impairments in ASD. They highlighted the finding that in the absence of a valid methodology adapted for the visually impaired population, diagnosis of ASD in children with VI is often based on non-objective clinical impression, with inconclusive prevalence data. The study of Valori and colleagues [21] assessed the feasibility and offered some early insights from a new paradigm for exploring how children and adults with ASD interact with Reality and Immersive Virtual Realities (IVR) when vision and proprioception are manipulated. The pilot indicates the good feasibility of the paradigm. Preliminary data visualisation suggests the importance of considering inter-individual variability.

5.5. Migrant Background

The study of Garcia-Primo and colleagues [22] explored (i) differences in age at ASD diagnosis between children with and without a migrant background in the main diagnostic centre for ASD in Upper Austria (ii) factors related to the age at diagnosis and (iii) whether specific factors differed between the two groups. No delay in diagnosing ASD in children with a migrant background in a country with universal health care and an established system of paediatric developmental surveillance was found. Awareness of ASD, including Asperger's syndrome, should be raised among families and healthcare professionals.

6. Treatment and Intervention

Fuller and the group of MIND Institute directed by Sally Rogers [23] conducted a meta-analysis in order to examine the effects of the Early Start Denver Model (ESDM) for young children with ASD on developmental outcome measures. Findings showed improvements in cognition and language. No significant effects were observed for measures of autism symptomology, adaptive behavior, social communication, or restrictive and repetitive behaviors. Marino and colleagues [24] presented an interesting RCT on telehealth. It was aimed at comparing the effect of a tele-assisted and in-person intervention based on a behavioral intervention protocol for families with children affected by ASDs.

Substantial improvements in the perception and management of children's behavior by parents, as well as in the influence of a reduction in parent stress levels on said children's behavior through the use of a tele-assisted intervention, were obtained. This trial demonstrated the evidence-based potential for telehealth to improve the treatment of ASDs. Bentenuto and colleagues [25] investigated intervention effects in terms of mediators and moderators in order to explain the variability and to highlight mechanisms of change in children with ASD. The findings support the importance of parental involvement in targeting ASD core symptoms. Further, results informed our understanding of early predictors in order to identify specific elements to be targeted in the individualized intervention design. Yazdani and colleagues [26] conducted an important review to evaluate the early behavioral intervention studies of ASD based on their participant exclusion criteria. Results indicated that studies that used restrictive exclusion criteria demonstrated greater differences in terms of outcomes between experimental and control groups in comparison to studies that used loosely defined exclusion criteria and/or did not define any exclusion criteria. The authors described implications for the generalizability of the studies' outcomes in relation to exclusion criteria. The study of Baker and colleagues [27] measured the reward positivity (RewP) in response to social and nonsocial stimuli in seven adolescents with ASD before and after participation in the Program for the Education and Enrichment of Relational Skills (PEERS®) intervention. Findings have implications for how neuroscience can be used as an objective outcome measure before and after intervention in ASD. Melongo and colleagues [28] reported a single case in which an intervention implemented to assist a 13.2-year-old boy with ASD without intellectual disability, aimed at improving his ability to compose persuasive texts was described. The Billeci and colleagues' paper [29] was aimed to evaluate the process applied in subjects with ASD to elaborate and communicate their experiences of daily life activities, as well as to assess the autonomic nervous system response that subtends such a process. This was a proof-of-concept study on the application of the cognitive–motivational–individualized (c.m.i.®), which needs to be extensively validated in the clinical setting. In terms of general care treatment, Narzisi and colleagues [30] described an experience of dental care supported by Information and Communication Technologies (ICT), for children with ASD in a public health service. The project demonstrated acceptability by parents, suggesting that public health dental care and prevention can be successfully implemented without resorting to costly pharmacological interventions (with potential side effects), taking better care of children's health.

7. Etiopathogenesis: Biomarkers, Biology, Genetic, Epigenetic and Risk Factor

Troisi and his group [31] described GEMMA (Genome, Environment, Microbiome and Metabolome in Autism), a prospective study supported by the European Commission, that follows at-risk infants from birth to identify potential biomarker predictors of ASD development followed by validation on large multi-omics datasets. The project includes clinical and pre-clinical studies in humanized murine models and in vitro colon models. This study will support the progress of a microbiome-wide association study (of human participants) to identify prognostic microbiome signatures and metabolic pathways underlying mechanisms for ASD progression and severity and potential treatment response.

Magdalena and colleagues [32] studied the preconception risk factors that are still poorly understood. The authors considered thirteen parameters for conception problems, conception with assisted reproductive techniques, the use and duration of oral contraception, the number of previous pregnancies and miscarriages, time since the previous pregnancy (in months), the history of mental illness in the family (including ASD), other chronic diseases in the mother or father and maternal and paternal treatment in specialist outpatient clinics. Findings showed that three factors statistically significantly increased the risk of developing ASD: mental illness in the mother/mother's family, maternal thyroid disease and maternal oral contraception. Pascucci and colleagues [33], coordinated by Antonio M. Persico from University Hospital of Messina (Italy), assessed the effects of a single acute injection of low- or high-dose of p-cresol in behavioral and neurochemical phenotypes of BTBR mice, a reliable animal model of human ASD. Findings support a gene–environment interaction model, whereby p-cresol, acting upon a susceptible genetic background, can acutely induce autism-like behaviors and produce abnormal dopamine metabolism in the reward circuitry. Lombardo and colleagues [34] aimed to evaluate markers of infections and immune activation in ASD by performing a meta-analysis of publicly available whole-genome transcriptomic datasets of brain samples from autistic patients and otherwise normal people. Overall, the data did not support an association between infection and ASD. Prosperi and his group [35] investigated the role of inflammatory biomarkers in ASD and their correlations with clinical phenotypes. The results did not highlight the presence of any systemic inflammatory state in ASD subjects neither disentangling children with/without GI symptoms. Lee and colleagues [36] aimed to verify noteworthy findings between genetic risk factors and ASD by employing the false-positive report probability (FPRP) and the Bayesian false-discovery probability (BFDP). In this study, the authors found noteworthy genetic comparisons highly related to an increased risk of ASD. Multiple genetic comparisons were shown to be associated with ASD risk. The Caria and colleagues' review [37] aimed to provide a critical synthesis of evidence linking alterations of the hypothalamus with impaired social cognition and behavior in ASD by integrating results of both anatomical and functional studies in individuals with ASD as well as in healthy carriers of oxytocin receptor (OXTR) genetic risk variant for ASD. Findings indicated that morphofunctional anomalies are implicated in the pathophysiology of ASD and call for further investigations aiming to elucidate anatomical and functional properties of hypothalamic nuclei underlying atypical socioemotional behavior in ASD. The review of Fusar-Poli and colleagues [38] was aimed to summarize the literature regarding the use of cannabinoids in ASD. The findings were promising, as cannabinoids appeared to improve some ASD-associated symptoms, such as problem behaviors, sleep problems, and hyperactivity, with limited cardiac and metabolic side effects. Conversely, the knowledge of their effects on ASD core symptoms is scarce. Tanaka and colleagues [39] in their pilot study focused on the neuroendocrinological response to participatory art activities, which are known to have a positive effect on emotion, self-expression, sociability, and physical wellbeing. These preliminary results suggested that the beneficial effects of participatory art activities may be partially mediated by oxytocin release, and may have therapeutic potential for disorders involving social dysfunction. The Stella Maris group [40] examined toddlers at their first diagnosis and after six months during two initiating joint attention (IJA) tasks using eye tracking. Findings suggest the potential use of eye-tracking technology as an objective, biological oriented marker, non-intrusive, adjunctive tool to measure developmental trajectories in toddlers with ASD.

8. Autism and Comorbidity

Masi and colleagues [41] conducted an exploratory study that addressed increased risk for suicidal ideation in high functioning autism spectrum disorders (HF-ASD). They studied this issue in a clinical group of 70 inpatient adolescents referred to a psychiatric emergency unit. Adolescents with Bipolar Disorder (BD) and HF-ASD and severe suicidal ideation or attempts (BD-ASD-S), were compared to adolescents with BD and HF-ASD without suicidal ideation or attempts (BD-ASD-noS), and to adolescents with BD and suicidal ideation or attempts without ASD (BD-noASD-S). Individuals with BD-ASD-S had a higher intelligence quotient, more severe clinical impairment, more lethality in suicide attempts, more internalizing symptoms, less impulsiveness, and lower social competence. The severity of ASD traits in individuals and parents did not correlate with suicidal risk. Some dimensions of resilience were protective in terms of repulsion by life and attraction to death. Gulisano and colleagues [42] aimed to identify the incidence of ASD in a large clinical sample of individuals affected by Gilles de la Tourette syndrome (GTS). Findings showed that the incidence of GTS with ASD was significantly lower in children than in adolescents. The incidence of GTS and ASD comorbidity in this study was high, and this has several implications in terms of treatment and prognosis.

9. Autism and Adulthood

Griffiths and colleagues [43] developed an online survey instrument to assess employers' perspectives on hiring job candidates with ASD. The cluster analysis indicated that company structures, policies and practices, and perceptions, as well as the needs of employers and employees, were important in determining who would successfully hire individuals with ASD. Key areas that require focused policies and practices include recruitment and hiring, training, accessibility and accommodations, and retention and advancement. Damiani and colleagues [44] aimed to test the association between epilepsy and regressive ASD. Secondly, they explored differences in behavioral and pharmacological profiles related to the presence of each of these conditions, as worse behavioral profiles have been separately associated with both epilepsy and regressive ASD in previous studies. The preliminary results suggested the presence of specific associations of different clinical conditions in subjects with rarely investigated phenotypes. In their paper, Keller and colleagues [45] described the experience of the Regional Center for Autism in Adulthood in Turin, Italy. It sought to develop a personalized rehabilitation and enablement program for people with ASD who received a diagnosis of autism in childhood/adolescence or for individuals with suspected adulthood ASD. This program is based on a Multistep Network Model involving people with ASD, family members, social workers, teachers, and clinicians. Findings indicated that the development of public centers specialized in assisting and treating people with autism (PWA) can improve the accuracy of ASD diagnosis in adulthood and foster specific habilitative interventions aimed to improve the quality of life of both PWA and their families. The study of Runge and colleagues [46] retrospectively analyzed the Cerebrospinal fluid (CSF) findings of adult patients with ASD. CSF basic measures (white blood cell count, total protein, albumin quotient, immunoglobulin G (IgG) index, and oligoclonal bands) and various antineuronal antibodies were compared with an earlier described mentally healthy control group of patients with idiopathic intracranial hypertension. The results of the study were limited by its retrospective and open design. The group differences in blood–brain barrier markers could be influenced by a different gender distribution between ASD patients and controls. The paper of Fusar-Poli and colleagues [47] was aimed to investigate self-reported autistic traits in individuals with ASD, schizophrenia spectrum disorders (SSD), and non-clinical controls (NCC), using the Autism-Spectrum Quotient (AQ) questionnaire. Findings showed that the AQ did not correlate with clinician-rated ADOS-2 scores in the ASD sample. Results confirmed that symptoms are partially overlapping in adults with ASD and psychosis. Moreover, they raise concerns regarding the usefulness of AQ as a screening tool in clinical populations

10. Broader Autism Phenotype (BAP)

Leonardi and colleagues [48] explored the construct of alexithymia in parents of children with and without ASD using a multi-method approach based on self-rated and external rater assessment. Results suggested the importance of using multi-method approaches to control for potential measurement bias and to detect psychological constructs such as alexithymia in subclinical samples such as parents of children with ASD. Riva and colleagues [49] conducted a prospective study of typically developing infants and measured frontal asymmetry in alpha oscillation (FAA) as a mediator between both maternal and paternal autistic traits and child ASD traits. Findings showed a potential cascade of effects whereby paternal autistic traits drive EEG markers contributing to ASD risk. Bianco and the group coordinated by Cosimo Urgesi [50] investigated whether the distribution of autistic traits in the general population, as measured through the Autistic Quotient (AQ), is associated with alterations of context-based predictions of social and non-social stimuli. Findings showed that the prediction of both social and non-social stimuli was facilitated when embedded in high-probability contexts. However, only the contextual modulation of non-social predictions was reduced in individuals with lower "Attention switching" abilities. The results provide evidence for an association between weaker context-based expectations of non-social events and higher autistic traits.

11. Conclusions

The published papers in this Special Issue (SI) testify to the complexity of performing research in the field of ASD. The multifactorial etiology inevitably calls different professional figures to a close collaboration. The published contributions underlined areas of progress and ongoing challenges which in the coming years could be able to give us more certain data.

To conclude, a special thank you to all authors who submitted their work to this Special Issue "Advances in Autism Research" and also the reviewers for dedicating their time and for helping to improve the quality of the published manuscripts.

Taking up the words of Andrew Meltzoff, who opened this editorial, the wish for this SI is that it might be, in its small way, *useful for society, as well as for psychology, neuroscience, and of course the children and families*.

Author Contributions: A.N. has conceptualized the Special Issue and wrote the Editorial. He read and agreed to the published version of the manuscript.

Funding: The writing of this editorial received no external funding.

Acknowledgments: I thank colleagues and friends worldwide who participated in making this Special Issue a concrete success. I would like to thank the colleagues of Department of Child Psychiatry and Psychopharmacology of IRCCS Stella Maris Foundation and especially Gabriele Masi, Head of Department, for supporting my research in the field of Autism Spectrum Disorder.

Conflicts of Interest: A.N. was the Guest Editor of the Special Issue "Advances in Autism Research".

Appendix A

Table A1. Authors, Countries, Institutions and Type of the papers included in the Special Issue "Advances in Autism Research".

Papers Reference	Authors	Country	Institutions	Type
[1]	Narzisi A.	Italy	IRCCS Stella Maris	Editorial
[2]	Colizzi, M.; Sironi, E.; Antonini, F.; Ciceri, M.L.; Bovo, C.; Zoccante, L.	Italy	University of Verona	Research
[3]	Brondino, N.; Damiani, S.; Politi, P.	Italy	University of Pavia	Research
[4]	Chiarotti, F.; Venerosi, A.	Italy	Italian National Institute of Health	Review
[5]	Petrocchi, S.; Levante, A.; Lecciso, F.	Switzerland; Italy	University of Salento/Università della Svizzera Italiana	Review
[6]	Levante, A.; Petrocchi, S.; Massagli, A.; Filograna, M.R.; De Giorgi, S.; Lecciso, F.	Italy; Switzerland	University of Salento/Università della Svizzera Italiana/IRCCS European Institute of Oncology	Research
[7]	Devescovi, R.; Monasta, L.; Bin, M.; Bresciani, G.; Mancini, A.; Carrozzi, M.; Colombi, C.	Italy; USA	IRCCS Burlo Garofalo/University of Michigan/IRCCS Stella Maris	Research
[8]	Taresh, S.; Ahmad, N.A.; Roslan, S.; Ma'rof, A.M.; Zaid, S.	Malaysia; Yemen	University Putra Malaysia/Sana'a University	Review
[9]	Baccinelli, W.; Bulgheroni, M.; Simonetti, V.; Fulceri, F.; Caruso, A.; Gila, L.; Scattoni, M.L.	Italy	Italian National Institute of Health	Research
[10]	Caruso, A.; Gila, L.; Fulceri, F.; Salvitti, T.; Micai, M.; Baccinelli, W.; Bulgheroni, M.; Scattoni, M.L.; on behalf of the NIDA Network Group	Italy	Italian National Institute of Health	Research
[11]	Alsaedi, R.H.	Australia; Saudi Arabia	Queensland University of Technology/Taibah University	Research
[12]	Barsotti, J.; Mangani, G.; Nencioli, R.; Pfanner, L.; Tancredi, R.; Cosenza, A.; Sesso, G.; Narzisi, A.; Muratori, F.; Cipriani, P.; Chilosi, A.M.	Italy	IRCCS Stella Maris	Research
[13]	Gladfelter, A.; Barron, K.L.	USA	Northern Illinois University	Research
[14]	Shield, A.; Igel, M.; Randall, K.; Meier, R.P.	USA	Miami University/University of Texas	Research
[16]	Andreou, M.; Skrimpa, V.	Germany	University of Cologne	Review

Table A1. *Cont.*

Papers Reference	Authors	Country	Institutions	Type
[17]	Papangelo, P.; Pinzino, M.; Pelagatti, S.; Fabbri-Destro, M.; Narzisi, A.	Italy	National Research Council	Research
[18]	Panerai, S.; Ferri, R.; Catania, V.; Zingale, M.; Ruccella, D.; Gelardi, D.; Fasciana, D.; Elia, M.	Italy	IRCCS Research Oasi	Research
[19]	Perin, C.; Valagussa, G.; Mazzucchelli, M.; Gariboldi, V.; Cerri, C.G.; Meroni, R.; Grossi, E.; Cornaggia, C.M.; Menant, J.; Piscitelli, D.	Italy; Luxemburg; Canada; Australia; USA	University of Milano Bicocca/Villa Santa Maria Foundation/ASST Rhodense, Ospedale "G. Salvini/LUNEX International University of Health, Exercise and Sports/University of New South Wales/McGill University/Pacific University	Research
[20]	Molinaro, A.; Micheletti, S.; Rossi, A.; Gitti, F.; Galli, J.; Merabet, L.B.; Fazzi, E.M.	Italy; USA	University of Brescia/ASST Spedali Civili of Brescia/Harvard Medical School	Review
[21]	Valori, L.; Bayramova, R.; McKenna-Plumley, P.E.; Farroni, T.	Italy; UK	University of Padova/Queen's University Belfast	Research
[22]	Garcia Primo, P.; Weber, C.; Posada de la Paz, M.; Fellinger, J.; Dirmhirn, A.; Holzinger, D.	Austria; Spain	Johannes Kepler University/University of Education Upper Austria/Instituto de Salud Carlos III/University of Vienna/University of Graz	Research
[23]	Fuller, E.A.; Oliver, K.; Vejnoska, S.F.; Rogers, S.J.	USA	University of California, Davis MIND Institute	Review
[24]	Marino, F.; Chilà, P.; Failla, C.; Crimi, I.; Minutoli, R.; Puglisi, A.; Arnao, A.A.; Tartarisco, G.; Ruta, L.; Vagni, D.; Pioggia, G.	Italy	National Research Council	Research
[25]	Bentenuto, A.; Bertamini, G.; Perzolli, S.; Venuti, P.	Italy	ODFLAB, University of Trento	Research
[26]	Yazdani, S.; Capuano, A.; Ghaziuddin, M.; Colombi, C.	Usa	Loyola University/University of Michigan	Review
[27]	Baker, E.; Veytsman, E.; Martin, A.M.; Blacher, J.; Stavropoulos, K.K.M.	Usa	University of California	Brief report
[28]	Melogno, S.; Pinto, M.A.; Ruzza, A.; Scalisi, T.G.	Italy	Sapienza University of Rome/Niccolò Cusano University of Rome	Case study
[29]	Billeci, L.; Caterino, E.; Tonacci, A.; Gava, M.L.	Italy	National Research Council	Research

Table A1. *Cont.*

Papers Reference	Authors	Country	Institutions	Type
[30]	Narzisi, A.; Bondioli, M.; Pardossi, F.; Billeci, L.; Buzzi, M.C.; Buzzi, M.; Pinzino, M.; Senette, C.; Semucci, V.; Tonacci, A.; Uscidda, F.; Vagelli, B.; Giuca, M.R.; Pelagatti, S.	Italy	National Research Council/IRCCS Stella Maris/University of Pisa	Research
[31]	Troisi, J.; Autio, R.; Beopoulos, T.; Bravaccio, C.; Carraturo, F.; Corrivetti, G.; Cunningham, S.; Devane, S.; Fallin, D.; Fetissov, S.; Gea, M.; Giorgi, A.; Iris, F.; Joshi, L.; Kadzielski, S.; Kraneveld, A.; Kumar, H.; Ladd-Acosta, C.; Leader, G.; Mannion, A.; Maximin, E.; Mezzelani, A.; Milanesi, L.; Naudon, L.; Peralta Marzal, L.N.; Perez Pardo, P.; Prince, N.Z.; Rabot, S.; Roeselers, G.; Roos, C.; Roussin, L.; Scala, G.; Tuccinardi, F.P.; Fasano, A.	Italy; Finland; France; Ireland; USA; Netherlands;	University of Salerno/Tampere University/Bio-Modeling System/University of Naples Federico II/Promete srl/ASL Salerno/University Road/Massachusetts General Hospital/John Hopkins School of Public Health/University of Normandy/Medinok Spa/Utrecht University/Danone Nutricia Research/Université Paris-Saclay/National Research Council/Euformatics/EBRI, Salerno	Research
[32]	Magdalena, H.; Beata, K.; Justyna, P.; Agnieszka, K.-G.; Szczepara-Fabian, M.; Buczek, A.; Ewa, E.-W.	Poland	University of Silesia	Research
[33]	Pascucci, T.; Colamartino, M.; Fiori, E.; Sacco, R.; Coviello, A.; Ventura, R.; Puglisi-Allegra, S.; Turriziani, L.; Persico, A.M.	Italy	University of Messina/Sapienza University of Rome/IRCCS Fondazione Santa Lucia/IRCCS Neuromed	Research
[34]	Lombardo, S.D.; Battaglia, G.; Petralia, M.C.; Mangano, K.; Basile, M.S.; Bruno, V.; Fagone, P.; Bella, R.; Nicoletti, F.; Cavalli, E.	Italy	University of Catania/University Sapienza/IRCCS Neuromed	Research
[35]	Prosperi, M.; Guiducci, L.; Peroni, D.G.; Narducci, C.; Gaggini, M.; Calderoni, S.; Tancredi, R.; Morales, M.A.; Gastaldelli, A.; Muratori, F.; Santocchi, E.	Italy	IRCCS Stella Maris	Research

Table A1. Cont.

Papers Reference	Authors	Country	Institutions	Type
[36]	Lee, J.; Son, M.J.; Son, C.Y.; Jeong, G.H.; Lee, K.H.; Lee, K.S.; Ko, Y.; Kim, J.Y.; Lee, J.Y.; Radua, J.; Eisenhut, M.; Gressier, F.; Koyanagi, A.; Stubbs, B.; Solmi, M.; Rais, T.B.; Kronbichler, A.; Dragioti, E.; Vasconcelos, D.F.P.; Silva, F.R.P.; Tizaoui, K.; Brunoni, A.R.; Carvalho, A.F.; Cargnin, S.; Terrazzino, S.; Stickley, A.; Smith, L.; Thompson, T.; Shin, J.I.; Fusar-Poli, P.	Italy; Korea; USA; UK; Spain; Sweden; France; Austria; Brazil; Tunisia; Germany; Canada; Japan;	University Wonju/Yonsei University/Washington University/Gyeongsang National University/Yonsei University/Hankuk University/King's College London/CIBERSAM/Karolinska Institute/IDIBAPS/Dunstable University/Bicêtre University Hospital/Universitat de Barcelona/ICREA/Instituto de Salud Carlos III/Maudsley NHS Foundation Trust/University of Padua/University of Toledo/University Innsbruck/Linköping University/Federal University of the Parnaiba Delta/Tunis El Manar University/University of São Paulo/University Hospital, LMU Munich/Centre for Addiction & Mental Health/University of Toronto/University of Piemonte Orientale/Södertörn University/National Institute of Mental Health, Tokyo/Anglia Ruskin University, Cambridge/University of Greenwich/OASIS Service, South London and Maudsley NHS Foundation Trust/University of Pavia	Research
[37]	Caria, A.; Ciringione, L.; de Falco, S.	Italy	University of Trento	Review
[38]	Fusar-Poli, L.; Cavone, V.; Tinacci, S.; Concas, I.; Petralia, A.; Signorelli, M.S.; Diaz-Caneja, C.M.; Aguglia, E.	Italy; Spain	University of Catania/Universidad Complutense	Review
[39]	Tanaka, S.; Komagome, A.; Iguchi-Sherry, A.; Nagasaka, A.; Yuhi, T.; Higashida, H.; Rooksby, M.; Kikuchi, M.; Arai, O.; Minami, K.; Tsuji, T.; Tsuji, C.	Japan; UK	Kanazawa University/Tokyo University/Kinjo University/University of Glasgow/University of Fukui	Research
[40]	Muratori, F.; Billeci, L.; Calderoni, S.; Boncoddo, M.; Lattarulo, C.; Costanzo, V.; Turi, M.; Colombi, C.; Narzisi, A.	Italy	IRCCS Stella Maris	Brief report
[41]	Masi, G.; Scullin, S.; Narzisi, A.; Muratori, P.; Paciello, M.; Fabiani, D.; Lenzi, F.; Mucci, M.; D'Acunto, G.	Italy	IRCCS Stella Maris	Research

Table A1. Cont.

Papers Reference	Authors	Country	Institutions	Type
[42]	Gulisano, M.; Barone, R.; Alaimo, S.; Ferro, A.; Pulvirenti, A.; Cirnigliaro, L.; Di Silvestre, S.; Martellino, S.; Maugeri, N.; Milana, M.C.; Scerbo, M.; Rizzo, R.	Italy	University of Catania	Research
[43]	Griffiths, A.J.; Hanson, A.H.; Giannantonio, C.M.; Mathur, S.K.; Hyde, K.; Linstead, E.	Usa	Chapman University	Research
[44]	Damiani, S.; Leali, P.; Nosari, G.; Caviglia, M.; Puci, M.V.; Monti, M.C.; Brondino, N.; Politi, P.	Italy	University of Pavia	Research
[45]	Keller, R.; Chieregato, S.; Bari, S.; Castaldo, R.; Rutto, F.; Chiocchetti, A.; Dianzani, U.	Italy	Adult Autism Center, Mental Health Department, Health Unit ASL Città di Torino/University of Turin	Research
[46]	Runge, K.; Tebartz van Elst, L.; Maier, S.; Nickel, K.; Denzel, D.; Matysik, M.; Kuzior, H.; Robinson, T.; Blank, T.; Dersch, R.; Domschke, K.; Endres, D.	Germany	University of Freiburg	Research
[47]	Fusar-Poli, L.; Ciancio, A.; Gabbiadini, A.; Meo, V.; Patania, F.; Rodolico, A.; Saitta, G.; Vozza, L.; Petralia, A.; Signorelli, M.S.; Aguglia, E.	Italy	University of Catania	Research
[48]	Leonardi, E.; Cerasa, A.; Famà, F.I.; Carrozza, C.; Spadaro, L.; Scifo, R.; Baieli, S.; Marino, F.; Tartarisco, G.; Vagni, D.; Pioggia, G.; Ruta, L.	Italy	National Research Council	Research
[49]	Riva, V.; Marino, C.; Piazza, C.; Riboldi, E.M.; Mornati, G.; Molteni, M.; Cantiani, C.	Italy; Canada	Scientific Institute IRCCS E. Medea/University of Toronto	Research
[50]	Bianco, V.; Finisguerra, A.; Betti, S.; D'Argenio, G.; Urgesi, C.	Italy	University of Udine	Research

References

1. Narzisi, A. Handle the Autism Spectrum Condition during Coronavirus (COVID-19) *Stay at Home* Period: Ten Tips for Helping Parents and Caregivers of Young Children. *Brain Sci.* **2020**, *10*, 207. [CrossRef]
2. Colizzi, M.; Sironi, E.; Antonini, F.; Ciceri, M.L.; Bovo, C.; Zoccante, L. Psychosocial and Behavioral Impact of COVID-19 in Autism Spectrum Disorder: An Online Parent Survey. *Brain Sci.* **2020**, *10*, 341. [CrossRef] [PubMed]
3. Brondino, N.; Damiani, S.; Politi, P. Effective Strategies for Managing COVID-19 Emergency Restrictions for Adults with Severe ASD in a Daycare Center in Italy. *Brain Sci.* **2020**, *10*, 436. [CrossRef] [PubMed]
4. Chiarotti, F.; Venerosi, A. Epidemiology of Autism Spectrum Disorders: A Review of Worldwide Prevalence Estimates Since 2014. *Brain Sci.* **2020**, *10*, 274. [CrossRef] [PubMed]
5. Petrocchi, S.; Levante, A.; Lecciso, F. Systematic Review of Level 1 and Level 2 Screening Tools for Autism Spectrum Disorders in Toddlers. *Brain Sci.* **2020**, *10*, 180. [CrossRef]
6. Levante, A.; Petrocchi, S.; Massagli, A.; Filograna, M.R.; De Giorgi, S.; Lecciso, F. Early Screening of the Autism Spectrum Disorders: Validity Properties and Cross-Cultural Generalizability of the First Year Inventory in Italy. *Brain Sci.* **2020**, *10*, 108. [CrossRef]
7. Devescovi, R.; Monasta, L.; Bin, M.; Bresciani, G.; Mancini, A.; Carrozzi, M.; Colombi, C. A Two-Stage Screening Approach with I-TC and Q-CHAT to Identify Toddlers at Risk for Autism Spectrum Disorder within the Italian Public Health System. *Brain Sci.* **2020**, *10*, 184. [CrossRef]
8. Taresh, S.; Ahmad, N.A.; Roslan, S.; Ma'rof, A.M.; Zaid, S. Pre-School Teachers' Knowledge, Belief, Identification Skills, and Self-Efficacy in Identifying Autism Spectrum Disorder (ASD): A Conceptual Framework to Identify Children with ASD. *Brain Sci.* **2020**, *10*, 165. [CrossRef]
9. Baccinelli, W.; Bulgheroni, M.; Simonetti, V.; Fulceri, F.; Caruso, A.; Gila, L.; Scattoni, M.L. Movidea: A Software Package for Automatic Video Analysis of Movements in Infants at Risk for Neurodevelopmental Disorders. *Brain Sci.* **2020**, *10*, 203. [CrossRef]
10. Caruso, A.; Gila, L.; Fulceri, F.; Salvitti, T.; Micai, M.; Baccinelli, W.; Bulgheroni, M.; Scattoni, M.L. on behalf of the NIDA Network Group; Early Motor Development Predicts Clinical Outcomes of Siblings at High-Risk for Autism: Insight from an Innovative Motion-Tracking Technology. *Brain Sci.* **2020**, *10*, 379. [CrossRef]
11. Masi, G.; Scullin, S.; Narzisi, A.; Muratori, P.; Paciello, M.; Fabiani, D.; Lenzi, F.; Mucci, M.; D'Acunto, G. Suicidal Ideation and Suicidal Attempts in Referred Adolescents with High Functioning Autism Spectrum Disorder and Comorbid Bipolar Disorder: A Pilot Study. *Brain Sci.* **2020**, *10*, 750. [CrossRef] [PubMed]
12. Gulisano, M.; Barone, R.; Alaimo, S.; Ferro, A.; Pulvirenti, A.; Cirnigliaro, L.; Di Silvestre, S.; Martellino, S.; Maugeri, N.; Milana, M.C.; et al. Disentangling Restrictive and Repetitive Behaviors and Social Impairments in Children and Adolescents with Gilles de la Tourette Syndrome and Autism Spectrum Disorder. *Brain Sci.* **2020**, *10*, 308. [CrossRef]
13. Troisi, J.; Autio, R.; Beopoulos, T.; Bravaccio, C.; Carraturo, F.; Corrivetti, G.; Cunningham, S.; Devane, S.; Fallin, D.; Fetissov, S.; et al. Genome, Environment, Microbiome and Metabolome in Autism (GEMMA) Study Design: Biomarkers Identification for Precision Treatment and Primary Prevention of Autism Spectrum Disorders by an Integrated Multi-Omics Systems Biology Approach. *Brain Sci.* **2020**, *10*, 743. [CrossRef] [PubMed]
14. Magdalena, H.; Beata, K.; Justyna, P.; Agnieszka, K.-G.; Szczepara-Fabian, M.; Buczek, A.; Ewa, E.-W. Preconception Risk Factors for Autism Spectrum Disorder—A Pilot Study. *Brain Sci.* **2020**, *10*, 293. [CrossRef] [PubMed]
15. Pascucci, T.; Colamartino, M.; Fiori, E.; Sacco, R.; Coviello, A.; Ventura, R.; Puglisi-Allegra, S.; Turriziani, L.; Persico, A.M. P-cresol Alters Brain Dopamine Metabolism and Exacerbates Autism-Like Behaviors in the BTBR Mouse. *Brain Sci.* **2020**, *10*, 233. [CrossRef] [PubMed]
16. Lombardo, S.D.; Battaglia, G.; Petralia, M.C.; Mangano, K.; Basile, M.S.; Bruno, V.; Fagone, P.; Bella, R.; Nicoletti, F.; Cavalli, E. Transcriptomic Analysis Reveals Abnormal Expression of Prion Disease Gene Pathway in Brains from Patients with Autism Spectrum Disorders. *Brain Sci.* **2020**, *10*, 200. [CrossRef] [PubMed]
17. Prosperi, M.; Guiducci, L.; Peroni, D.G.; Narducci, C.; Gaggini, M.; Calderoni, S.; Tancredi, R.; Morales, M.A.; Gastaldelli, A.; Muratori, F.; et al. Inflammatory Biomarkers are Correlated with Some Forms of Regressive Autism Spectrum Disorder. *Brain Sci.* **2019**, *9*, 366. [CrossRef]
18. Lee, J.; Son, M.J.; Son, C.Y.; Jeong, G.H.; Lee, K.H.; Lee, K.S.; Ko, Y.; Kim, J.Y.; Lee, J.Y.; Radua, J.; et al. Genetic Variation and Autism: A Field Synopsis and Systematic Meta-Analysis. *Brain Sci.* **2020**, *10*, 692. [CrossRef]
19. Caria, A.; Ciringione, L.; de Falco, S. Morphofunctional Alterations of the Hypothalamus and Social Behavior in Autism Spectrum Disorders. *Brain Sci.* **2020**, *10*, 435. [CrossRef]

20. Fusar-Poli, L.; Cavone, V.; Tinacci, S.; Concas, I.; Petralia, A.; Signorelli, M.S.; Díaz-Caneja, C.M.; Aguglia, E. Cannabinoids for People with ASD: A Systematic Review of Published and Ongoing Studies. *Brain Sci.* **2020**, *10*, 572. [CrossRef]
21. Tanaka, S.; Komagome, A.; Iguchi-Sherry, A.; Nagasaka, A.; Yuhi, T.; Higashida, H.; Rooksby, M.; Kikuchi, M.; Arai, O.; Minami, K.; et al. Participatory Art Activities Increase Salivary Oxytocin Secretion of ASD Children. *Brain Sci.* **2020**, *10*, 680. [CrossRef] [PubMed]
22. Muratori, F.; Billeci, L.; Calderoni, S.; Boncoddo, M.; Lattarulo, C.; Costanzo, V.; Turi, M.; Colombi, C.; Narzisi, A. How Attention to Faces and Objects Changes Over Time in Toddlers with Autism Spectrum Disorders: Preliminary Evidence from An Eye Tracking Study. *Brain Sci.* **2019**, *9*, 344. [CrossRef] [PubMed]
23. Alsaedi, R.H. An Assessment of the Motor Performance Skills of Children with Autism Spectrum Disorder in the Gulf Region. *Brain Sci.* **2020**, *10*, 607. [CrossRef] [PubMed]
24. Barsotti, J.; Mangani, G.; Nencioli, R.; Pfanner, L.; Tancredi, R.; Cosenza, A.; Sesso, G.; Narzisi, A.; Muratori, F.; Cipriani, P.; et al. Grammatical Comprehension in Italian Children with Autism Spectrum Disorder. *Brain Sci.* **2020**, *10*, 510. [CrossRef]
25. Gladfelter, A.; Barron, K.L. How Children with Autism Spectrum Disorder, Developmental Language Disorder, and Typical Language Learn to Produce Global and Local Semantic Features. *Brain Sci.* **2020**, *10*, 231. [CrossRef]
26. Shield, A.; Igel, M.; Randall, K.; Meier, R.P. The Source of Palm Orientation Errors in the Signing of Children with ASD: Imitative, Motoric, or Both? *Brain Sci.* **2020**, *10*, 268. [CrossRef]
27. Cristofani, C.; Sesso, G.; Cristofani, P.; Fantozzi, P.; Inguaggiato, E.; Muratori, P.; Narzisi, A.; Pfanner, C.; Pisano, S.; Polidori, L.; et al. The Role of Executive Functions in the Development of Empathy and Its Association with Externalizing Behaviors in Children with Neurodevelopmental Disorders and Other Psychiatric Comorbidities. *Brain Sci.* **2020**, *10*, 489. [CrossRef]
28. Andreou, M.; Skrimpa, V. Theory of Mind Deficits and Neurophysiological Operations in Autism Spectrum Disorders: A Review. *Brain Sci.* **2020**, *10*, 393. [CrossRef]
29. Papangelo, P.; Pinzino, M.; Pelagatti, S.; Fabbri-Destro, M.; Narzisi, A. Human Figure Drawings in Children with Autism Spectrum Disorders: A Possible Window on the Inner or the Outer World. *Brain Sci.* **2020**, *10*, 398. [CrossRef]
30. Panerai, S.; Ferri, R.; Catania, V.; Zingale, M.; Ruccella, D.; Gelardi, D.; Fasciana, D.; Elia, M. Sensory Profiles of Children with Autism Spectrum Disorder with and without Feeding Problems: A Comparative Study in Sicilian Subjects. *Brain Sci.* **2020**, *10*, 336. [CrossRef]
31. Perin, C.; Valagussa, G.; Mazzucchelli, M.; Gariboldi, V.; Cerri, C.G.; Meroni, R.; Grossi, E.; Cornaggia, C.M.; Menant, J.; Piscitelli, D. Physiological Profile Assessment of Posture in Children and Adolescents with Autism Spectrum Disorder and Typically Developing Peers. *Brain Sci.* **2020**, *10*, 681. [CrossRef] [PubMed]
32. Molinaro, A.; Micheletti, S.; Rossi, A.; Gitti, F.; Galli, J.; Merabet, L.B.; Fazzi, E.M. Autistic-Like Features in Visually Impaired Children: A Review of Literature and Directions for Future Research. *Brain Sci.* **2020**, *10*, 507. [CrossRef] [PubMed]
33. Valori, I.; Bayramova, R.; McKenna-Plumley, P.E.; Farroni, T. Sensorimotor Research Utilising Immersive Virtual Reality: A Pilot Study with Children and Adults with Autism Spectrum Disorders. *Brain Sci.* **2020**, *10*, 259. [CrossRef] [PubMed]
34. Garcia Primo, P.; Weber, C.; Posada de la Paz, M.; Fellinger, J.; Dirmhirn, A.; Holzinger, D. Explaining Age at Autism Spectrum Diagnosis in Children with Migrant and Non-Migrant Background in Austria. *Brain Sci.* **2020**, *10*, 448. [CrossRef]
35. Fuller, E.A.; Oliver, K.; Vejnoska, S.F.; Rogers, S.J. The Effects of the Early Start Denver Model for Children with Autism Spectrum Disorder: A Meta-Analysis. *Brain Sci.* **2020**, *10*, 368. [CrossRef]
36. Marino, F.; Chilà, P.; Failla, C.; Crimi, I.; Minutoli, R.; Puglisi, A.; Arnao, A.A.; Tartarisco, G.; Ruta, L.; Vagni, D.; et al. Tele-Assisted Behavioral Intervention for Families with Children with Autism Spectrum Disorders: A Randomized Control Trial. *Brain Sci.* **2020**, *10*, 649. [CrossRef]
37. Bentenuto, A.; Bertamini, G.; Perzolli, S.; Venuti, P. Changes in Developmental Trajectories of Preschool Children with Autism Spectrum Disorder during Parental Based Intensive Intervention. *Brain Sci.* **2020**, *10*, 289. [CrossRef]
38. Yazdani, S.; Capuano, A.; Ghaziuddin, M.; Colombi, C. Exclusion Criteria Used in Early Behavioral Intervention Studies for Young Children with Autism Spectrum Disorder. *Brain Sci.* **2020**, *10*, 99. [CrossRef]
39. Baker, E.; Veytsman, E.; Martin, A.M.; Blacher, J.; Stavropoulos, K.K.M. Increased Neural Reward Responsivity in Adolescents with ASD after Social Skills Intervention. *Brain Sci.* **2020**, *10*, 402. [CrossRef]

40. Melogno, S.; Pinto, M.A.; Ruzza, A.; Scalisi, T.G. Improving the Ability to Write Persuasive Texts in a Boy with Autism Spectrum Disorder: Outcomes of an Intervention. *Brain Sci.* **2020**, *10*, 264. [CrossRef]
41. Billeci, L.; Caterino, E.; Tonacci, A.; Gava, M.L. Behavioral and Autonomic Responses in Treating Children with High-Functioning Autism Spectrum Disorder: Clinical and Phenomenological Insights from Two Case Reports. *Brain Sci.* **2020**, *10*, 382. [CrossRef] [PubMed]
42. Narzisi, A.; Bondioli, M.; Pardossi, F.; Billeci, L.; Buzzi, M.C.; Buzzi, M.; Pinzino, M.; Senette, C.; Semucci, V.; Tonacci, A.; et al. "Mom Let's Go to the Dentist!" Preliminary Feasibility of a Tailored Dental Intervention for Children with Autism Spectrum Disorder in the Italian Public Health Service. *Brain Sci.* **2020**, *10*, 444. [CrossRef] [PubMed]
43. Griffiths, A.J.; Hanson, A.H.; Giannantonio, C.M.; Mathur, S.K.; Hyde, K.; Linstead, E. Developing Employment Environments Where Individuals with ASD Thrive: Using Machine Learning to Explore Employer Policies and Practices. *Brain Sci.* **2020**, *10*, 632. [CrossRef] [PubMed]
44. Damiani, S.; Leali, P.; Nosari, G.; Caviglia, M.; Puci, M.V.; Monti, M.C.; Brondino, N.; Politi, P. Association of Autism Onset, Epilepsy, and Behavior in a Community of Adults with Autism and Severe Intellectual Disability. *Brain Sci.* **2020**, *10*, 486. [CrossRef] [PubMed]
45. Keller, R.; Chieregato, S.; Bari, S.; Castaldo, R.; Rutto, F.; Chiocchetti, A.; Dianzani, U. Autism in Adulthood: Clinical and Demographic Characteristics of a Cohort of Five Hundred Persons with Autism Analyzed by a Novel Multistep Network Model. *Brain Sci.* **2020**, *10*, 416. [CrossRef]
46. Runge, K.; Tebartz van Elst, L.; Maier, S.; Nickel, K.; Denzel, D.; Matysik, M.; Kuzior, H.; Robinson, T.; Blank, T.; Dersch, R.; et al. Cerebrospinal Fluid Findings of 36 Adult Patients with Autism Spectrum Disorder. *Brain Sci.* **2020**, *10*, 355. [CrossRef]
47. Fusar-Poli, L.; Ciancio, A.; Gabbiadini, A.; Meo, V.; Patania, F.; Rodolico, A.; Saitta, G.; Vozza, L.; Petralia, A.; Signorelli, M.S.; et al. Self-Reported Autistic Traits Using the AQ: A Comparison between Individuals with ASD, Psychosis, and Non-Clinical Controls. *Brain Sci.* **2020**, *10*, 291. [CrossRef]
48. Leonardi, E.; Cerasa, A.; Famà, F.I.; Carrozza, C.; Spadaro, L.; Scifo, R.; Baieli, S.; Marino, F.; Tartarisco, G.; Vagni, D.; et al. Alexithymia Profile in Relation to Negative Affect in Parents of Autistic and Typically Developing Young Children. *Brain Sci.* **2020**, *10*, 496. [CrossRef]
49. Riva, V.; Marino, C.; Piazza, C.; Riboldi, E.M.; Mornati, G.; Molteni, M.; Cantiani, C. Paternal—But Not Maternal—Autistic Traits Predict Frontal EEG Alpha Asymmetry in Infants with Later Symptoms of Autism. *Brain Sci.* **2019**, *9*, 342. [CrossRef]
50. Bianco, V.; Finisguerra, A.; Betti, S.; D'Argenio, G.; Urgesi, C. Autistic Traits Differently Account for Context-Based Predictions of Physical and Social Events. *Brain Sci.* **2020**, *10*, 418. [CrossRef]

Publisher's Note: MDPI stays neutral with regard to jurisdictional claims in published maps and institutional affiliations.

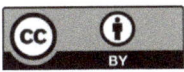

© 2020 by the author. Licensee MDPI, Basel, Switzerland. This article is an open access article distributed under the terms and conditions of the Creative Commons Attribution (CC BY) license (http://creativecommons.org/licenses/by/4.0/).

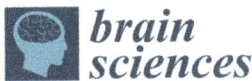 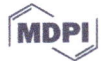

Editorial

Handle the Autism Spectrum Condition during Coronavirus (COVID-19) *Stay at Home* Period: Ten Tips for Helping Parents and Caregivers of Young Children

Antonio Narzisi

Department of Child Psychiatry and Psychopharmacology, IRCCS Stella Maris Foundation, 56018 Pisa, Italy; antonio.narzisi@fsm.unipi.it

Received: 24 March 2020; Accepted: 31 March 2020; Published: 1 April 2020

1. Introduction

COVID-19 has become pandemic [1] and many government decrees have declared restrictive measures in order to prevent its wider spread. For parents and children, staying at home is one of these measures. In this situation the handling of young children with special needs such as autism spectrum condition (ASC) could be challenging for families and caregivers. Usually these children have interventions for several hours a week at home with special therapists or in dedicated hospitals and institutes. However at the moment, due to contagion containment measures, both the families and the ASC children are not physically supported by their therapists and they cannot attend the outside interventions. These measures, necessary for the health of all of us, need to be carefully handled to avoid an increase in parental stress and an exacerbation of children's behavioral problems. ASC is a severe multifactorial disorder characterized by an umbrella of specific peculiarities in the areas of the social communication, restricted interests, and repetitive behaviours [2]. The incidence of ASC is worldwide and recent epidemiological data estimated it to be higher than 1/100 [3,4]. The main aim of this editorial is to give some advice, summarized in 10 tips, to help families to handle children with ASC during this period.

2. The 10 Tips for Helping Parents and Caregivers of Young Children

2.1. Explain to Your Child What COVID-19 Is

Children with ASC have a concrete cognitive style and some of them can have serious verbal issues and show difficulties in phenomenological perception [5]. It is important to explain what COVID-19 is and why we all have to stay at home. The explanation has to be simple and concrete. For this purpose it is possible to appeal to augmentative alternative communication (AAC). It is also possible to ask for help from therapists in preparing a brief pamphlet titled 'What is COVID-19?' using individualized AAC strategies. For verbal young children the explanation should be supported with concept mapping to make it easier for the child to understand.

2.2. Structure Daily Life Activities

It is widely reported that children with ASC have executive functioning deficits [6] and they could show issues in planning their daily life activities, especially when their routine is broken. For this reason it is important, especially now, to structure daily life activities. The home is the unique setting in which activities take place. It would be useful to subdivide the daily activities, assigning a different room for each one of them. This structure can be useful not only for children with ASC who are low and/or middle functioning but also for those who are high functioning. This can be an activity to share with the entire family as a type of game. Using a blackboard, each member of the family can have his space to write the planned activities.

2.3. Handle Semi-Structured Play Activities

Children with ASC enjoy playing, but they can find some types of play difficult because of sensory issues or because they prefer structured or semi-structured activities [7].

During the day it will be important to handle play activities. These can be individual and/or shared. Choose activities that your child prefers. For example, LEGO therapy [8,9] could be a good solution for children with ASC who are low or high functioning. LEGO-based therapy is an increasingly popular social skills programme for children and young people with social communication problems such as ASC. It can be a semi-structured play activity shared with parents or siblings in a home setting [10].

2.4. Use of Serious Games

Serious games can be useful to improve social cognition and to recognize facial emotions, emotional gestures, and emotional situations in children with ASC [11]. Serious games can be a fundamental resource for ASC children. Many serious games are free and can be downloaded as an App for tablet and/or PC from specialized sites. Serious games could be an educational alternative to video games or the internet tout-court.

2.5. Shared Video Game and/or Internet Sessions with Parents

Video games and the internet are extremely attractive for children with ASC but they could become an absorbent interest [12], especially in this period when children are called to stay at home. It is not possible to avoid children playing with the computer but at the moment, when parents are also at home, it could be useful establish a rule whereby children are expected to share the video games/internet (with parents, siblings, or other caregiver). This could avoid a potential risk of isolation of the child and an internet addiction.

2.6. Implement and Share Special Interests with Parents

Special interests can be a characteristic of the people with ASC. There is a growing amount of evidence recognizing the potential benefits that special interests can bring [13]. Special interests have to be supported from parents and/or caregivers. Trains, maps, animals, comic books, geography, electronics, and history can be just a few of potential special interests. In this period in which parents and children stay at home they could plan some activities sharing these special interests.

2.7. Online Therapy for High-Functioning Children

It is well recognized that psychiatric vulnerabilities and/or comorbidities are high in children with ASC. Among these comorbidities anxiety disorder is one of the most reported [14]. Psychiatric comorbidities could contribute to a developmental breakdown especially in adolescence age. The actual state of alert for COVID-19 could be an event that is difficult to mentalize for children with ASC. For this reason, if the children were engaged in psychotherapy before the COVID-19 alert, it is very important that they continue it. Since many therapists have stopped their face-to-face therapy, it is strongly advised to continue the psychotherapy in an online video or audio modality with the same weekly appointments. It could reduce the anxiety, check the mood, and offer to the children a private space in which to talk with a specialist.

2.8. Weekly Online Consultations for Parents and Caregivers

Parents of children with autism experience more stress and are more susceptible than parents of children with other disabilities [15]. At the moment, parents are alone in the handling of their children with ASD. This can represent a further high risk for their stress levels, which are already severely tried.

For this reason it can be very useful to have the opportunity for a weekly online consultation with the therapists of their children. It is valid for parents of both low- and high-functioning children. In the case of low functioning, parents could share a brief home video with the therapists about the behavior of the children during free play or structured sessions at home. In the case of children who are high functioning the consultation could be a dialogical exchange focused on the most appropriate ways to manage this difficult time of COVID-19 alert and to update parents about the degree of coping strategies of the children.

2.9. Maintain Contact with the School

A growing body of research supports the suggestion that the relationships which children form with their teachers and classmates have an impact on learning [16]. It is very important to dedicate a time slot for the homework. This is a routine that has to be maintained. For the maintenance of social contacts with the school companions it is suggested to have at least a weekly contact with one of the class companions. The modality of this contact should depend from the child's preferences. It could be an online video for those that prefer it. For children with ASC who do not prefer to use video for online contacts they could be encouraged to write a letter to one of their school companions or to call them via phone [17]. For both children and parents, it is strongly encouraged to maintain contact with a special teacher online or by phone.

2.10. Leave Spare Time

Children with ASC have to be stimulated, as pointed in tips 1–9, but it is also possible be leave them a proper quota of spare time during the day (e.g., take a short walk near the house).

In this period children could have an increase in stereotypies. This does not need to be a particular concern. At the moment, when habits are changing, the stress levels can be elevated for children with ASC and the increase of stereotypies could be the behavioral result of perceived stress. They will certainly not regress.

3. Conclusions

These suggestions are obviously not exhaustive but they could represent a useful help for parents and/or caregiver of children with ASC to handle the severe situation caused COVID-19 and to optimize the person–environment fit.

COVID-19 is questioning the routine of our young children with ASC and they are called to respect rules and habits that are not always understandable for them (i.e., disinfect your hands, do not touch your eyes or nose, and cover your mouth. They are also not able to see people they would like to meet and must stay at home). These changing routines could cause them profound suffering. For this reason we all (parents, therapists, and researchers) must be united and quickly establish new and functional routines to allow our young children to be safe and peaceful. As ASC experts we have to find different ways to be close to our patients and their families.

I wish to conclude this editorial by citing and sharing a sentence from Italian colleagues currently engaged in the emergency medical system in Milano: "The Italian public health authorities has just started to fight a battle that must be won" [18].

Conflicts of Interest: The author declare no conflicts of interest.

References

1. Nelson, C.W. COVID-19: Time for WHO to reconsider its stance towards Taiwan. *Nature* **2020**, *579*, 193. [CrossRef] [PubMed]
2. Psychiatric Association. *Diagnostic and Statistical Manual of Mental Disorders*, 5th ed.; Psychiatric Association: Washington, DC, USA, 2013.

3. Maenner, M.J.; Shaw, K.A.; Baio, J.; Washington, A.; Patrick, M.; DiRienzo, M.; Christensen, D.L.; Wiggins, L.D.; Pettygrove, S.; Andrews, J.G.; et al. Prevalence of Autism Spectrum Disorder Among Children Aged 8 Years—Autism and Developmental Disabilities Monitoring Network, 11 Sites, United States, 2016. *MMWR Surveill. Summ.* **2020**, *69*, 1–12. [CrossRef] [PubMed]
4. Narzisi, A.; Posada, M.; Barbieri, F.; Chericoni, N.; Ciuffolini, D.; Pinzino, M.; Romano, R.; Scattoni, M.L.; Tancredi, R.; Calderoni, S.; et al. Prevalence of Autism Spectrum Disorder in a large Italian catchment area, A school-based population study within the ASDEU project. *Epidemiol. Psychiatr. Sci.* **2018**, *29*, e5. [CrossRef] [PubMed]
5. Pellicano, E.; Burr, D. When the world becomes 'too real': A Bayesian explanation of autistic perception. *Trends. Cogn. Sci.* **2012**, *16*, 504–510. [CrossRef] [PubMed]
6. Narzisi, A.; Muratori, F.; Calderoni, S.; Fabbro, F.; Urgesi, C. Neuropsychological profile in high functioning autism spectrum disorders. *J. Autism. Dev. Disord.* **2013**, *43*, 1895–1909. [CrossRef] [PubMed]
7. Kojovic, N.; Ben Hadid, L.; Franchini, M.; Schaer, M. Sensory Processing Issues and Their Association with Social Difficulties in Children with Autism Spectrum Disorders. *J Clin Med.* **2019**, *8*, 10. [CrossRef] [PubMed]
8. Lai, M.C.; Anagnostou, E.; Wiznitzer, M.; Allison, C.; Baron-Cohen, S. Evidence-based support for autistic people across the lifespan: Maximising potential, minimising barriers, and optimising the person-environment fit. *Lancet Neurol.* **2020**, *3*. [CrossRef]
9. LeGoff, D.B. Use of LEGO as a therapeutic medium for improving social competence. *J. Autism. Dev. Disord.* **2004**, *34*, 557–571. [CrossRef] [PubMed]
10. Peckett, H.; MacCallum, F.; Knibbs, J. Maternal experience of Lego Therapy in families with children with autism spectrum conditions: What is the impact on family relationships? *Autism* **2016**, *20*, 879–887. [CrossRef] [PubMed]
11. Boucenna, S.; Narzisi, A.; Tilmont, E.; Muratori, F.; Pioggia, G.; Cohen, D.; Chetouani, M. Interactive Technologies for autistic childre: A Review. *Cogn. Comput.* **2014**, *6*, 722–740. [CrossRef]
12. Fineberg, N.A.; Demetrovics, Z.; Stein, D.J.; Ioannidis, K.; Potenza, M.N.; Grünblatt, E.; Brand, M.; Billieux, J.; Carmi, L.; King, D.L.; et al. COST Action Network, Chamberlain SR. Manifesto for a European research network into problematic Usage of the Internet. *Eur. Neuropsychopharmacol.* **2018**, *28*, 1232–1246. [CrossRef] [PubMed]
13. Lee, E.A.L.; Black, M.H.; Falkmer, M.; Tan, T.; Sheehy, L.; Bölte, S.; Girdler, S. "We Can See a Bright Future": Parents' Perceptions of the Outcomes of Participating in a Strengths-Based Program for Adolescents with Autism Spectrum Disorder. *J. Autism. Dev. Disord.* **2020**, *19*. [CrossRef] [PubMed]
14. Lai, M.C.; Kassee, C.; Besney, R.; Bonato, S.; Hull, L.; Mandy, W.; Szatmari, P.; Ameis, S.H. Prevalence of co-occurring mental health diagnoses in the autism population: A systematic review and meta-analysis. *Lancet Psychiatry* **2019**, *6*, 819–829. [CrossRef]
15. Drogomyretska, K.; Fox, R.; Colbert, D. Brief Report: Stress and Perceived Social Support in Parents of Children with ASD. *J. Autism. Dev. Disord.* **2020**, *21*. [CrossRef] [PubMed]
16. Roorda, D.L.; Koomen, H.M.; Spilt, J.L.; Thijs, J.T.; Oort, F.J. Interpersonal behaviors and complementarity in interactions between teachers and kindergartners with a variety of externalizing and internalizing behaviors. *J. Sch. Psychol.* **2013**, *51*, 143–158. [CrossRef] [PubMed]
17. Kumazaki, H.; Muramatsu, T.; Kobayashi, K.; Watanabe, T.; Terada, K.; Higashida, H.; Yuhi, T.; Mimura, M.; Kikuchi, M. Feasibility of autism-focused public speech training using a simple virtual audience for autism spectrum disorder. *Psychiatry Clin. Neurosci.* **2020**, *74*, 124–131. [CrossRef] [PubMed]
18. Spina, S.; Marrazzo, F.; Migliari, M.; Stucchi, R.; Sforza, A.; Fumagalli, R. The response of Milan's Emergency Medical System to the COVID-19 outbreak in Italy. *Lancet* **2020**, *14*, 395. [CrossRef]

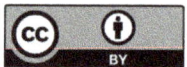 © 2020 by the author. Licensee MDPI, Basel, Switzerland. This article is an open access article distributed under the terms and conditions of the Creative Commons Attribution (CC BY) license (http://creativecommons.org/licenses/by/4.0/).

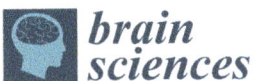

Article

Suicidal Ideation and Suicidal Attempts in Referred Adolescents with High Functioning Autism Spectrum Disorder and Comorbid Bipolar Disorder: A Pilot Study

Gabriele Masi [1,*], Silvia Scullin [1], Antonio Narzisi [1], Pietro Muratori [1], Marinella Paciello [2], Deborah Fabiani [1], Francesca Lenzi [1], Maria Mucci [1] and Giulia D'Acunto [1]

1. IRCCS Stella Maris, Scientific Institute of Child Neurology and Psychiatry, Calambrone, 56018 Pisa, Italy; silviascullin@gmail.com (S.S.); antonio.narzisi@fsm.unipi.it (A.N.); pmuratori@fsm.unipi.it (P.M.); deborah.fabiani@gmail.com (D.F.); flenzi@fsm.unipi.it (F.L.); mmucci@fsm.unipi.it (M.M.); gdacunto@fsm.unipi.it (G.D.)
2. Faculty of Psychology, Università Telematica Internazionale Uninettuno, 00186 Rome, Italy; m.paciello@uninettunouniversity.net
* Correspondence: gabriele.masi@fsm.unipi.it

Received: 3 September 2020; Accepted: 14 October 2020; Published: 17 October 2020

Abstract: Suicidal ideation and attempts in adolescents are closely associated to bipolar disorders (BD). Growing evidence also suggests that high functioning autism spectrum disorders (HF-ASD) are at increased risk for suicidal ideation and behaviors. Although BD and HF-ASD are frequently comorbid, no studies explored suicidality in these individuals. This exploratory study addressed this issue in a clinical group of inpatient adolescents referred to a psychiatric emergency unit. Seventeen adolescents with BD and HF-ASD and severe suicidal ideation or attempts (BD-ASD-S), were compared to 17 adolescents with BD and HF-ASD without suicidal ideation or attempts (BD-ASD-noS), and to 18 adolescents with BD and suicidal ideation or attempts without ASD (BD-noASD-S), using a structured assessment methodology. Individuals with BD-ASD-S had a higher intelligence quotient, more severe clinical impairment, more lethality in suicide attempts, more internalizing symptoms, less impulsiveness, and lower social competence. Severity of ASD traits in individuals and parents did not correlate with suicidal risk. Some dimensions of resilience were protective in terms of repulsion by life and attraction to death. Main limitations are the small sample size, the lack of a control group of typically developing adolescents. However, a better understanding of the specificities of bipolar HF-ASD individuals with suicidality may improve prevention and treatment strategies.

Keywords: autism spectrum disorder; bipolar disorder; suicidal ideation; suicidal attempts; adolescence

1. Introduction

The concept of suicidality includes both suicidal ideation, with or without a plan, and with a wide range of severity, and suicidal attempts, that is self-injurious behaviors intended to kill oneself, with or without medical implications, but nonfatal, while completed suicides are fatal [1]. The term suicidality has long fallen out of favor with psychiatrists and psychologists, due to its imprecision, as it includes heterogeneous clinical conditions, not only in terms of presentation, but also in etiology, diagnosis, prognosis, and treatment. Disentangling this wide range of individuals in more specific subgroups, according to age and gender, psychiatric diagnoses, neurodevelopmental pathways, personality traits, psychiatric familial load, previous traumatic experiences, and social difficulties, may favor a more precise definition of risk factors, and more focused and appropriate prevention and treatment strategies [2,3].

There is growing evidence that a diagnosis of Autism Spectrum Disorders (ASD) is one of the risk factors for suicide [4,5]. In a population-based cohort of ASD probands ($n = 27,122$, all diagnosed between 1987 and 2009) compared with gender-, age-, and county of residence-matched controls ($n = 2,672,185$), Hirvikoski et al. [6] reported a probability for ASD to die by suicide 10 times greater than in the general population. In a clinical cohort study, including 367 high functioning individuals with ASD, 243 (66%) presented self-reported suicidal ideation, and 127 (35%) self-reported plans or attempts at suicide. They more likely reported lifetime experience of suicidal ideation than the UK population sample (odds ratio 9.6 (95% CI 7.6–11.9), $p < 0.0001$), than people with one, two, or more medical illnesses ($p < 0.0001$), or with psychotic illness ($p = 0.019$) [7].

Suicidality in high functioning (HF)-ASD can present with specific features [4]. Thoughts can become easily ruminative, not only in terms of triggering situations for suicidal ideation (i.e., impaired interpretation of social relationships), but also in methods of searching information aimed at planning a suicide attempt [8]. Furthermore, the high lethality and violence of the suicidal methods in ASD individuals (such as hanging, gunshot, railway hitting, or jumping off a bridge) increases the risk of a completed suicide during an attempt, compared to other psychiatric populations [9]. This evidence suggests that ASD should be considered a specific and independent risk factor for suicide [10,11].

Studies specifically addressing suicidal risk factors in youth with ASD have underlined the role of extreme loneliness [12,13], social adverse experiences [14,15], previous traumas [16], internalizing symptoms (anxiety/mood disorders), low emotional regulation, and ADHD [16,17], particularly in HF-ASD individuals [18–20]. Some cognitive features, such as decreased cognitive flexibility, insight of disease, and communication skills may flatten the expression of subjective suffering [21,22]. This is particularly true in adolescence, the age range with the highest suicidal risk [4]. HF-ASD adolescents are mostly exposed to increased social pressure, they can become more acutely aware of their disability, and they have to face the unbridgeable gap between themselves and neurotypical peers [22].

Among the factor increasing suicide risk, mood disorders, have been shown to be strongly related to suicidal outcomes [23]. Even if depressive disorders have been traditionally linked to the concept of suicidality [24], bipolar disorder (BD) has increasingly become, in the last decades, even more closely related to suicidal risk [25]. A systematic review (1970–2017) including articles on completed suicide in individuals with BD showed that suicide rates in BD are approximately 20- to 30-fold greater than in general population, with higher risk in BD-II individuals, and with a heritability of completed suicide of about 40%. Factors related to completed suicide are early onset, family history of suicide among first-degree relatives, previous attempted suicides, type of treatment, somatic, and psychiatric comorbidities [25].

Psychiatric comorbidity in ASD is still under-investigated, even if nearly 70% of people with ASD, including children and adolescents, experience at least one comorbid psychiatric disorder, and around 40% may have two or more psychiatric disorders [9,26,27]. Regarding the different comorbidities in ASD, the prevalence of mood disorder among 21,797 participants with ASD has been reported as 18.8% (95% CI: 10.6–31.1) [28]. The prevalence of depressive disorders has been reported by Lai and colleagues as 11% (95% CI: 9–13) in children and adults [29], and by Hudson and colleagues (meta-analysis including 66 studies) as 12.3% (95% CI: 9.7–15.5) and 14.4% (95% CI: 10.3–19.8) (current and lifetime prevalence, respectively) [30].

The BD-ASD association has been more recently highlighted, along with its important clinical and therapeutic implications [31]. Two reviews assessed the co-occurrence of bipolar disorders in ASD [29,32]. Vannucchi and colleagues found that the prevalence of bipolar disorders ranged from 6% to 21.4% across studies [32], whereas Lai and colleagues reported a prevalence of 5% (95% CI: 3–6) among 153,192 ASD individuals [29]. Regarding only children and adolescents, Joshi and colleagues [31] found that 30% (47/155) of bipolar I probands met criteria for ASD (diagnosis based on DSM-III-R criteria).

While both BD and HF-ASD represent independent risk factors for suicidal ideation and behavior, their association in terms of increased suicidal risk is strongly under-explored in clinical samples. Dell'Osso and colleagues [33] investigated the prevalence of suicidal ideation in 34 adult individuals with ASD without intellectual disability, 68 with subthreshold ASD ("autistic traits"), and 160 healthy controls. Individuals with ASD reported significantly higher scores than the other two groups in mood disorders and depression, while the subthreshold autistic individuals presented higher scores than the heathy control group. Of note, both individuals with ASD and subthreshold ASD scored higher in suicidality, compared to healthy controls, without significant differences between clinical and subthreshold ASD individuals. The depressive score and the restricted interests and rumination domain score were the strongest predictors of suicidality. These results underline the association between mood spectrum and suicidality in adult individuals with ASD, including those with subthreshold forms. These correlations have not been explored in adolescents with ASD, albeit the high rates of suicidal ideation and attempts in this age range.

Among the different personality features possibly related to suicidal risk in adolescents, three domains were considered as particularly significant, according to the available literature, the attitude to life and death, the impulsivity, and the resilience to life stressors. The repulsion by life and the attraction (or low fearlessness) about death have been proved to be related to suicidality in adolescents with psychiatric diagnoses [34,35]. Highly impulsive adolescents tend to act rashly in the context of negative emotions, because long-term benefits are less important than the immediate short-term gains of emotion regulation [36]. Finally, life adversities or stressful life events increase the risk of suicidal ideation and behaviors) [3], and low adaptive resilience abilities after stressful life events are a further vulnerability factor and a possible target for interventions [37].

The aim of our study is to explore if within the bipolar spectrum, adolescents with ASD and suicidality may present specificities in three personality dimensions usually related to suicidality in adolescence (resilience, impulsivity, and attitude to life and death). We compared subjects with BD, ASD, and suicidality (Group 1), with BD; and suicidality, but without ASD (Group 2); and BD and ASD, but without suicidality (Group 3), in order to possibly disentangle the role of autism and suicidality in bipolarity. We hypothesized that bipolar adolescents with HF-ASD could present specific clinical characteristics in their suicidal manifestations, including clinical severity, cognitive abilities, psychiatric comorbidities, and personality features, compared to those without suicidality or without ASD, which may represent possible targets for the diagnostic procedures and treatment plans. Given the exploratory design of the study, we investigated these psychological features without a-priori hypotheses.

2. Materials and Methods

2.1. Sample

This was a naturalistic study based on a clinical database of 52 adolescents (age range 11 to 18 years) with BD, all referred as individuals to our psychiatric emergency unit between January 2018 and July 2019. Seventeen individuals (age range 11 to 18 years) had a comorbid HF-ASD and severe suicidal ideation or suicide attempt(s) (BD-ASD-S group), 17 (age range 11 to 18 years) a comorbid HF-ASD, but without suicidal ideation or suicidal attempt(s) (BD-ASD-noS group), and 18 (age range 11 to 18 years) with severe suicidal ideation or suicide attempts, but not ASD (BD-NoASD-S). The diagnosis of BD was based on DSM 5 criteria, and a diagnostic interview, the Kiddie Schedule for Affective Disorders and Schizophrenia for School-Aged Children-Present and Lifetime Version (K-SADS-PL) [38], administered to the patient and at least one parent.

The diagnosis of ASD was based on the DSM 5 diagnostic criteria [39], and confirmed with the module 3 of Autism Diagnostic Observation Schedule—Second Version (ADOS-2) [40]. Only a minority of individuals' caregivers were interviewed with the Autism Diagnostic Interview-Revised (ADI-R) [41]. The ADI-R is less effective in the diagnosis of HF-ASDA and it may not recognize more subtle forms of ASD [42]. It is therefore possible that, in these individuals with HF-ASD, the symptoms may not be evident at 4 to 5 years of age (developmental period investigated in the ADI-R), but could emerge only when social demands exceed these individuals' limited capacities [39].

The diagnosis of severe suicidal ideation or suicide attempt was based on a score 3 or above at the Columbia–Suicide Severity Rating Scale [CSSRS] [43]. All the individuals presented normal intelligence (Full scale IQ above 85), based on the Wechsler Intelligence Scale for Children—Fourth Edition (WISC-IV) [44].

2.2. Measures

All the individuals received a diagnostic assessment with the K-SADS-PL, a semi-structured interview to diagnose childhood mental disorders in children aged 6 to 18, administered by trained child psychiatrists, in order to diagnose BD (including Type I, Type II, and type NOS), ASD, and comorbidities. All the individuals were assessed with the WISC-IV, to exclude an Intellectual Disability.

The ADOS-2 was administered to support the diagnosis of ASD to all the individuals with first diagnosis of ASD based on historical information and the diagnostic interview K-SADS-PL. The ADOS-2 is a semi-structured interaction that measures symptoms of autism through a standard set of probes. It provides an empirically derived algorithm that differentiates children with ASDs from those with other delays or with typical development. The ADOS-Calibrated Severity Score was used to assess the severity of autistic symptoms [45].

The global clinical severity was assessed with the Clinical Global Impression Severity (CGI-S) [46], while the functional impairment with the Child Global Assessment Scale (C-GAS) [47].

For a dimensional assessment of psychopathology, all individuals were assessed with the Child Behavior Checklist (CBCL) [42,48], a 118-item scale, completed by parents, assessing how often a certain behavior applies to their offspring, on a three-point scale (0 = absent, 1 = occurs sometimes, 2 = occurs often), clustered in two broad-band scores, designated as Internalizing Problems and Externalizing Problems, a Total Problem Score, and with 8 different syndromes scales (Withdrawal, Somatic complaints, Anxiety/depression, Social problems, Thought problems, Attention, Rule-breaking behavior, Aggressive behavior). In the current study, we assessed the presence of Emotional Dysregulation using the CBCL Dysregulation Profile (CBCL-DP), based on the sum of t-scores of the three CBCL subscales, Anxious/depression, Attention problems, and Aggressive behaviors [43,49]. The reliability coefficients (Cronbach) of CBCL Attention Problems, Aggression, and Anxious/Depressed subscales were 0.82, 0.81, and 0.82, respectively.

Type of suicidality and severity of suicidal ideation and behavior were assessed using the Columbia–Suicide Severity Rating Scale (CSSRS), (score 3 or higher), recommended by the Center for Disease Control and Prevention and Food and Drug Administration for the assessment of adolescents at high suicidal risk.

In order to explore further psychological features possibly related to suicidal risk, that is attitude to life and death, impulsivity, and resilience abilities facing life adversities, three specific measures were included in the assessment for all the individuals included in the study.

The Multi-Attitude Suicide Tendency Scale (MAST) [50] was used to assess attitude for life and death, related to the fearlessness about death, and to the capability for suicide. This measure, designed to assess suicidal tendencies in youth, is a 30-item scale exploring four types of attitudes: attraction to life, repulsion by life, attraction to death, and repulsion by death. All four factor scales showed good reliability estimates, as well as relationships with measures of suicidal behavior and ideation and general psychopathology [50,51].

Impulsivity was assessed with the Barratt Impulsiveness Scale-11 (BIS-11) [52,53], including 30 items that are scored to yield second-order factors, Attentional, Motor, and Non-planning impulsiveness.

Resilience was explored with the Resilience scale for Adolescent (READ) [54–56], a self-administered 28-item questionnaire, with a score for each item ranging from 1 (totally disagree) to 5 (totally agree), which incorporates intrapersonal and interpersonal protective factors mapping onto the three salient domains of resilience, including individual, family, and external environment. Confirmatory factor analysis validated the original five-factor structure of the READ, including Personal Competence,

Social Competence, Structured Style, Family Cohesion, and Social Resources. The measures showed good reliability and validity in adolescents [57].

All participants and parents were informed about the assessment instruments. Written informed consent was obtained from participants and parents. The study conformed to Declaration of Helsinki; the Ethics Committee of the Hospital approved the methodology of the study (Identification Code 2014/0001507).

2.3. Statistical Analyses

Descriptive analyses were used to describe demographic and clinical characteristics of the whole sample. Chi-square analyses were performed on categorical variables, and a t-test or one-way ANOVA on continuous variables, with statistical significance set at 0.05. The Bonferroni–Holm method was used for multiple comparisons. The Student's t-test, with Bonferroni correction, was used in order to compare the calibrated severity score of ADOS-2 between BD-ASD-S and BD-ASD-noS.

A structural equation modeling (SEM) was conducted to examine the association between resilience protective factors measured by READ scales and suicide tendency measured by the MAST (attraction and/or repulsion to life and/or death) in all individuals. The SEM model has been tested using the maximum likelihood (ML) method since none of the variables exceed the value of |1| for univariate skewness and kurtosis. To examine model fit, several goodness-of-fit indices were used: the comparative fit index (CFI), the Tucker and Lewis index (TLI), the standardized root mean square residual (SRMR), and the root mean square error of approximation (RMSEA).

3. Results

The three groups BD-ASD-S, BD-noASD—S, and BD-ASD-noS did not differ according to mean age (14.53 ± 2.03 years, 14.78 ± 1.86 years and 14.94 ± 2.22 years, respectively, F = 0.175, df = 51, p = 0.840), while gender ratio was uneven, as in the BD-ASD-S the male/female was 14/3, in BD-noASD-S 6/12, and in BD-ASD-noS 10/7, (χ^2 = 8.62, df = 2, p = 0.013). Regarding the frequency of the BD types (BD I, BD II, and BD Not Otherwise Specified) in the three groups, they were respectively, six, seven, and five in the BD-ASD-S; six, eight, and three in the BD-noASD—S; and seven, five, and five in the BD-ASD-noS. Differences among groups were not statistically significant (χ^2 = 0.92, df = 4, p = 0.921, ns).

The intellectual quotient, measured with the WISC-IV, was significantly higher in the BD-ASD-S group than in the other two groups for the full scale IQ and for the verbal comprehension index, while for the perceptual reasoning and working memory indices, BD-ASD-S scored significantly higher than BD-ASD-NoS. The processing speed index did not differ among groups (Table 1).

Regarding clinical severity, assessed with the CGI-S, the BD-ASD-S group was the most severely impaired (6.41 ± 0.71), compared to the BD-noASD-S (6.00 ± 0.68), and BD-ASD-noS (4.82 ± 0.95) (F = 18.5, p < 0.001). Similarly, the BD-ASD-S group presented the greatest functional impairment, assessed with the C-GAS (28.76 ± 7.35), compared to the BD-noASD-S (35.06 ± 7.11), and the BD-ASD-noS (41.47 ± 7.97) (F = 12.25, p < 0.001).

According to the type of suicidality, assessed with the CSSI-R, types of suicidal ideation, frequency of ideation, control over ideation, deterrents from suicide behavior, and reasons for ideation did not differ among groups. Preparatory acts did not differ, but potential lethality higher than 1 was more frequent in the BD-ASD-S group (41.2%), compared to the BD-noASD-S group (11.1%) (p = 0.042).

Regarding psychiatric diagnoses, according the K-SADS-PL, only obsessive compulsive disorder was more frequently reported in individuals with BD-ASD-S (70.6%), and with BD-ASD-noS (41.2%), compared to those with BD-noASD-S (5.6%) (χ^2 = 15.70, df = 2, p < 0.001 for both BD- ASD-S and BD-ASD-noS after Bonferroni–Helm method). All the other categorical diagnoses (ADHD, anxiety disorders, depression, and disruptive behavior disorders) did not differ among groups.

Regarding the comparison among groups according to the CBCL, individuals with BD-ASD-S presented higher scores in the internalizing problems, and, among the syndrome scales, in the thought disorders scale, while the anxiety-depressed and the withdrawal scales only approached statistical significance, and the three groups did not differ according to the dysregulation profile score (Table 2).

Table 1. Wechsler Intelligence Scale for Children—Fourth Edition (WISC-IV) (Wechsler, 2003). Comparisons among groups. Legenda; BD-ASD-S = Bipolar Disorder + High Functioning Autism Spectrum Disorder + Severe Suicide Ideation or Attempt; BD-noASD-S = Bipolar Disorder + Severe Suicide Ideation or Attempt, without High Functioning Autism Spectrum Disorder; BD-ASD-noS = Bipolar Disorder + High Functioning Autism Spectrum Disorder, without Severe Suicide Ideation or Attempt; SD: Standard Deviations; FSIQ: Total Intellectual Quotient; VCI: Verbal Comprehension Index; PRI: Perceptual Reasoning Index; WMI: Working Memory Index; PSI: Processing Speed Index. Statistical significance at $p < 0.05$.

	Group 1 BD-ASD-S Mean; SD	Group 2 BD-no ASD-S Mean; SD	Group 3 BD-ASD-NoS Mean; SD	One-Way ANOVA (F); p	Bonferroni–Holm Gr1 vs. Gr.2 p	Gr.1 vs. Gr.3 p	Gr.2 vs. Gr.3 p
FSIQ	112.9; 16.2	97.3; 13.2	84.8; 18.8	(9.43); 0.001	0.041	0.000	ns
VCI	116.6; 18.4	99.8; 15.1	91.0; 17.1	(7.67); 0.002	0.029	0.002	ns
PRI	115.5; 16.9	104.2; 13.2	96.9; 19.8	(4.12); 0.024	Ns	0.023	ns
WMI	102.4; 14.1	91.4; 11.7	80.0; 12.1	(7.59); 0.002	Ns	0.001	ns
PSI	92.3; 10.7	94.94; 18.4	80.0; 18.4	(2.43); ns	Ns	ns	ns

Table 2. Child Behavior Checklist (CBCL): Comparisons among groups. Legenda: BD-ASD-S = Bipolar Disorder + High Functioning Autism Spectrum Disorder + Severe Suicide Ideation or Attempt; BD-noASD-S = Bipolar Disorder + Severe Suicide Ideation or Attempt, without High Functioning Autism Spectrum Disorder; BD-ASD-noS = Bipolar Disorder + High Functioning Autism Spectrum Disorder, without Severe Suicide Ideation or Attempt. Statistical significance at $p < 0.05$.

	Group 1 BD-ASD-S Mean; SD	Group 2 BD-no ASD-S Mean; SD	Group 3 BD-ASD-NoS Mean; SD	One-Way ANOVA (F); p	Gr1 vs. Gr.2 p	Gr.1 vs. Gr.3 p	Gr.2 vs. Gr.3 p
Internalizing	72.7; 7.6	69.9; 4.8	66.4;9.1	(3.1); ns	ns	0.049	ns
Externalizing	60.8; 7.9	63.2; 9.1	60.7; 6.4	(0.57); ns	ns	ns	ns
Total	68.1; 6.2	67.6; 5.6	65.6; 6.7	(0.79); ns	ns	ns	ns
Anxious/Depressed	75.1; 9.8	72.9; 9.2	66.9; 10.8	(3.1); ns	ns	ns	ns
Withdrawn	75.7; 9.3	73.2; 11.3	67.3; 9,9	(3.0); ns	ns	ns	ns
Somatic Complaints	62.8; 9.9	59.3; 7.0	59.2; 9.3	(0.93); ns	ns	ns	ns
Social Problems	65.9; 8.2	64.9; 7.6	67.4; 7.4	(0.46); ns	ns	ns	ns
Thought Problems	70.9; 9.3	70.2; 5.3	63.28: 9.2	(4.7); 0.013	ns	0.023	0.042
Attention	59.4.; 4.9	62.9; 8.9	64.2; 7.9	(1.9); ns	ns	ns	ns
Rule Breaking Problems	59.5; 6.2	627; 8.8	58,8; 5.83	(1.5); ns	ns	ns	ns
Aggressive behavior	61.9; 9.4	64.8; 9.5	60.9; 6.1	(1.0); ns	ns	ns	ns
Dysregulation Profile	196.4; 16.0	200.7; 19.1	192.1; 19.7	(0.96); ns	ns	ns	ns

Autism severity according to ADOS-Calibrated Severity Score, did not differ significantly between suicidal and non-suicidal individuals with ASD (BD-ASD-S: M = 5.85, SD = 1.15 versus BD-ASD-noS: M = 5.59, SD = 0.76 t = 0.701, $p = 0.243$).

All the four scales of the prevalent attitude (repulsion or attraction) for life and death (attraction to life, repulsion by life, attraction to death, and repulsion by death) failed to reach statistical difference among groups.

Similarly, the attentional and motor impulsivity, as well as the total score of the BIS, did not differ in the three groups. On the contrary, the non-planned impulsivity was higher in the BD-noASD-S group, compared to BD-ASD-S and BD-ASD-noS groups (F = 3.85, $p = 0.028$). More specifically, in multiple comparisons, ASD suicidal individuals presented less non planned impulsivity than individuals without ASD ($p = 0.040$).

On the Resilience test (READ), only Personal Competence differed among groups (F = 6.85, $p = 0.004$), as, after multiple comparisons, individuals with BD-ASD-noS significantly outscored those with BD-noASD-S ($p = 0.003$). All the other four dimensions of the scale (Social Competence, Structured Style, Family Cohesion, and Social Resources), as well as total score, were similar among groups.

Results of the path analysis (χ^2 (7) = 6.232, p = ns, CFI = 1, TLI = 1; SRMR = 0.057, RMSEA = 0.000 (0.000–0.164), p = ns) attest that some resilience dimensions were significantly associated with suicide tendency. In particular, personal competences (unstandardized coefficient: −0.19, S.E. = 0.09) and structured style (unstandardized coefficient: −0.29, S.E. = 0.10) were negatively associated with repulsion by life, and social resource (unstandardized coefficient: −0.24, S.E. = 0.12) was negatively associated with attraction to death. The model explained the 25% of repulsion by life variance, and 0.05% of attraction to death variance (Figure 1).

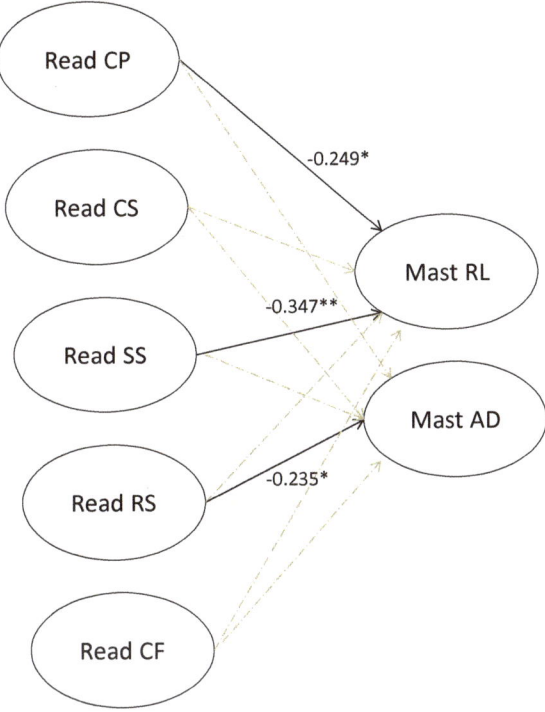

Figure 1. Relationships between Resiliency and Suicide Tendency. Note: READ CP = Personal Competence, READ CS = Social Competence, READ SS = Structured Style, READ RS = Social Resources, READ CF = Family Cohesion, Mast RL = repulsion by life, Mast AD = attraction to death. *: $p < 0.05$, **: $p < 0.01$.

4. Discussion

If BD is a well-known risk factor for suicide ideation and behavior, this risk may be markedly increased in bipolar individuals with HF-ASD. In fact, persons with HF-ASD experience the world in a specific way, compared with typically developing individuals, from basic information processing and attribution processing patterns, to social perspectives, such as the difficulties in expressing feelings and communicating with others [4,8,32,53,54,58]. A better comprehension of possible peculiarities in a very special population with both BD and HF-ASD may improve our understanding on how suicidal behaviors may be recognized, managed and treated. In our study, suicidal bipolar individuals with ASD were more frequently males, and presented greater clinical severity and functional impairment. Furthermore, they presented higher potential lethality of their suicidality, compared to the group without ASD, consistently with literature findings [17,32,55,56,59,60]. These differences were not accounted for by the type of BD, which did not differ among groups.

The suicidal individuals with ASD presented also a higher IQ, suggesting that the psychopathological severity has a greater impact on global functioning than their cognitive functioning [57,61]. Consistently, studies on populations with neurodevelopmental disorders reported that individuals with intellectual disabilities show a lower suicide rate than general population [57,58,61,62]. A high IQ may represent a specific risk factor [59,60,63,64], as it may imply an increased self-consciousness of one's own disability, leading to painful feelings of inadequacy, guilt, and exclusion from peer groups. Such aspects may be more evident during adolescence, when heightened social requests can easily go beyond the individual's coping abilities, further worsening the social withdrawal [58,61–63,65–68].

Regarding psychiatric diagnoses, only OCD differed among groups, and was more frequently reported in ASD individuals, irrespective of the presence of suicidality. However, a recent study showed that rumination was significantly associated with a history of attempted suicide in a sample of 75 adults with ASD [8,16].

Suicidal individuals with BD-ASD individuals presented at the CBCL (completed by parents) significantly more internalizing problems and thought problems. Internalized symptoms can represent a risk factor for suicide in individuals with ASD [16,24]. Hence, investigating symptoms with standardized scales with both individuals and caregivers, including direct psychiatric interviews, is crucial, given that many individuals with HF-ASD are able to "camouflage" internalized symptoms.

The severity of autistic traits in individuals with or without suicidality, according to ADOS-2, did not differ between the two groups, suggesting that this feature does not affect the suicidal risk. Available evidence on this topic is inconsistent. While a number of studies on "Asperger syndrome" populations have shown a negative correlation between suicidal ideation and autistic traits [15,23,67,69], on the contrary Cassidy et al. [7,15] reported that persons diagnosed with Asperger syndrome with previous suicide attempts showed significantly higher autistic traits than individuals with this diagnosis without a history of attempted suicide.

In our study, the three groups did not differ according to repulsion or attraction for life and death. On the contrary, non-planned impulsivity was highest in the BD-noASD-S group, compared to both the ASD groups (with or without suicidality), suggesting that in individuals with ASD the suicidality may be less impulsive than in individuals without ASD, although both the groups have a diagnosis of BD This could imply a "colder" transition from ideation to suicide attempt, leading to more lethal strategies [68,70].

Regarding resilience, personal competence was lowest in individuals with BD-noASD-S individuals, and highest in those with BD-non suicidal ASD, with intermediate scores in the BD-ASD-S group, suggesting that the feeling of a low personal competence is more urgent in non-autistic individuals, and namely in those who present suicidal ideation or behavior, in whom it may have a triggering role in their suicidality.

A structural equation modeling was applied to examine the influences among variables that may interact, namely, between resilience protective factors, and suicide tendency, in terms of attraction and/or repulsion to life and/or death. Some dimensions of resilience, particularly personal competences and structured style were protective in terms of repulsion by life, while social resource was protective in terms of attraction to death. This information may guide possible therapeutic interventions aimed at reinforcing specific areas of resilience in order to improve some risk factors related to suicide vulnerability in adolescence.

Our study shows a number of limitations that could limit the generalization of the results. Major limitations of the study are the small sample size, and the lack of a control group of typically developing adolescents. Furthermore, these groups were not recruited through an age- and gender-matching protocol design, although no statistically significant age difference emerged, and the female component was only scarcely represented. Finally, only a selected number of features were considered as relevant, and the diagnostic exploration did not include other potentially important elements.

Our study provides a first, exploratory contribution for better understanding the peculiarities of adolescents with BD and ASD and severe suicide ideation or suicide attempts, helpful for subsequent targeted examination of suicidality in autism/bipolar disorder. These specificities may help clinicians not only in the diagnostic process, focusing investigations on specific areas, but also in the prevention and treatment strategies, for planning timely and finely customized educational and therapeutic approaches, at the individual level, contributing to a precision medicine even in these complex and often misunderstood individuals.

Author Contributions: Conceptualization: G.M., S.S., M.M., G.D.; Methodology: G.M., G.D., A.N., P.M., M.P.; Data collection: S.S, D.F., F.L., G.D.; Statistical analyses: P.M. and M.P.; Writing first draft: G.M.; Discussion on the first draft and conclusions: S.S., A.N., P.M., M.P., D.F., F.L., M.M., G.D.; All authors have read and agreed to the published version of the manuscript.

Funding: This research was funded by the Italian Ministry of the Health RC2019 and 5 × 1000 founds.

Acknowledgments: The authors wish to thank all the participants, the adolescent and their parents

Conflicts of Interest: Gabriele Masi was in advisory boards for Angelini, received grants from Lundbeck and Humana, and was speaker for Angelini, FB Health, Janssen, Lundbeck, and Otsuka. The other authors report no other conflicts of interest.

References

1. Nock, M.W.; Green, J.G.; Hwang, I.; Mclaughlin, K.A.; Sampson, M.A.; Zaslavsky, A.M.; Kessler, R.C. Prevalence, correlates and treatment of lifetime suicidal behavior among adolescents: Results from the National Comorbidity Survey Replication –Adolescent Supplement (NCSA). *JAMA Psychiatry* **2013**, *70*, 300–310. [CrossRef] [PubMed]
2. Glenn, C.R.; Kleiman, E.M.; Kellerman, J.; Pollak, O.; Cha, C.B.; Esposito, E.C.; Porter, A.C.; Wyman, P.A.; Boatman, A.E. Annual Research Review: A meta-analytic review of worldwide suicide rates in adolescents. *J. Child Psychol. Psychiatry* **2020**, *61*, 294–308. [CrossRef] [PubMed]
3. Hawton, K.; Saunders, K.E.; O'Connor, R.C. Self-harm and suicide in adolescents. *Lancet* **2012**, *379*, 2373–2382. [CrossRef]
4. Oliphant, R.Y.K.; Smith, E.M.; Grahame, V. What is the Prevalence of Self-harming and Suicidal Behaviour in Under 18s with ASD, with or Without an Intellectual Disability? *J. Autism. Dev. Disord.* **2020**. [CrossRef] [PubMed]
5. Wijnhoven, L.A.; Niels-Kessels, H.; Creemers, D.H.; Verhulst, A.A.; Otten, R.; Engels, R.C. Prevalence of comorbid depressive symptoms and suicidal ideation in children with autism spectrum disorder and elevated anxiety symptoms. *J. Child Adolesc. Mental Health* **2019**, *31*, 77–84. [CrossRef]
6. Hirvikoski, T.; Mittendorfer-Rutz, E.; Boman, M.; Larsson, H.; Lichtenstein, P.; Bölte, S. Premature mortality in autism spectrum disorder. *Br. J. Psychiatry* **2016**, *208*, 232–238. [CrossRef]
7. Cassidy, S.; Bradley, P.; Robinson, J.; Allison, C.; McHugh, M.; Baron-Cohen, S. Suicidal ideation and suicide plans or attempts in adults with Asperger's syndrome attending a specialist diagnostic clinic: A clinical cohort study. *Lancet Psychiatry* **2014**, *1*, 142–147. [CrossRef]
8. Arwert, T.G.; Sizoo, B.B. Self-reported Suicidality in Male and Female Adults with Autism Spectrum Disorders: Rumination and Self-esteem. *J. Autism Dev. Disord.* **2020**. [CrossRef]
9. Fitzgerald, M. Suicide and Asperger's syndrome. *Crisis* **2007**, *28*, 1–3. [CrossRef]
10. Cassidy, S.; Bradley, L.; Shaw, R. Baron-Cohen, S. Risk markers for suicidality in autistic adults. *Mol. Autism.* **2018**, *31*, 9–42.
11. Chen, M.H.; Pan, T.L.; Lan, W.H.; Hsu, J.W.; Huang, K.L.; Su, T.P.; Li, C.T.; Lin, W.C.; Wei, H.T.; Chen, T.J.; et al. Risk of Suicide Attempts among Adolescents and Young Adults with Autism Spectrum Disorder: A Nationwide Longitudinal Follow-Up Study. *J. Clin. Psychiatry* **2017**, *78*, e1174–e1179. [CrossRef] [PubMed]
12. Culpin, I.; Mars, B.; Pearson, R.M.; Golding, J.; Heron, J.; Bubak, I.; Carpenter, P.; Magnusson, C.; Gunnell, D.; Rai, D. Autistic Traits and Suicidal Thoughts, Plans, and Self-Harm in Late Adolescence: Population-Based Cohort Study. *J. Am. Acad. Child Adolesc. Psychiatry* **2018**, *57*, 313–320. [CrossRef]
13. Veenstra-VanderWeele, J. Recognizing the Problem of Suicidality in Autism Spectrum Disorder. *J. Am. Acad. Child Adolesc. Psychiatry* **2018**, *57*, 302–303. [CrossRef] [PubMed]

14. Cappadocia, M.C.; Weiss, J.A.; Pepler, D. Bullying experiences among children and youth with autism spectrum disorders. *J. Autism Dev. Disord.* **2012**, *42*, 266–277. [CrossRef] [PubMed]
15. Shtayermman, O. Peer victimization in adolescents and young adults diagnosed with Asperger's Syndrome: A link to depressive symptomatology, anxiety symptomatology and suicidal ideation. *Issues Compr. Pediatr. Nurs.* **2007**, *30*, 87–107. [CrossRef]
16. Storch, E.A.; Sulkowski, M.L.; Nadeau, J.; Lewin, A.B.; Arnold, E.B.; Mutch, P.J.; Jones, A.M.; Murphy, T.K. The phenomenology and clinical correlates of suicidal thoughts and behaviors in youth with autism spectrum disorders. *J. Autism. Dev. Disord.* **2013**, *43*, 2450–2459. [CrossRef] [PubMed]
17. Hedley, D.; Uljarević, M.; Foley, K.R.; Richdale, A.; Trollor, J. Risk and protective factors underlying depression and suicidal ideation in Autism Spectrum Disorder. *Depress. Anxiety* **2018**, *35*, 648–657. [CrossRef]
18. Leyfer, O.T.; Folstein, S.E.; Bacalman, S.; Davis, N.O.; Dinh, E.; Morgan, J.; Tager-Flusberg, H.; Lainhart, J.E. Comorbid psychiatric disorders in children with autism: Interview development and rates of disorders. *J. Autism Dev. Disord.* **2006**, *36*, 849–861. [CrossRef]
19. van Steensel, F.J.; Bögels, S.M.; Perrin, S. Anxiety disorders in children and adolescents with autistic spectrum disorders: A meta-analysis. *Clin. Child Fam. Psychol. Rev.* **2011**, *14*, 302–317. [CrossRef] [PubMed]
20. Ben-Sasson, A.; Hen, L.; Fluss, R.; Cermak, S.A.; Engel-Yeger, B.; Gal, E. A meta-analysis of sensory modulation symptoms in individuals with autism spectrum disorders. *J. Autism Dev. Disord.* **2009**, *39*, 1–11. [CrossRef]
21. Foley Nicpon, M.; Doobay, A.F.; Assouline, S.G. Parent, teacher, and self-perceptions of psychosocial functioning in intellectually gifted children and adolescents with autism spectrum disorder. *J. Autism Dev. Disord.* **2010**, *40*, 1028–1038. [CrossRef] [PubMed]
22. Meyer, J.A.; Mundy, P.C.; Vaughan Van Hecke, A.; Durocher, J.S. Social attribution processes and comorbid psychiatric symptoms in children with Asperger syndrome. *Autism* **2006**, *10*, 383–402. [CrossRef]
23. Twenge, J.M.; Cooper, A.B.; Joiner, T.E.; Duffy, M.E.; Binau, S.G. Age, period, and cohort trends in mood disorder indicators and suicide-related outcomes in a nationally representative dataset, 2005–2017. *J. Abnorm. Psychol.* **2019**, *128*, 185–199. [CrossRef] [PubMed]
24. Rao, U.; Weissman, M.M.; Martin, J.A.; Hammond, R.W. Childhood depression and risk of suicide: A preliminary report of a longitudinal study. *J. Am. Acad. Child Adolesc. Psychiatry* **1993**, *32*, 21–27. [CrossRef] [PubMed]
25. Plans, L.; Barrot, C.; Nieto, E.; Rios, J.; Schulze, T.G.; Papiol, S.; Mitjans, M.; Vieta, E.; Benabarre, A. Association between completed suicide and bipolar disorder: A systematic review of the literature. *J. Affect. Disord.* **2019**, *242*, 111–122. [CrossRef] [PubMed]
26. Hossain, M.M.; Khan, N.; Sultana, A.; Ma, P.; McKyer, E.L.J.; Ahmed, H.U.; Purohit, N. Prevalence of comorbid psychiatric disorders among people with autism spectrum disorder: An umbrella review of systematic reviews and meta-analyses. *Psychiat. Res.* **2020**, *18*, 112922. [CrossRef]
27. Simonoff, E.; Pickels, A.; Charman, T.; Chandler, S.; Loucas, T.; Baird, G. Psychiatric disorders in children and adolescents with autism spectrum disorders: Prevalence, comorbidity, and associated factors in a population-derived sample. *J. Am. Acad. Child Adolesc. Psychiatry* **2008**, *47*, 921–929. [CrossRef]
28. Lugo Marín, J.; Alviani Rodríguez-Franco, M.; Mahtani Chugani, V.; Magán Maganto, M.; Díez Villoria, E.; Canal Bedia, R. Prevalence of schizophrenia spectrum disorders in average-iq adults with autism spectrum disorders: A meta-analysis. *J. Autism Dev. Disord.* **2018**, *48*, 239–250. [CrossRef]
29. Lai, M.-C.; Kassee, C.; Besney, R.; Bonato, S.; Hull, L.; Mandy, W.; Szatmari, P.; Ameis, S.H. Prevalence of co-occurring mental health diagnoses in the autism population: A systematic review and meta-analysis. *Lancet Psychiatry* **2019**. [CrossRef]
30. Hudson, C.C.; Hall, L.; Harkness, K.L. Prevalence of depressive disorders in individuals with autism spectrum disorder: A meta-analysis. *J. Abnorm. Child Psychol.* **2019**, *47*, 165–175. [CrossRef]

31. Joshi, G.; Biederman, J.; Petty, C.; Goldin, R.I.; Eurtak, S.L.; Wozniak, J. Examining the comorbidity of bipolar disorder and autism spectrum disorders: A large controlled analysis of phenotypic and familial correlates in a referred population of youth with bipolar I disorder with and without autism spectrum disorders. *J. Clin. Psychiatry* **2013**, *74*, 578–586. [CrossRef] [PubMed]
32. Vannucchi, G.; Masi, G.; Toni, C.; Dell'Osso, L.; Erfurth, A.; Perugi, G. Bipolar disorder in adults with Asperger's Syndrome: A systematic review. *J. Affect. Disord.* **2014**, *168*, 151–160. [CrossRef] [PubMed]
33. Dell'Osso, L.; Carpita, B.; Muti, D.; Morelli, V.; Salarpi, G.; Salerni, A.; Scotto, J.; Massimetti, C.; Gesi, C.; Ballerio, M.; et al. Mood symptoms and suicidality across the autism spectrum. *Compr. Psychiatry* **2019**, *91*, 34–38. [CrossRef]
34. Osman, A.; Gilpin, A.R.; Kopper, B.A.; Barrios, F.X.; Gutierrez, P.M.; Chiros, C.E. The Multi Attitude Suicide Tendency Scale: Further Validation with Adolescent Psychiatric Inpatients. *Suicide Life Threat Behav.* **2000**, *30*, 377–385. [PubMed]
35. Klomek, A.B.; Orbach, I.; Sher, L.; Sommerfeld, E.; Diller, R.; Apter, A.; Shahar, G.; Zalsman, G. Quality of depression among suicidal inpatient youth. *Arch. Suicide Res.* **2008**, *12*, 133–140. [CrossRef]
36. Park, C.H.K.; Lee, J.W.; Lee, S.Y.; Shim, S.H.; Moon, J.J.; Paik, J.W.; Cho, S.J.; Kim, S.G.; Kim, M.H.; Kim, S.; et al. Implications of Increased Trait Impulsivity on Psychopathology and Experienced Stress in the Victims of Early Trauma With Suicidality. *J. Nerv. Ment. Dis.* **2018**, *206*, 840–849. [CrossRef]
37. Jakobsen, I.S.; Larsen, K.J.; Horwood, J.L. Suicide Risk Assessment in Adolescents -C-SSRS, K10, and READ. *Crisis* **2017**, *38*, 247–254. [CrossRef]
38. Kaufman, J.; Birmaher, B.; Brent, D.; Rao, U.; Flynn, C.; Moreci, P.; Williamson, D.; Ryan, N. Schedule for Affective Disorders and Schizophrenia for School-Age Children-Present and Lifetime Version (K-SADS-PL): Initial reliability and validity data. *J. Am. Acad. Child Adolesc. Psychiatry* **1997**, *36*, 980–988. [CrossRef]
39. American Psychiatric Association. *Diagnostic and Statistical Manual for Mental Disorders – Fifth Edition (DSM 5)*; American Psychiatric Association: Arlington, VA, USA, 2013.
40. Lord, C.; Rutter, M.; DiLavore, P.C.; Risi, S.; Gotham, K.; Bishop, S. *Autism Diagnostic Observation Schedule*, 2nd ed.; Western Psychological Services: Torrance, CA, USA, 2012.
41. Rutter, M.; Le Couteur, A.; Lord, C. *Autism Diagnostic Interview – Revised*; Western Psychological Services: Torrance, CA, USA, 2003.
42. Saemundsen, E.; Magnússon, P.; Smári, J.; Sigurdardóttir, S. Autism Diagnostic Interview-Revised and the Childhood Autism Rating Scale: Convergence and discrepancy in diagnosing autism. *J. Autism Dev. Disord.* **2003**, *33*, 319–328. [CrossRef]
43. Posner, K.; Brown, G.K.; Stanley, B.; Brent, D.A.; Yershova, K.V.; Oquendo, M.A.; Currier, G.W.; Melvin, G.A.; Greenhill, L.; Shen, S.; et al. The Columbia-Suicide Severity Rating Scale: Initial validity and internal consistency findings from three multisite studies with adolescents and adults. *Am. J. Psychiatry* **2011**, *168*, 1266–1277. [CrossRef]
44. Wechsler, D. *The Wechsler Intelligence Scale for Children*, 4th ed.; Pearson: London, UK, 2003.
45. Gotham, K.; Pickles, A.; Lord, C. Standardizing ADOS scores for a measure of severity in autism spectrum disorders. *J. Autism Dev. Disord.* **2009**, *39*, 693–705. [CrossRef] [PubMed]
46. Guy, W. *ECDEU Assessment Manual for Psychopharmacology, Revised*; US Department of Health, Education and Welfare: Rockville, MD, USA, 1976.
47. Shaffer, D.; Gould, M.S.; Brasic, J.; Ambrosini, P.; Fisher, P.; Bird, H.; Aluwahlia, S.A. Children's Global Assessment Scale (CGAS). *Arch. Gen. Psychiatry* **1983**, *40*, 1228–1231. [CrossRef] [PubMed]
48. Achenbach, T.M.; Rescorla, L.A. *Manual for the ASEBA School-Age Forms and Profiles. Burlington, VT: University of Vermont Research Center for Children, Youth, & Families*; University of Vermont: Burlington, VT, USA, 2001.
49. Deutz, M.H.; Geeraerts, S.B.; van Baar, A.L.; Deković, M.; Prinzie, P. The Dysregulation Profile in middle childhood and adolescence across reporters: Factor structure, measurement invariance, and links with self-harm and suicidal ideation. *Eur. Child Adolesc. Psychiatry* **2016**, *25*, 431–442. [CrossRef] [PubMed]
50. Orbach, I.; Milstein, I.; Har-Even, D.; Apter, A.; Tiano, S.; Elizur, A. A Multi-Attitude Suicide Tendency Scale for adolescents. *J. Consult. Clin. Psychol.* **1991**, *3*, 398–404. [CrossRef]
51. Osman, A.; Barrios, F.X.; Panak, W.F.; Osman, J.R.; Hoffman, J.; Hammer, R. Validation of the Multi-Attitude Suicide Tendency scale in adolescent samples. *J. Clin. Psychol.* **1994**, *50*, 847–855. [CrossRef]
52. Patton, J.H.; Stanford, M.S.; Barratt, E.S. Factor structure of the Barratt impulsiveness scale. *J. Clin. Psychol.* **1995**, *51*, 768–774. [CrossRef]

53. Fossati, A.; Di Ceglie, A.; Acquarini, E.; Barratt, E.S. Psychometric properties of an Italian version of the Barratt Impulsiveness Scale-11 (BIS-11) in nonclinical subjects. *J. Clin. Psychol.* **2001**, *57*, 815–828. [CrossRef] [PubMed]
54. Hjemdal, O.; Friborg, O.; Stiles, T.C.; Martinussen, M.; Rosenvinge, J. A new scale for adolescent resilience: Grasping the central protective resources behind healthy development. *Measur. Eval. Couns. Dev.* **2006**, *39*, 84–96. [CrossRef]
55. Stratta, P.; Riccardi, I.; Di Cosimo, A.; Rossi, A.; Rossi, A. A validation study of the italian version of the resilience scale for adolescents (READ). *J. Commun. Psychol.* **2012**, *40*. [CrossRef]
56. von Soest, T.; Mossige, S.; Stefansen, K.; Hjemdal, O.A. Validation Study of the Resilience Scale for Adolescents (READ). *J. Psychopathol. Behav. Assess.* **2010**, *32*, 215–225. [CrossRef]
57. Hjemdal, O.; Vogel, P.A.; Solem, S.; Hagan, K.; Stiles, T.C. The relationship between resilience and levels of anxiety, depression and obsessive-compulsive symptoms in adolescents. *Clin. Psychol. Psychother.* **2011**, *18*, 314–321. [CrossRef] [PubMed]
58. Lai, M.C.; Anagnostou, E.; Wiznitzer, M.; Allison, C.; Baron-Cohen, S. Evidence-based support for autistic people across the lifespan: Maximising potential, minimising barriers, and optimising the person-environment fit. *Lancet Neurol.* **2020**. [CrossRef]
59. Kato, K.; Mikami, K.; Akama, F.; Yamada, K.; Maehara, M.; Kimoto, K.; Kimoto, K.; Sato, R.; Takahashi, Y.; Fukushima, R.; et al. Clinical features of suicide attempts in adults with autism spectrum disorders. *Gen. Hosp. Psychiatry* **2013**, *35*, 50–53. [CrossRef] [PubMed]
60. Hannon, G.; Taylor, E.P. Suicidal behaviour in adolescents and young adults with ASD: Findings from a systematic review. *Clin. Psychol. Rev.* **2013**, *33*, 1197–1204. [CrossRef]
61. Howlin, P.; Asgharian, A. The diagnosis of autism and Asperger syndrome: Findings from a survey of 770 families. *Dev. Med. Child Neurol.* **1999**, *41*, 834–839. [CrossRef]
62. Huband, N.; Tantam, D. Attitudes to self-injury within a group of mental health staff. *Br. J. Med. Psychol.* **2000**, *73*, 495–504. [CrossRef]
63. Myriam De-la-Iglesia, M.; Olivar, J.S. Risk factors for depression in children and adolescents with high functioning autosm spectrum disorders. *Sci. World J.* **2015**, 127853. [CrossRef]
64. Balfe, M.; Tantam, D. A descriptive social and health profile of a community sample of adults and adolescents with Asperger syndrome. *BMC Res. Notes* **2010**, *3*, 300. [CrossRef]
65. Gotham, K.; Bishop, S.L.; Brunwasser, S.; Lord, C. Rumination and perceived impairment associated with depressive symptoms in a verbal adolescent-adult ASD sample. *Autism Res.* **2014**, *7*, 381–391. [CrossRef]
66. Hedley, D.; Young, R. Social comparison processes and depressive symptoms in children and adolescents with Asperger syndrome. *Autism* **2006**, *10*, 139–153. [CrossRef]
67. Turecki, G. Preventing suicide: Where are we? *Lancet Psychiatry* **2016**, *3*, 597–598. [CrossRef]
68. Brent, D.A.; Perper, J.; Goldstein, C.; Kolko, D.J.; Allan, M.J.; Allman, C.J.; Zelenak, J.P. Risk factor for adolescent suicide. A comparison of adolescent suicide victims with suicidal in patients. *Arch. Gen. Psychiatry.* **1988**, *45*, 581–588. [CrossRef] [PubMed]
69. Demirkaya Karakoç, S.; Tutkunkardaş, M.D.; Mukaddes, N.M. Assessment of suicidality in children and adolescents with diagnosis of high functioning autism spectrum disorder in a Turkish clinical sample. *Neuropsychiatr. Dis. Treat.* **2016**, *11*, 2921–2926. [CrossRef] [PubMed]
70. McDonnell, C.G.; Bradley, C.C.; Kanne, S.M.; Lajonchere, C.; Warren, Z.; Carpenter, L.A. When Are We Sure? Predictors of Clinician Certainty in the Diagnosis of Autism Spectrum Disorder. *J. Autism Dev. Disord.* **2019**, *49*, 1391–1401. [CrossRef]

Publisher's Note: MDPI stays neutral with regard to jurisdictional claims in published maps and institutional affiliations.

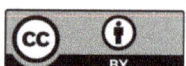

© 2020 by the authors. Licensee MDPI, Basel, Switzerland. This article is an open access article distributed under the terms and conditions of the Creative Commons Attribution (CC BY) license (http://creativecommons.org/licenses/by/4.0/).

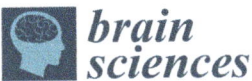 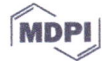

Article

Genome, Environment, Microbiome and Metabolome in Autism (GEMMA) Study Design: Biomarkers Identification for Precision Treatment and Primary Prevention of Autism Spectrum Disorders by an Integrated Multi-Omics Systems Biology Approach

Jacopo Troisi [1,*], Reija Autio [2], Thanos Beopoulos [3], Carmela Bravaccio [4], Federica Carraturo [5], Giulio Corrivetti [6], Stephen Cunningham [7], Samantha Devane [8], Daniele Fallin [9], Serguei Fetissov [10], Manuel Gea [3], Antonio Giorgi [11], François Iris [3], Lokesh Joshi [7], Sarah Kadzielski [8], Aletta Kraneveld [12], Himanshu Kumar [13], Christine Ladd-Acosta [9], Geraldine Leader [7], Arlene Mannion [7], Elise Maximin [14], Alessandra Mezzelani [15], Luciano Milanesi [15], Laurent Naudon [14], Lucia N. Peralta Marzal [12], Paula Perez Pardo [12], Naika Z. Prince [12], Sylvie Rabot [14], Guus Roeselers [13], Christophe Roos [16], Lea Roussin [14], Giovanni Scala [1], Francesco Paolo Tuccinardi [5] and Alessio Fasano [17]

1. Theoreo srl spin off company of the University of Salerno, Via degli Ulivi, 3, 84090 Montecorvino Pugliano (SA), Italy; scala@theoreosrl.com
2. Faculty of Social Sciences, Health Sciences Unit, Tampere University, Arvo Ylpön Katu 34, 33014 Tampere, Finland; reija.autio@tuni.fi
3. Bio-Modeling System, 3, Rue De L'arrivee. 75015 Paris, France; thanos.beopoulos@bmsystems.org (T.B.); manuel.gea@bmsystems.org (M.G.); francois.iris@bmsystems.org (F.I.)
4. Department of science medicine translational, University of Naples Federico II, Via Pansini 5, 80131 Naples, Italy; carmela.bravaccio@unina.it
5. Promete srl, Piazzale Tecchio 45, 80125 Napoli, Italy; federica.carraturo@unina.it (F.C.); tuccinardi@promete.it (F.P.T.)
6. Azienda Sanitaria Locale (ASL) Salerno, Via Nizza, 146, 84125 Salerno (SA), Italy; corrivetti@gmail.com
7. National University of Ireland Galaway, University Road, Galaway, Ireland; stephen.cunningham@nuigalway.ie (S.C.); lokesh.joshi@nuigalway.ie (L.J.); geraldine.leader@nuigalway.ie (G.L.); arlene.mannion@nuigalway.ie (A.M.)
8. Massachusetts General Hospital, Fruit Street, 55, Boston, MA 02114, USA; SDEVANE@mgh.harvard.edu (S.D.); smkadzielski@mgh.harvard.edu (S.K.)
9. John Hopkins School of Public Health and the Wendy Klag Center for Autism and Developmental Disabilities, 615 N. Wolfe St, Baltimore, MD 21205, USA; dfallin@jhu.edu (D.F.); claddac1@jhu.edu (C.L.-A.)
10. Laboratory of Neuronal and Neuroendocrine Differentiation and Communication, Inserm UMR 1239, Rouen University of Normandy, 25 rue Tesnière, 76130 Mont-Saint-Aignan, France; Serguei.Fetissov@univ-rouen.fr
11. Medinok Spa, Via Palazziello, 80040 Volla (NA), Italy; a.giorgi@perfexia.it
12. Division of Pharmacology, Utrecht Institute for Pharmaceutical Sciences, Faculty of Science, Utrecht University, Universiteitsweg 99, 3508 TB Utrecht, The Netherlands; a.d.kraneveld@uu.nl (A.K.); l.n.peraltamarzal@uu.nl (L.N.P.M.); p.perezpardo@uu.nl (P.P.P.); n.z.prince@uu.nl (N.Z.P.)
13. Danone Nutricia Research, Uppsalalaan, 12, 3584 CT Utrecht, The Netherlands; Himanshu.KUMAR@nutricia.com (H.K.); Guus.ROESELERS@danone.com (R.G.)
14. Institut National de Recherche Pour L'agriculture, L'alimentation et L'environnement (INRAE), AgroParisTech, Micalis Institute, Université Paris-Saclay, 78350 Jouy-en-Josas, France; Elise.Maximin@inrae.fr (E.M.); laurent.naudon@inrae.fr (L.N.); sylvie.rabot@inrae.fr (S.R.); lea.roussin@inrae.fr (L.R.)
15. Consiglio Nazionale delle Ricerche (CNR), Piazzale Aldo Moro, 7, 00185 Roma, Italy; alessandra.mezzelani@itb.cnr.it (A.M.); luciano.milanesi@itb.cnr.it (L.M.)
16. Euformatics, Tekniikantie, 02150 Espoo, Finland; christophe.roos@euformatics.com
17. European Biomedical Research Institute of Salerno (EBRIS), Via S. de Renzi, 3, 84125 Salerno (SA), Italy; afasano@mgh.harvard.edu

*   Correspondence: troisi@theoreosrl.com; Tel./Fax: +39-089-0977-435

Received: 29 August 2020; Accepted: 14 October 2020; Published: 16 October 2020

Abstract: Autism Spectrum Disorder (ASD) affects approximately 1 child in 54, with a 35-fold increase since 1960. Selected studies suggest that part of the recent increase in prevalence is likely attributable to an improved awareness and recognition, and changes in clinical practice or service availability. However, this is not sufficient to explain this epidemiological phenomenon. Research points to a possible link between ASD and intestinal microbiota because many children with ASD display gastro-intestinal problems. Current large-scale datasets of ASD are limited in their ability to provide mechanistic insight into ASD because they are predominantly cross-sectional studies that do not allow evaluation of perspective associations between early life microbiota composition/function and later ASD diagnoses. Here we describe GEMMA (Genome, Environment, Microbiome and Metabolome in Autism), a prospective study supported by the European Commission, that follows at-risk infants from birth to identify potential biomarker predictors of ASD development followed by validation on large multi-omics datasets. The project includes clinical (observational and interventional trials) and pre-clinical studies in humanized murine models (fecal transfer from ASD probands) and in vitro colon models. This will support the progress of a microbiome-wide association study (of human participants) to identify prognostic microbiome signatures and metabolic pathways underlying mechanisms for ASD progression and severity and potential treatment response.

Keywords: microbiome; metabolomics; autism; study design; biomarker discovery; precise medicine

1. Introduction

Autism Spectrum Disorder (ASD) is a lifelong neurodevelopmental disorder characterized by deficits in social communication and social interaction, in addition to restricted, repetitive patterns of behavior, interests, or activities [1]. As a spectrum disorder, its symptoms may range from mild to severe. Some children may have strong language and intellectual abilities whereas others may not be verbal and may require lifelong care. Globally, ASD incidence has shown a 35-fold increase compared to the 1960s and 1970s, when the first epidemiological studies were conducted [2–6]. As documented by the Centers for Disease Control and Prevention, ASD affects 1 in 54 children in USA [7] and 1 in 89 in Europe [8].

Children born in a family with an affected sibling show a ten-fold higher risk of developing the condition [9]. These data, including a large-scale exome sequencing study [10], suggest a combination of non-Mendelian genetic and environmental factors in ASD pathogenesis [11,12]. One environmental factor that is emerging as important for ASD risk is the immune system [13–16]. Indeed, individuals with ASD show increased expression of genes encoding mediators of the innate immune response [15]. Low-grade systemic inflammatory events [17,18], combined with the hypofunction of protective, anti-inflammatory mechanisms [19], lead to mechanisms related to the biochemical and neuroanatomical characteristics associated with autism pathogenesis [20–22]. Immunoregulation, in addition to dysregulated immunoregulation, particularly during the first 1000 days of life [23], are guided by the gut microbiome. Low-grade systemic inflammatory responses can lead to psychiatric disorders, such as ASD and psychological stress, which leads to further inflammation through pathways involved in the intestinal microbiota homeostasis [24,25].

Many individuals with ASD have symptoms of associated comorbidities. These include medical comorbidities, such as gastrointestinal (GI) and immune system disorders (namely gut dysbiosis, susceptibility to infections, and increased prevalence of autoimmune disorders), sleep problems, feeding problems and epilepsy; comorbid psychopathology, including Attention-Deficit/Hyperactivity

Disorder (AD/HD), anxiety, mood problems, disruptive behavior; and developmental comorbidity, namely the presence of an intellectual disability.

A large number of individuals are living with ASD. Thus, ASD is a serious public health concern. The medical expenditure for ASD is higher than that for cancer, heart disease, and stroke combined [26,27]. Blumberg et al. [28] suggested that the recent increase in prevalence could be in part attributed to greater recognition and awareness, or changes in clinical practice or service availability. However, these changes are not sufficient to explain this phenomenon [6]. ASD is a multifactorial disorder; therefore, the contribution of environmental factors could explain its development in addition to why different therapeutic approaches, based on gene/environment interaction theory, have achieved conflicting results [29–31]. The GEMMA (Genome, Environment, Microbiome and Metabolome in Autism) team hypothesizes that many environmental factors can alter intestinal microbiota composition and activity, causing epigenetic modifications, changes in the metabolome profile, and increases in intestinal barrier permeability and macromolecule trafficking with the alteration of immune responses, thus contributing to the progression and development of ASD. Furthermore, it is hypothesized that the genome/metagenome interaction determines the switch from immune tolerance to immune response. Environmental stimuli, including dietary and microbial factors, can trigger an immune response, such as the neuroinflammation responsible for the behavioral changes that characterize ASD and intestinal inflammation causing its GI comorbidity.

The existence of a gut–brain axis was hypothesized by Bolte in the late 1990s [32]. This was one of the first reports of unhealthy changes in the intestinal tract's resident community (microbiome), driving both behavioral and GI problems in babies with ASD. Finegold et al. [33] showed that the increase in toxin-producing gut bacteria populations directly affects the brain via the vagus nerve. Currently, changes in gut microbiota of ASD patients with and without GI symptoms are well established [34–36], suggesting the potential beneficial effect of fecal transplantation [37,38].

Unfortunately, current large-scale studies of ASD are mainly of cross-sectional study design, which can provide information about associations between microbiome changes and ASD diagnoses but lack the information regarding the temporality of these changes. This limits inferences about causality or utility as an early life biomarker. Indeed, currently, there are no established biomarkers for ASD to enable its clinical diagnosis, which relies on behavioral evaluations. In addition, no medications are currently available to treat the core symptoms of ASD and results from intervention research are mixed [39].

2. Study Design

GEMMA is a multi-center, prospective, open-label, uncontrolled study with an observational and an interventional arm, comprised of collaborators in the European Union and the United States. It is coordinated by the European Biomedical Research Institute of Salerno (EBRIS), in Campania, Italy. GEMMA aims to study genomic, environmental, microbiome, and metabolomic factors that, via the immune system, may contribute to the development of ASD longitudinally. This study offers the potential to identify the mechanisms and/or biomarkers involved in either development or exacerbation of ASD signs and symptoms, which will potentially broaden the range of available therapeutic interventions (Figure 1).

The project includes clinical (observational and interventional trials) and pre-clinical studies. Several pre-clinical studies in humanized murine models (fecal transfer from ASD probands) and in vitro colon models will be performed simultaneously with clinical studies from the moment of recruitment of at-risk infants and their affected ASD sibling. This will support the progress of a microbiome-wide association study (of human participants) to identify prognostic microbiome signatures and metabolic pathways underlying mechanisms for ASD progression and severity and potential treatment response. The preclinical work will provide valuable information regarding validation of specific biomarkers mechanistically linked to the onset of ASD, which will be used to rationalize future patient stratification for primary intervention.

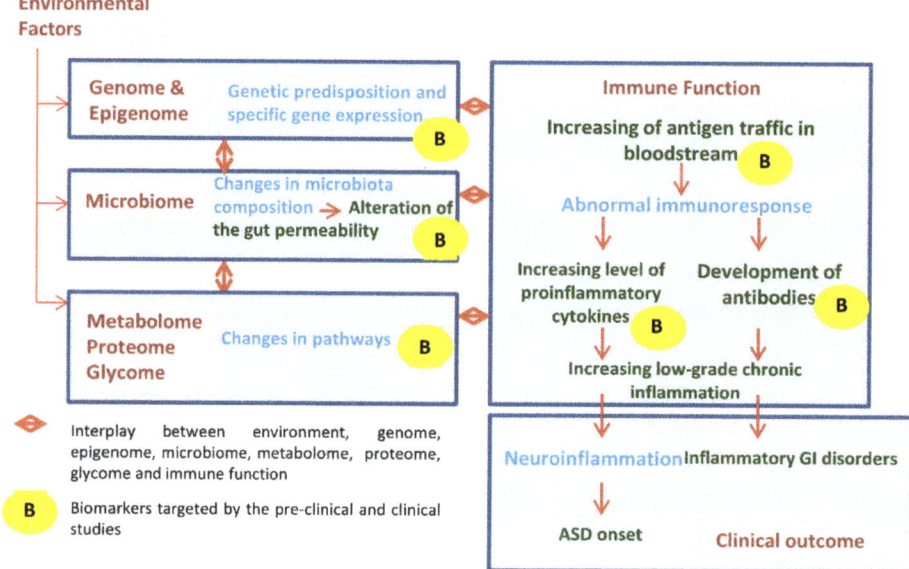

Figure 1. GEMMA (Genome, Environment, Microbiome and Metabolome in Autism) study design.

2.1. Pre-Clinical Studies

An in vitro micro-scale colon microbiota model or "colon microcosm" that mimics the microbiota of the human colon will be used to investigate effects of various combinations of prebiotic fiber types and probiotics on microbiota composition and functionality. The colon microcosms will be inoculated with fecal samples collected from children diagnosed with ASD with and without a history of GI problems, and from healthy siblings (controls) between the ages of 3 and 14. Samples will be excluded if the participants have used psychotropic medications in the previous 6 months and antibiotics and/or probiotics in the previous 2 months (Figure 2).

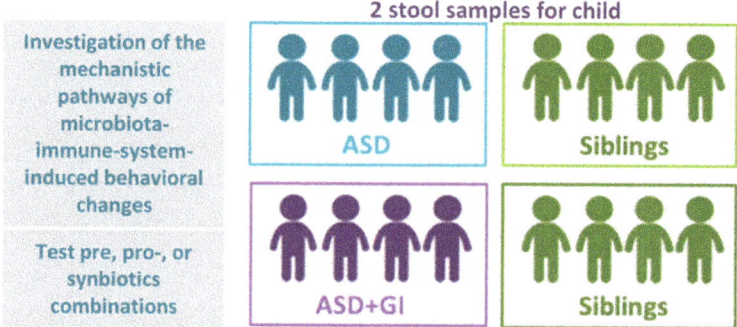

Figure 2. Preclinical studies—development of humanized mouse models by transplanting fecal samples from a well-characterized ASD diagnosed proband (and sibling controls). Four groups of children, each with 4 children, recruited in one center in Europe (Italy): autistic with no GI problems, autistic with GI problems, controls without or with GI problems. Ongoing.

The impact of pre- and probiotic combinations on microbiota composition and function will be measured by 16S rRNA gene sequencing, metagenomics, and targeted and untargeted metabolites analyses.

The preclinical studies in murine models will be carried out simultaneously with the other studies for two reasons: to provide further information on validation of specific biomarkers mechanistically linked to the onset of ASD and, consequently, to treat future patients primarily with a more precise intervention.

The preclinical studies in murine models include the development of humanized mouse models through transplanting fecal samples from a well-characterized ASD diagnosed proband (and sibling controls) in the families included in the clinical observational study. The fecal samples will be the same as those collected for the in vitro studies described above. In addition to wild type naïve mice, fecal transplantation will be conducted in genetically vulnerable (PCDH-KO), food allergic (CMA), and valproate-treated (VPA) male mice which have been previously demonstrated to show ASD-like behavior [40–43]. The natural gut microbiota of these mice will be depleted before transplantation with the human fecal samples. This will be achieved at the age of 3 weeks, with antibiotic treatment followed by a bowel cleansing according to procedures described by Le Roy and coworkers [44]. Fecal transplantation will also be conducted in germ-free male mice, which have abnormal development of the nervous system and show deficits in cognition, social behavior, and stress-related behaviors [45–51]. The microbial content of human donors will be orally administered to recipient microbiota-depleted or germ-free mice. Behavior, microbiota composition, gut permeability, metabolites, mucosal and systemic immune profiles (intestinal tract, mesenteric lymph nodes, blood, and spleen), neurotransmitters, and neuroinflammation in the brain will be evaluated to investigate the mechanistic evidence of the intestinal microbiota–brain axis in ASD. In addition, ASD-humanized VPA and CMA male mice will be suitable splenocyte donors for transferring their behavioral phenotype to naïve mice to reveal whether the ASD-like phenotype is microbiome-immune system-dependent. A second series of preclinical studies will establish whether correction of intestinal microbial dysbiosis by pre/pro/synbiotic intervention prevents and/or treats ASD-like behavior in ASD murine models. Selected ASD humanized murine models will be fed diets supplemented with selected pre/pro/synbiotics, which will be prescreened using microcosms systems as described above. Those that affect neurodevelopment, behavior, and the GI tract positively will be used in the clinical intervention trial.

2.2. Clinical Study

2.2.1. Participants

GEMMA aims to enroll 600 infants younger than 6 months/26 weeks of age, who have an older sibling with ASD for the observational trial. The recruitment will be carried out in three different centers: Irish Center for Autism and Neurodevelopmental Research (ICAN) at the National University of Ireland, Galway, Azienda Sanitaria Locale Salerno (ASL), and satellite centers in Italy, and Mass General Hospital for Children (MGHFC) Lurie Center for Autism in USA. The first study samples must be collected prior to the introduction of solid foods. Children who have started any other therapeutic intervention for ASD will also be excluded from the study. According to our previous experience with similar projects involving two cohorts of infants at-risk of celiac disease [52,53], enrollment will be performed by inviting parents' of the autistic patients who are followed by the recruitment clinics to participate in the study in the case of newborns, and advertising the study among ASD support and ASD patients' groups. Moreover, a traditional and social media diffusion plan was created to increase the project knowledge and support. No compensation will be provided to the participant.

Infants aged 18–36 months who were recruited, completed the observational study, developed clinical signs and symptoms of ASD, and whose parents permit the intervention of solely dietary and oral therapy in this study, will be invited to enroll for a follow-on dietary interventional trial.

2.2.2. Observational Trial

This study phase will evaluate infants at high risk of ASD. To achieve the sample size needed for clinical and biological comparisons, and ensure there is a reasonable representation across study sites, each site will target recruitment of 200 infants at high risk of developing ASD, over a 3 year period. All recruited children will undergo regular clinical and laboratory evaluations for 36 months, or more in the case of ASD development based on the annual intermediate clinical data check. Blood, urine, stools, and saliva samples will be collected every 6 months until 36 months of age.

Regarding GI symptoms, children will be evaluated for chronic irregular bowel movements (constipation, diarrhea), encopresis, recurrent abdominal pain, gastroesophageal reflux, and vomiting or food aversion. On these bases, the evaluable target study population (see Table 1 for inclusion/exclusion criteria) will be divided into four groups (depending on their clinical outcome: neuro competent at-risk infants with (NC-GI) and without GI symptoms (NC), ASD infants with GI symptoms (ASD-GI) and ASD infants without GI symptoms (ASD)). Maternal and paternal genomic samples will be taken from parents of infants at the time of enrollment and analyzed to examine inherited and de novo genetic traits.

Table 1. Inclusion and exclusion criteria for the observational trial.

Inclusion Criteria (All Must be Met)	Exclusion Criteria (Participant Will be Excluded from the Study if Any of the Criteria are Met)
1. Healthy newborns or infants 2. First-degree relatives of ASD participant (at least one sibling affected by ASD) 3. Younger than 6 months/26 weeks 4. Have never received solid food (elementary formula feeding permitted)	1. Newborns with significant health issues that require surgical treatments or continuous medical treatments and/or surgical treatments 2. Infants older than 6 months/26 weeks 3. Infants who have been introduced to solid food (including occasional use) 4. Severe GI problems requiring immediate treatment (life-threatening) 5. Severely underweight/malnourished children 6. Dietary restriction in the previous 3 months 7. Tube feeding 8. Drugs since birth which may affect the biomarkers being assessed, for example 9. Antibiotics within one month prior to enrollment; antibiotics used as a continuous course for ≥28 days prior to enrolment

Autism Diagnostic Observation Schedule (ADOS Toddler) evaluation [54] will be conducted every 6 months by a trained physician, starting at 12 months of age. For children younger than 24 months who test positive in the ADOS Toddler evaluation, the evaluation will be repeated one month later to confirm diagnosis to enroll the infant in an interventional study, and will be used to divide the participants into two groups: ASD children or non-ASD children (typically developing). Typically developing children will be followed until 36 months (see Figure 3) of age and their data will be selected at the end of the study to provide the information for the matched control comparisons.

Additional behavioral assessments include Early Screening for Autism and Communication Disorders and Repetitive Behavior Scale [55,56], Mullen Scales of Early Learning (MSEL) [57], and Vineland Adaptive Behavior Scales (VABS) [58]. These assessments will take place at 24 and 36 months of age.

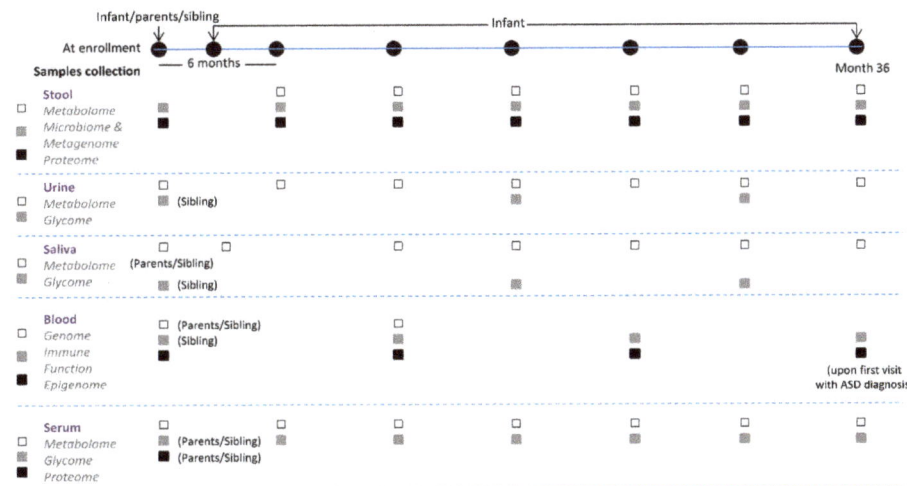

Figure 3. Clinical trials—prospective multi-center observational study evaluating infants at risk of ASD. 600 infants—newborns, less than 6 months of age—at risk, i.e., first-degree relatives of ASD individuals, recruited in US, Italy, and Ireland (200 infants at each site, over a 3-year period). Ongoing.

2.2.3. Interventional Trial

This prospective, multi-center, open-label, uncontrolled study (Figure 4) evaluates the effects of pre/pro/synbiotics supplementation started in infants between the ages of 18 and 36 months with a diagnosis of ASD.

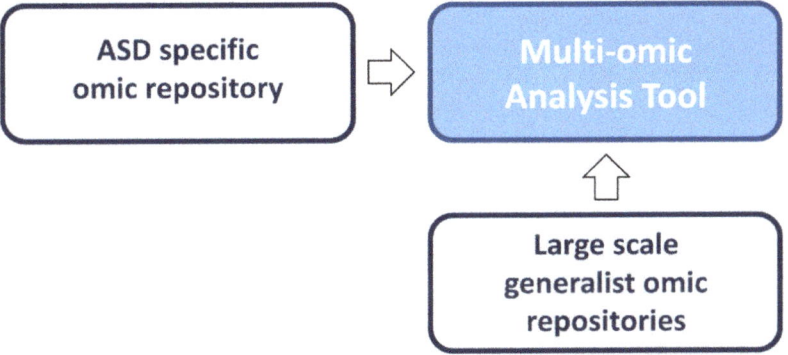

Figure 4. Interventional trial—prospective, multi-center, open-label, uncontrolled study to evaluate the effects of pre/pro/synbiotics supplementation in infants with a diagnosis of ASD. Forty children between the ages of 18 and 36 months diagnosed with ASD from the observational trial will be recruited (with parental consent).

A minimum of 40 children diagnosed with ASD from the observational trial will be recruited to the interventional trial, subject to parental consent. Each ASD infant will undergo a Positron Emission Tomography (PET) scan of their brain, at the beginning and end of the interventional study, to obtain information on the degree of neuro-inflammation and the potential effect of the intervention. The presence/absence of GI symptoms will also be evaluated.

Clinical and laboratory assessments will be made at the time of enrollment, monthly for 3 months, and then at the conclusion of the 6 month study.

The study was approved by the relevant ethics committee of each enrolling country. In particular: CE Campania Sud (IRB n.30/2019) for Italy; Partners Human Research (IRB ver.01/04/2019) for USA; and Clinical Research Ethics Committee of Galway University Hospital (IRB n. C.A. 2127/19) for Ireland. A written consent form will be signed by each participant or their legal representative. The clinical trial was registered with the access number: NCT04271774 (https://clinicaltrials.gov).

2.3. Data Collection

The timetables of data and sample collection are shown in Supplementary Tables S1–S3 and in Figure 3. Pre-screening may occur verbally via a telephone call or in person at a hospital clinic. Parents who wish to enroll their infant in the study will provide proof of ASD diagnosis for the child with the condition. Each clinical site will be responsible for its own data collection and management. Data will be monitored remotely for completeness and coherence by the project management team. All data will be collected through a secure, internet-based electronic capture system (REDCap) [59]. Participating institutions will be granted access to the electronic storage module with all appropriate forms and schedules pre-loaded. Each institution will only be able to view data for participants enrolled at their site. The coordinating center will be granted access to unidentified data from all sites through the electronic data capture system.

Parental and Child Questionnaires

An online questionnaire will be filled out by the family every month during the 6 months of intervention. Moreover, it will be filled out by the family at 9, 15, 21, 27, and 33 months of age and will include infant dietary data and the use of concomitant medication (vaccinations and antibiotics), demographics, infant clinical history including but not limited to infections, onset of food intolerance, and chronic stress. Parents will also be requested to complete the Aberrant Behavior Checklist (ABC) at all visits and at 9 months. Assessment scales for infant development (Rome 3 Criteria GSRS, ADOS-Toddler, Mullen scale, CGI-S, CGI-I) will be assessed, during the interventional trial, every month for the first three months of the study, and three months later at the final 6-month study visit.

2.4. Serological Markers

2.4.1. Whole Blood

Blood sampling will take place at enrollment, 0–6 months post birth, and at 12, 18, 24, 30, and 36 months of age. Blood for hematology, biochemistry evaluation, biomarker identification, and genetic assays will be collected from infants fasting for at least 3 h. The blood collection procedure is as follows: via umbilical cord for infants enrolled during gestation, or by heel sampling at enrollment (at 0–6 months of at-risk infant age), 1 mL every 6 months from 12 months of age, and finally at development of ASD or at the 36-month (observational study termination visit). The assays that will be performed on blood include whole genome sequencing on infants that develop ASD. Furthermore, DNA methylation (DNAm) will be measured among infants that develop ASD using samples obtained at three time points: (1) enrollment, (2) the time of ASD diagnosis, and (3) the completion of the interventional trial. In preparation for future testing, a biorepository will be established. A blood sample will be taken after 12 months for peripheral blood mononuclear cell (PBMC) isolation and immune profiling analysis.

Moreover, serum testing will take place at enrollment of the clinical study, 0–6 months post birth, and at 12, 18, 24, 30, and 36 months of age. A quantity of 500 uL of serum will be taken from the infant fasting for 3 h to evaluate serum zonulin (20 µL); serum IgA and IgG anti-gliadin and anti-casein antibody determination (40 µL) by the ELISA method; serum pro-inflammatory cytokines, including cIL-1, TNF-α, IFN-, IL-10, IL-12, IL-6, IL15, and IL-8 by Bioplex assay (75 µL) [60]; and cytokine gene expression by RT-PCR.

If ASD is developed, whole genome sequencing of the infant and of both parents will be performed.

2.4.2. Stool, Urine, and Saliva Samples

Every 3 months after enrollment, urine and stool samples will be collected at home and shipped to the laboratory for biomarker assay. Because patient samples are divided according to the presence and absence of a history of GI problems with an onset earlier than the initiation of toilet training, the aim is to select children with a biological rather than psychological etiology of GI discomfort. The control group includes fecal samples from age- and gender-matched control participants without previous diagnosis of a neurodevelopmental disorder and without a history of GI problems. Exclusion criteria for the use of patients and control samples include the use of psychotropic medication for the previous 6 months and antibiotics and/or probiotics for the previous 2 months.

Saliva samples will be taken for microbiome and glycome (the whole set of carbohydrates) analysis. Moreover, when possible subsequent analysis/correlation with blood biomarker levels either within this protocol or at a later timepoint will be performed. The saliva samples will be analyzed for pro-inflammatory markers and for six inflammatory markers selected from a previous study [61].

3. Factor of Interest

3.1. Environmental

Birthing delivery mode, method of infant feeding, and introduction of solid food and allergen to the infant diet could represent potential environmental factors causing ASD, so these will be recorded for each enrolled participant [53,62,63]. A diary of antibiotic usage will be completed by the parents monthly for the first year of life, and food diaries completed at the same time points will assess duration of breastfeeding (or other preferred feeding mode).

After the first year of life, detailed, although less frequent, records of antibiotic use will be obtained with each stool sample for the remaining duration of the study. Although the food diary will be discontinued at this time, pertinent dietary habits of both the mother and child will continue to be carefully recorded approximately every six months.

Moreover, details such as antibiotic exposure in early infancy, family living address, exposure to pets, and gastrointestinal sporadic symptoms will also be recorded.

3.2. Genetics

Currently, ASD heritability based on mono- and dizygotic twins is estimated to be about 79–80% [64,65]. Concordance is higher in monozygotic twins than dizygotic twins.

First-degree relatives of ASD probands show behavioral or cognitive features associated with autism intensification, such as language and social dysfunction, albeit in lesser forms [66], known as "broader phenotype" [67–70].

ASD-related social impairments are heritable [71] and increase in unaffected parents and children of autistic probands [72]. Several studies evaluating sub-threshold ASD traits in population cohorts suggested that different components, separately representing language, social function, and repetitive or stereotyped behaviors contribute to ASD [73–75]. Globally, these results suggest that ASD features represent a continuum of function that may be inherited in distinct patterns. This is consistent with the knowledge that specific genetic factors contribute to the development and function of specific brain structures, and that distinct brain circuits may underlie different components of autism [76].

Moreover, several genetic syndromes, including Fragile X, Tuberous Sclerosis, Joubert Syndrome and Smith Lemli Opitz, are known to cause, although with low penetrance, ASD-like symptoms [76,77]. This evidence further favors a genetic cause for ASD [78].

To assess the contribution of genetic risk factors, in combination with exposure and other omics data, we will perform whole genome sequencing in all participants with ASD, in addition to their parents. This will enable investigation of both common and rare variants that contribute to ASD risk.

3.3. GI Microbiome and Metabolome

The complete understanding of the host-GI microbiome genomics is necessary for the prediction of the activation of metabolic pathways linked with functional and clinical outcomes. Urine and stool samples will be collected and analyzed for a metabolomic phenotype of the GI microbiota and metabolomics profiles, including metabolites linked to bacterial activity in ASD. The metabolomic profiles, exploratory semi-quantitative assays, and targeted quantitative assays will be conducted throughout the study. Systems models of integrated metabolomic phenotypes will be created with the statistically linked data between the microbiota and immune function. By conjoining microbiota data and metabolomic data we will be able to understand the functions associated with GI comorbidity of children with ASD and the ASD patient-derived microbiota. Dietary interventions with pre/pro/synbiotics will be created based on the results found in the humanized mouse models undergoing fecal transplantation with ASD-specific microbiota.

3.4. Immune Function

The peripheral blood mononuclear cells (PBMCs) will be harvested and studied for immune functions. Standard flow cytometry will be used to measure monocyte and T-cell intracellular cytokine patterns. By looking at the T cell populations in children with ASD with and without GI symptoms we will be able to understand what cellular activation and functional alterations are present. Assays performed on serum samples collected at clinical visits include: serum zonulin determination; serum IgA and IgG anti-gliadin and anti-casein determination by the ELISA method; serum pro-inflammatory cytokines, including IL-1, TNF, IFN, IL-10, IL-12, IL-6, IL-15, and IL-8 by Bioplex assay; and cytokine gene expression by RT-PCR. Protein glycosylation is directly involved in nearly every biological process presenting altered glycosylation as potential biomarkers in many human conditions including inflammation, diabetes, rheumatism, cancer, and neurological disorders [79]. Serum immunoglobulin glyco-signaturing will be performed using lectin microarrays and anti-glycan ELISA profiling. Saliva samples will also be analyzed for proinflammatory cytokines and inflammatory markers selected from a previous study [61], and altered glycan and glycation products.

4. Statistical Approach

4.1. Statistical Methods

Categorical data will be described using frequency counts and percentages, and continuous data with mean, standard deviation, median, minimum, and maximum. Both parametric and non-parametric methods will be used to analyze the data. All omics data will be preprocessed with appropriate methods. The multi-omics analyses will be performed with statistical tests, regression models, and more advanced methods such as sparse canonical correlation analysis and random forest analysis. The false discovery rate (FDR) method will be used to adjust the *p*-values for multiple comparisons. Statistical significance will be set at $p < 0.05$.

4.2. Power Analysis

We estimated a conservative drop-off of 20% based on our previous experience with similar projects involving two cohorts of infants at-risk of celiac disease, one that has been followed for 10 years with a 20% drop-off [52] and a second that has been followed up to 7 years with a 12% drop-off [53]. The final cohort will comprise approximately 500 at-risk infants. Expected prevalence of ASD at 18–24 months in first-degree relatives is 14.7% [9], so in this study we estimate 73 ASD diagnoses. The expected prevalence of GI symptoms in an ASD population is 60% [80], so we anticipate 44 of the 73 ASD diagnosed infants to also present GI symptoms.

4.3. Developing an Integrative Multilevel Model to Predict ASD

Path a: A causal path between the genetics and the final effect on the onset of ASD, with the microbiome as the mediator (a1 × a2), so that the intestinal microbiome will be altered for the genetics to ultimately influence the development of the disorder (microbiome-mediated epigenetic pressure).

Path b: A causal path of the microbiome's effect on ASD mediated (b1 × b2) by the metabolic activity of intestinal bacteria, which, through the production of metabolites, affects the intestinal transcriptome and proteome. Including a bidirectional path between microbiome and metabolomics to capture how metabolism could alter the microbial metabolism and ultimately the risk for ASD.

Path c: A bidirectional path between the transcriptome and the microbiome because their causal relationship will depend on each other.

Path d: A direct relationship between lifestyle factors and the onset of the disorder mediated (d1 × d2) by alterations in the microbiome.

Path e: The environment affecting the onset of the disorder as a mediator and affecting the composition of the microbiome and resulting metabolome, in turn, influencing gene and protein expression.

Full Model: Time points will be clustered within individual characteristics; analyzing all of the paths listed above, individuals will be clustered within families, and families within regions.

5. Discussions and Conclusions

The implementation of primary prevention strategies for ASD via manipulation of the intestinal microbiota represents a complete paradigm shift of treatment and prevention of ASD. The identification of specific ASD metagenomics and metabolomics phenotypes can also help to define additional biomarker-based diagnostic tools and therapeutic interventions. Additionally, GEMMA's biorepository will encourage future epigenetic studies and validation of biomarkers. Our findings may also impact the prevention and treatment of other neuroinflammatory conditions.

Supplementary Materials: The following are available online at http://www.mdpi.com/2076-3425/10/10/743/s1, Table S1: Information that will be collected from the enrolled participant during the project. Table S2: Samples that will be collected from the enrolled participants divided for project time. Table S3: Psychiatric evaluation of the enrolled participants.

Author Contributions: Conceptualization, A.F., A.K., C.L.-A., G.C., G.L., J.T., M.G., R.A. and S.R.; methodology, A.G., A.M. (Alessandra Mezzelani), A.M. (Arlene Mannion), C.B., C.R., D.F., E.M., F.I., G.R., H.K., L.J., L.M., L.N., N.Z.P., P.P.P., S.C., S.D., S.F., S.K. and T.B.; writing—original draft preparation, J.T.; writing—review and editing, A.F., A.K., C.L.-A., G.C., G.L., M.G., R.A., S.R., A.G., A.M. (Alessandra Mezzelani), A.M. (Arlene Mannion), C.B., C.R., D.F., E.M., F.C., F.I., F.P.T., G.R., G.S., H.K., L.J., L.M., L.N., L.N.P.M., L.R., N.Z.P., P.P.P., S.C., S.D., S.F., S.K. and T.B.; supervision, A.F.; project administration, F.C., F.P.T. All authors have read and agreed to the published version of the manuscript.

Funding: GEMMA project was funded by the European Commission by means of the Horizon 2020 program (call H2020-SC1-BHC-03-2018) with the project ID 825033.

Acknowledgments: This work is conducted with support from the Advisory Board Members (California Institute of Technology, Winclove Probiotics, University of California Davis, Center for Autism and the Developing Brain, Ohio State University, the Autism Speaks Autism Treatment Network, Arizona State University, University College Cork), from the Consortium Partners: Fondazione EBRIS, in charge of project management and coordination and providing the gut permeability and immunological evaluation of the enrolled subjects; Nutricia Research Bv in charge of nutritional formulation development for interventional trial; Medinok Spa and Consiglio Nazionale Delle Ricerche (CNR) in charge of data analysis and multi-omics platform development; Bio Modeling Systems in charge of the mechanistic pathway hypothesis development; Euformatics in charge of analysis and the interpretation of the genomic variants of the patient material, and for the comparison of the variants from the different patient cohorts, Theoreo Srl and Imperial College Of Science in charge of metabolomics analysis and interpretation; National University of Ireland Galway, Azienda Sanitaria, Locale (ASL) Salerno and Massachusettse General Hospital for Children, in charge of enrollments for observation and interventional trials; Institut National de Recherche pour l'Agriculture, l'Alimentation et l'Environnement in charge of analyzing the genomic and transcriptomic profiles of the host microbiota; Institut National de la Santé et de la Recherche Médicale, in charge of proteomics analysis; Utrecht University, in charge of pre-clinical studies; Tampereen Yliopisto, in charge of experimental design; Johns Hopkins University in charge of epigenomic evaluation and interpretation. Financial contributions were made by European Union.

Conflicts of Interest: The authors declare no conflict of interest.

References

1. Evans, B. How autism became autism: The radical transformation of a central concept of child development in Britain. *Hist. Hum. Sci.* **2013**, *26*, 3–31. [CrossRef] [PubMed]
2. Elsabbagh, M.; Divan, G.; Koh, Y.-J.; Kim, Y.S.; Kauchali, S.; Marcín, C.; Montiel-Nava, C.; Patel, V.; Paula, C.S.; Wang, C.; et al. Global prevalence of autism and other pervasive developmental disorders. *Autism Res.* **2012**, *5*, 160–179. [CrossRef]
3. Newschaffer, C.J.; Croen, L.A.; Daniels, J.; Giarelli, E.; Grether, J.K.; Levy, S.E.; Mandell, D.S.; Miller, L.A.; Pinto-Martin, J.; Reaven, J.; et al. The epidemiology of autism spectrum disorders. *Annu. Rev. Public Health* **2007**, *28*, 235–258. [CrossRef] [PubMed]
4. Wing, L.; Potter, D. The epidemiology of autistic spectrum disorders: Is the prevalence rising? *Ment. Retard. Dev. Disabil. Res. Rev.* **2002**, *8*, 151–161. [CrossRef]
5. Fombonne, E. The prevalence of autism. *JAMA* **2003**, *289*, 87–89. [CrossRef] [PubMed]
6. Centers for Disease Control and Prevention. *(CDC) Prevalence of Autism Spectrum Disorders—Autism and Developmental Disabilities Monitoring Network, 14 Sites USA, 2008*; Centers for Disease Control and Prevention: Atlanta, GA, USA, 2012.
7. Maenner, M.J. Prevalence of Autism Spectrum Disorder Among Children Aged 8 Years—Autism and Developmental Disabilities Monitoring Network, 11 Sites, United States, 2016. *MMWR Surveill. Summ.* **2020**, *69*, 1–12. [CrossRef] [PubMed]
8. Autism Spectrum Disorders in the European Union (ASDEU). Consortium Autism Spectrum Disorders in the European Union (ASDEU): Final Report: Main Results of the ASDEU Project, ASDEU, Madrid: 28 August 2018. Available online: http://repositorio.insa.pt/handle/10400.18/6188 (accessed on 15 October 2020).
9. Ozonoff, S.; Young, G.S.; Carter, A.; Messinger, D.; Yirmiya, N.; Zwaigenbaum, L.; Bryson, S.; Carver, L.J.; Constantino, J.N.; Dobkins, K.; et al. Recurrence risk for autism spectrum disorders: A Baby Siblings Research Consortium study. *Pediatrics* **2011**, *128*, e488–e495. [CrossRef]
10. Satterstrom, F.K.; Kosmicki, J.A.; Wang, J.; Breen, M.S.; De Rubeis, S.; An, J.-Y.; Peng, M.; Collins, R.; Grove, J.; Klei, L.; et al. Large-Scale Exome Sequencing Study Implicates Both Developmental and Functional Changes in the Neurobiology of Autism. *Cell* **2020**, *180*, 568–584.e23. [CrossRef] [PubMed]
11. Bai, D.; Yip, B.H.K.; Windham, G.C.; Sourander, A.; Francis, R.; Yoffe, R.; Glasson, E.; Mahjani, B.; Suominen, A.; Leonard, H.; et al. Association of Genetic and Environmental Factors With Autism in a 5-Country Cohort. *JAMA Psychiatry* **2019**, *76*, 1035–1043. [CrossRef]
12. Sandin, S.; Lichtenstein, P.; Kuja-Halkola, R.; Larsson, H.; Hultman, C.M.; Reichenberg, A. The familial risk of autism. *JAMA* **2014**, *311*, 1770–1777. [CrossRef]
13. Brucato, M.; Ladd-Acosta, C.; Li, M.; Caruso, D.; Hong, X.; Kaczaniuk, J.; Stuart, E.A.; Fallin, M.D.; Wang, X. Prenatal exposure to fever is associated with autism spectrum disorder in the boston birth cohort. *Autism Res.* **2017**, *10*, 1878–1890. [CrossRef]
14. Croen, L.A.; Qian, Y.; Ashwood, P.; Zerbo, O.; Schendel, D.; Pinto-Martin, J.; Daniele Fallin, M.; Levy, S.; Schieve, L.A.; Yeargin-Allsopp, M.; et al. Infection and Fever in Pregnancy and Autism Spectrum Disorders: Findings from the Study to Explore Early Development. *Autism Res.* **2019**, *12*, 1551–1561. [CrossRef] [PubMed]
15. DiStasio, M.M.; Nagakura, I.; Nadler, M.J.; Anderson, M.P. T-lymphocytes and Cytotoxic Astrocyte Blebs Correlate Across Autism Brains. *Ann. Neurol.* **2019**, *86*, 885–898. [CrossRef] [PubMed]
16. Hornig, M.; Bresnahan, M.A.; Che, X.; Schultz, A.F.; Ukaigwe, J.E.; Eddy, M.L.; Hirtz, D.; Gunnes, N.; Lie, K.K.; Magnus, P.; et al. Prenatal fever and autism risk. *Mol. Psychiatry* **2018**, *23*, 759–766. [CrossRef] [PubMed]
17. Nankova, B.B.; Agarwal, R.; MacFabe, D.F.; La Gamma, E.F. Enteric bacterial metabolites propionic and butyric acid modulate gene expression, including CREB-dependent catecholaminergic neurotransmission, in PC12 cells–possible relevance to autism spectrum disorders. *PLoS ONE* **2014**, *9*, e103740. [CrossRef]
18. Macfabe, D. Autism: Metabolism, mitochondria, and the microbiome. *Glob. Adv. Health Med.* **2013**, *2*, 52–66. [CrossRef] [PubMed]
19. Scumpia, P.O.; Kelly-Scumpia, K.; Stevens, B.R. Alpha-lipoic acid effects on brain glial functions accompanying double-stranded RNA antiviral and inflammatory signaling. *Neurochem. Int.* **2014**, *64*, 55–63. [CrossRef]

20. Zielinski, B.A.; Prigge, M.B.D.; Nielsen, J.A.; Froehlich, A.L.; Abildskov, T.J.; Anderson, J.S.; Fletcher, P.T.; Zygmunt, K.M.; Travers, B.G.; Lange, N.; et al. Longitudinal changes in cortical thickness in autism and typical development. *Brain* **2014**, *137*, 1799–1812. [CrossRef]
21. Stoner, R.; Chow, M.L.; Boyle, M.P.; Sunkin, S.M.; Mouton, P.R.; Roy, S.; Wynshaw-Boris, A.; Colamarino, S.A.; Lein, E.S.; Courchesne, E. Patches of Disorganization in the Neocortex of Children with Autism. *N. Engl. J. Med.* **2014**, *370*, 1209–1219. [CrossRef]
22. Rossignol, D.A.; Frye, R.E. A review of research trends in physiological abnormalities in autism spectrum disorders: Immune dysregulation, inflammation, oxidative stress, mitochondrial dysfunction and environmental toxicant exposures. *Mol. Psychiatry* **2012**, *17*, 389–401. [CrossRef]
23. Kostic, A.D.; Gevers, D.; Siljander, H.; Vatanen, T.; Hyotylainen, T.; Hamalainen, A.-M.; Peet, A.; Tillmann, V.; Poho, P.; Mattila, I.; et al. The dynamics of the human infant gut microbiome in development and in progression toward type 1 diabetes. *Cell Host Microbe* **2015**, *17*, 260–273. [CrossRef] [PubMed]
24. Rook, G.A.; Raison, C.L.; Lowry, C.A. Microbiota, immunoregulatory old friends and psychiatric disorders. In *Microbial Endocrinology: The Microbiota-Gut-Brain Axis in Health and Disease*; Springer: Berlin/Heidelberg, Germany, 2014; pp. 319–356.
25. Borre, Y.E.; Moloney, R.D.; Clarke, G.; Dinan, T.G.; Cryan, J.F. The impact of microbiota on brain and behavior: Mechanisms & therapeutic potential. In *Microbial Endocrinology: The Microbiota-Gut-Brain Axis in Health and Disease*; Springer: Berlin/Heidelberg, Germany, 2014; pp. 373–403.
26. Shimabukuro, T.T.; Grosse, S.D.; Rice, C. Medical expenditures for children with an autism spectrum disorder in a privately insured population. *J. Autism Dev. Disord.* **2008**, *38*, 546–552. [CrossRef] [PubMed]
27. Peacock, G.; Amendah, D.; Ouyang, L.; Grosse, S.D. Autism spectrum disorders and health care expenditures: The effects of co-occurring conditions. *J. Dev. Behav. Pediatr.* **2012**, *33*, 2–8. [CrossRef]
28. Blumberg, S.J.; Bramlett, M.D.; Kogan, M.D.; Schieve, L.A.; Jones, J.R.; Lu, M.C. Changes in prevalence of parent-reported autism spectrum disorder in school-aged U.S. children: 2007 to 2011–2012. *Natl. Health Stat. Rep.* **2013**, *65*, 1–11.
29. Fletcher-Watson, S.; McConnell, F.; Manola, E.; McConachie, H. Interventions based on the Theory of Mind cognitive model for autism spectrum disorder (ASD). *Cochrane Database Syst. Rev.* **2014**, *3*, CD008785. [CrossRef]
30. Sukhodolsky, D.G.; Bloch, M.H.; Panza, K.E.; Reichow, B. Cognitive-behavioral therapy for anxiety in children with high-functioning autism: A meta-analysis. *Pediatrics* **2013**, *132*, e1341–e1350. [CrossRef] [PubMed]
31. Millward, C.; Ferriter, M.; Calver, S.; Connell-Jones, G. Gluten- and casein-free diets for autistic spectrum disorder. *Cochrane Database Syst. Rev.* **2008**, *2*, CD003498. [CrossRef] [PubMed]
32. Bolte, E.R. Autism and Clostridium tetani. *Med. Hypotheses* **1998**, *51*, 133–144. [CrossRef]
33. Finegold, S.M.; Molitoris, D.; Song, Y.; Liu, C.; Vaisanen, M.-L.; Bolte, E.; McTeague, M.; Sandler, R.; Wexler, H.; Marlowe, E.M.; et al. Gastrointestinal Microflora Studies in Late-Onset Autism. *Clin. Infect. Dis.* **2002**, *35*, S6–S16. [CrossRef]
34. Pulikkan, J.; Mazumder, A.; Grace, T. Role of the Gut Microbiome in Autism Spectrum Disorders. In *Reviews on Biomarker Studies in Psychiatric and Neurodegenerative Disorders*; Guest, P.C., Ed.; Springer International Publishing: Cham, Switzerland, 2019; pp. 253–269, ISBN 978-3-030-05542-4.
35. Sharon, G.; Cruz, N.J.; Kang, D.-W.; Gandal, M.J.; Wang, B.; Kim, Y.-M.; Zink, E.M.; Casey, C.P.; Taylor, B.C.; Lane, C.J.; et al. Human Gut Microbiota from Autism Spectrum Disorder Promote Behavioral Symptoms in Mice. *Cell* **2019**, *177*, 1600–1618.e17. [CrossRef]
36. Strati, F.; Cavalieri, D.; Albanese, D.; De Felice, C.; Donati, C.; Hayek, J.; Jousson, O.; Leoncini, S.; Renzi, D.; Calabrò, A.; et al. New evidences on the altered gut microbiota in autism spectrum disorders. *Microbiome* **2017**, *5*, 24. [CrossRef] [PubMed]
37. Kang, D.-W.; Adams, J.B.; Gregory, A.C.; Borody, T.; Chittick, L.; Fasano, A.; Khoruts, A.; Geis, E.; Maldonado, J.; McDonough-Means, S.; et al. Microbiota Transfer Therapy alters gut ecosystem and improves gastrointestinal and autism symptoms: An open-label study. *Microbiome* **2017**, *5*, 10. [CrossRef]
38. Kang, D.-W.; Adams, J.B.; Coleman, D.M.; Pollard, E.L.; Maldonado, J.; McDonough-Means, S.; Caporaso, J.G.; Krajmalnik-Brown, R. Long-term benefit of Microbiota Transfer Therapy on autism symptoms and gut microbiota. *Sci. Rep.* **2019**, *9*, 5821. [CrossRef] [PubMed]
39. Masi, A.; DeMayo, M.M.; Glozier, N.; Guastella, A.J. An overview of autism spectrum disorder, heterogeneity and treatment options. *Neurosci. Bull.* **2017**, *33*, 183–193. [CrossRef]

40. de Theije, C.G.M.; Wu, J.; Koelink, P.J.; Korte-Bouws, G.A.H.; Borre, Y.; Kas, M.J.H.; da Silva, S.L.; Korte, S.M.; Olivier, B.; Garssen, J.; et al. Autistic-like behavioural and neurochemical changes in a mouse model of food allergy. *Behav. Brain Res.* **2014**, *261*, 265–274. [CrossRef] [PubMed]
41. de Theije, C.G.M.; van den Elsen, L.W.J.; Willemsen, L.E.M.; Milosevic, V.; Korte-Bouws, G.A.H.; da Silva, S.L.; Broersen, L.M.; Korte, S.M.; Olivier, B.; Garssen, J.; et al. Dietary long chain n-3 polyunsaturated fatty acids prevent impaired social behaviour and normalize brain dopamine levels in food allergic mice. *Neuropharmacology* **2015**, *90*, 15–22. [CrossRef]
42. Saunders, J.M.; Moreno, J.L.; Ibi, D.; Sikaroodi, M.; Kang, D.J.; Muñoz-Moreno, R.; Dalmet, S.S.; García-Sastre, A.; Gillevet, P.M.; Dozmorov, M.G.; et al. Gut microbiota manipulation during the prepubertal period shapes behavioral abnormalities in a mouse neurodevelopmental disorder model. *Sci. Rep.* **2020**, *10*, 4697. [CrossRef]
43. Wu, J.; de Theije, C.G.M.; da Silva, S.L.; Abbring, S.; van der Horst, H.; Broersen, L.M.; Willemsen, L.; Kas, M.; Garssen, J.; Kraneveld, A.D. Dietary interventions that reduce mTOR activity rescue autistic-like behavioral deficits in mice. *Brain Behav. Immun.* **2017**, *59*, 273–287. [CrossRef]
44. Le Roy, T.; Debédat, J.; Marquet, F.; Da-Cunha, C.; Ichou, F.; Guerre-Millo, M.; Kapel, N.; Aron-Wisnewsky, J.; Clément, K. Comparative Evaluation of Microbiota Engraftment Following Fecal Microbiota Transfer in Mice Models: Age, Kinetic and Microbial Status Matter. *Front. Microbiol.* **2019**, *9*, 3289. [CrossRef]
45. Stilling, R.M.; Moloney, G.M.; Ryan, F.J.; Hoban, A.E.; Bastiaanssen, T.F.; Shanahan, F.; Clarke, G.; Claesson, M.J.; Dinan, T.G.; Cryan, J.F. Social interaction-induced activation of RNA splicing in the amygdala of microbiome-deficient mice. *eLife* **2018**, *7*, e33070. [CrossRef]
46. Hoban, A.E.; Stilling, R.M.; Moloney, G.; Shanahan, F.; Dinan, T.G.; Clarke, G.; Cryan, J.F. The microbiome regulates amygdala-dependent fear recall. *Mol. Psychiatry* **2018**, *23*, 1134–1144. [CrossRef] [PubMed]
47. Luczynski, P.; Whelan, S.O.; O'Sullivan, C.; Clarke, G.; Shanahan, F.; Dinan, T.G.; Cryan, J.F. Adult microbiota-deficient mice have distinct dendritic morphological changes: Differential effects in the amygdala and hippocampus. *Eur. J. Neurosci.* **2016**, *44*, 2654–2666. [CrossRef]
48. Desbonnet, L.; Clarke, G.; Shanahan, F.; Dinan, T.G.; Cryan, J.F. Microbiota is essential for social development in the mouse. *Mol. Psychiatry* **2014**, *19*, 146–148. [CrossRef]
49. Buffington, S.A.; Di Prisco, G.V.; Auchtung, T.A.; Ajami, N.J.; Petrosino, J.F.; Costa-Mattioli, M. Microbial Reconstitution Reverses Maternal Diet-Induced Social and Synaptic Deficits in Offspring. *Cell* **2016**, *165*, 1762–1775. [CrossRef] [PubMed]
50. Neufeld, K.M.; Kang, N.; Bienenstock, J.; Foster, J.A. Reduced anxiety-like behavior and central neurochemical change in germ-free mice. *Neurogastroenterol. Motil.* **2011**, *23*, 255–264.e119. [CrossRef] [PubMed]
51. Arentsen, T.; Raith, H.; Qian, Y.; Forssberg, H.; Diaz Heijtz, R. Host microbiota modulates development of social preference in mice. *Microb. Ecol. Health Dis.* **2015**, *26*, 29719. [CrossRef]
52. Lionetti, E.; Castellaneta, S.; Francavilla, R.; Pulvirenti, A.; Tonutti, E.; Amarri, S.; Barbato, M.; Barbera, C.; Barera, G.; Bellantoni, A. Introduction of gluten, HLA status, and the risk of celiac disease in children. *N. Engl. J. Med.* **2014**, *371*, 1295–1303. [CrossRef]
53. Leonard, M.M.; Camhi, S.; Huedo-Medina, T.B.; Fasano, A. Celiac Disease Genomic, Environmental, Microbiome, and Metabolomic (CDGEMM) Study Design: Approach to the Future of Personalized Prevention of Celiac Disease. *Nutrients* **2015**, *7*, 9325–9336. [CrossRef]
54. Gotham, K.; Pickles, A.; Lord, C. Standardizing ADOS Scores for a Measure of Severity in Autism Spectrum Disorders. *J. Autism Dev. Disord.* **2009**, *39*, 693–705. [CrossRef]
55. Guthrie, W.; Swineford, L.B.; Nottke, C.; Wetherby, A.M. Early diagnosis of autism spectrum disorder: Stability and change in clinical diagnosis and symptom presentation. *J. Child. Psychol. Psychiatry* **2013**, *54*, 582–590. [CrossRef]
56. Wetherby, A.; Lord, C.; Woods, J.; Guthrie, W.; Pierce, K.; Shumway, S.; Thurm, A.; Ozonoff, S. The Early Screening for Autism and Communication Disorders (ESAC): Preliminary Field-Testing of An. Autism-Specific Screening Tool for Children 12 to 36 Months of Age. In Proceedings of the International Meeting for Autism Research, Chicago, IL, USA, 7–9 May 2009. Available online: https://www.researchgate.net/publication/268144139_The_Early_Screening_for_Autism_and_Communication_Disorders_ESAC_Preliminary_Field-Testing_of_An_Autism-Specific_Screening_Tool_for_Children_12_to_36_Months_of_Age (accessed on 15 October 2020).

57. Akshoomoff, N. Use of the Mullen Scales of Early Learning for the assessment of young children with Autism Spectrum Disorders. *Child. Neuropsychol.* **2006**, *12*, 269–277. [CrossRef] [PubMed]
58. Freeman, B.J.; Del'Homme, M.; Guthrie, D.; Zhang, F. Vineland Adaptive Behavior Scale Scores as a Function of Age and Initial IQ in 210 Autistic Children. *J. Autism Dev. Disord.* **1999**, *29*, 379–384. [CrossRef]
59. Harris, P.A.; Taylor, R.; Thielke, R.; Payne, J.; Gonzalez, N.; Conde, J.G. Research Electronic Data Capture (REDCap)-A metadata-driven methodology and workflow process for providing translational research informatics support. *J. Biomed. Inform.* **2009**, *42*, 377–381. [CrossRef] [PubMed]
60. Houser, B. Bio-Rad's Bio-Plex® suspension array system, xMAP technology overview. *Arch. Physiol. Biochem.* **2012**, *118*, 192–196. [CrossRef] [PubMed]
61. Wetie, A.G.N.; Wormwood, K.L.; Russell, S.; Ryan, J.P.; Darie, C.C.; Woods, A.G. A Pilot Proteomic Analysis of Salivary Biomarkers in Autism Spectrum Disorder. *Autism Res.* **2015**, *8*, 338–350. [CrossRef]
62. Curran, E.A.; Dalman, C.; Kearney, P.M.; Kenny, L.C.; Cryan, J.F.; Dinan, T.G.; Khashan, A.S. Association Between Obstetric Mode of Delivery and Autism Spectrum Disorder: A Population-Based Sibling Design Study. *JAMA Psychiatry* **2015**, *72*, 935–942. [CrossRef]
63. Tseng, P.-T.; Chen, Y.-W.; Stubbs, B.; Carvalho, A.F.; Whiteley, P.; Tang, C.-H.; Yang, W.-C.; Chen, T.-Y.; Li, D.-J.; Chu, C.-S.; et al. Maternal breastfeeding and autism spectrum disorder in children: A systematic review and meta-analysis. *Nutr. Neurosci.* **2019**, *22*, 354–362. [CrossRef]
64. Bailey, A.; Le Couteur, A.; Gottesman, I.; Bolton, P.; Simonoff, E.; Yuzda, E.; Rutter, M. Autism as a strongly genetic disorder: Evidence from a British twin study. *Psychol. Med.* **1995**, *25*, 63–77. [CrossRef]
65. Rosenberg, R.E.; Law, J.K.; Yenokyan, G.; McGready, J.; Kaufmann, W.E.; Law, P.A. Characteristics and concordance of autism spectrum disorders among 277 twin pairs. *Arch. Pediatrics Adolesc. Med.* **2009**, *163*, 907–914. [CrossRef]
66. Losh, M.; Adolphs, R.; Poe, M.D.; Couture, S.; Penn, D.; Baranek, G.T.; Piven, J. Neuropsychological profile of autism and the broad autism phenotype. *Arch. Gen. Psychiatry* **2009**, *66*, 518–526. [CrossRef]
67. Warren, Z.E.; Foss-Feig, J.H.; Malesa, E.E.; Lee, E.B.; Taylor, J.L.; Newsom, C.R.; Crittendon, J.; Stone, W.L. Neurocognitive and behavioral outcomes of younger siblings of children with autism spectrum disorder at age five. *J. Autism Dev. Disord.* **2012**, *42*, 409–418. [CrossRef]
68. Constantino, J.N. The quantitative nature of autistic social impairment. *Pediatric Res.* **2011**, *69*, 55R–62R. [CrossRef] [PubMed]
69. Gamliel, I.; Yirmiya, N.; Jaffe, D.H.; Manor, O.; Sigman, M. Developmental trajectories in siblings of children with autism: Cognition and language from 4 months to 7 years. *J. Autism Dev. Disord.* **2009**, *39*, 1131–1144. [CrossRef]
70. Pickles, A.; Starr, E.; Kazak, S.; Bolton, P.; Papanikolaou, K.; Bailey, A.; Goodman, R.; Rutter, M. Variable expression of the autism broader phenotype: Findings from extended pedigrees. *J. Child. Psychol. Psychiatry Allied Discip.* **2000**, *41*, 491–502. [CrossRef]
71. Constantino, J.N.; Todd, R.D. Intergenerational transmission of subthreshold autistic traits in the general population. *Biol. Psychiatry* **2005**, *57*, 655–660. [CrossRef]
72. Constantino, J.N.; Lajonchere, C.; Lutz, M.; Gray, T.; Abbacchi, A.; McKenna, K.; Singh, D.; Todd, R.D. Autistic social impairment in the siblings of children with pervasive developmental disorders. *Am. J. Psychiatry* **2006**, *163*, 294–296. [CrossRef] [PubMed]
73. Steer, C.D.; Golding, J.; Bolton, P.F. Traits contributing to the autistic spectrum. *PLoS ONE* **2010**, *5*, e12633. [CrossRef] [PubMed]
74. Ronald, A.; Happé, F.; Bolton, P.; Butcher, L.M.; Price, T.S.; Wheelwright, S.; Baron-Cohen, S.; Plomin, R. Genetic heterogeneity between the three components of the autism spectrum: A twin study. *J. Am. Acad. Child Adolesc. Psychiatry* **2006**, *45*, 691–699. [CrossRef] [PubMed]
75. Ronald, A.; Larsson, H.; Anckarsäter, H.; Lichtenstein, P. A twin study of autism symptoms in Sweden. *Mol. Psychiatry* **2011**, *16*, 1039. [CrossRef]
76. Geschwind, D.H. Autism: Many genes, common pathways? *Cell* **2008**, *135*, 391–395. [CrossRef]
77. Coleman, M.; Gillberg, C. *The Biology of the Autistic Syndromes*; Praeger: Westport, NY, USA, 1985; ISBN 0-275-91309-0.
78. Abrahams, B.S.; Geschwind, D.H. Advances in autism genetics: On the threshold of a new neurobiology. *Nat. Rev. Genet.* **2008**, *9*, 341. [CrossRef] [PubMed]

79. Hart, G.W.; Copeland, R.J. Glycomics hits the big time. *Cell* **2010**, *143*, 672–676. [CrossRef] [PubMed]
80. Wasilewska, J.; Klukowski, M. Gastrointestinal symptoms and autism spectrum disorder: Links and risks-a possible new overlap syndrome. *Pediatric Health Med. Ther.* **2015**, *6*, 153–166. [CrossRef] [PubMed]

Publisher's Note: MDPI stays neutral with regard to jurisdictional claims in published maps and institutional affiliations.

 © 2020 by the authors. Licensee MDPI, Basel, Switzerland. This article is an open access article distributed under the terms and conditions of the Creative Commons Attribution (CC BY) license (http://creativecommons.org/licenses/by/4.0/).

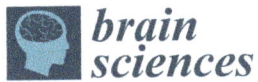 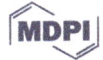

Article

Genetic Variation and Autism: A Field Synopsis and Systematic Meta-Analysis

Jinhee Lee [1,†], Min Ji Son [2,†], Chei Yun Son [3,†], Gwang Hun Jeong [4,†], Keum Hwa Lee [5,†], Kwang Seob Lee [6], Younhee Ko [7], Jong Yeob Kim [2], Jun Young Lee [8], Joaquim Radua [9,10,11,12], Michael Eisenhut [13], Florence Gressier [14], Ai Koyanagi [15,16,17], Brendon Stubbs [18,19], Marco Solmi [9,20,21], Theodor B. Rais [22], Andreas Kronbichler [23], Elena Dragioti [24], Daniel Fernando Pereira Vasconcelos [25], Felipe Rodolfo Pereira da Silva [25], Kalthoum Tizaoui [26], André Russowsky Brunoni [27,28,29,30], Andre F. Carvalho [31,32], Sarah Cargnin [33], Salvatore Terrazzino [33], Andrew Stickley [34,35], Lee Smith [36], Trevor Thompson [37], Jae Il Shin [5,*] and Paolo Fusar-Poli [9,38,39,*]

1. Department of Psychiatry, Yonsei University Wonju College of Medicine, Wonju 26426, Korea; jinh.lee95@yonsei.ac.kr
2. Yonsei University College of Medicine, Seoul 03722, Korea; minji9144@hanmail.net (M.J.S.); crossing96@yonsei.ac.kr (J.Y.K.)
3. Department of Psychological & Brain Sciences, Washington University in St. Louis, St. Louis, MO 63130, USA; hy321321@naver.com
4. College of Medicine, Gyeongsang National University, Jinju 52727, Korea; gwangh.jeong@gmail.com
5. Department of Pediatrics, Yonsei University College of Medicine, Seoul 03722, Korea; AZSAGM@yuhs.ac
6. Severance Hospital, Yonsei University College of Medicine, Seoul 03722, Korea; kwangseob@yuhs.ac
7. Division of Biomedical Engineering, Hankuk University of Foreign Studies, Gyeonggi-do 17035, Korea; younko@hufs.ac.kr
8. Department of Nephrology, Yonsei University Wonju College of Medicine, Wonju 26426, Korea; junyoung07@yonsei.ac.kr
9. Early Psychosis: Interventions and Clinical-detection (EPIC) Lab, Department of Psychosis Studies, Institute of Psychiatry, Psychology & Neuroscience, King's College London, London SE5 8AB, UK; radua@clinic.cat (J.R.); marco.solmi83@gmail.com (M.S.)
10. Mental Health Networking Biomedical Research Centre (CIBERSAM), 08036 Barcelona, Spain
11. Centre for Psychiatry Research, Department of Clinical Neuroscience, Karolinska Institute, 11330 Stockholm, Sweden
12. Institut d'Investigacions Biomèdiques August Pi i Sunyer (IDIBAPS), 08036 Barcelona, Spain
13. Department of Pediatrics, Luton & Dunstable University Hospital NHS Foundation Trust, Luton LU4ODZ, UK; michael_eisenhut@yahoo.com
14. CESP, Inserm UMR1178, Department of Psychiatry, Assistance Publique-Hôpitaux de Paris, Bicêtre University Hospital, 94275 Le Kremlin Bicêtre, France; florence.gressier@aphp.fr
15. Research and Development Unit, Parc Sanitari Sant Joan de Déu, Universitat de Barcelona, Fundació Sant Joan de Déu, CIBERSAM, 08830 Barcelona, Spain; a.koyanagi@pssjd.org
16. ICREA, Pg. Lluis Companys 23, 08010 Barcelona, Spain
17. Instituto de Salud Carlos III, Centro de Investigación Biomédica en Red de Salud Mental, CIBERSAM, 28029 Madrid, Spain
18. Physiotherapy Department, South London and Maudsley NHS Foundation Trust, London SE5 8AZ, UK; brendon.stubbs@kcl.ac.uk
19. Department of Psychological Medicine, Institute of Psychiatry, Psychology and Neuroscience, King's College London, London SE5 8AF, UK
20. Department of Neurosciences, University of Padua, 90133 Padua, Italy
21. Neurosciences Center, University of Padua, 90133 Padua, Italy
22. Department of Psychiatry, University of Toledo Medical Center, Toledo, OH 43614, USA; Theodor.Rais@utoledo.edu
23. Department of Internal Medicine IV, Medical University Innsbruck, Anichstraße 35, 6020 Innsbruck, Austria; andreas.kronbichler@i-med.ac.at

24 Pain and Rehabilitation Centre, and Department of Health, Medicine and Caring Sciences, Linköping University, SE-581 85 Linköping, Sweden; elena.dragioti@liu.se
25 Laboratory of Histological Analysis and Preparation (LAPHIS), Federal University of the Parnaiba Delta, Parnaiba 64202-020, Brazil; vasconcelos@ufpi.edu.br (D.F.P.V.); feliperodolfo.15@hotmail.com (F.R.P.d.S.)
26 Department of Basic Sciences, Medicine Faculty of Tunis, Tunis El Manar University, 15 Rue Djebel Lakdar, Tunis 1007, Tunisia; kalttizaoui@gmail.com
27 University Hospital, University of São Paulo, São Paulo CEP 05508-000, Brazil; brunowsky@gmail.com
28 Service of Interdisciplinary Neuromodulation, Department and Institute of Psychiatry, University of São Paulo Medical School, São Paulo CEP 01246-903, Brazil
29 Laboratory of Neuroscience and National Institute of Biomarkers in Neuropsychiatry, Department and Institute of Psychiatry, University of São Paulo Medical School, São Paulo CEP 01246-903, Brazil
30 Department of Psychiatry and Psychotherapy, University Hospital, LMU Munich, 80336 Munich, Germany
31 Centre for Addiction & Mental Health, Toronto, ON M6J 1H4, Canada; andre.carvalho@camh.ca
32 Department of Psychiatry, University of Toronto, Toronto, ON M5T 1R8, Canada
33 Department of Pharmaceutical Sciences and Interdepartmental Research Center of Pharmacogenetics and Pharmacogenomics (CRIFF), University of Piemonte Orientale, 28100 Novara, Italy; sarah.cargnin@uniupo.it (S.C.); salvatore.terrazzino@uniupo.it (S.T.)
34 The Stockholm Center for Health and Social Change (SCOHOST), Södertörn University, 141 89 Huddinge, Sweden; amstick66@gmail.com
35 Department of Preventive Intervention for Psychiatric Disorders, National Institute of Mental Health, National Center of Neurology and Psychiatry, 4-1-1 Ogawahigashicho, Kodaira, Tokyo 187-8553, Japan
36 The Cambridge Centre for Sport and Exercise Sciences, Anglia Ruskin University, Cambridge CB1 1PT, UK; lee.smith@anglia.ac.uk
37 Department of Psychology, University of Greenwich, London SE10 9LS, UK; T.Thompson@greenwich.ac.uk
38 OASIS Service, South London and Maudsley NHS Foundation Trust, London SE8 5HA, UK
39 Department of Brain and Behavioral Sciences, University of Pavia, 27100 Pavia, Italy
* Correspondence: shinji@yuhs.ac (J.I.S.); paolo.fusar-poli@kcl.ac.uk (P.F.-P.)
† These authors contributed equally.

Received: 19 August 2020; Accepted: 14 September 2020; Published: 30 September 2020

Abstract: This study aimed to verify noteworthy findings between genetic risk factors and autism spectrum disorder (ASD) by employing the false positive report probability (FPRP) and the Bayesian false-discovery probability (BFDP). PubMed and the Genome-Wide Association Studies (GWAS) catalog were searched from inception to 1 August, 2019. We included meta-analyses on genetic factors of ASD of any study design. Overall, twenty-seven meta-analyses articles from literature searches, and four manually added articles from the GWAS catalog were re-analyzed. This showed that five of 31 comparisons for meta-analyses of observational studies, 40 out of 203 comparisons for the GWAS meta-analyses, and 18 out of 20 comparisons for the GWAS catalog, respectively, had noteworthy estimations under both Bayesian approaches. In this study, we found noteworthy genetic comparisons highly related to an increased risk of ASD. Multiple genetic comparisons were shown to be associated with ASD risk; however, genuine associations should be carefully verified and understood.

Keywords: autism spectrum disorder; false positive report probability (FPRP); Bayesian false-discovery probability (BFDP); meta-analysis; Genome-Wide Association Studies (GWAS)

1. Introduction

Autism spectrum disorder (ASD) is a brain-based neurodevelopmental disorder characterized by pervasive impairments in reciprocal social communication, social interaction, and restricted and repetitive behaviors or interests, resulting in a substantial burden of individuals, families, and society [1,2]. The repeated reports of recent increase in the prevalence of ASD have raised substantial public concerns. For example, in large, nationwide population-based studies, the estimated ASD prevalence was reported to be 2.47% among U.S. children and adolescents in 2014–2016 [3–5].

Although the full range of etiologies underlying ASD remain largely unexplained, progress has been made in the past decade in identifying some neurobiological and genetic risk factors, and it has been well established that combination of genetic and environmental factors is involved in the etiopathogenesis of autism [1,6]. There is a strong genetic background of ASD, which was demonstrated by the fact that heritability is as high as 80–90% [7,8]. It is possible to estimate the heritability of ASD by taking into the account its covariance within twins, as twins are matched for many characteristics, including in utero and family environment, as well as other developmental aspects [7,9,10].

ASD is polygenic and genetic variants contribute to ASD risk and phenotypic variability. The results of previous studies showed genome-wide genetic links between ASD [11,12]. They indicated that typical variation in social behavior and adaptive functioning and multiple types of genetic risk for ASD influence a continuum of behavioral and developmental traits.

To the best of our knowledge, this is the comprehensive study to summarize the loci that are associated with ASD among the several known loci reported to be related with ASD. We have synthesized all available susceptibility loci for ASD retrieved from meta-analyses regarding the association between the individual polymorphisms and ASD. For the study, we reviewed observational studies, Genome-Wide Association Studies (GWAS) meta-analyses, the combined analysis of GWAS discovery and replication cohorts, the GWAS catalog and GWAS data from GWAS meta-analyses [13]. Furthermore, we applied a Bayesian approaches including false positive report probability (FPRP) and Bayesian false discovery probability (BFDP) to estimate the noteworthiness of the evidence [14,15]. Using these popular Bayesian statistics (i.e., FPRP and BFDP), our study shows that the results of genotype associations between the gene variant and disease were found to be noteworthy (genuine associations). Through these methods, we selected only statistically meaningful values excluding false-positive values and analyzed them again. We aimed to provide an overview to interpret the statistical significance of reported findings and discuss the identified associations in the suggested genetic risk factors for ASD.

2. Materials and Methods

This review was conducted following a registered protocol. The specified methods are available on the PROSPERO database with the registration number CRD42018091704. The Preferred Reporting Items for Systematic Reviews and Meta-Analyses (PRISMA) guidelines of this review are shown in Supplementary Table S1.

2.1. Experimental Section

2.1.1. Inclusion and Exclusion Criteria

Studies were included if they satisfied the following conditions: (1) estimated the risk of ASD in humans using meta-analyses in terms of odds ratio (OR) and 95% confidence interval (CI); (2) published in English. Articles were excluded if (1) they did not cover the subject of genetic polymorphism or ASD; (2) did not have individual results for ASD; (3) did not use statistical methods of meta-analysis.

2.1.2. Search Strategy

A PubMed search was performed to extract data from meta-analyses regarding the gene polymorphisms of ASD published until 1 August, 2019. Two of the authors (MJ Son and CY Son) used the search terms (autism AND meta OR meta-analysis) and obtained relevant articles, first, by scanning the titles and abstracts and, second, by reviewing the full-text (Figure 1). During the selection process, all genetic, gen*, and related terms were included in the relevant articles. Any disagreements were resolved by discussion and consensus. In the case of GWAS, the GWAS catalog was additionally used, as well as PubMed, for a more precise search.

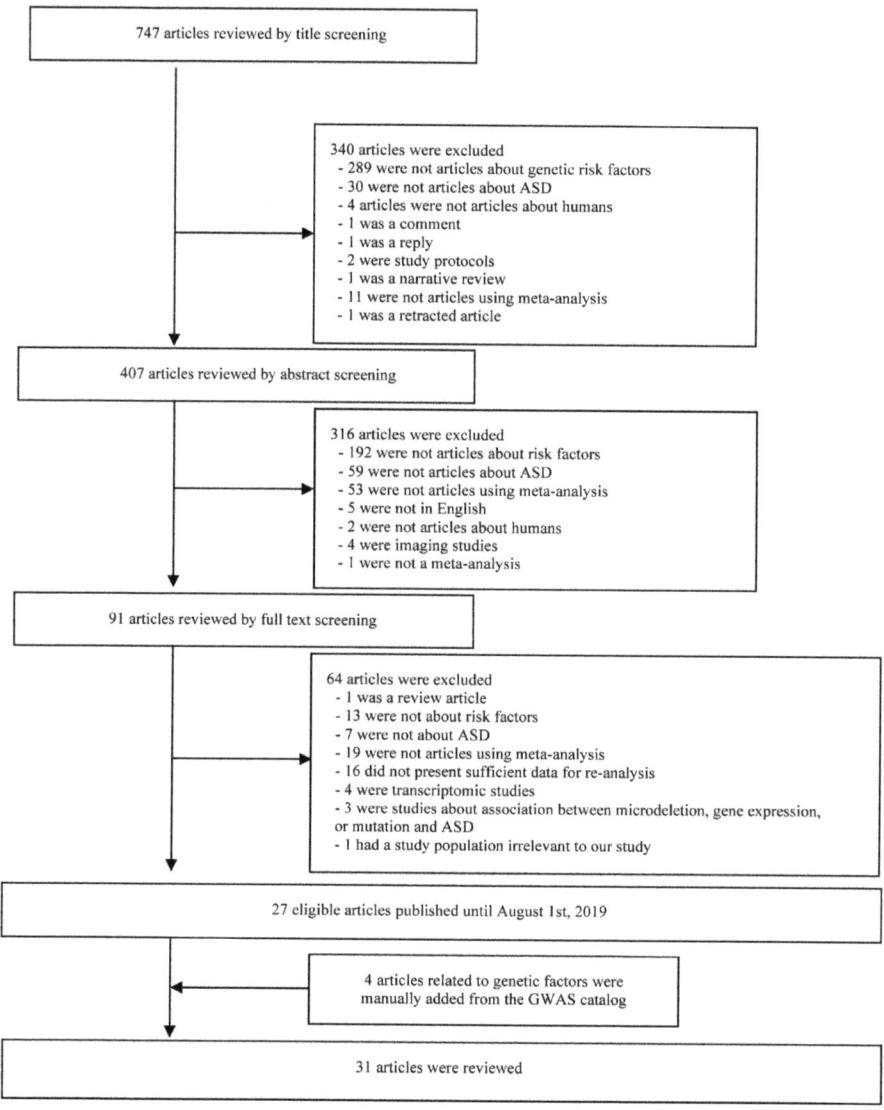

Figure 1. Flow chart of literature search.

2.1.3. Data Extraction

From each article, we extracted the first author, year of publication, the number of individual studies included, the number of cases and controls, and the number of families if a meta-analysis included family-based studies, the type of statistical model (fixed or random) and study design. We also recorded gene name, gene variants, genotypic comparison, OR with 95% CI, and the corresponding p-value. We retrieved all the main data (preferably adjusted), and, for comprehensiveness we additionally extracted subgroup analysis data if the main data were not statistically significant. When data were incomplete, we contacted the corresponding authors for additional information.

Reported association was considered statistically significant if p-value < 0.05 for meta-analyses of observational studies, and $<5 \times 10^{-8}$ for GWAS or meta-analyses of GWAS. Meanwhile, genetic associations with a $5 \times 10^{-8} < p$-value < 0.05 were defined as being of borderline significance in GWAS or meta-analyses of GWAS. In addition, we recorded genetic comparisons with p-value $< 5 \times 10^{-8}$ for our gene network, even when they were not re-analyzable due to insufficient raw data.

2.2. Statistical Analysis

Evaluations of the statistical significance of studies about genetic polymorphisms too often inferred false positives, when the evaluations were solely based on p-value [15]. Therefore, to clarify "noteworthy" association between re-analyzable genetic variants and ASD, we employed the two Bayesian approaches: FPRP and BFDP [15]. We used the Excel spreadsheets created by Wacholder et al. [15] and Wakefield [14] to calculate FPRP and BFDP, respectively. We computed FPRP at two prior probability levels of 10^{-3} and 10^{-6} and used statistical power to detect two OR levels, 1.2 and 1.5, so that readers can make their own judgment about the evidence for each genetic variant. BFDP is similar to FPRP but uses more information than FPRP [14]. Both prior probability levels were chosen as one of the low and very low values of levels, respectively. We computed BFDP at two prior probabilities levels, 10^{-3} and 10^{-6}. We set the thresholds of noteworthiness of FPRP and BFDP to be <0.2 and <0.8, respectively, as recommended by the original papers and highlighted corresponding results in bold type [14,15]. Gene variants were determined to have a noteworthy association with ASD if they satisfied both thresholds.

2.3. Construction of Protein-Protein Interaction (PPI) Network

We collected genetic comparisons either with noteworthy results under both FPRP and BFDP or with p-value $< 5 \times 10^{-8}$ to establish a network of genes using STRING 9.1 (protein-protein interaction network, PPI network) related to ASD [16]. Genetic comparison results, which show genome-wide significance (p-value $< 5 \times 10^{-8}$) or borderline significance (p-value < 0.05) with a noteworthy association under both Bayesian approaches, were included. Any results with a p-value $< 5 \times 10^{-8}$ that were not re-analyzable were also added in the network analysis. PPI networks provide a critical assessment of protein function on ASD including direct (physical) as well as indirect (functional) associations.

3. Results

3.1. Study Characteristics

The initial PubMed literature search yielded 747 articles. Out these, 656 articles were excluded after screening the title and abstract, and 64 articles were omitted after reviewing the full-text. Twenty-seven studies were finally included for the re-analysis of observational studies, GWAS, and meta-analyses of GWAS (Figure 1).

Additionally, 25 articles were searched on the GWAS catalog, but 14 articles did not meet the criteria were excluded. Among the remaining 11 articles, five articles were not re-analyzable due to insufficient raw data. Moreover, five articles were already included in our dataset from the PubMed search. However, we retained three of the non-re-analyzable articles [17–19] since they satisfied the cut-off value of statistical significance for our PPI network (p-value $< 5 \times 10^{-8}$). Out of the remaining six articles, two were already in our dataset from the literature search from PubMed. Finally, four articles from the GWAS catalog were manually added to 27 articles previously screened from PubMed, leading to a total of 31 eligible articles [17–47] being included in the systematic review (Figure 1).

3.2. Re-Analysis of Meta-Analyses

This paper is divided into two parts: (1) the observational studies part, and (2) the GWAS part. In the observational studies, all statistics were collected considering the overlapping, and results of gene variants with/without statistical significance (Table 1, Supplementary Table S2). Even though genetic variants examined in several studies, we excluded the studies if the data were not significant performed by FPRP or BFDP. In the GWAS part, data from previously published meta-analyses and newly added data from the GWAS catalog were re-analyzed.

3.2.1. Re-Analysis of Meta-Analyses of Observational Studies

Among the 31 eligible studies, 19 were meta-analyses of observational studies, which corresponded to 125 genetic comparisons. Thirty one out of 125 genotype comparisons were reported as being statistically significant using the criteria of p-value < 0.05 as listed in Table 1.

Out of the 31 genotype comparisons (Table 1), three (9.7%), and two (6.5%) were verified to be noteworthy (<0.2) using FPRP estimation, at a prior probability of 10^{-3} and 10^{-6} with a statistical power to detect an OR of 1.2; seven (22.6%) and two (6.5%) were verified to be noteworthy (<0.2) using FPRP estimation, at a prior probability of 10^{-3} and 10^{-6} with a statistical power to detect an OR of 1.5. In terms of BFDP, five (16.1%) and two (6.5%) comparisons had noteworthy findings (<0.8) at a prior probability of 10^{-3} and 10^{-6}. Two single nucleotide polymorphisms (SNPs) were found to be noteworthy under FPRP estimation only, and not under BFDP (Comparison T vs. C, SLC25A12/rs2292813 [20]; C vs. T, SLC25A12/rs2292813 [24]). In contrast, none of the SNPs were identified to be noteworthy exclusively under BFDP. Consequently, five out of 31 SNPs were found noteworthy using both FPRP and BFDP (T vs. C, MTHFR C677T; T (minor), MTHFR C677T; Comparison G vs. A, DRD3/rs167771; C vs. G, RELN/rs362691; A (minor), OXTR/rs7632287).

3.2.2. Re-Analysis of Meta-Analyses of GWAS

Seven GWAS meta-analyses and one study with a combined analysis of GWAS discovery and replication added up to 203 genetic comparisons [30–34,46–48] with statistical or borderline significant results. Out of 277 comparisons, 44 had p-value ≥ 0.05 (Table S2), none of which showed noteworthy estimation of FPRP and BFDP with statistical or borderline significant results. From the 203 comparisons, only one (0.5%), MACROD2/rs4141463 A (minor allele), was statistically significant under the genome-wide significance threshold (p-value $< 5 \times 10^{-8}$), while the remaining 202 comparisons (99.5%) satisfied the criteria of borderline significance ($5 \times 10^{-8} < p$-value < 0.05) previously defined.

We examined the 203 genetic comparisons with a genome-wide or borderline significance using both FPRP and BFDP estimation. With FPRP estimation, forty-one (20.2%) and four (2.0%) were assessed to be noteworthy at a prior probability of 10^{-3} and 10^{-6} with statistical power to detect an OR of 1.2. Moreover, fifty-four (26.6%) and eight (3.9%) were identified as noteworthy at a prior probability of 10^{-3} and 10^{-6} with statistical power to detect an OR of 1.5. Overall, forty genetic comparisons (19.7%) were found noteworthy under both Bayesian approaches, which included a single genetic comparison satisfying the conventional significance threshold of p-value < 0.05 (Table 2).

3.2.3. Re-Analysis of Results from the GWAS Catalog and GWAS Datasets Included in the GWAS Meta-Analyses

Genetic comparisons additionally extracted from the GWAS catalog were also re-analyzed (Table 3). Among the 20 included comparisons, two (10.0%) genotype comparisons, MACROD2/rs4141463 and LOCI105370358-LOCI107984602/rs4773054, extracted from the GWAS catalog were reported to be significant with a p-value $< 5 \times 10^{-8}$. The remaining 18 comparisons were of borderline statistical significance (p-value between 0.05 and 5×10^{-8}).

While assessing noteworthiness, five (25.0%) and three (15.0%) were verified as being noteworthy using FPRP estimation, at a prior probability of 10^{-3} and 10^{-6}, respectively, with the statistical power to detect a 1.2 OR. In addition, eighteen (90.0%) and four (25.0%) showed noteworthiness at a prior probability of 10^{-3} and 10^{-6} with the statistical power to detect a 1.5 OR, respectively. In the BFDP estimation, nineteen (95.0%) and two (10.0%) were assessed as being noteworthy at a prior probability of 10^{-3} and 10^{-6}, respectively. Finally, 18 genetic associations (95%) of both significant and borderline statistically significant results were verified as being noteworthy under both the FPRP and BFDP approaches. The total number of associations included two comparisons with genome-wide significance (p-value $< 5 \times 10^{-8}$) and sixteen comparisons with borderline significance (p-value between 0.05 and 5×10^{-8}).

In order to develop the analysis further, we extracted the GWAS data that was both statistically significant and noteworthy under both Bayesian approaches, from the GWAS meta-analysis and GWAS catalog. They were extracted from five articles [30–34], with 70 of the GWAS data being noteworthy under both FPRP and BFDP. Results with noteworthy association are summarized in Table 4.

Table 1. Re-analysis results of gene variants with statistical significance (p-value < 0.05) from observational studies.

Author, Year	Gene/Variant	Comparison	OR (95% CI)	p-Value	Model	No. of Studies	Power OR 1.2	Power OR 1.5	FPRP Values at Prior Probability				BFDP	BFDP
									OR 1.2		OR 1.5		0.001	0.000001
									0.001	0.000001	0.001	0.000001		
Gene variants with statistically significance (p-value < 0.05), FPRP < 0.2 and BFDP < 0.8 from observational studies														
Rai 2016 [21]	MTHFR C677T	T vs. C	1.37 (1.25, 1.50)	<0.0001	Fixed	Overall (13)	0.002	0.975	0.000	0.005	0.000	0.000	0.000	0.001
Mohammad et al. 2016 [23]	MTHFR C677T	T (minor)	1.47 (1.31, 1.65)	<0.0001	Fixed	Overall (8)	0.000	0.634	0.000	0.179	0.000	0.000	0.000	0.009
Warrier et al. 2015 [24]	DRD3/rs167771	G vs. A	1.822 (1.398, 2.375)	9.08×10^{-6}	Fixed	Overall (2)	0.001	0.075	0.901	1.000	0.108	0.992	0.649	0.999
Warrier et al. 2015 [24]	RELN/rs362691	C vs. G	0.832 (0.763, 0.908)	3.93×10^{-5}	Fixed	Overall (6)	0.486	1.000	0.071	0.987	0.036	0.974	0.584	0.999
LoParo et al. 2015 [26]	OXTR/rs7632287	A (minor)	1.43 (1.23, 1.68)	0.000005	Random	Caucasian (2)	0.016	0.720	0.451	0.999	0.018	0.950	0.432	0.999
Gene variants with statistically significance (p-value < 0.05), FPRP > 0.2 or BFDP > 0.8 from observational studies														
Liu et al. 2015 [20]	SLC25A12/rs2056202	T vs. C	0.809 (0.713, 0.917)	0.001	Fixed	Overall (8)	0.321	0.999	0.740	1.000	0.478	0.999	0.957	1.000
Liu et al. 2015 [20]	SLC25A12/rs2292813	T vs. C	0.752 (0.649, 0.871)	<0.001	Fixed	Overall (7)	0.085	0.946	0.626	0.999	0.131	0.993	0.831	1.000
Pu et al. 2013 [2]	MTHFR C677T	TT+CT vs. CC	1.56 (1.12, 2.18)	0.009	Random	Overall (8)	0.062	0.409	0.993	1.000	0.957	1.000	0.995	1.000
Pu et al. 2013 [2]	MTHFR A1298C	CC vs. AA+AC	0.73 (0.56, 0.97)	0.03	Fixed	Overall (5)	0.181	0.734	0.994	1.000	0.976	1.000	0.997	1.000
Warrier et al. 2015 [24]	SLC25A12/rs2292813	C vs. T	1.372 (1.161, 1.621)	1.97×10^{-4}	Fixed	Overall (6)	0.058	0.853	0.777	1.000	0.191	0.996	0.877	1.000
Warrier et al. 2015 [24]	CNTNAP2/rs7794745	A vs. T	0.887 (0.828, 0.950)	1.00×10^{-3}	Fixed	Overall (3)	0.963	1.000	0.389	0.998	0.380	0.998	0.952	1.000
Warrier et al. 2015 [24]	SLC25A12/rs2056202	T vs. C	1.227 (1.079, 1.396)	2.00×10^{-3}	Fixed	Overall (8)	0.368	0.999	0.837	1.000	0.654	0.999	0.976	1.000
Warrier et al. 2015 [24]	OXTR/rs2268491	T vs. C	1.31 (1.092, 1.572)	4.00×10^{-3}	Fixed	Overall (2)	0.173	0.927	0.955	1.000	0.799	1.000	0.987	1.000
Warrier et al. 2015 [24]	EN2/rs1861972	A vs. G	1.125 (1.035, 1.224)	6.00×10^{-3}	Fixed	Overall (8)	0.933	1.000	0.869	1.000	0.861	1.000	0.993	1.000
Warrier et al. 2015 [24]	MTHFR/rs1801133	T vs. C	1.370 (1.079, 1.739)	1.00×10^{-2}	Random	Overall (10)	0.138	0.772	0.986	1.000	0.926	1.000	0.994	1.000
Warrier et al. 2015 [24]	ASMT/rs4446909	G vs. A	1.195 (1.038, 1.375)	1.30×10^{-2}	Fixed	Overall (3)	0.523	0.999	0.961	1.000	0.928	1.000	0.995	1.000
Warrier et al. 2015 [24]	MET/rs38845	A vs. G	1.322 (1.013, 1.724)	1.60×10^{-2}	Random	Overall (3)	0.237	0.824	0.994	1.000	0.979	1.000	0.998	1.000
Warrier et al. 2015 [24]	SLC6A4/rs2020936	T vs. C	1.244 (1.036, 1.492)	1.90×10^{-2}	Fixed	Overall (4)	0.349	0.978	0.982	1.000	0.950	1.000	0.996	1.000
Warrier et al. 2015 [24]	SLC6A4/5Htnr VNTR	12 vs. 9/10	1.492 (1.068, 2.083)	1.90×10^{-2}	Fixed	Caucasian (4)	0.100	0.513	0.995	1.000	0.973	1.000	0.997	1.000
Warrier et al. 2015 [24]	STX1A/rs4717806	A vs. T	0.851 (0.741, 0.978)	2.30×10^{-2}	Fixed	Overall (4)	0.616	1.000	0.974	1.000	0.958	1.000	0.997	1.000
Warrier et al. 2015 [24]	RELN/rs736707	T vs. C	1.269 (1.030, 1.563)	2.50×10^{-2}	Random	Overall (7)	0.299	0.942	0.988	1.000	0.964	1.000	0.997	1.000
Warrier et al. 2015 [24]	PON1/rs662	A vs. G	0.794 (0.642, 0.983)	3.40×10^{-2}	Fixed	Overall (2)	0.329	0.946	0.990	1.000	0.973	1.000	0.997	1.000
Warrier et al. 2015 [24]	OXTR/rs237887	G vs. A	1.163 (1.002, 1.349)	4.70×10^{-2}	Fixed	Overall (2)	0.660	1.000	0.986	1.000	0.979	1.000	0.998	1.000
Warrier et al. 2015 [24]	EN2/rs1861973	T vs. C	0.86 (0.791, 0.954)	3.00×10^{-3}	Fixed	TDT (3)	0.724	1.000	0.858	1.000	0.814	1.000	0.989	1.000
Aoki et al., 2016 [25]	SCL25A12/rs2292813	G (risk allele)	1.190 (1.052, 1.346)	0.006	Random	Overall (9)	0.553	1.000	0.911	1.000	0.849	1.000	0.990	1.000
Aoki et al., 2016 [25]	SCL25A12/rs2056202	G (risk allele)	1.206 (1.035, 1.405)	0.016	Random	Overall (10)	0.474	0.997	0.972	1.000	0.942	1.000	0.996	1.000
LoParo et al., 2015 [26]	OXTR/rs237887	G (minor allele)	0.89 (0.79, 0.98)	0.0239	Random	Overall (3)	0.910	1.000	0.951	1.000	0.947	1.000	0.997	1.000
LoParo et al., 2015 [26]	OXTR/rs2268491	T (minor allele)	1.20 (1.05, 1.35)	0.0075	Random	Overall (3)	0.500	1.000	0.828	1.000	0.707	1.000	0.981	1.000
Wang et al., 2014 [27]	RELN/rs362691	R vs. NR	0.69 (0.56, 0.86)	0.001	Fixed	Overall (7)	0.047	0.620	0.954	1.000	0.607	0.999	0.969	1.000
Torrico et al., 2015 [28]	PTCHD1/rs7052177	T (major allele)	0.58 (0.45, 0.76)	6.8×10^{-5}	Fixed	European (4) [†]	0.004	0.156	0.948	1.000	0.333	0.998	0.890	1.000
Kranz et al., 2016 [29]	OXTR/rs237889	A vs. G	1.12 (1.01, 1.24)	0.0365	Random	Overall (3)	0.908	1.000	0.970	1.000	0.967	1.000	0.998	1.000

Abbreviations: A, Adenine; C, Cytosine; G, Guanine; T, Thymine; R, Risk allele; NR, Non-risk allele; CI, confidence interval; NA, not available; The bold in the table means significant results by FPRP and BFDP. [†] This article reported only the number of datasets not the number of individual studies included in the meta-analysis. Thus, we wrote the number of datasets in the parenthesis.

Table 2. Re-analysis results of gene variants with genome wide statistical significance (p-value $< 5 \times 10^{-8}$) and borderline statistical significance ($5 \times 10^{-8} \leq p$-value < 0.05) in GWAS meta-analyses.

Author, Year	Gene	Variant	Comparison	OR (95% CI)	p-Value	Power OR 1.2	Power OR 1.5	FPRP Values at Prior Probability						BFDP 0.001	BFDP 0.000001
								OR 1.2		OR 1.5					
								0.001	0.000001	0.001	0.000001				

Gene variants with statistically significance (p-value $< 5 \times 10^{-8}$), FPRP < 0.2 and BFDP < 0.8 from meta-analysis of GWAS

Author, Year	Gene	Variant	Comparison	OR (95% CI)	p-Value	Power OR 1.2	Power OR 1.5	FPRP 0.001	FPRP 0.000001	FPRP 0.001	FPRP 0.000001	BFDP 0.001	BFDP 0.000001
Anney et al., 2010 [30]	MACROD2	rs4141463	A (minor allele)	0.73 (0.66–0.82)	3.7×10^{-8}	0.013	0.937	0.009	0.898	0.000	0.107	0.008	0.891

Gene variants with statistically borderline significance ($5 \times 10^{-8} \leq p$-value < 0.05), FPRP < 0.2 and BFDP < 0.8 from meta-analyses of GWAS

Author, Year	Gene	Variant	Comparison	OR (95% CI)	p-Value	Power OR 1.2	Power OR 1.5	FPRP 0.001	FPRP 0.000001	FPRP 0.001	FPRP 0.000001	BFDP 0.001	BFDP 0.000001
Anney et al., 2017 [31]	ALPK3 NMB SCAND2P SEC11A SLC28A1 WDR73 ZNF592	rs4842996	T vs. C	1.08 (1.05–1.12)	0.00001044	1.000	1.000	0.032	0.971	0.032	0.971	0.688	1.000
	EXOC4	rs6467494	T vs. C	1.07 (1.04–1.09)	0.0000172	1.000	1.000	0.000	0.000	0.000	0.000	0.000	0.000
	NA	rs13233145	A vs. C	1.07 (1.04–1.10)	0.00002906	1.000	1.000	0.002	0.618	0.002	0.618	0.136	0.994
	NA	rs7684366	T vs. C	0.93 (0.90–0.96)	0.00003137	1.000	1.000	0.007	0.882	0.007	0.882	0.373	0.998
	MEGF10	rs73785549	C vs. G	1.15 (1.08–1.21)	0.0001308	0.950	1.000	0.000	0.070	0.000	0.067	0.005	0.835
	ANO4	rs2055471	A vs. T	1.07 (1.03–1.10)	0.0001334	1.000	1.000	0.002	0.618	0.002	0.618	0.136	0.994
	BNC2	rs7860276	A vs. G	1.10 (1.05–1.15)	0.0003196	1.000	1.000	0.026	0.964	0.026	0.964	0.598	0.999
	NA	rs2293280	C vs. G	1.12 (1.06–1.18)	0.0003606	0.995	1.000	0.020	0.954	0.020	0.954	0.514	0.999
	NA	rs16975940	T vs. C	1.07 (1.03–1.10)	0.0004742	1.000	1.000	0.002	0.618	0.002	0.618	0.136	0.994
	NA	rs10169115	C vs. G	1.06 (1.02–1.09)	0.004465	1.000	1.000	0.041	0.977	0.041	0.977	0.778	1.000
	C10orf76 CUEDC2 ELOVL3 FBXL15 GBF1 HPS6 LDB1 MIR146B NFKB2 NOLC1 PITX3 PPRC1 PSD	rs1409313	T vs. C	1.10 (1.06–1.14)	1.467×10^{-6}	1.000	1.000	0.000	0.145	0.000	0.145	0.014	0.936
	ESRRG	rs12725407	C vs. G	1.10 (1.06–1.14)	2.115×10^{-6}	1.000	1.000	0.000	0.145	0.000	0.145	0.014	0.936
	HDAC4 MIR2467 MIR4269	rs2931203	A vs. T	0.92 (0.88–0.95)	4.243×10^{-6}	1.000	1.000	0.000	0.261	0.000	0.261	0.031	0.970
Ma et al., 2009 [32]	NA	rs7704909	C(minor)/T(major)	1.30 (1.15–1.46)	1.53×10^{-5}	0.088	0.992	0.096	0.991	0.009	0.905	0.295	0.998
	NA	rs1896731	C(minor)/T(major)	0.76 (0.67–0.85)	1.90×10^{-5}	0.053	0.989	0.028	0.966	0.002	0.609	0.076	0.988
	NA	rs12518194	G(minor)/A(major)	1.31 (1.16–1.49)	8.34×10^{-6}	0.091	0.980	0.302	0.998	0.039	0.976	0.605	0.999
	NA	rs4307059	C(minor)/T(major)	1.31 (1.16–1.48)	1.29×10^{-5}	0.079	0.985	0.153	0.995	0.014	0.936	0.383	0.998
	NA	rs4327572	T(minor)/C(major)	1.32 (1.17–1.49)	4.05×10^{-5}	0.062	0.981	0.103	0.991	0.007	0.878	0.249	0.997
Anney et al., 2010 [30]	NA	rs4078417	C (minor allele)	1.19 (1.10–1.30)	5.6×10^{-5}	0.574	1.000	0.167	0.995	0.103	0.991	0.795	1.000
	PPP2R5C	rs7142002	G (minor allele)	0.64 (0.53–0.78)	2.9×10^{-6}	0.004	0.343	0.687	1.000	0.028	0.966	0.459	0.999
Kuo et al., 2015 [33]	NAALADL2	rs3914502	A (minor allele)	1.4 (1.2–1.6)	3.5×10^{-6}	0.012	0.844	0.062	0.985	0.001	0.482	0.051	0.982
	NAALADL2	rs2222447	A (minor allele)	0.7 (0.6–0.8)	5.3×10^{-5}	0.005	0.763	0.030	0.969	0.000	0.178	0.013	0.932
	NA	rs12543592	G (minor allele)	0.7 (0.6–0.8)	3.2×10^{-6}	0.005	0.763	0.030	0.969	0.000	0.178	0.013	0.932
	NA	rs7026342	C (minor allele)	1.6 (1.2–2.0)	1.8×10^{-4}	0.006	0.285	0.864	1.000	0.113	0.992	0.749	1.000
	NA	rs7030851	A (minor allele)	1.6 (1.3–2.0)	1.4×10^{-4}	0.006	0.285	0.864	1.000	0.113	0.992	0.749	1.000

Table 2. Cont.

Author, Year	Gene	Variant	Comparison	OR (95% CI)	p-Value	Power OR 1.2	Power OR 1.5	FPRP Values at Prior Probability						BFDP 0.001	BFDP 0.000001
								OR 1.2		OR 1.5					
								0.001	0.000001	0.001	0.000001				
Anney et al., 2012 [34]	RASSF5	rs11118968	A	0.44 (0.32–0.61)	2.452×10^{-7}	0.000	0.006	0.930	1.000	0.117	0.993			0.504	0.999
	DNER	rs6752370	G	1.62 (1.33–1.96)	8.526×10^{-7}	0.001	0.214	0.407	0.999	0.003	0.764			0.089	0.990
	YEATS2	rs263035	G	1.39 (1.22–1.57)	2.258×10^{-7}	0.009	0.890	0.013	0.928	0.000	0.115			0.009	0.898
	None	rs29456	A	1.65 (1.37–1.99)	1.226×10^{-7}	0.000	0.159	0.272	0.997	0.001	0.504			0.028	0.967
	None	rs1936295	A	1.69 (1.37–2.09)	6.636×10^{-7}	0.001	0.136	0.620	0.999	0.009	0.905			0.179	0.995
	None	rs4761371	A	0.46 (0.34–0.63)	3.914×10^{-7}	0.000	0.010	0.924	1.000	0.111	0.992			0.521	0.999
	None	rs288604	G	1.58 (1.32–1.88)	2.975×10^{-7}	0.001	0.279	0.207	0.996	0.001	0.473			0.032	0.971
	MACROD2	rs6110458	A	1.46 (1.27–1.69)	1.806×10^{-7}	0.004	0.641	0.084	0.989	0.001	0.383			0.033	0.971
	MACROD2 NCRNA00186	rs14135	G	1.49 (1.28–1.74)	1.778×10^{-7}	0.003	0.534	0.130	0.993	0.001	0.467			0.042	0.977
	NCRNA00186 MACROD2	rs1475531	C	1.53 (1.30–1.79)	2.011×10^{-7}	0.001	0.402	0.083	0.989	0.000	0.213			0.013	0.929
	PARD3B	rs4675502	NA	1.28 (1.16–1.41)	4.34×10^{-7}	0.095	0.999	0.006	0.856	0.001	0.362			0.030	0.969
	NA	rs7711337	NA	0.82 (0.76–0.89)	8.25×10^{-7}	0.350	1.000	0.006	0.854	0.002	0.672			0.091	0.990
	NA	rs7834018	NA	0.64 (0.53–0.77)	7.54×10^{-7}	0.003	0.333	0.465	0.999	0.007	0.871			0.186	0.996
	TAF1C	rs4150167	NA	0.51 (0.39–0.66)	2.91×10^{-7}	0.000	0.021	0.764	1.000	0.015	0.937			0.142	0.994

Gene variants with statistically borderline significance ($5 \times 10^{-8} \leq p$-value < 0.05), FPRP > 0.2 or BFDP > 0.2 from meta-analyses of GWAS

Waltes, 2014 [46]	CYFIP1 [c]	rs7170637	G > A	0.85 (0.75, 0.96)	0.007	0.625	1.000	0.934	1.000	0.898	1.000			0.993	1.000
	CAMK4 [c]	rs25925	C > G	1.31 (1.04, 1.64)	0.021	0.222	0.881	0.988	1.000	0.954	1.000			0.996	1.000
Anney et al., 2017 [31]	NA	rs1436358	T vs. C	0.86 (0.79–0.93)	0.00001473	0.785	1.000	0.168	0.995	0.137	0.994			0.844	1.000
	MACROD2 MACROD2-AS1	rs6079556	A vs. C	0.94 (0.91–0.97)	0.00001731	1.000	1.000	0.102	0.991	0.102	0.991			0.887	1.000
	LINC00635	chr8_94389815_I	I vs. D	0.92 (0.89–0.96)	0.00002102	1.000	1.000	0.109	0.992	0.109	0.992			0.867	1.000
	LINCR-0001 PRSS55	rs4840484	T vs. C	1.07 (1.04–1.11)	0.00002307	1.000	1.000	0.232	0.997	0.232	0.997			0.945	1.000
Anney et al., 2017 (continued)	ADTRP	rs10947543	C vs. G	0.94 (0.91–0.97)	0.000031	1.000	1.000	0.102	0.991	0.102	0.991			0.887	1.000
	LRRC4 MIR593 SND1 SND1-IT1	chr7_127644308_D	D vs. I	0.93 (0.90–0.97)	0.00003235	1.000	1.000	0.422	0.999	0.422	0.999			0.972	1.000
	CCDC93 DDX18 INSIG2	chr2_118616767_D	I vs. D	0.85 (0.78–0.93)	0.00003531	0.667	1.000	0.374	0.998	0.285	0.997			0.921	1.000
	NA	chr14_99235398_I	I vs. D	0.87 (0.81–0.94)	0.00003765	0.862	1.000	0.327	0.998	0.296	0.998			0.930	1.000
	TTBK1	rs2756174	A vs. C	0.94 (0.91–0.97)	0.00005245	1.000	1.000	0.102	0.991	0.102	0.991			0.887	1.000
	HCG4B HLA-A HLA-H	rs115254791	T vs. G	0.94 (0.90–0.97)	0.00005321	1.000	1.000	0.102	0.991	0.102	0.991			0.887	1.000
	MIR2113	rs9482120	A vs. C	0.94 (0.91–0.97)	0.00009513	1.000	1.000	0.102	0.991	0.102	0.991			0.887	1.000
	CRTAP SUSD5	chr3_33191013_D	I vs. D	0.93 (0.89–0.97)	0.0000957	1.000	1.000	0.422	0.999	0.422	0.999			0.972	1.000
	NA	rs9285005	A vs. G	0.91 (0.86–0.96)	0.0001147	0.999	1.000	0.354	0.998	0.354	0.998			0.956	1.000
	LOC100505609	rs73065342	T vs. G	0.89 (0.83–0.95)	0.0001169	0.976	1.000	0.322	0.998	0.317	0.998			0.941	1.000
	DCAF4 DPF3 PAPLN PSEN1 RBM25 ZFYVE1	rs1203311	A vs. C	0.86 (0.79–0.94)	0.0001394	0.756	1.000	0.540	0.999	0.470	0.999			0.960	1.000
	MACROD2	rs192259652	A vs. T	0.91 (0.85–0.96)	0.0001438	0.999	1.000	0.354	0.998	0.354	0.998			0.956	1.000
	FOXP1	rs76188283	T vs. C	1.09 (1.05–1.14)	0.0002093	1.000	1.000	0.142	0.994	0.142	0.994			0.892	1.000
	CCDC38 NTN4 SNRPF	chr12_96221819_D	I vs. D	0.94 (0.91–0.97)	0.0002128	1.000	1.000	0.102	0.991	0.102	0.991			0.887	1.000
	NA	chr3_182308608_I	D vs. I	0.94 (0.90–0.97)	0.0002755	1.000	1.000	0.102	0.991	0.102	0.991			0.887	1.000
	ASTN2 PAPPA PAPPA-AS1	rs7026354	A vs. G	1.05 (1.03–1.08)	0.0003018	1.000	1.000	0.407	0.999	0.407	0.999			0.979	1.000
	NA	rs2368140	A vs. G	0.94 (0.91–0.98)	0.0003049	1.000	1.000	0.783	1.000	0.783	1.000			0.993	1.000
	NA	rs13016472	T vs. C	0.94 (0.91–0.98)	0.0003629	1.000	1.000	0.783	1.000	0.783	1.000			0.993	1.000
	DSCAM	rs62235658	T vs. C	0.92 (0.87–0.97)	0.0004132	1.000	1.000	0.668	1.000	0.668	1.000			0.986	1.000
	NA	rs3113169	C vs. G	0.93 (0.90–0.97)	0.0004234	1.000	1.000	0.422	0.999	0.422	0.999			0.972	1.000

Table 2. Cont.

Author, Year	Gene	Variant	Comparison	OR (95% CI)	p-Value	Power OR 1.2	Power OR 1.5	FPRP Values at Prior Probability OR 1.2 0.001	OR 1.2 0.000001	OR 1.5 0.001	OR 1.5 0.000001	BFDP 0.001	BFDP 0.000001
	CASKIN2 CGA3 GRB2 LOC100287042 MIF4GD MIR3678 MIR6785 MRPS7 NUP85 SLC25A19 TMEM94 TSEN54	rs12950709	A vs. G	0.92 (0.87–0.97)	0.0004387	1.000	1.000	0.668	1.000	0.668	1.000	0.986	1.000
	CAMP CDC25A CSPG5 DHX30 MAP4 MIR1226 MIR4443 SMARCC1 ZNF589	rs7429990	A vs. C	0.94 (0.91–0.97)	0.0004525	1.000	1.000	0.102	0.991	0.102	0.991	0.887	1.000
	NA	chr8_84959513_D	D vs. I	0.89 (0.83–0.96)	0.0004634	0.956	1.000	0.728	1.000	0.718	1.000	0.985	1.000
	ACTN2	rs4659712	A vs. G	0.95 (0.92–0.98)	0.0004976	1.000	1.000	0.550	0.999	0.550	0.999	0.986	1.000
	ASB4	rs113706540	T vs. C	0.93 (0.88–0.97)	0.0005006	1.000	1.000	0.422	0.999	0.422	0.999	0.972	1.000
	GJD4	rs7897060	C vs. G	0.95 (0.91–0.98)	0.0005789	1.000	1.000	0.550	0.999	0.550	0.999	0.986	1.000
	AK5 DNAJB4 FAM73A FUBP1 GIPC2 MGC27382 NEXN NEXN-AS1 USP33 ZJZ3	rs12126604	T vs. C	0.92 (0.87–0.97)	0.0006161	1.000	1.000	0.668	1.000	0.668	1.000	0.986	1.000
	SEMA6D	rs17387110	T vs. G	0.95 (0.92–0.98)	0.0006996	1.000	1.000	0.550	0.999	0.550	0.999	0.986	1.000
	NA	chr16_62649826_D	D vs. I	0.87 (0.80–0.95)	0.0007369	0.831	1.000	0.697	1.000	0.657	0.999	0.979	1.000
	NA	rs4239875	A vs. G	1.06 (1.03–1.10)	0.0008018	1.000	1.000	0.672	1.000	0.672	1.000	0.990	1.000
	CTNNA3 DNAJC12 HERC4 MYPN POU5F1P5 SIRT1	chr10_69763783_D	I vs. D	0.91 (0.86–0.97)	0.0008401	0.997	1.000	0.792	1.000	0.791	1.000	0.991	1.000
	CLIC5 ENPP4 ENPP5	rs7762549	A vs. G	0.95 (0.92–0.98)	0.000885	1.000	1.000	0.550	0.999	0.550	0.999	0.986	1.000
	NA	chr18_76035713_D	D vs. I	0.93 (0.88–0.97)	0.000884	1.000	1.000	0.422	0.999	0.422	0.999	0.972	1.000
	BRICD5 CASKIN1 DNASE1L2 E4F1 MIR3180-5 MIR4516 MLST8 PGP PKD1 RAB26 SNHG19 SNORD60 TRAF7	rs2078282	A vs. G	0.94 (0.91–0.98)	0.0009187	1.000	1.000	0.783	1.000	0.783	1.000	0.993	1.000
	OPCML	rs7952100	C vs. G	1.06 (1.03–1.10)	0.0009399	1.000	1.000	0.672	1.000	0.672	1.000	0.990	1.000
	LOC101927907 LRRTM4	rs58500924	A vs. G	0.90 (0.84–0.96)	0.0009721	0.990	1.000	0.581	0.999	0.579	0.999	0.977	1.000
	RNGTT	rs35675874	A vs. G	0.94 (0.91–0.98)	0.001031	1.000	1.000	0.783	1.000	0.783	1.000	0.993	1.000
	LOC101928505 LOC101928539	chr5_570079215_I	D vs. I	1.07 (1.03–1.11)	0.001076	1.000	1.000	0.232	0.997	0.232	0.997	0.945	1.000
	DPP4 SLC4A10	rs2909451	T vs. C	0.94 (0.90–0.98)	0.001078	1.000	1.000	0.783	1.000	0.783	1.000	0.993	1.000
	ERAP2 LNPEP	rs55767008	T vs. C	0.89 (0.82–0.96)	0.001182	0.956	1.000	0.728	1.000	0.718	1.000	0.985	1.000
	C2orf15 KIAA1211L LIPT1 LOC101927070 TSGA10	rs10202643	A vs. T	0.95 (0.92–0.98)	0.001269	1.000	1.000	0.550	0.999	0.550	0.999	0.986	1.000
	AUTS2	rs2293507	T vs. G	0.88 (0.81–0.96)	0.001337	0.890	1.000	0.817	1.000	0.799	1.000	0.989	1.000
	NA	rs138457704	A vs. G	1.07 (1.03–1.11)	0.001357	1.000	1.000	0.232	0.997	0.232	0.997	0.945	1.000
	GLDC	rs13288399	C vs. G	0.95 (0.91–0.98)	0.001357	1.000	1.000	0.550	0.999	0.550	0.999	0.986	1.000
	MTFR1 PDE7A	rs1513723	C vs. G	0.95 (0.92–0.98)	0.001447	1.000	1.000	0.550	0.999	0.550	0.999	0.986	1.000
	ASTN2 ASTN2-AS1 PAPPA TRIM32	rs146737360	T vs. G	0.95 (0.92–0.98)	0.001534	1.000	1.000	0.550	0.999	0.550	0.999	0.986	1.000
	NA	chr6_45726254_D	D vs. I	0.90 (0.83–0.96)	0.001606	0.990	1.000	0.581	0.999	0.579	0.999	0.977	1.000
	NA	rs6742513	C vs. G	1.07 (1.03–1.11)	0.001611	1.000	1.000	0.232	0.997	0.232	0.997	0.945	1.000
	NA	rs73204738	A vs. C	0.92 (0.88–0.97)	0.001617	1.000	1.000	0.668	1.000	0.668	1.000	0.986	1.000
	LINC01553	rs11817353	A vs. C	0.95 (0.92–0.98)	0.001678	1.000	1.000	0.550	0.999	0.550	0.999	0.986	1.000

Table 2. Cont.

Author, Year	Gene	Variant	Comparison	OR (95% CI)	p-Value	Power OR 1.2	Power OR 1.5	FRP Values at Prior Probability						BFDP 0.001	BFDP 0.000001
								OR 1.2		OR 1.5					
								0.001	0.000001	0.001	0.000001				
Anney et al., 2017 (continued)	RAD51B	rs2842330	A vs. C	1.10 (1.04–1.16)	0.001845	0.999	1.000	0.303	0.998	0.303	0.998			0.946	1.000
	RBFOX1	rs12930616	C vs. G	1.05 (1.02–1.09)	0.001985	1.000	1.000	0.913	1.000	0.913	1.000			0.998	1.000
	GRID2	rs6811974	T vs. G	0.95 (0.93–0.98)	0.001995	1.000	1.000	0.550	0.999	0.550	0.999			0.986	1.000
	NA	rs7135621	T vs. C	0.96 (0.93–0.98)	0.002059	1.000	1.000	0.094	0.991	0.094	0.991			0.915	1.000
	GFER NOXO1 NPW RNF151 RPS2 SNHG9 SNORA78 SYNGR3 TBL3 ZNF598	rs55742253	T vs. C	0.93 (0.88–0.98)	0.002075	1.000	1.000	0.868	1.000	0.868	1.000			0.995	1.000
	PTPRB	rs10784860	T vs. C	0.95 (0.91–0.98)	0.002211	1.000	1.000	0.550	0.999	0.550	0.999			0.986	1.000
	LOC101927768	rs9387201	C vs. G	1.09 (1.03–1.14)	0.002427	1.000	1.000	0.142	0.994	0.142	0.994			0.892	1.000
	BTBD11 LOC101929162 PRDM4 PWP1	rs4964602	T vs. G	0.95 (0.91–0.98)	0.00256	1.000	1.000	0.550	0.999	0.550	0.999			0.986	1.000
	NA	rs1376888	T vs. C	1.05 (1.02–1.08)	0.002668	1.000	1.000	0.407	0.999	0.407	0.999			0.979	1.000
	KLHL29	rs10182178	A vs. G	1.05 (1.02–1.08)	0.003508	1.000	1.000	0.407	0.999	0.407	0.999			0.979	1.000
	UBE2H	rs78661858	A vs. G	0.91 (0.85–0.97)	0.003665	0.997	1.000	0.792	1.000	0.792	1.000			0.991	1.000
	VAPA	rs29063	A vs. G	1.04 (1.01–1.07)	0.004075	1.000	1.000	0.873	1.000	0.873	1.000			0.997	1.000
	NA	rs190401890	A vs. T	1.12 (1.04–1.20)	0.004114	0.975	1.000	0.568	0.999	0.562	0.999			0.975	1.000
	LOC102723427	rs192668887	T vs. C	0.91 (0.84–0.97)	0.004205	0.997	1.000	0.792	1.000	0.791	1.000			0.991	1.000
	SLC12A7	rs73031119	A vs. G	0.91 (0.84–0.97)	0.004399	0.997	1.000	0.792	1.000	0.791	1.000			0.991	1.000
	ADGRL2	rs75695875	A vs. G	0.93 (0.87–0.98)	0.004715	1.000	1.000	0.868	1.000	0.868	1.000			0.995	1.000
	NA	rs1943999	C vs. G	0.96 (0.92–0.99)	0.004915	0.999	1.000	0.903	1.000	0.903	1.000			0.998	1.000
	DNAH6	rs2222734	A vs. G	0.92 (0.87–0.98)	0.005058	1.000	1.000	0.906	1.000	0.906	1.000			0.996	1.000
	OR8A1 OR8B12	rs2226753	T vs. C	0.96 (0.93–0.99)	0.005074	1.000	1.000	0.903	1.000	0.903	1.000			0.998	1.000
	TUSC5	rs35713482	A vs. G	1.05 (1.01–1.08)	0.005154	1.000	1.000	0.407	0.999	0.407	0.999			0.979	1.000
	C5orf15 VDAC1	rs67120295	T vs. G	1.06 (1.02–1.10)	0.005745	1.000	1.000	0.672	1.000	0.672	1.000			0.990	1.000
	NA	rs76010911	A vs. G	1.11 (1.04–1.19)	0.006255	0.986	1.000	0.769	1.000	0.767	1.000			0.989	1.000
	MTMR9 SLC35G5 TDH	rs6601581	T vs. C	1.06 (1.02–1.11)	0.006463	1.000	1.000	0.930	1.000	0.930	1.000			0.998	1.000
	HSDL2 MIR3134 PTBP3 SUSD1 CRTC3 GABARAPL3 IQGAP1	rs7024761	A vs. G	1.05 (1.02–1.09)	0.00648	1.000	1.000	0.913	1.000	0.913	1.000			0.998	1.000
	ZNF774	rs2601187	A vs. G	1.05 (1.01–1.08)	0.006859	1.000	1.000	0.407	0.999	0.407	0.999			0.979	1.000
	LOC101927189 LRRC1	rs4715431	A vs. G	1.04 (1.01–1.08)	0.007007	1.000	1.000	0.977	1.000	0.977	1.000			0.999	1.000
	NA	rs646680	A vs. G	0.95 (0.92–0.99)	0.00723	1.000	1.000	0.937	1.000	0.937	1.000			0.998	1.000
	CCNE1	rs12609867	A vs. G	0.95 (0.91–0.99)	0.00743	1.000	1.000	0.937	1.000	0.937	1.000			0.998	1.000
	NOS1AP OLFML2B KDM4A KDM4A-AS1 LOC101929592	rs75192393	T vs. C	1.07 (1.02–1.12)	0.007697	1.000	1.000	0.787	1.000	0.787	1.000			0.993	1.000
	MIR6079 PTPRF ST3GAL3	rs79857083	T vs. C	1.04 (1.01–1.08)	0.007758	1.000	1.000	0.977	1.000	0.977	1.000			0.999	1.000
	NA	rs142968358	T vs. G	1.04 (1.01–1.07)	0.007789	1.000	1.000	0.873	1.000	0.873	1.000			0.997	1.000
	C3orf80 IGSF11 IGSF11-AS1 UPK1B	rs1102586	A vs. G	1.06 (1.02–1.10)	0.007844	1.000	1.000	0.672	1.000	0.672	1.000			0.990	1.000
	NA	chr11_98107192_D	D vs. I	1.04 (1.01–1.08)	0.00785	1.000	1.000	0.977	1.000	0.977	1.000			0.999	1.000
	C9orf135	rs76014157	A vs. G	0.90 (0.82–0.98)	0.007946	0.962	1.000	0.941	1.000	0.939	1.000			0.997	1.000
	NA	rs6437449	A vs. G	1.07 (1.02–1.11)	0.008708	1.000	1.000	0.232	0.997	0.232	0.997			0.945	1.000
	MYO5A	chr15_52811815_D	I vs. D	0.90 (0.81–0.98)	0.008799	0.962	1.000	0.941	1.000	0.939	1.000			0.997	1.000
	NA	rs9466619	A vs. G	0.95 (0.92–0.99)	0.009071	1.000	1.000	0.937	1.000	0.937	1.000			0.998	1.000

Table 2. Cont.

Author, Year	Gene	Variant	Comparison	OR (95% CI)	p-Value	Power OR 1.2	Power OR 1.5	FPRP Values at Prior Probability				BFDP 0.001	BFDP 0.000001
								OR 1.2		OR 1.5			
								0.001	0.000001	0.001	0.000001		
	NA	rs6117854	A vs. G	0.96 (0.93–0.99)	0.01012	1.000	1.000	0.903	1.000	0.903	1.000	0.998	1.000
	C7orf33	rs6955951	A vs. T	1.04 (1.01–1.07)	0.01015	1.000	1.000	0.873	1.000	0.873	1.000	0.997	1.000
	LHX6	rs72767788	A vs. C	0.95 (0.91–0.99)	0.01093	1.000	1.000	0.937	1.000	0.937	1.000	0.998	1.000
	NA	rs2028664	A vs. C	1.04 (1.01–1.07)	0.01095	1.000	1.000	0.873	1.000	0.873	1.000	0.997	1.000
	ELAVL2	rs180861134	A vs. T	1.05 (1.01–1.09)	0.01104	1.000	1.000	0.913	1.000	0.913	1.000	0.998	1.000
	RASGEF1C	rs12659560	T vs. C	1.04 (1.01–1.07)	0.0112	1.000	1.000	0.873	1.000	0.873	1.000	0.997	1.000
	MIR548AZ SYNE2	rs2150291	T vs. C	1.05 (1.01–1.09)	0.0113	1.000	1.000	0.913	1.000	0.913	1.000	0.998	1.000
	WDFY4	rs118059975	A vs. C	0.95 (0.91–0.99)	0.01146	1.000	1.000	0.937	1.000	0.937	1.000	0.998	1.000
	LINC01525 MAN1A2	rs3820500	A vs. G	1.04 (1.01–1.07)	0.0116	1.000	1.000	0.873	1.000	0.873	1.000	0.997	1.000
	GALNT10	rs17629195	T vs. C	1.04 (1.01–1.07)	0.012	1.000	1.000	0.873	1.000	0.873	1.000	0.997	1.000
	MIR597 TNKS	rs78853604	T vs. C	1.05 (1.01–1.08)	0.01256	1.000	1.000	0.407	0.999	0.407	0.999	0.979	1.000
	EXT1	rs7835763	A vs. T	1.04 (1.01–1.08)	0.01283	1.000	1.000	0.977	1.000	0.977	1.000	0.999	1.000
	NA	rs4652928	A vs. G	0.96 (0.92–0.99)	0.01384	1.000	1.000	0.903	1.000	0.903	1.000	0.998	1.000
	PDE1C	rs11976985	T vs. C	0.95 (0.92–0.99)	0.0141	1.000	1.000	0.937	1.000	0.937	1.000	0.998	1.000
	BAX FTL GYS1	rs2230267	T vs. C	1.04 (1.01–1.07)	0.01429	1.000	1.000	0.873	1.000	0.873	1.000	0.997	1.000
Amey et al., 2017 (continued)	GRID2	rs6854329	C vs. G	0.92 (0.86–0.99)	0.01486	0.996	1.000	0.963	1.000	0.963	1.000	0.998	1.000
	NA	rs1926229	C vs. G	1.05 (1.01–1.08)	0.01496	1.000	1.000	0.407	0.999	0.407	0.999	0.979	1.000
	NA	rs261351	T vs. C	0.96 (0.93–0.99)	0.01498	1.000	1.000	0.903	1.000	0.903	1.000	0.998	1.000
	RAPGEF2	rs4440173	A vs. G	1.04 (1.01–1.07)	0.01564	1.000	1.000	0.873	1.000	0.873	1.000	0.997	1.000
	MIR4650-1 MIR4650-2 POM121 SBDSP1 SPDYE7P TYW1B	rs4392770	T vs. C	1.05 (1.01–1.09)	0.01564	1.000	1.000	0.913	1.000	0.913	1.000	0.998	1.000
	NA	rs138493916	C vs. G	1.08 (1.02–1.14)	0.01783	1.000	1.000	0.840	1.000	0.840	1.000	0.994	1.000
	NA	rs615512	A vs. G	1.08 (1.02–1.14)	0.01811	1.000	1.000	0.840	1.000	0.840	1.000	0.994	1.000
	EP400 EP400NL PUS1 SNORA49	rs11608890	T vs. G	0.94 (0.88–0.99)	0.0187	1.000	1.000	0.951	1.000	0.951	1.000	0.998	1.000
	DIAPH3	chr13_60161890_I	I vs. D	1.05 (1.01–1.09)	0.01984	1.000	1.000	0.913	1.000	0.913	1.000	0.998	1.000
	ADAM12	rs1674923	T vs. C	0.96 (0.93–0.99)	0.0203	1.000	1.000	0.903	1.000	0.903	1.000	0.998	1.000
	ATP2B2 GHRL GHRLOS IRAK2 LINC00852 MIR378B MIR885 SEC13 TATDN2	rs7619985	A vs. G	1.04 (1.01–1.07)	0.02102	1.000	1.000	0.873	1.000	0.873	1.000	0.997	1.000
	UNC13C	rs75099274	A vs. G	1.08 (1.01–1.14)	0.02123	1.000	1.000	0.840	1.000	0.840	1.000	0.994	1.000
	Z5WIM6	rs10053166	A vs. G	0.95 (0.90–0.99)	0.02226	1.000	1.000	0.937	1.000	0.937	1.000	0.998	1.000
	HIVEP3	rs2786484	T vs. C	0.93 (0.86–0.99)	0.0237	1.000	1.000	0.958	1.000	0.958	1.000	0.998	1.000
	FJX1 TRIM44	rs76847144	T vs. C	0.93 (0.86–0.99)	0.02643	1.000	1.000	0.958	1.000	0.958	1.000	0.998	1.000
	WB5CR17	rs148521358	C vs. G	0.94 (0.88–0.99)	0.02731	1.000	1.000	0.951	1.000	0.951	1.000	0.998	1.000
	MIR3134 SUSD1	rs2564899	T vs. C	0.97 (0.94–1.00)	0.02735	1.000	1.000	0.980	1.000	0.980	1.000	0.999	1.000
	NA	chr8_138837351_I	I vs. D	1.05 (1.01–1.09)	0.0284	1.000	1.000	0.913	1.000	0.913	1.000	0.998	1.000
	LINC01393 MDFIC	rs7799732	A vs. G	1.03 (1.00–1.06)	0.03114	1.000	1.000	0.978	1.000	0.978	1.000	0.999	1.000
	TBX18 TBX18-AS1	rs76397051	A vs. G	1.05 (1.01–1.10)	0.034	1.000	1.000	0.975	1.000	0.975	1.000	0.999	1.000
	NA	rs171794	T vs. C	1.06 (1.01–1.12)	0.03587	1.000	1.000	0.974	1.000	0.974	1.000	0.999	1.000
	GDA	rs4327921	A vs. G	0.97 (0.94–1.00)	0.03938	1.000	1.000	0.980	1.000	0.980	1.000	0.999	1.000
	NA	rs2167941	T vs. G	1.05 (1.00–1.10)	0.04203	1.000	1.000	0.975	1.000	0.975	1.000	0.999	1.000

Table 2. Cont.

Author, Year	Gene	Variant	Comparison	OR (95% CI)	p-Value	Power OR 1.2	Power OR 1.5	FRPR Values at Prior Probability							BFDP 0.001	BFDP 0.000001
								OR 1.2		OR 1.5						
								0.001	0.000001	0.001	0.000001					
	EVA1C	rs62216215	A vs. C	1.04 (1.00-1.08)	0.04598	1.000	1.000	0.977	1.000	0.977	1.000				0.999	1.000
	LINC01036	rs17589281	T vs. C	0.95 (0.89-1.00)	0.04716	1.000	1.000	0.980	1.000	0.980	1.000				0.999	1.000
	LOC283585	rs61979775	T vs. C	0.97 (0.93-1.00)	0.04813	1.000	1.000	0.980	1.000	0.980	1.000				0.999	1.000
	CHMP4A GMPR2 MDP1 NEDD8 NEDD8-MDP1 TM9SF1 TSSK4	rs72694312	T vs. G	1.06 (1.00-1.11)	0.04814	1.000	1.000	0.930	1.000	0.930	1.000				0.998	1.000
Ma et al., 2009 [32]	NA	rs10065041	T(minor)/C(major)	1.21 (1.08-1.36)	3.24 × 10⁻⁴	0.445	1.000	0.757	1.000	0.581	0.999				0.970	1.000
	NA	rs10038113	C(minor)/T(major)	0.75 (0.70-0.90)	3.40 × 10⁻⁶	0.129	0.897	0.939	1.000	0.688	1.000				0.979	1.000
	NA	rs6894838	T(minor)/C(major)	1.26 (1.12-1.42)	8.00 × 10⁻⁵	0.212	0.998	0.416	0.999	0.131	0.993				0.827	1.000
Anney et al., 2010 [30]	HAT1	rs6731562	G (minor allele)	1.25 (1.11-1.41)	2.0 × 10⁻⁴	0.253	0.998	0.527	0.999	0.220	0.996				0.891	1.000
	POU6F2	rs10258862	G (minor allele)	1.09 (1.00-1.18)	4.6 × 10⁻²	0.991	1.000	0.971	1.000	0.971	1.000				0.998	1.000
	NA	rs6557675	A (minor allele)	0.84 (0.76-0.93)	1.0 × 10⁻³	0.561	1.000	0.583	0.999	0.440	0.999				0.953	1.000
	MYH11	rs17284809	A (minor allele)	0.63 (0.50-0.79)	5.7 × 10⁻⁵	0.008	0.312	0.891	1.000	0.168	0.995				0.821	1.000
	G5G1L	rs205409	G (minor allele)	0.91 (0.84-0.99)	2.8 × 10⁻²	0.980	1.000	0.966	1.000	0.966	1.000				0.998	1.000
	TAF1C	rs4150167	A (minor allele)	0.54 (0.40-0.73)	2.1 × 10⁻⁵	0.002	0.085	0.963	1.000	0.420	0.999				0.905	1.000
Kuo et al., 2015 [33]	GLIS1	rs12082358	C (minor allele)	1.3 (1.1-1.5)	2.2 × 10⁻⁴	0.136	0.975	0.705	1.000	0.251	0.997				0.906	1.000
	GLIS1	rs12080993	A (minor allele)	1.3 (1.1-1.5)	1.5 × 10⁻⁴	0.136	0.975	0.705	1.000	0.251	0.997				0.906	1.000
	GPD2	rs3916984	A (minor allele)	1.3 (1.1-1.5)	3.1 × 10⁻⁴	0.136	0.975	0.705	1.000	0.251	0.997				0.906	1.000
	LRP2/BBS5	rs13014164	C (minor allele)	1.7 (1.3-2.3)	8.6 × 10⁻⁵	0.012	0.209	0.980	1.000	0.735	1.000				0.974	1.000
	PDGFRA	rs7697680	G (minor allele)	1.5 (1.2-1.9)	9.2 × 10⁻⁴	0.032	0.500	0.960	1.000	0.607	0.999				0.967	1.000
	FSTL4	rs11741756	A (minor allele)	1.3 (1.1-1.5)	1.2 × 10⁻²	0.136	0.975	0.705	1.000	0.251	0.997				0.906	1.000
	NA	rs13211684	G (minor allele)	1.3 (1.1-1.5)	2.5 × 10⁻³	0.136	0.975	0.705	1.000	0.251	0.997				0.906	1.000
	NA	rs10966205	T (minor allele)	1.3 (1.2-1.5)	2.9 × 10⁻⁵	0.136	0.975	0.705	1.000	0.251	0.997				0.906	1.000
	C10orf68	rs10763893	A (minor allele)	1.6 (1.2-2.2)	6.1 × 10⁻⁴	0.038	0.346	0.990	1.000	0.917	1.000				0.992	1.000
	NA	rs12366025	A (minor allele)	1.3 (1.1-1.6)	3.8 × 10⁻³	0.225	0.912	0.983	1.000	0.936	1.000				0.995	1.000
	NA	rs11030597	G (minor allele)	1.3 (1.1-1.6)	4.1 × 10⁻³	0.225	0.912	0.983	1.000	0.936	1.000				0.995	1.000
	NA	rs7933990	A (minor allele)	1.3 (1.1-1.6)	2.5 × 10⁻³	0.225	0.912	0.983	1.000	0.936	1.000				0.995	1.000
	NA	rs11030606	A (minor allele)	1.3 (1.1-1.6)	5.6 × 10⁻³	0.225	0.912	0.983	1.000	0.936	1.000				0.995	1.000
	MACROD2	rs17263514	A (minor allele)	1.2 (1.0-1.4)	1.4 × 10⁻²	0.500	0.998	0.976	1.000	0.953	1.000				0.996	1.000
	BCAS1/CYP24A1	rs12479663	C (minor allele)	1.5 (1.3-1.9)	4.0 × 10⁻⁵	0.032	0.500	0.960	1.000	0.607	0.999				0.967	1.000

Abbreviations: A, Adenine; C, Cytosine; G, Guanine; T, Thymine; D, Deletion; I, Insertion; R, Risk allele; NR, Non-risk allele; FPRP, false positive rate probability; BFDP, Bayesian false discovery probability; OR, odds ratio; CI, confidence interval; NA, not available.

Table 3. Re-analysis results of gene variants with genome wide statistical significance (p-value $< 5 \times 10^{-8}$, FPRP < 0.2 and BFDP < 0.8 from GWAS catalog) and borderline statistical significance ($5 \times 10^{-8} \leq p$-value < 0.05) in the genome-wide association studies (GWAS) catalog.

Author, Year	Gene	Variant	Comparison	OR (95% CI)	p-Value	Power OR 1.2	Power OR 1.5	FPRP Values at Prior Probability				BFDP 0.001	BFDP 0.000001
								OR 1.2		OR 1.5			
								0.001	0.000001	0.001	0.000001		
Gene variants with statistically significance (p-value $< 5 \times 10^{-8}$, FPRP < 0.2 and BFDP < 0.8 from GWAS catalog)													
Anney et al., 2010 [30]	MACROD2	rs4141463	NA	1.37 (1.22–1.52)	4.00×10^{-8}	0.006	0.956	0.000	0.316	0.000	0.003	0.000	0.208
Chaste et al., 2014 [35]	AL163541.1	rs4773054	NA	2.66 (1.83–3.86)	5.00×10^{-8}	0.000	0.001	0.949	1.000	0.169	0.995	0.526	0.999
Gene variants with statistically borderline significance ($5 \times 10^{-8} \leq p$-value < 0.05, FPRP < 0.2 and BFDP < 0.8 from GWAS catalog)													
Anney et al., 2010 [30]	PPP2R5C	rs7142002	NA	1.56 (1.28–1.89)	3.00×10^{-6}	0.004	0.344	0.602	0.999	0.016	0.942	0.338	0.998
Anney et al., 2012 [34]	TAF1C	rs4150167	NA	1.96 (1.52–2.56)	3.00×10^{-7}	0.000	0.025	0.832	1.000	0.031	0.969	0.269	0.997
Anney et al., 2012 [34]	PARD3B	rs4675502	NA	1.28 (1.16–1.41)	4.00×10^{-7}	0.095	0.999	0.006	0.856	0.001	0.362	0.030	0.969
Anney et al., 2012 [34]	AC113414.1	rs7711337	NA	1.22 (1.12–1.32)	8.00×10^{-7}	0.340	1.000	0.002	0.689	0.001	0.429	0.038	0.975
Anney et al., 2012 [34]	AC009446.1, EYA1	rs7834018	NA	1.56 (1.3–1.89)	8.00×10^{-7}	0.004	0.344	0.602	0.999	0.016	0.942	0.338	0.998
Anney et al., 2017 [31]	AL133270.1, AL139093.1	rs142968358	T (risk allele)	1.1 (1.06–1.14)	1.00×10^{-6}	1.000	1.000	0.000	0.145	0.000	0.145	0.014	0.936
Anney et al., 2017 [31]	EXT1	rs7835763	A (risk allele)	1.1 (1.06–1.14)	2.00×10^{-6}	1.000	1.000	0.000	0.145	0.000	0.145	0.014	0.936
Chaste et al., 2014 [35]	INHCAP	rs1867503	NA	1.55 (1.30–1.84)	4.00×10^{-7}	0.002	0.354	0.241	0.997	0.002	0.608	0.058	0.984
Chaste et al., 2014 [35]	CUEDC2	rs1409313	NA	1.75 (1.40–2.18)	4.00×10^{-7}	0.000	0.085	0.610	0.999	0.007	0.876	0.121	0.993
Chaste et al., 2014 [35]	CTU2	rs11641365	NA	2.06 (1.54–2.76)	3.00×10^{-7}	0.000	0.017	0.897	1.000	0.071	0.987	0.433	0.999
Chaste et al., 2014 [35]	AC067752.1, AC024598.1, ZNF365	rs93895	NA	1.91 (1.48–2.47)	2.00×10^{-7}	0.000	0.033	0.804	1.000	0.024	0.961	0.241	0.997
Kuo et al., 2015 [33]	LINC01151, AC108136.1	rs12543592	G (risk allele)	1.43 (1.25–1.67)	3.00×10^{-6}	0.013	0.727	0.318	0.998	0.008	0.895	0.275	0.997
Kuo et al., 2015 [33]	NAALADL2	rs3914502	A (risk allele)	1.4 (1.20–1.60)	4.00×10^{-6}	0.012	0.844	0.062	0.985	0.001	0.482	0.051	0.982
Kuo et al., 2015 [33]	OR2M4	rs10888329	NA	1.82 (1.29–2.33)	8.00×10^{-6}	0.000	0.062	0.809	1.000	0.031	0.970	0.338	0.998
Kuo et al., 2015 [33]	5GSM2	rs2447097	A (risk allele)	1.53 (1.27–1.85)	9.00×10^{-6}	0.006	0.419	0.652	0.999	0.026	0.965	0.467	0.999
Ma et al., 2009 [32]	Intergenic (RNU6-374P - MSNP1)	rs10038113	T (risk allele)	1.33 (1.11–1.43)	3.00×10^{-6}	0.003	0.999	0.000	0.000	0.000	0.000	0.000	0.000
Gene variants with statistically borderline significance ($5 \times 10^{-8} \leq p$-value < 0.05), FPRP > 0.2 or BFDP > 0.8 from GWAS catalog													
Chaste et al., 2014 [35]	AL163541.1	rs4773054	NA	2.9 (1.91–4.39)	7.00×10^{-8}	0.000	0.001	0.970	1.000	0.345	0.998	0.741	1.000
Anney et al., 2017 [31]	HLA-A, AL671277.1	rs115254791	G (risk allele)	1.0869565 (1.05–1.14)	4.00×10^{-6}	1.000	1.000	0.376	0.998	0.376	0.998	0.963	1.000

Abbreviations: A, Adenine; G, Guanine; T, Thymine; FPRP, false positive rate probability; BFDP, Bayesian false discovery probability; OR, odds ratio; CI, confidence interval; F, fixed effects model; R, random effects model; NA, not available; ASD, autism spectrum disorder.

Table 4. Re-analysis results of gene variants with genome wide statistical significance (p-value $< 5 \times 10^{-8}$) and borderline statistical significance ($5 \times 10^{-8} \leq p$-value < 0.05) in the GWAS datasets included in GWAS meta-analyses (results of FPRP < 0.2 and BFDP < 0.8).

Author, Year	Trait	Gene(s)	Variant	Comparison	OR (95% CI)	p-Value	Power OR 1.2	Power OR 1.5	FPRP Values at Prior Probability						BFDP 0.001	BFDP 0.000001
									OR 1.2			OR 1.5				
									0.001	0.000001	0.001	0.000001				
Anney et al., 2012 [34]	ASD (European)	ERBB4	rs1879532	A	2.02 (1.57–2.59)	1.55×10^{-8}	0.000	0.009	0.595	0.999	0.003	0.757			0.026	0.964
Anney et al., 2012 [34]	Autism (European)	None	rs289932	A	0.49 (0.38–0.64)	5.04×10^{-8}	0.000	0.012	0.772	1.000	0.014	0.932			0.114	0.992
Anney et al., 2012 [34]	ASD	TMEM132B	rs16919315	A	0.53 (0.42–0.67)	5.12×10^{-8}	0.000	0.028	0.589	0.999	0.004	0.800			0.049	0.981
Anney et al., 2012 [34]	Autism (European)	ERBB4	rs1879532	A	1.72 (1.39–2.11)	1.66×10^{-7}	0.000	0.095	0.416	0.999	0.002	0.676			0.044	0.979
Anney et al., 2010 [30]	Autism	NA	rs6557675	A (minor allele)	0.61 (0.51–0.71)	2.20×10^{-7}	0.000	0.126	0.006	0.861	0.000	0.001			0.000	0.048
Anney et al., 2012 [34]	Autism (European)	None	rs289858	A	0.52 (0.40–0.67)	2.81×10^{-7}	0.000	0.027	0.762	1.000	0.015	0.940			0.161	0.995
Anney et al., 2012 [34]	ASD	SYNE2	rs2150291	A	1.72 (1.40–2.13)	2.83×10^{-7}	0.000	0.105	0.579	0.999	0.006	0.864			0.119	0.993
Anney et al., 2012 [34]	ASD (European)	RPH3AL	rs7207517	A	1.97 (1.51–2.57)	3.05×10^{-7}	0.000	0.022	0.817	1.000	0.025	0.963			0.226	0.997
Anney et al., 2012 [34]	Autism (European)	None	rs4761371	A	0.46 (0.34–0.63)	3.91×10^{-7}	0.000	0.010	0.924	1.000	0.111	0.992			0.521	0.999
Anney et al., 2012 [34]	ASD (European)	PRAMEF12	rs1812242	A	1.44 (1.25–1.66)	4.29×10^{-7}	0.006	0.713	0.077	0.988	0.001	0.411			0.038	0.975
Anney et al., 2012 [34]	ASD	None	rs10904487	G	0.63 (0.52–0.75)	4.29×10^{-7}	0.001	0.262	0.198	0.996	0.001	0.440			0.028	0.966
Anney et al., 2012 [34]	Autism (European)	None	rs289932	A	0.67 (0.57–0.79)	5.42×10^{-7}	0.005	0.524	0.286	0.998	0.004	0.784			0.135	0.994
Anney et al., 2010 [30]	Autism	MACROD2	rs4141463	A (minor allele)	0.62 (0.52–0.73)	5.50×10^{-7}	0.000	0.192	0.047	0.980	0.000	0.048			0.002	0.655
Anney et al., 2012 [34]	Autism	None	rs9608521	A	1.46 (1.25–1.69)	7.62×10^{-7}	0.004	0.641	0.084	0.989	0.001	0.383			0.033	0.971
Anney et al., 2012 [34]	ASD	None	rs1408744	A	0.65 (0.54–0.77)	8.06×10^{-7}	0.002	0.385	0.235	0.997	0.002	0.618			0.062	0.985
Anney et al., 2017 [31]	ASD	LINC00535	chr8_94389815_I	I vs. D	1.14 (1.09–1.19)	9.47×10^{-7}	0.990	1.000	0.000	0.002	0.000	0.002			0.686	1.000
Anney et al., 2012 [34]	ASD (European)	PC	rs7122539	A	0.60 (0.49–0.74)	9.64×10^{-7}	0.001	0.162	0.628	0.999	0.011	0.917			0.213	0.996
Anney et al., 2010 [30]	Autism	MACROD2	rs4814324	A (minor allele)	1.58 (1.34–1.86)	9.80×10^{-7}	0.000	0.266	0.076	0.988	0.000	0.128			0.006	0.859
Anney et al., 2010 [30]	Autism	MACROD2	rs6079544	A (minor allele)	1.57 (1.33–1.84)	1.20×10^{-6}	0.000	0.287	0.053	0.982	0.000	0.081			0.004	0.797
Anney et al., 2017 [31]	ASD	EXOC4	rs6467494	T vs. C	1.12 (1.07–1.16)	1.43×10^{-6}	1.000	1.000	0.000	0.000	0.000	0.000			0.197	0.996
Anney et al., 2010 [30]	Autism	MACROD2	rs6079536	A (minor allele)	0.64 (0.54–0.75)	1.60×10^{-6}	0.001	0.307	0.059	0.984	0.000	0.102			0.005	0.837
Anney et al., 2010 [30]	ASD	MYH11	rs17284809	A (minor allele)	0.52 (0.30–0.69)	1.70×10^{-6}	0.001	0.043	0.915	1.000	0.121	0.993			0.636	0.999
Anney et al., 2010 [30]	Autism	MACROD2	rs6079553	A (minor allele)	1.55 (1.31–1.82)	2.10×10^{-6}	0.001	0.344	0.090	0.990	0.000	0.204			0.011	0.920
Anney et al., 2010 [30]	Autism	MACROD2	rs6074798	A (minor allele)	1.56 (1.32–1.84)	2.10×10^{-6}	0.001	0.321	0.123	0.993	0.000	0.287			0.017	0.945
Anney et al., 2017 [31]	ASD	OPCML	rs7952100	C vs.G	1.14 (1.09–1.19)	2.49×10^{-6}	0.990	1.000	0.000	0.002	0.000	0.002			0.686	1.000
Anney et al., 2010 [30]	Autism	MACROD2	rs10446030	G (minor allele)	1.54 (1.30–1.81)	3.20×10^{-6}	0.001	0.375	0.116	0.992	0.000	0.301			0.019	0.951
Kuo et al., 2015 [33]	ASD	STYK1	rs16922945	C (minor allele)	1.86 (1.43–2.43)	3.43×10^{-6}	0.001	0.057	0.891	1.000	0.085	0.989			0.572	0.999
Anney et al., 2010 [30]	Autism	POU5F2	rs10258862	G (minor allele)	1.41 (1.23–1.61)	3.70×10^{-6}	0.009	0.820	0.043	0.978	0.000	0.319			0.027	0.966
Anney et al., 2010 [30]	Autism	MACROD2	rs6079540	A (minor allele)	0.65 (0.55–0.77)	3.70×10^{-6}	0.002	0.385	0.235	0.997	0.002	0.618			0.062	0.985
Anney et al., 2010 [30]	Autism	MACROD2	rs6074787	A (minor allele)	1.53 (1.30–1.80)	4.10×10^{-6}	0.002	0.406	0.147	0.994	0.001	0.418			0.031	0.970
Anney et al., 2010 [30]	ASD	MACROD2	rs6074798	A (minor allele)	1.38 (1.22–1.56)	4.80×10^{-6}	0.013	0.909	0.020	0.954	0.000	0.224			0.018	0.948
Anney et al., 2010 [30]	Autism	MACROD2	rs980319	G (minor allele)	1.52 (1.29–1.79)	5.10×10^{-6}	0.002	0.437	0.184	0.996	0.001	0.543			0.050	0.981

Table 4. Cont.

Author, Year	Trait	Gene(s)	Variant	Comparison	OR (95% CI)	p-Value	Power OR 1.2	Power OR 1.5	FPRP Values at Prior Probability						
									OR 1.2			OR 1.5		BFDP	BFDP
									0.001	0.000001	0.001	0.000001		0.001	0.000001
Anney et al., 2010 [30]	Autism	MACROD2	rs6079537	G (minor allele)	1.52 (1.29–1.79)	6.00×10^{-6}	0.002	0.437	0.184	0.996	0.001	0.543		0.050	0.981
Kuo et al., 2015 [33]	ASD	NA	rs10966205	A (minor allele)	1.52 (1.27–1.83)	6.25×10^{-6}	0.006	0.444	0.609	0.999	0.022	0.957		0.426	0.999
Kuo et al., 2015 [33]	ASD	OR2M4	rs10888329	T (minor allele)	0.55 (0.43–0.72)	8.05×10^{-6}	0.001	0.081	0.916	1.000	0.144	0.994		0.718	1.000
Anney et al., 2010 [30]	ASD	MACROD2	rs6079536	A (minor allele)	0.73 (0.65–0.83)	8.50×10^{-6}	0.022	0.917	0.067	0.986	0.002	0.628		0.084	0.989
Anney et al., 2010 [30]	ASD	NA	rs6657675	A (minor allele)	0.72 (0.63–0.82)	8.70×10^{-6}	0.014	0.877	0.051	0.982	0.001	0.457		0.047	0.980
Kuo et al., 2015 [33]	ASD	NA	rs7933990	A (minor allele)	1.72 (1.35–2.19)	9.40×10^{-6}	0.002	0.133	0.861	1.000	0.075	0.988		0.606	0.999
Kuo et al., 2015 [33]	ASD	MNT	rs2447097	A (minor allele)	1.53 (1.27–1.85)	9.45×10^{-6}	0.006	0.419	0.652	0.999	0.026	0.965		0.467	0.999
Kuo et al., 2015 [33]	ASD	GSG1L	rs205409	G (minor allele)	0.72 (0.64–0.82)	9.60×10^{-6}	0.014	0.877	0.051	0.982	0.001	0.457		0.047	0.980
Anney et al., 2010 [30]	ASD	OR2M4	rs6672981	C (minor allele)	0.55 (0.42–0.72)	9.64×10^{-6}	0.001	0.081	0.916	0.982	0.144	0.994		0.718	1.000
Kuo et al., 2015 [33]	ASD	OR2M4	rs4397683	C (minor allele)	0.55 (0.42–0.72)	9.86×10^{-6}	0.001	0.081	0.916	1.000	0.144	0.994		0.718	1.000
Anney et al., 2010 [30]	ASD	MACROD2	rs980319	G (minor allele)	1.36 (1.20–1.54)	1.00×10^{-5}	0.024	0.939	0.049	0.981	0.001	0.570		0.068	0.987
Kuo et al., 2015 [33]	ASD	BCAS1/CYP24A1	rs12479663	G (minor allele)	1.81 (1.38–2.36)	1.08×10^{-5}	0.001	0.083	0.907	1.000	0.124	0.993		0.687	1.000
Anney et al., 2010 [30]	ASD	MACROD2	rs4814324	A (minor allele)	1.36 (1.20–1.54)	1.10×10^{-5}	0.024	0.939	0.049	0.981	0.001	0.570		0.068	0.987
Kuo et al., 2015 [33]	ASD	KRR1	rs3741496	C (minor allele)	1.49 (1.24–1.78)	1.15×10^{-5}	0.009	0.529	0.565	0.999	0.020	0.954		0.430	0.999
Kuo et al., 2015 [33]	ASD	OR2M4	rs4642918	C (minor allele)	0.56 (0.43–0.73)	1.24×10^{-5}	0.002	0.099	0.917	1.000	0.155	0.995		0.745	1.000
Anney et al., 2010 [30]	ASD	MACROD2	rs6079544	A (minor allele)	1.35 (1.20–1.53)	1.30×10^{-5}	0.033	0.951	0.074	0.988	0.003	0.733		0.124	0.993
Kuo et al., 2015 [33]	ASD	NA	rs13211684	G (minor allele)	1.56 (1.28–1.91)	1.36×10^{-5}	0.006	0.352	0.750	1.000	0.045	0.979		0.572	0.999
Kuo et al., 2015 [33]	ASD	MNT	rs2447095	A (minor allele)	1.52 (1.26–1.84)	1.45×10^{-5}	0.008	0.446	0.695	1.000	0.038	0.975		0.552	0.999
Kuo et al., 2015 [33]	ASD	NA	rs12543592	A (minor allele)	0.67 (0.56–0.81)	1.63×10^{-5}	0.012	0.521	0.744	1.000	0.063	0.985		0.678	1.000
Anney et al., 2010 [30]	ASD	MACROD2	rs6079553	A (minor allele)	1.35 (1.19–1.52)	1.70×10^{-5}	0.026	0.959	0.027	0.965	0.001	0.424		0.041	0.977
Kuo et al., 2015 [33]	ASD	KRR1	rs1051446	C (minor allele)	1.47 (1.23–1.76)	1.77×10^{-5}	0.014	0.587	0.669	1.000	0.045	0.979		0.614	0.999
Anney et al., 2010 [30]	ASD	NA	rs4078417	C (minor allele)	1.38 (1.21–1.57)	1.90×10^{-5}	0.017	0.897	0.055	0.983	0.001	0.524		0.059	0.984
Anney et al., 2010 [30]	ASD	MACROD2	rs10446030	G (minor allele)	1.34 (1.19–1.52)	2.20×10^{-5}	0.043	0.960	0.110	0.992	0.006	0.847		0.210	0.996
Kuo et al., 2015 [33]	ASD	GPD2	rs3916984	T (minor allele)	0.62 (0.49–0.77)	2.25×10^{-5}	0.004	0.256	0.804	1.000	0.056	0.984		0.595	0.999
Kuo et al., 2015 [33]	ASD	NA	rs12366025	T (minor allele)	1.67 (1.31–2.11)	2.49×10^{-5}	0.003	0.184	0.860	1.000	0.086	0.989		0.662	0.999
Ma et al., 2009 [32]	Autism	NA	rs10038113	C (minor)/T(major)	0.67 (0.56–0.81)	2.75×10^{-5}	0.012	0.521	0.744	1.000	0.063	0.985		0.678	1.000
Anney et al., 2010 [30]	ASD	MACROD2	rs6079540	G (minor allele)	0.75 (0.66–0.84)	2.90×10^{-5}	0.034	0.979	0.019	0.950	0.001	0.399		0.037	0.975
Anney et al., 2010 [30]	Autism	HAT1	rs6731562	G (minor allele)	1.51 (1.27–1.81)	3.30×10^{-5}	0.006	0.471	0.562	0.999	0.017	0.946		0.383	0.998
Anney et al., 2010 [30]	ASD	MACROD2	rs6074787	A (minor allele)	1.33 (1.18–1.50)	3.40×10^{-5}	0.047	0.975	0.067	0.986	0.003	0.776		0.147	0.994
Kuo et al., 2015 [33]	ASD	GLIS1	rs12080933	A (minor allele)	1.48 (1.23–1.78)	3.57×10^{-5}	0.013	0.557	0.707	1.000	0.053	0.983		0.648	0.999
Kuo et al., 2015 [33]	ASD	FSTL4	rs11741756	T (minor allele)	1.67 (1.31–2.13)	3.64×10^{-5}	0.004	0.194	0.903	1.000	0.157	0.995		0.785	1.000
Kuo et al., 2015 [33]	ASD	STYK1	rs7953930	T (minor allele)	1.65 (1.30–2.09)	3.83×10^{-5}	0.004	0.215	0.888	1.000	0.133	0.994		0.761	1.000
Anney et al., 2010 [30]	Autism	NA	rs4078417	C (minor allele)	1.50 (1.26–1.79)	4.10×10^{-5}	0.007	0.500	0.509	0.999	0.014	0.933		0.339	0.998
Anney et al., 2010 [30]	ASD	MACROD2	rs4141463	A (minor allele)	0.75 (0.66–0.85)	4.30×10^{-5}	0.049	0.967	0.118	0.993	0.007	0.873		0.243	0.997
Kuo et al., 2015 [33]	ASD	OR2M3	rs11204613	G (minor allele)	0.58 (0.45–0.75)	4.60×10^{-5}	0.003	0.144	0.920	1.000	0.185	0.996		0.799	1.000
Anney et al., 2010 [30]	ASD	MACROD2	rs6079537	G (minor allele)	1.32 (1.17–1.49)	5.40×10^{-5}	0.062	0.981	0.103	0.991	0.007	0.878		0.249	0.997
Anney et al., 2010 [30]	Autism	GSG1L	rs205409	G (minor allele)	0.69 (0.58–0.81)	1.10×10^{-4}	0.011	0.663	0.353	0.998	0.009	0.896		0.271	0.997
Anney et al., 2010 [30]	Autism	POU5F2	rs10258862	G (minor allele)	1.43 (1.21–1.71)	1.80×10^{-4}	0.027	0.700	0.764	1.000	0.112	0.992		0.799	1.000

Abbreviations: ASD, Autism spectrum disorders; A, Adenine; C, Cytosine; G, Guanine; T, Thymine; D, Deletion; I, Insertion; FPRP, false positive rate probability; BFDP, Bayesian false discovery probability; OR, odds ratio; CI, confidence interval; GWAS, Genome-Wide Association Studies; NA, not available.

3.3. Protein-Protein Interaction (PPI) Network

We established PPI networks related to the risk of ASD by filtering genes noteworthy under both FPRP and BFDP or genes with a p-value $< 5 \times 10^{-8}$. We included the results of both re-analyzed and non-re-analyzable genetic comparisons from meta-analyses of observational studies and GWAS, GWAS included in meta-analyses of GWAS, and the GWAS catalog. The statistically significant results of non-re-analyzable studies are presented in the Supplement Table S3.

The major genes that included a strong genetic connection were the myc-associated factor X (MAX) network transcriptional repressor (MNT), oxytocin receptor (OXTR), nucleolar and coiled-body phosphoprotein (NOLC1), peroxisome proliferator-activated receptor gamma related coactivator-related 1 (PPRC1), pyruvate carboxylase (PC), methylenetetrahydrofolate reductase (MTHFR), multiple epidermal growth factor like domains 10 (MEGF10), nuclear factor kappa B subunit 2 (NFKB2), histone deacetylase 4 (HDAC4), etc. (Figure 2 and Table 5).

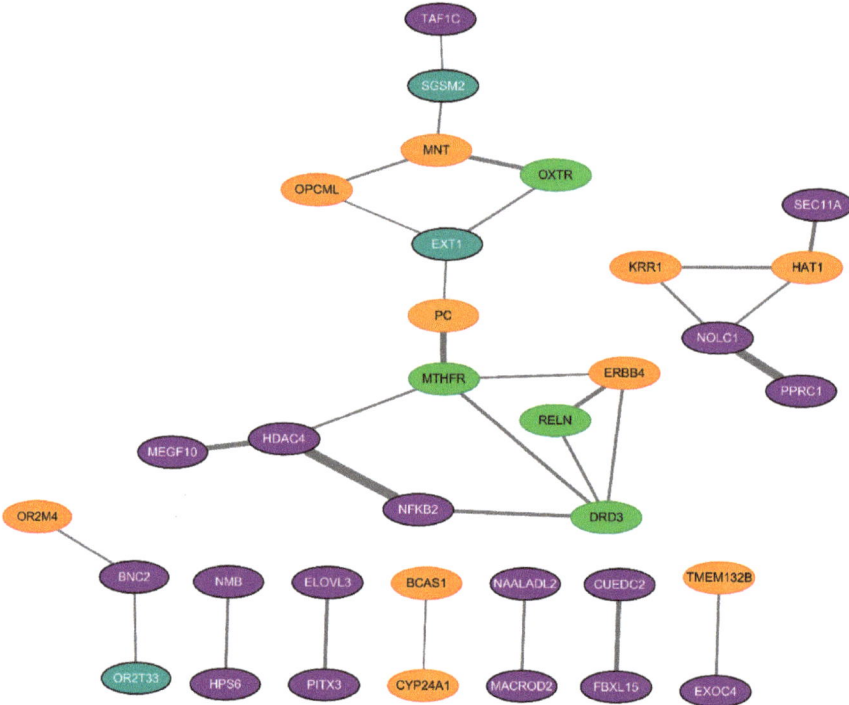

Figure 2. Protein-protein interaction network of ASD. There were 34 distinct genes with about 30 genetic connections among them. The thickness of the line connecting genes represents the score of PPI interaction using STRING9.1 and the color of each gene represents the source of the data; orange, GWAS data: green, GWAS catalog: purple, meta-analysis of GWAS: light green, meta-analysis of observational studies.

Table 5. Lists of genes involved in the PPI network.

Gene	Function of the Encoding Proteins
OXTR	Receptor for oxytocin associated with social recognition and emotion processing
MTHFR	Influences susceptibility to neural tube defect by changing folate metabolism
RELN	Control cell positioning and neural migration during brain development
DRD3	D3 subtype of the five dopamine receptors; localized to the limbic areas of the brain
MNT	Protein member of the Myc/Max/Mad network; transcriptional repressor and an antagonist of Myc-dependent transcriptional activation and cell growth
OPCML	Member of the IgLON subfamily in the immunoglobulin protein superfamily of proteins; localized in the plasma membrane; accessory role in opioid receptor function
PC	Pyruvate carboxylase; gluconeogenesis, lipogenesis, insulin secretion and synthesis of neurotransmitter glutamate
ERBB4	Tyr protein kinase family and the epidermal growth factor receptor subfamily; binds to and is activated by neuregulins, and induces mitogenesis and differentiation
OR2M4	Members of a large family of GPCR; olfactory receptors initiating a neuronal response that triggers the perception of a smell
BCAS1	Oncogene; highly expressed in three amplified breast cancer cell lines and in one breast tumor without amplification at 20q13.2.
CYP24A1	Cytochrome P450 superfamily of enzymes; drug metabolism and synthesis of cholesterol, steroids and other lipids
TMEM132B	The function remains poorly understood despite their mutations associated with non-syndromic hearing loss, panic disorder, and cancer
KRR1	Nucleolar protein; 18S rRNA synthesis and 40S ribosomal assembly
HAT1	Type B histone acetyltransferase; rapid acetylation of newly synthesized cytoplasmic histones; replication-dependent chromatin assembly
SGSM2	GTPase activator; regulators of membrane trafficking
EXT1	Endoplasmic reticulum-resident type II transmembrane glycosyltransferase; involved in the chain elongation step of heparan sulfate biosynthesis
OR2T33	Members of a large family of GPCR; share a 7-transmembrane domain structure with many neurotransmitter and hormone receptors
TAF1C	Binds to the core promoter of ribosomal RNA genes to position the polymerase properly; acts as a channel for regulatory signals
HDAC4	Class II of the histone deacetylase/acuc/apha family; represses transcription when tethered to a promoter
MEGF10	Member of the multiple epidermal growth factor-like domains protein family; cell adhesion, motility and proliferation; critical mediator of apoptotic cell phagocytosis; amyloid-beta peptide uptake in brain
NFKB2	Subunit of the transcription factor complex nuclear factor-kappa-B; central activator of genes involved in inflammation and immune function
BNC2	Conserved zinc finger protein; skin color saturation
NMB	Member of the bombesin-like family of neuropeptides; negatively regulate eating behavior; regulate colonic smooth muscle contraction
HPS6	Organelle biogenesis associated with melanosomes, platelet dense granules, and lysosomes
ELOVL3	GNS1/SUR4 family; elongation of long chain fatty acids to provide precursors for synthesis of sphingolipids and ceramides
PITX3	Member of the RIEG/PITX homeobox family; transcription factors; lens formation during eye development
NAALADL2	Not well-known, but diseases associated with NAALADL2 include Chromosome 6Pter-P24 Deletion Syndrome and Cornelia De Lange Syndrome.
MACROD2	Deacetylase removing ADP-ribose from mono-ADP-ribosylated proteins; translocate from the nucleus to the cytoplasm upon DNA damage

Table 5. Cont.

Gene	Function of the Encoding Proteins
CUEDC2	CUE domain-containing protein; down-regulate ESR1 protein levels through progesterone-induced and degradation of receptors
FBXL15	Substrate recognition component of SCF E3 ubiquitin-protein ligase complex; mediates the ubiquitination and subsequent proteasomal degradation of SMURF1
EXOC4	Component of the exocyst complex; targeting exocytic vesicles to specific docking sites on the plasma membrane
NOLC1	Nucleolar protein; act as a regulator of RNA polymerase I; neural crest specification; nucleologenesis
PPRC1	Similar to PPAR–gamma coactivator 1; activate mitochondrial biogenesis through NRF1 in response to proliferative signals
SEC11A	Member of the peptidase S26B family; subunit of the signal peptidase complex; cell migration and invasion, gastric cancer and lymph node metastasis

Abbreviations: OXTR, Oxytocin Receptor; MTHFR, Methylene tetrahydrofolate reductase; RELN, reelin, DRD3, Dopamine Receptor D3; MNT, Myc-associated factor X (MAX) Network Transcriptional Repressor; OPCML, opioid binding protein/cell adhesion molecule-like; PC, Pyruvate carboxylase; ERBB4, Erb-B2 Receptor Tyrosine Kinase 4; OR2M4, olfactory receptor family 2 subfamily M member 4; GPCR, G protein-coupled receptor; BCAS1, Breast Carcinoma Amplified Sequence 1; CYP24A1, Cytochrome P450 Family 24 Subfamily A Member 1; TMEM132B, transmembrane protein 132B; KRR1, KRR1 small subunit processome component homolog; HAT1, histone acetyltransferase 1; SGSM2, small G protein signaling modulator 2; EXT1, Exostosin-1; OR2T33, Olfactory receptor 2T33; TAF1C, TATA-Box Binding Protein Associated Factor, RNA Polymerase I Subunit C; HDAC4, Histone deacetylase 4; MEGF10, Multiple Epidermal Growth Factor Like Domains 10; NFKB2, Nuclear Factor Kappa B Subunit 2; BNC2, basonuclin 2; NMB, Neuromedin B; HPS6, Hermansky–Pudlak syndrome 6; ELOVL3, Elongation Of Very Long Chain Fatty Acids Protein 3, PITX3, Pituitary homeobox 3; NAALADL2, N-Acetylated Alpha-Linked Acidic Dipeptidase Like 2; MACROD2, Mono-ADP Ribosylhydrolase 2; CUEDC2, CUE domain containing 2; FBXL15, F-Box And Leucine Rich Repeat Protein 15; EXOC4, Exocyst Complex Component 4; NOLC1, Nucleolar And Coiled-Body Phosphoprotein 1; PPRC1, peroxisome proliferator-activated receptor gamma, coactivator-related 1; SEC11A, SEC11 Homolog A, Signal Peptidase Complex Subunit.

4. Discussion

To our knowledge, this study is the first study of ASD genetic risk factors, which assessed the levels of evidence of the published meta-analyses showing the association between susceptible loci and ASD. Overall, genetic comparisons with noteworthy results were confirmed as risk factors for ASD. The genetic comparisons highly related to an increased risk of ASD might reflect the implication in neurodevelopment and specific synaptogenesis of ASD.

According to the PPI network, composed of noteworthy results obtained when using both Bayesian approaches, multiple genes were included as a risk factor for ASD. Investigating the lists genes as a risk factor, promising candidates encoded the protein associated with neural development and specification, and also with neurotransmitters and its receptors. These genes were RELN and DRD3 from observational studies, and PC, OPCML, ERBB4, OR2M4, MEGF10, OR2T33, NMB, and NOLC1, from GWAS. In line with our findings, previous reports have supported that the migration and proliferation of neuronal cells is essential to understanding neurodevelopmental disorders such as ASD or schizophrenia [49,50]. In addition, apart from anatomical approaches, genes correlated with neuropeptides and receptors, such as those in the brain or hippocampus, also explain the pathophysiology of the disease at a molecular level [51]. The list of genes included is presented in Table 5.

The present comprehensive re-analyses shows that, although a large number of studies have suggested numerous possible genetic risk factors for ASD, truly significant results are small and a partial part of whole results. For instance, we detected false positive results in 26 out of 31 (83.9%) meta-analyses of observational studies and 163 out of 203 (80.3%) in meta-analyses of GWAS, respectively. However, only a small portion of genetic comparisons with a p-value < 0.05 exhibited noteworthy associations with ASD under both Bayesian approaches (Tables 1–4).

Moreover, we also detected that genetic comparisons with borderline statistical significance ($5 \times 10^{-8} < p$-value < 0.05) accounted for 53 out of 126 (42%) noteworthy comparisons from GWAS or meta-analyses of GWAS. These genetic comparisons might have been neglected if the p-value alone was considered to determine noteworthiness. Using the two Bayesian approaches as we did, or relaxing the current GWAS threshold as Panagiotou et al. suggests, might enable better interpretation of GWAS results [48].

Based on the observational studies, out of 31 statistically significant genotype comparisons, five (16.1%) were found noteworthy under both FPRP and BFDP: T vs. C, MTHFR C677T; T (minor), MTHFR C677T; G vs. A, DRD3/rs167771; C vs. G, RELN/rs362691; A (minor), OXTR/rs7632287. From the meta-analyses of GWAS, we could confirm that 34 distinct genes are noteworthy under both Bayesian approaches with about 30 genetic connections. However, the fact that all three comparisons with a p-value $< 5 \times 10^{-8}$—rs1879532 (Table S3), rs4773054 (Table 2), rs4141463 (Table 2)—displayed noteworthiness may indicate that the stringent threshold of $p < 5 \times 10^{-8}$ is a good tool for verification of the true noteworthiness of genetic risk factors.

There are several limitations in our review. First, we did not include studies that have not been meta-analyzed, or meta-analyses that had insufficient data in our review. Secondly, we only included the single findings of a meta-analysis with the lowest p-value per genetic variant. Therefore, we could not consider potentially meaningful subgroup analyses for different ethnicity, location, gender, and type of genotype comparison (i.e., random or fixed) when selecting a certain outcome. We focused on whether the individual genotype variant was truly associated with ASD or not, regardless of the specific type of the genotype comparison or ethnicity.

Our study has several strengths and implications. For example, to our knowledge, this is the first study that simultaneously analyzed a sizeable amount of data about genetic factors including not only GWAS but also the GWAS catalog. Despite the known high heritability of ASD and abundant research in ASD that has focused on the underlying genetic causes, the literature on genetic risk factors for ASD has not fully reached a consensus. This comprehensive review of genetic associations linked to ASD may improve understanding of the strengths and limitations of each form of research, and advance better and novel approaches for examining ASD in the field of genetic research. The findings of this study could provide mechanisms that may be explored for the development of novel neurotherapeutic agents both for the prevention and treatment of ASD.

5. Conclusions

In conclusion, we synthesized published meta-analyses on risk factors of ASD to acquire noteworthy findings and false positive results by adopting two Bayesian approaches for genetic factors. We attempted to synthesize all meta-analyses on genetic polymorphisms linked to ASD and found noteworthy genetic factors highly related to an increased risk of ASD. We also investigated their validity by discovering false positive results under Bayesian methods. To verify results obtained from genetic analyses, both approaches may have advantages, especially for interpretation of results obtained from observational studies. We found noteworthy results from GWAS, not only with p-value ranging between 0.05 and 5×10^{-8}, but also from genetic variants within borderline significance rage which were almost half of the genetic variants. This finding speculates that the genetic variants with borderline significance needs to be further analyzed to determine what associations are genuine.

Supplementary Materials: The following are available online at http://www.mdpi.com/2076-3425/10/10/692/s1, Supplementary Table S1. PRISMA 2009 Checklist; Supplementary Table S2. Gene variants without statistical significance (p-value $\geq$ 0.05) in meta-analyses of observational studies; Supplementary Table S3. Non-re-analyzable gene variants with genome wide statistical significance (p-value $< 5 \times 10^{-8}$) from the GWAS catalog, meta-analyses of GWAS and the GWAS datasets included in the GWAS meta-analysis.

Author Contributions: J.L., M.J.S., J.I.S. and P.F.-P. designed the study. J.L., M.J.S., C.Y.S., G.H.J., K.H.L., K.S.L. and J.I.S. collected the data and M.J.S., G.H.J., K.H.L. and Y.K. did the analysis. J.L., M.J.S., C.Y.S., G.H.J., K.H.L., K.S.L., Y.K., J.Y.K., J.Y.L., J.R., M.E., F.G., A.K. (Ai Koyanagi), B.S., M.S., T.B.R., A.K. (Andreas Kronbichler), E.D., D.F.P.V., F.R.P.d.S., K.T., A.R.B., A.F.C., S.C., S.T., A.S., L.S., T.T., J.I.S., and P.F.-P. wrote the first draft of the manuscript and gave critical comments on manuscript draft. All authors have read and agreed to the published version of the manuscript.

Funding: This research received no external funding.

Conflicts of Interest: The authors declare no conflict of interest.

References

1. Lyall, K.; Croen, L.; Daniels, J.; Fallin, M.D.; Ladd-Acosta, C.; Lee, B.K.; Park, B.Y.; Snyder, N.W.; Schendel, D.; Volk, H.; et al. The changing epidemiology of autism spectrum disorders. *Annu. Rev. Public Health* **2017**, *38*, 81–102. [CrossRef] [PubMed]
2. American Psychiatric Association. *Diagnostic and Statistical Manual of Mental Disorders (dsm-5®)*, 5th ed.; American Psychiatric Pub.: Arlington, VA, USA, 2013.
3. Xu, G.; Strathearn, L.; Liu, B.; Bao, W. Prevalence of autism spectrum disorder among us children and adolescents, 2014–2016. *JAMA* **2018**, *319*, 81–82. [CrossRef] [PubMed]
4. Zablotsky, B.; Black, L.I.; Maenner, M.J.; Schieve, L.A.; Blumberg, S.J. Estimated prevalence of autism and other developmental disabilities following questionnaire changes in the 2014 national health interview survey. *Natl. Health Stat. Rep.* **2015**, *87*, 1–20.
5. Christensen, D.L.; Baio, J.; Van Naarden Braun, K.; Bilder, D.; Charles, J.; Constantino, J.N.; Daniels, J.; Durkin, M.S.; Fitzgerald, R.T.; Kurzius-Spencer, M.; et al. Prevalence and characteristics of autism spectrum disorder among children aged 8 years—Autism and developmental disabilities monitoring network, 11 sites, united states, 2012. *MMWR Surveill. Summ.* **2016**, *65*, 1–23. [CrossRef]
6. Kim, J.Y.; Son, M.J.; Son, C.Y.; Radua, J.; Eisenhut, M.; Gressier, F.; Koyanagi, A.; Carvalho, A.F.; Stubbs, B.; Solmi, M.; et al. Environmental risk factors and biomarkers for autism spectrum disorder: An umbrella review of the evidence. *Lancet Psychiatry* **2019**, *6*, 590–600. [CrossRef]
7. Ronald, A.; Hoekstra, R.A. Autism spectrum disorders and autistic traits: A decade of new twin studies. *Am. J. Med. Genet. B Neuropsychiatr. Genet.* **2011**, *156B*, 255–274. [CrossRef]
8. Bai, D.; Yip, B.H.K.; Windham, G.C.; Sourander, A.; Francis, R.; Yoffe, R.; Glasson, E.; Mahjani, B.; Suominen, A.; Leonard, H.; et al. Association of genetic and environmental factors with autism in a 5-country cohort. *JAMA Psychiatry* **2019**. [CrossRef]

9. MacGregor, A.J.; Snieder, H.; Schork, N.J.; Spector, T.D. Twins: Novel uses to study complex traits and genetic diseases. *Trends Genet* **2000**, *16*, 131–134. [CrossRef]
10. Modabbernia, A.; Velthorst, E.; Reichenberg, A. Environmental risk factors for autism: An evidence-based review of systematic reviews and meta-analyses. *Mol. Autism.* **2017**, *8*, 13. [CrossRef]
11. Robinson, E.B.; St Pourcain, B.; Anttila, V.; Kosmicki, J.A.; Bulik-Sullivan, B.; Grove, J.; Maller, J.; Samocha, K.E.; Sanders, S.J.; Ripke, S.; et al. Genetic risk for autism spectrum disorders and neuropsychiatric variation in the general population. *Nat. Genet.* **2016**, *48*, 552–555. [CrossRef]
12. State, M.W.; Levitt, P. The conundrums of understanding genetic risks for autism spectrum disorders. *Nat. Neurosci.* **2011**, *14*, 1499–1506. [CrossRef] [PubMed]
13. MacArthur, J.; Bowler, E.; Cerezo, M.; Gil, L.; Hall, P.; Hastings, E.; Junkins, H.; McMahon, A.; Milano, A.; Morales, J. The new nhgri-ebi catalog of published genome-wide association studies (gwas catalog). *Nucleic Acids Res.* **2016**, *45*, D896–D901. [CrossRef] [PubMed]
14. Wakefield, J. A bayesian measure of the probability of false discovery in genetic epidemiology studies. *Am. J. Hum. Genet.* **2007**, *81*, 208–227. [CrossRef] [PubMed]
15. Wacholder, S.; Chanock, S.; Garcia-Closas, M.; El Ghormli, L.; Rothman, N. Assessing the probability that a positive report is false: An approach for molecular epidemiology studies. *J. Natl. Cancer Inst.* **2004**, *96*, 434–442. [CrossRef] [PubMed]
16. Szklarczyk, D.; Franceschini, A.; Wyder, S.; Forslund, K.; Heller, D.; Huerta-Cepas, J.; Simonovic, M.; Roth, A.; Santos, A.; Tsafou, K.P.; et al. String v10: Protein-protein interaction networks, integrated over the tree of life. *Nucleic Acids Res.* **2015**, *43*, D447–D452. [CrossRef]
17. Wang, K.; Zhang, H.; Ma, D.; Bucan, M.; Glessner, J.T.; Abrahams, B.S.; Salyakina, D.; Imielinski, M.; Bradfield, J.P.; Sleiman, P.M.; et al. Common genetic variants on 5p14.1 associate with autism spectrum disorders. *Nature* **2009**, *459*, 528–533. [CrossRef]
18. Xia, K.; Guo, H.; Hu, Z.; Xun, G.; Zuo, L.; Peng, Y.; Wang, K.; He, Y.; Xiong, Z.; Sun, L.; et al. Common genetic variants on 1p13.2 associate with risk of autism. *Mol. Psychiatry* **2014**, *19*, 1212–1219. [CrossRef]
19. Grove, J.; Ripke, S.; Als, T.D.; Mattheisen, M.; Walters, R.K.; Won, H.; Pallesen, J.; Agerbo, E.; Andreassen, O.A.; Anney, R.; et al. Identification of common genetic risk variants for autism spectrum disorder. *Nat. Genet.* **2019**, *51*, 431–444. [CrossRef]
20. Liu, J.; Yang, A.; Zhang, Q.; Yang, G.; Yang, W.; Lei, H.; Quan, J.; Qu, F.; Wang, M.; Zhang, Z. Association between genetic variants in slc25a12 and risk of autism spectrum disorders: An integrated meta-analysis. *Am. J. Med Genet. Part B Neuropsychiatr. Genet.* **2015**, *168*, 236–246. [CrossRef]
21. Rai, V. Association of methylenetetrahydrofolate reductase (mthfr) gene c677t polymorphism with autism: Evidence of genetic susceptibility. *Metab. Brain Dis.* **2016**, *31*, 727–735. [CrossRef]
22. Pu, D.; Shen, Y.; Wu, J. Association between mthfr gene polymorphisms and the risk of autism spectrum disorders: A meta-analysis. *Autism Res.* **2013**, *6*, 384–392. [CrossRef] [PubMed]
23. Shaik Mohammad, N.; Sai Shruti, P.; Bharathi, V.; Krishna Prasad, C.; Hussain, T.; Alrokayan, S.A.; Naik, U.; Radha Rama Devi, A. Clinical utility of folate pathway genetic polymorphisms in the diagnosis of autism spectrum disorders. *Psychiatr. Genet.* **2016**, *26*, 281–286. [CrossRef] [PubMed]
24. Warrier, V.; Chee, V.; Smith, P.; Chakrabarti, B.; Baron-Cohen, S. A comprehensive meta-analysis of common genetic variants in autism spectrum conditions. *Mol. Autism* **2015**, *6*, 49. [CrossRef] [PubMed]
25. Aoki, Y.; Cortese, S. Mitochondrial aspartate/glutamate carrier slc25a12 and autism spectrum disorder: A meta-analysis. *Mol. Neurobiol.* **2016**, *53*, 1579–1588. [CrossRef]
26. LoParo, D.; Waldman, I.D. The oxytocin receptor gene (oxtr) is associated with autism spectrum disorder: A meta-analysis. *Mol. Psychiatr.* **2015**, *20*, 640–646. [CrossRef]
27. Wang, Z.; Hong, Y.; Zou, L.; Zhong, R.; Zhu, B.; Shen, N.; Chen, W.; Lou, J.; Ke, J.; Zhang, T.; et al. Reelin gene variants and risk of autism spectrum disorders: An integrated meta-analysis. *Am. J. Med. Genet. B Neuropsychiatr. Genet.* **2014**, *165B*, 192–200. [CrossRef]
28. Torrico, B.; Fernandez-Castillo, N.; Hervas, A.; Mila, M.; Salgado, M.; Rueda, I.; Buitelaar, J.K.; Rommelse, N.; Oerlemans, A.M.; Bralten, J.; et al. Contribution of common and rare variants of the ptchd1 gene to autism spectrum disorders and intellectual disability. *Eur. J. Hum. Genet.* **2015**, *23*, 1694–1701. [CrossRef]
29. Kranz, T.M.; Kopp, M.; Waltes, R.; Sachse, M.; Duketis, E.; Jarczok, T.A.; Degenhardt, F.; Gorgen, K.; Meyer, J.; Freitag, C.M.; et al. Meta-analysis and association of two common polymorphisms of the human oxytocin receptor gene in autism spectrum disorder. *Autism Res.* **2016**, *9*, 1036–1045. [CrossRef]

30. Anney, R.; Klei, L.; Pinto, D.; Regan, R.; Conroy, J.; Magalhaes, T.R.; Correia, C.; Abrahams, B.S.; Sykes, N.; Pagnamenta, A.T.; et al. A genome-wide scan for common alleles affecting risk for autism. *Hum. Mol. Genet.* **2010**, *19*, 4072–4082. [CrossRef]

31. The Autism Spectrum Disorders Working Group of The Psychiatric Genomics Consortium. Meta-analysis of gwas of over 16,000 individuals with autism spectrum disorder highlights a novel locus at 10q24.32 and a significant overlap with schizophrenia. *Mol. Autism* **2017**, *8*, 21. [CrossRef]

32. Ma, D.; Salyakina, D.; Jaworski, J.M.; Konidari, I.; Whitehead, P.L.; Andersen, A.N.; Hoffman, J.D.; Slifer, S.H.; Hedges, D.J.; Cukier, H.N.; et al. A genome-wide association study of autism reveals a common novel risk locus at 5p14.1. *Ann. Hum. Genet.* **2009**, *73*, 263–273. [CrossRef] [PubMed]

33. Kuo, P.H.; Chuang, L.C.; Su, M.H.; Chen, C.H.; Chen, C.H.; Wu, J.Y.; Yen, C.J.; Wu, Y.Y.; Liu, S.K.; Chou, M.C.; et al. Genome-wide association study for autism spectrum disorder in taiwanese han population. *PLoS ONE* **2015**, *10*, e0138695. [CrossRef] [PubMed]

34. Anney, R.; Klei, L.; Pinto, D.; Almeida, J.; Bacchelli, E.; Baird, G.; Bolshakova, N.; Bolte, S.; Bolton, P.F.; Bourgeron, T.; et al. Individual common variants exert weak effects on the risk for autism spectrum disorders. *Hum. Mol. Genet.* **2012**, *21*, 4781–4792. [CrossRef] [PubMed]

35. Chaste, P.; Klei, L.; Sanders, S.J.; Hus, V.; Murtha, M.T.; Lowe, J.K.; Willsey, A.J.; Moreno-De-Luca, D.; Timothy, W.Y.; Fombonne, E. A genome-wide association study of autism using the simons simplex collection: Does reducing phenotypic heterogeneity in autism increase genetic homogeneity? *Biol. Psychiatry* **2015**, *77*, 775–784. [CrossRef]

36. Main, P.A.; Angley, M.T.; O'Doherty, C.E.; Thomas, P.; Fenech, M. The potential role of the antioxidant and detoxification properties of glutathione in autism spectrum disorders: A systematic review and meta-analysis. *Nutr. Metab.* **2012**, *9*, 35. [CrossRef]

37. Huang, C.H.; Santangelo, S.L. Autism and serotonin transporter gene polymorphisms: A systematic review and meta-analysis. *Am. J. Med. Genet. B Neuropsychiatr. Genet.* **2008**, *147B*, 903–913. [CrossRef]

38. Curran, S.; Bolton, P.; Rozsnyai, K.; Chiocchetti, A.; Klauck, S.M.; Duketis, E.; Poustka, F.; Schlitt, S.; Freitag, C.M.; Lee, I.; et al. No association between a common single nucleotide polymorphism, rs4141463, in the macrod2 gene and autism spectrum disorder. *Am. J. Med Genet. Part B: Neuropsychiatr. Genet.* **2011**, *156*, 633–639. [CrossRef]

39. Yang, P.Y.; Menga, Y.J.; Li, T.; Huang, Y. Associations of endocrine stress-related gene polymorphisms with risk of autism spectrum disorders: Evidence from an integrated meta-analysis. *Autism Res.* **2017**, *10*, 1722–1736. [CrossRef]

40. Song, R.R.; Zou, L.; Zhong, R.; Zheng, X.W.; Zhu, B.B.; Chen, W.; Liu, L.; Miao, X.P. An integrated meta-analysis of two variants in hoxa1/hoxb1 and their effect on the risk of autism spectrum disorders. *PLoS ONE* **2011**, *6*, e25603. [CrossRef]

41. Chen, N.; Bao, Y.; Xue, Y.; Sun, Y.; Hu, D.; Meng, S.; Lu, L.; Shi, J. Meta-analyses of reln variants in neuropsychiatric disorders. *Behav. Brain Res.* **2017**, *332*, 110–119. [CrossRef]

42. Werling, A.M.; Bobrowski, E.; Taurines, R.; Gundelfinger, R.; Romanos, M.; Grunblatt, E.; Walitza, S. Cntnap2 gene in high functioning autism: No association according to family and meta-analysis approaches. *J. Neural. Transm.* **2016**, *123*, 353–363. [CrossRef] [PubMed]

43. Zhang, T.; Zhang, J.; Wang, Z.; Jia, M.; Lu, T.; Wang, H.; Yue, W.; Zhang, D.; Li, J.; Wang, L. Association between cntnap2 polymorphisms and autism: A family-based study in the chinese han population and a meta-analysis combined with gwas data of psychiatric genomics consortium. *Autism Res.* **2019**, *12*, 553–561. [CrossRef] [PubMed]

44. Noroozi, R.; Taheri, M.; Ghafouri-Fard, S.; Bidel, Z.; Omrani, M.D.; Moghaddam, A.S.; Sarabi, P.; Jarahi, A.M. Meta-analysis of gabrb3 gene polymorphisms and susceptibility to autism spectrum disorder. *J. Mol. Neurosci.* **2018**, *65*, 432–437. [CrossRef] [PubMed]

45. Mahdavi, M.; Kheirollahi, M.; Riahi, R.; Khorvash, F.; Khorrami, M.; Mirsafaie, M. Meta-analysis of the association between gaba receptor polymorphisms and autism spectrum disorder (ASD). *J. Mol. Neurosci.* **2018**, *65*, 1–9. [CrossRef] [PubMed]

46. Waltes, R.; Duketis, E.; Knapp, M.; Anney, R.J.; Huguet, G.; Schlitt, S.; Jarczok, T.A.; Sachse, M.; Kampfer, L.M.; Kleinbock, T.; et al. Common variants in genes of the postsynaptic fmrp signalling pathway are risk factors for autism spectrum disorders. *Hum. Genet.* **2014**, *133*, 781–792. [CrossRef] [PubMed]

47. Torrico, B.; Chiocchetti, A.G.; Bacchelli, E.; Trabetti, E.; Hervas, A.; Franke, B.; Buitelaar, J.K.; Rommelse, N.; Yousaf, A.; Duketis, E.; et al. Lack of replication of previous autism spectrum disorder gwas hits in european populations. *Autism Res.* **2017**, *10*, 202–211. [CrossRef] [PubMed]
48. Panagiotou, O.A.; Ioannidis, J.P.A.; Genome-Wide Significance Project. What should the genome-wide significance threshold be? Empirical replication of borderline genetic associations. *Int. J. Epidemiol.* **2011**, *41*, 273–286. [CrossRef]
49. Skaar, D.A.; Shao, Y.; Haines, J.L.; Stenger, J.E.; Jaworski, J.; Martin, E.R.; DeLong, G.R.; Moore, J.H.; McCauley, J.L.; Sutcliffe, J.S.; et al. Analysis of the reln gene as a genetic risk factor for autism. *Mol. Psychiatry* **2005**, *10*, 563–571. [CrossRef]
50. Glessner, J.T.; Wang, K.; Cai, G.; Korvatska, O.; Kim, C.E.; Wood, S.; Zhang, H.; Estes, A.; Brune, C.W.; Bradfield, J.P.; et al. Autism genome-wide copy number variation reveals ubiquitin and neuronal genes. *Nature* **2009**, *459*, 569–573. [CrossRef]
51. Purcell, A.E.; Jeon, O.H.; Zimmerman, A.W.; Blue, M.E.; Pevsner, J. Postmortem brain abnormalities of the glutamate neurotransmitter system in autism. *Neurology* **2001**, *57*, 1618–1628. [CrossRef]

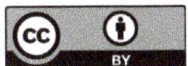

© 2020 by the authors. Licensee MDPI, Basel, Switzerland. This article is an open access article distributed under the terms and conditions of the Creative Commons Attribution (CC BY) license (http://creativecommons.org/licenses/by/4.0/).

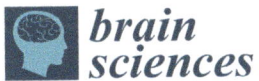 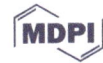

Article

Physiological Profile Assessment of Posture in Children and Adolescents with Autism Spectrum Disorder and Typically Developing Peers

Cecilia Perin [1],*, Giulio Valagussa [1,2], Miryam Mazzucchelli [1], Valentina Gariboldi [1,3], Cesare Giuseppe Cerri [1], Roberto Meroni [4], Enzo Grossi [2], Cesare Maria Cornaggia [1], Jasmine Menant [5] and Daniele Piscitelli [1,6,7]

1. School of Medicine and Surgery, University of Milano Bicocca, 20126 Milan, Italy; giulio.valagussa@gmail.com (G.V.); miryam.mazzucchelli@gmail.com (M.M.); valentina.gariboldi@gmail.com (V.G.); cesare.cerri@unimib.it (C.G.C.); cesaremaria.cornaggia@unimib.it (C.M.C.); daniele.piscitelli@mcgill.ca (D.P.)
2. Autism Research Unit, "Villa Santa Maria" Foundation, 22038 Como, Italy; Enzo.Grossi@bracco.com
3. ASST Rhodense, Ospedale "G. Salvini", 20024 Milan, Italy
4. Department of Physiotherapy, LUNEX International University of Health, Exercise and Sports, Differdange, 4671 Luxembourg, Luxembourg; roberto.meroni@lunex-university.net
5. Neuroscience Research Australia and School of Public Health and Community Medicine, University of New South Wales, Sydney, NSW 2052, Australia; j.menant@neura.edu.au
6. School of Physical and Occupational Therapy, McGill University, Montreal, QC H3G 1Y5, Canada
7. School of Physical Therapy and Athletic Training, Pacific University, Hillsboro, OR 97123, USA
* Correspondence: cecilia.perin@unimib.it; Tel.: +39-0362-986-446; Fax: +39-0362-986-439

Received: 15 September 2020; Accepted: 25 September 2020; Published: 27 September 2020

Abstract: A sound postural system requires sensorimotor integration. Evidence suggests that individuals with Autism Spectrum Disorder (ASD) present sensorimotor integration impairments. The Physiological Profile Assessment (PPA) can be used to evaluate postural capacity assessing five physiological subsets (i.e., vision, reaction time, peripheral sensation, lower limb strength, balance); however, no studies applied the PPA in young individuals. Therefore, this study aimed to investigate the PPA in children and adolescents with ASD compared with age-matched typically developing (TD) individuals and examine the relationship between the PPA subset within the ASD and TD participants according to different age groups. Percentiles from the PPA were obtained from the TD children and adolescents ($n = 135$) for each test. Performances of the individuals with ASD ($n = 18$) were examined relative to the TD percentiles. ASD participants' scores were above the 90th percentile (i.e., poor performance) in most sensory, motor and balance parameters. Performance in most of the PPA tests significantly improved with older age in the TD group but not in the ASD group. The study findings support the use of the PPA in TD children and adolescents while further research should investigate postural capacity in a larger ASD sample to enhance the understanding of sensorimotor systems contributing to compromised postural control.

Keywords: autism spectrum disorder; neurodevelopmental disorders; assessment; sensorimotor integration; postural balance

1. Introduction

Autism spectrum disorder (ASD) is a neurodevelopmental disorder affecting ~1 in 59 with four males diagnosed for each female in North America [1] and 1 in 87 children aged 7–9 years in Italy [2]. According to the Diagnostic and Statistical Manual of Mental Disorders fifth edition (DSM-5) [3], individuals with ASD are diagnosed based on some core features that manifest during the early developmental years. Deficits in social communication and social interaction are associated with repetitive patterns of behavior, interests or activities that cause significant impairment in social, occupational or other areas of functioning. In addition to these characteristic features, several motor dysfunctions have been described in ASD children and teenagers including disruptions in motor milestone development [4,5], clumsiness, impaired motor coordination, disturbance in reach-to-grasp movements [6–8], deficits in gross and fine motor skills [9] and abnormal gait patterns [10,11] Postural control impairments have also been reported in ASD individuals [12–17].

Postural control is a fundamental skill in daily human life for the ability to plan the coordination of movement and in maintaining dynamic and static balance for social interactions [18]. Postural control relies on the sensorimotor integration of various sources such as vestibular, visual and somatosensory pathways and actual states [19]. Interestingly, children and adolescents with ASD appear to have sensory processing that differentiate them from typically developing (TD) peers [20–22]. Individuals with ASD exhibited deficits in functional balance and motor performance [14].

To date, studies of postural control in children with ASD have used standardized clinical tests to assess gross motor proficiency in children such as the Movement Assessment Battery for Children-2 (MABC-2) [23] and the Test of Gross Motor Development [24], the Zurich Neuromotor Assessment [25] and the Physical Neurological Examination of Subtle Signs (PANESS) [26] or force platform instrumental approaches [13,27–29]. However, these tests have not integrated the multiple features of sensorimotor parameters involved in postural control for the maintenance of balance.

Lord et al. [30] developed the Physiological Profile Assessment (PPA) for a comprehensive assessment of sensorimotor functions related to postural capacity. The PPA assesses five physiological systems, i.e., vestibular function, peripheral sensation, muscle force, vision and reaction time, which are involved in the maintenance of stable and dynamic balance.

The PPA has been used on healthy individuals [31], subjects with neurological disorders to assess postural impairments [32–34] and the elderly with musculoskeletal disorders [35]. This instrument, based on interval scales [36], has been demonstrated to have psychometrically sound proprieties with a lower administrative burden compared with biomechanical assessments using motion capture and force platforms [30,33].

Although the PPA was successfully administered in the adult population, no studies investigated its applicability in younger individuals. Therefore, the first aim of this cross-sectional study was to examine the sensory and motor functions involved in postural control in TD children and adolescents and in age-matched individuals with ASD using the PPA. The second aim was to investigate the relationship between each PPA subset within ASD and TD participants for each age group. The preliminary results were presented in abstract form [37].

2. Materials and Methods

2.1. Participants

TD individuals were recruited from three public schools in the suburbs of a metropolitan city in northern Italy. Children and adolescents with ASD were recruited from a Neuropsychiatric Institute where ASD patients were followed. Inclusion criteria were as follows: age between 6 and 18 years and an ASD diagnosis according to the DSM-5 criteria [3] confirmed through an Autism Diagnostic Observation Schedule (ADOS-2) [38]. Exclusion criteria were neurological or orthopedic co-morbidities that might influence the test performances, lack of compliance with the PPA, interruption of the assessments and/or showing signs of irritation. Control participants (TD) were typically developing children and adolescents aged between 6 and 18 years. Exclusion criteria were neurological, cognitive or orthopedic impairments that might influence performance in the sensorimotor and balance tests (e.g., the ability to sit, stand and ambulate independently).

The study was conducted following the declaration of Helsinki and was approved by the local Ethics Committee (Protocol Number: 3532017). All parents provided written, informed consent to allow their child's participation in the study.

2.2. Physiological Profile Assessment

All ASD and TD children and adolescents were assessed using the PPA [30]. The PPA is a multi-item instrument that evaluates physiological domains contributing to postural control. The PPA includes tests of vision, peripheral sensation, lower limb muscle strength, simple reaction time and balance, which are detailed below. The assessment for ASD children was performed by two residents in physical medicine and a rehabilitation clinician. TD children were assessed by six trained residents in physical medicine and a rehabilitation clinician. All assessors were trained to administer the PPA. The clinicians were not blind when performing the PPA with ASD and TD participants. The researchers involved in the data analysis were blind.

2.2.1. Vision

Visual acuity was measured using a letter chart with high- and low-contrast (10%) letters. Acuity was assessed binocularly with participants wearing their distance glasses (if applicable) at a test distance of 3 m and measured in terms of the logarithm of the minimum angle resolvable in minutes of arc (logMAR). Edge contrast sensitivity was assessed using the Melbourne Edge Test, which presents 20 circular patches containing edges with reducing contrast. The lowest contrast patch correctly identified was recorded as the participant's contrast sensitivity in decibel units where one dB = 10 log10 contrast. Depth perception was measured using a Howard-Dohlman depth perception apparatus. This device presents two vertical rods; one is fixed and the other one can move forward and back along a track using two strings. Participants are required to pull on the strings to adjust the position of the movable rod to align it to the fixed one. Participants are seated three meters away from the apparatus. The error in aligning the rods is recorded in centimeters. The average of four trials was computed.

2.2.2. Peripheral Sensation

Tactile sensitivity on the dominant ankle was measured with a Semmes-Weinstein-type pressure aesthesiometer. The filaments were applied to the center of the lateral malleolus of the ankle. Participants were instructed that the filament would be placed on their ankle when the examiner said "A" or "B." If they felt the filament in contact with their skin, they had to report to the examiner whether they felt it on "A" or "B." The finest filament correctly detected was identified. Pressure (in grams) exerted by this filament was converted to log10 0.1 mg, yielding a scale of approximately equal intensity intervals between filaments. Proprioception was measured using a lower limb matching test that recorded the difference (in degrees) in matching the great toes on either side of a vertical transparent acrylic sheet inscribed with a protractor and placed between the legs. Participants were required to perform the test with their eyes closed. The mean error of five trials was computed.

2.2.3. Reaction Time

Simple reaction time was assessed in milliseconds using a hand-held electronic timer and a light as the stimulus and depression of a switch by the finger and the foot as the responses. A modified computer mouse was used as the response box for the finger press task and a pedal switch was used for the foot press task. Five practice trials were undertaken followed by 10 experimental trials. The mean of these 10 trials was computed.

2.2.4. Lower Limb Muscle Strength

Isometric knee extensor and flexor muscle strength were assessed on the dominant leg using a spring gauge. The force of the knee extensor and flexor muscles was measured with the participant sitting in a tall chair with a strap around the leg 10 cm above the ankle joint and the hip and knee joint angles positioned at approximately 90 degrees. In three trials per muscle group, the subject attempted to push/pull against the strap assembly with maximal force for 2 to 3 s; the greatest force for each muscle group was recorded in kilograms. Ankle isometric dorsiflexion strength was assessed using a footplate attached to a spring gauge. Participants were seated in a standard chair and their dominant foot was secured to the footplate with the angle of the knee at approximately 110 degrees. The greatest maximal dorsiflexion force (in kilograms) measured out of three trials was recorded.

2.2.5. Balance

Participants performed the balance tests barefoot using a swaymeter that measured displacements of the body at the level of the waist. The device consisted of a 40 cm-long rod with a vertically mounted pen at its end. The rod was attached to the subject by a firm belt and extended posteriorly for the tests of postural sway and anteriorly for the tests of maximal balance range and coordinated stability. Postural sway was assessed with eyes open and closed; first on a firm surface then on a medium density foam rubber mat (15 cm thick). In each of the four conditions, the pen on the extremity of the swaymeter recorded the subject's sway on a sheet of millimeter graph paper fastened to the top of an adjustable-height table as the subject attempted to stand as still as possible for 30 s. For each trial, anteroposterior and mediolateral sway were recorded in mm and the sway area (anteroposterior x mediolateral distances) was calculated in mm^2. Limits of stability and control of the center of mass (COM) movements were assessed using the maximal balance range and coordinated stability tests. The maximum balance range test measured the limits of stability in the anteroposterior plane as the participants were instructed to lean as far forward and as far back as possible without moving the feet or bending at the hips. The test was repeated three times with the highest anteroposterior range taken as the test result. The score was obtained by multiplying the distance in mm by a factor that considered the average height per age [39] and the age of the subject. The coordinated stability test required each participant to adjust their balance by leaning or rotating the body without moving the feet so that the pen followed and remained within the borders of a 1.5 cm-wide convoluted track. A total error score was calculated by summing the number of occasions that the pen failed to stay within the path; five points were accrued for a cut corner and one for a crossed side. Participants performed one practice trial before the experimental trial. A score corresponding to mean plus three standard deviations calculated per age was attributed to the subjects unable to perform some subsets of the PPA according to Lord, Menz and Tiedemann [30].

2.3. Statistical Analysis

The TD participants were divided into eight age groups (i.e., one group per year) that matched the individual ages of the ASD participants: 6 years, 8 years, 11 years, 12 years, 13 years, 14 years, 16 years and 18 years old. Data normality was confirmed through the visual inspection of quantile-quantile (Q-Q) plots and Kolmogorov–Smirnov tests. Given the skewness of the data distribution, we used percentiles for each PPA item and age group to obtain a reference database of TD children and adolescents. We calculated the 10th, 50th and 90th percentiles for each performance and each age range. For some parameters (edge contrast sensitivity, lower limb strength, maximum balance range test), the scale was inverted so that all items scoring over the 90th percentile indicated poorer performance and those scoring under the 10th percentile indicated better performance. For each test, we compared scores of single ASD subjects with the scores obtained by TD subjects in the age-matched group. Spearman correlations were used to assess correlations between the PPA performance scores and age in each group separately. Data were analyzed using SPSS version 25 for Windows (SPSS, Inc., Chicago, IL, USA) and the *p*-value was set at <0.05.

3. Results

One hundred and thirty-five (100/35 male/female) TD children and adolescents were recruited according the following age groups: 6 years ($n = 11$), 8 years ($n = 16$), 11 years ($n = 21$), 12 years ($n = 12$), 13 years ($n = 14$), 14 years ($n = 24$), 16 years ($n = 18$) and 18 years ($n = 19$).

Eighteen age-matched children and adolescents with ASD were enrolled (age: 12.4 ± 3.7 years; 16/2 male/female). Participants with ASD were age-matched according the following groups: 6 years ($n = 2$), 8 years ($n = 3$), 11 years ($n = 2$), 12 years ($n = 2$), 13 years ($n = 1$), 14 years ($n = 4$), 16 years ($n = 3$) and 18 years ($n = 1$) old. Their intellectual disability ranged from mild ($n = 5$), moderate ($n = 11$) to severe ($n = 2$). Eight participants had an ASD severity level of 1, nine participants of 2 and one participant of 3. Analysis of the Autism Diagnostic Observation Schedule Calibrated Severity Score (ADOS CSS) showed five participants had a score in the Autism Spectrum Disorder range and 13 participants in Autism range. Detailed characteristics are shown in Table 1.

Table 1. Demographic and clinical characteristics of ASD subjects.

ID	Age (yrs)	Sex	Intellectual Disability [†]	ASD Severity Level [†]	ADOS CSS
1	6	F	mild	1	4
2	6	F	mild	1	4
3	8	M	mild	1	8
4	8	M	mild	1	7
5	8	M	moderate	2	6
6	11	M	moderate	2	8
7	11	M	moderate	2	7
8	12	M	moderate	1	5
9	12	M	moderate	2	7
10	13	M	moderate	1	4
11	14	M	moderate	1	4
12	14	M	mild	1	6
13	14	M	moderate	2	6
14	14	M	moderate	2	6
15	16	M	moderate	2	7
16	16	M	severe	3	8
17	16	M	severe	2	7
18	18	M	moderate	2	6

Note: ADOS CSS = Autism Diagnostic Observation Schedule Calibrated Severity Score; M = male; F = female; ASD = autism spectrum disorder; [†] = intellectual disability and level of severity of autism according to DSM-5 criteria.

The test took between 60 and 90 min; two participants (ID 16 and 17) completed the assessment in two sessions. No TD participants or individuals with ASD reported fatigue during the assessment.

Figures 1–4 present performances of the ASD participants relative to the reference values (percentiles) of age-matched TD participants for vision, sensation, reaction time, force and balance tests, respectively. All percentiles for TD children and adolescents divided according to age groups can be found in Supplementary Table S1.

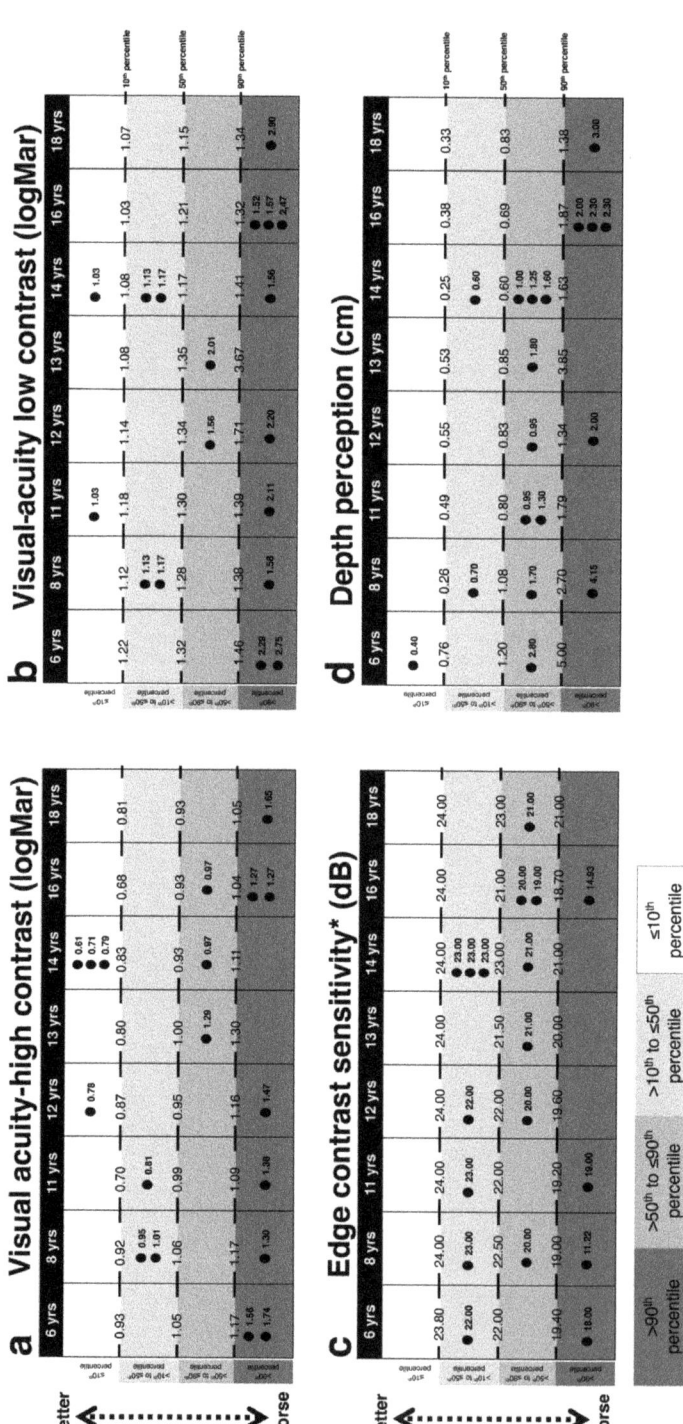

Figure 1. Comparison between each ASD subject's performance in the Physiological Profile Assessment (PPA) vision tests and age-matched reference values (percentiles) for typically developing (TD) subjects. Light gray to dark gray corresponds with better to worse performance. In (**a**) visual acuity high-contrast, in (**b**) visual acuity low-contrast, in (**c**) edge contrast sensitivity, in (**d**) depth perception. The reference value of the 10th, 50th and 90th percentiles and each ASD subject values are reported. Intervals for each performance represent: ≤10th, 10th < x ≤ 50th, 50th < x ≤ 90th, >90th percentile from the top to the bottom, respectively. Abbreviations: yrs, years; LogMar, minutes of arc; dB, decibel units; cm, centimeters. * indicates the percentile scale was inverted, i.e., for all items a score over the 90th percentile is an indicator of a worse performance.

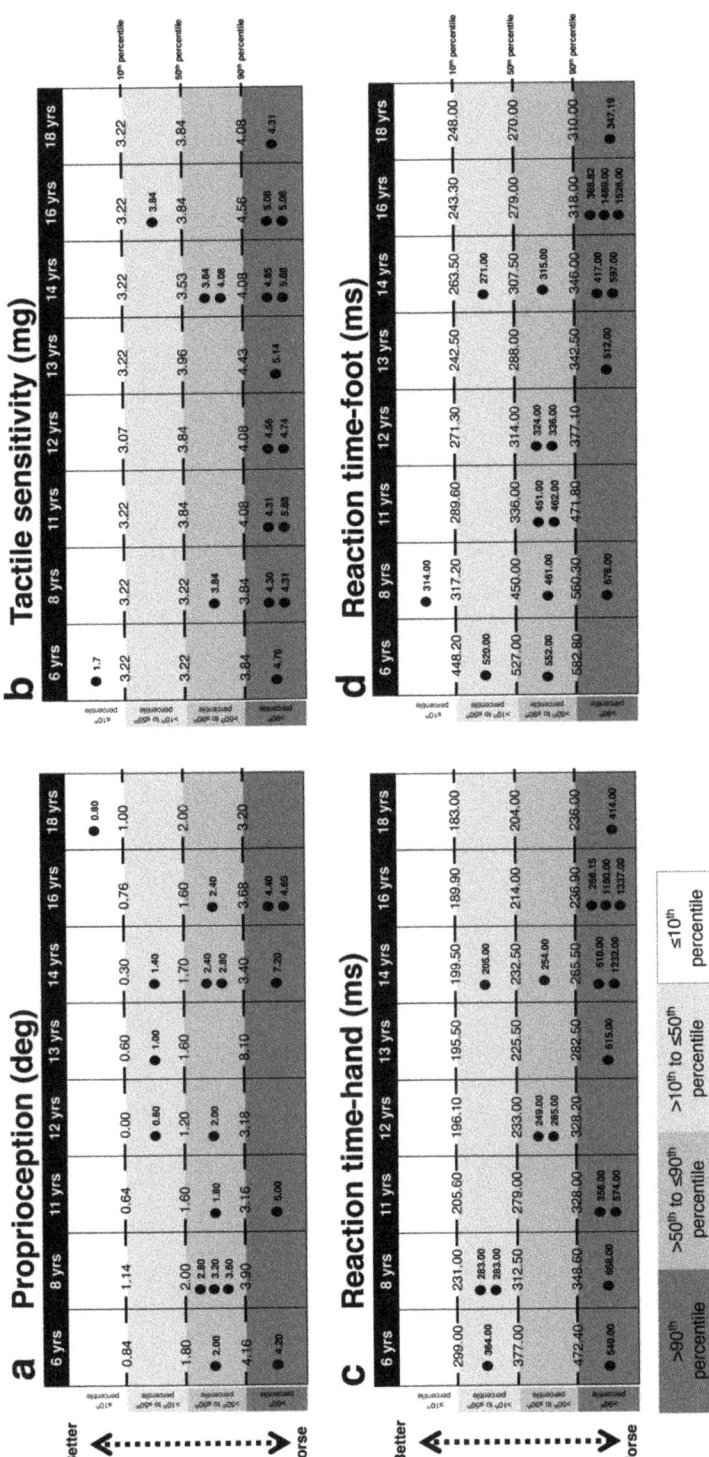

Figure 2. Comparison between each ASD subject's performance in the PPA peripheral sensation and reaction time tests and age-matched reference values (percentiles) for TD subjects. Light gray to dark gray corresponds with better to worse performance. In (**a**) proprioception, in (**b**) tactile sensitivity, in (**c**) reaction time on hand, in (**d**) reaction time on foot. The reference value of the 10th, 50th and 90th percentiles and each ASD subject values are reported. Intervals for each performance represent: ≤10th, 10th < x ≤ 50th, 50th < x ≤ 90th, >90th percentile from the top to the bottom, respectively. Abbreviations: yrs, years; deg, degree; mg, milligrams; ms, milliseconds.

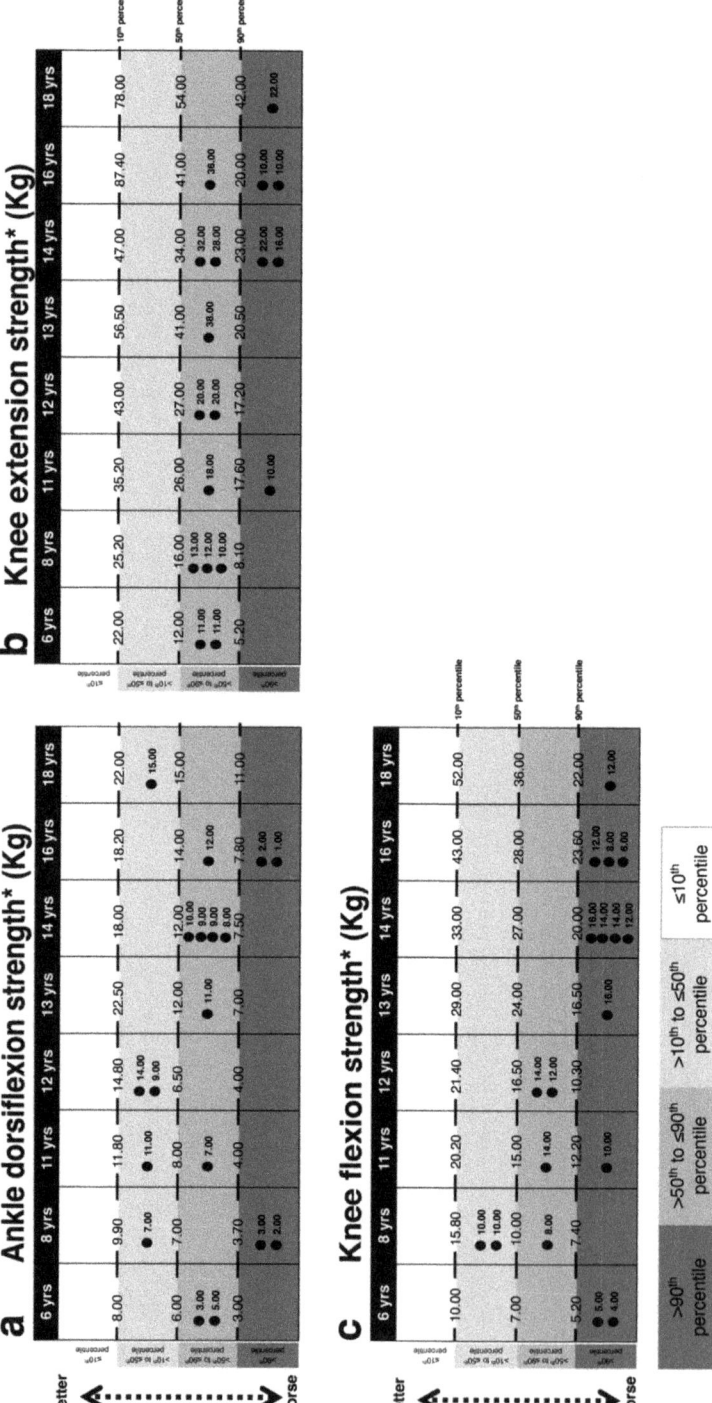

Figure 3. Comparison between each ASD subject's performance in the PPA tests of lower limb strength and age-matched reference values (percentiles) for TD subjects. Light gray to dark gray corresponds with better to worse performance. In (**a**) ankle dorsiflexion force, in (**b**) knee extension force, in (**c**) knee flexion force. The reference value of the 10th, 50th and 90th percentiles and each ASD subject values are reported. Intervals for each performance represent: ≤ 10th, 10th < x ≤ 50th, 50th < x ≤ 90th, >90th percentile from the top to the bottom, respectively. * indicates the percentile scale was inverted, i.e., for all items a score over the 90th percentile is an indicator of a worse performance. Abbreviations: yrs, years; kg, kilograms.

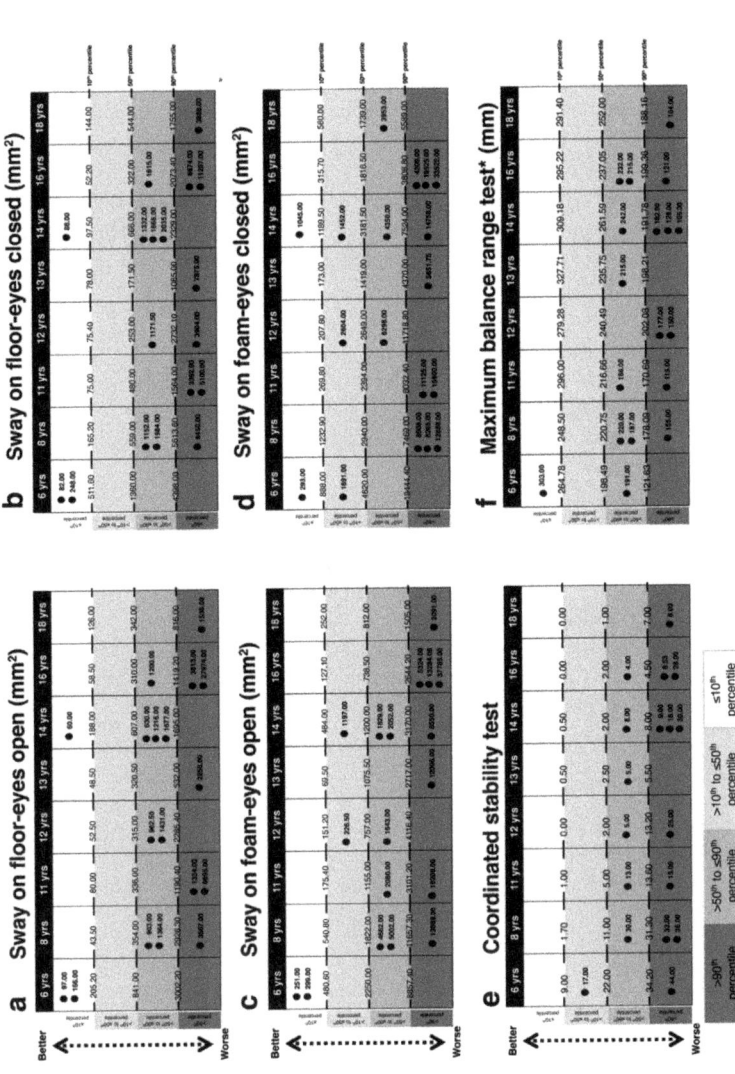

Figure 4. Comparison between each ASD subject's performance in the PPA balance tests and age-matched reference value (percentiles) for TD subjects. Light gray to dark gray corresponds with better to worse performance. In (**a**) sway on floor eyes open, in (**b**) sway on floor eyes closed, in (**c**) sway on foam eyes open, in (**d**) sway on foam eyes closed, in (**e**) coordinated stability test, in (**f**) maximum balance range test. The reference value of the 10th, 50th and 90th percentiles and each ASD subject values are reported. Intervals for each performance represent: ≤10th, 10th < x ≤ 50th, 50th < x ≤ 90th, >90th percentile from the top to the bottom, respectively. * indicates the percentile scale was inverted, i.e., for all items a score over the 90th percentile is an indicator of a worse performance. Abbreviations: yrs, years; mm2, millimeters square; mm, millimeters.

3.1. Vision

As shown in Figure 1, up to half of the ASD participants performed over the 90th percentile corresponding with a worse performance in the following tests: visual acuity high-contrast ($n = 8$), visual acuity low-contrast ($n = 10$), edge contrast sensitivity ($n = 4$) and depth perception ($n = 6$). Conversely, only a few ASD participants performed below the 10th percentile, indicating better performance in the following tests: visual acuity high-contrast ($n = 4$), visual acuity low-contrast ($n = 2$) and depth perception ($n = 1$).

Three-quarters of ASD subjects ($n = 13$) scored above the 90th percentile in the test of tactile sensitivity and one subject under the 10th percentile. In the test of proprioception, five subjects scored over the 90th percentile and one under the 10th percentile (See Figure 2).

3.2. Reaction Time

Eleven ASD individuals had prolonged hand reaction time over the 90th percentile relative to TD individuals and eight ASD individuals performed over the 90th percentile in the foot reaction time test. Of note though, one child with ASD had foot reaction times under the 10th percentile (Figure 2).

3.3. Lower Limb Muscle Strength

As displayed in Figure 3 regarding ankle dorsiflexor muscle strength, four subjects scored over the 90th percentile. For knee strength, six subjects scored over the 90th percentile for the knee extensor muscles and 12 subjects for the knee flexor muscles.

3.4. Balance

As shown in Figure 4, between seven and 10 subjects performed over the 90th percentile in the balance tests: sway on floor eyes open ($n = 7$), sway on floor eyes closed ($n = 8$), sway on foam eyes open ($n = 8$), sway on foam eyes closed ($n = 10$), coordinated stability test ($n = 11$) and maximum balance range test ($n = 9$). Conversely, three children performed under the 10th percentile for age in both tests of sway on the floor, two children in the test of sway on the foam with eyes open and two children in the test of sway on the foam with eyes closed and one child in the maximum balance range test. Figure 5 depicts the subjects' profile according to the percentile for each of the PPA subtests. Notably, all ASD subjects showed poor performance at least in three subtests and all participants showed poor performance in one of the balance tests.

3.5. Relationships between Test Performance and Age

In TD participants, all items of the PPA significantly correlated with age except for edge contrast sensitivity, proprioception and sway on floor with eyes open and closed. In ASD participants, only performance in the test of coordinated stability was significantly correlated with age. Correlations are shown in Table 2.

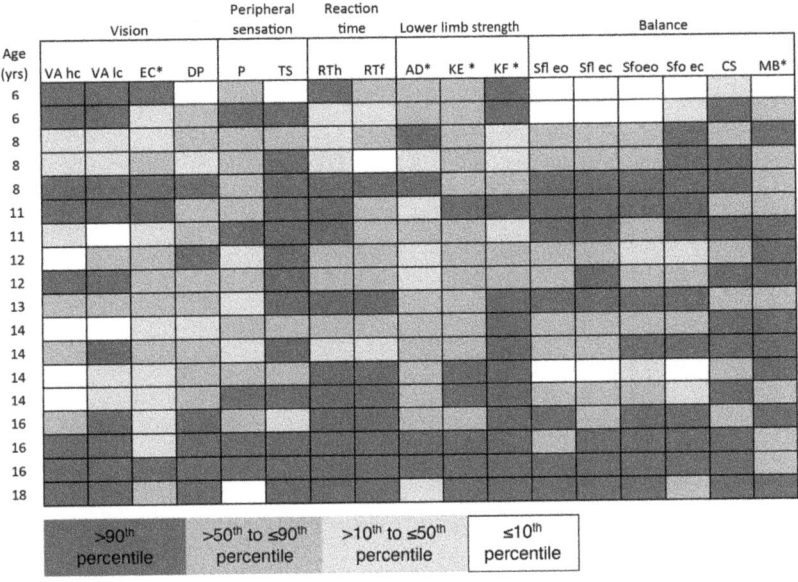

Figure 5. ASD subjects' profile. Each ASD subject's PPA performance box is colored with the correspondence of range percentile. Light gray to dark gray corresponds with better to worse performance. Abbreviations: yrs, years; VAhc, visual acuity high-contrast; VAlc, visual acuity low-contrast; EC, edge contrast sensitivity; DP, deep perception; P, proprioception; TS, tactile sensitivity; RTh, hand reaction time; RTf, foot reaction time; AD, ankle dorsiflexors force; KE, knee extensors force; KF, knee flexors force; Sfl eo, sway on floor eyes open; Sfl ec, sway on floor eyes closed; Sfo eo, sway on foam eyes open; Sfo ec, sway on foam eyes closed; CS, coordinated stability test; MB, maximum balance range test. * indicates the percentile scale was inverted so that all items scoring over the 90th percentile indicated poorer performance.

Table 2. Correlations between individual test performance and age.

	ASD	TD
	Rho Spearman	Rho Spearman
Visual acuity high-contrast	−0.254	−0.415 **
Visual acuity low-contrast	−0.021	−0.455 **
Edge contrast sensitivity	0.069	0.066
Depth perception	0.273	−0.294 **
Proprioception	−0.072	−0.053
Tactile sensitivity	0.219	0.275 **
Ankle dorsiflexion force	0.338	0.677 **
Knee extensor muscle force	0.383	0.765 **
Knee flexors muscle force	0.361	0.883 **
Reaction time: hand	0.105	−0.698 **
Reaction time: foot	−0.058	−0.770 **
Sway floor eyes open	0.320	−0.040
Sway floor eyes closed	0.330	−0.123
Sway foam eyes open	0.317	−0.319 **
Sway foam eyes closed	0.140	−0.218 *
Coordinated stability test	−0.565 *	−0.596 **
Maximum balance range test	−0.298	0.288 **

Note: ASD = autism spectrum disorder; TD = typically developing; * = correlation significant with $p < 0.05$; ** = correlation significant with $p < 0.01$.

4. Discussion

The results support the use of the five physiological measures of the PPA in TD children and adolescents. The PPA was also successfully administered to a subset of individuals with ASD during developmental ages. No fatigue and adverse events were reported from both groups.

We compared each PPA subtest between ASD and TD participants across age groups. Postural impairments might have a significant impact on the development of perceptual motor skills and social functioning in individuals with ASD [14]. According to Mergner's multisensorial feedback model [40], an efficient postural control system requires the interaction of sensory, motor and integration systems. The central nervous system (CNS) integrates multiple inputs from visual, vestibular, proprioceptive and tactile somatosensory systems. The CNS includes both predictive and adaptive components whose regulation depends on a sensory reweight of the feedbacks enabling the human body to function correctly against gravity and environmental perturbation forces [19]. A marked deficit in any one of the feedback systems or a combination of mild impairments in multiple sensorimotor physiological domains may lead to postural disorders [18]. Sensorimotor organization mutates during human development [41] due to a variety of reasons including learning and aging processes that make individuals reach adult assets at around the age of 13–14 years old [42]. However, individuals with ASD appear to have patterns of sensory processing that differentiate them from TD peers [20–22].

As performances of the TD population in the sensory, motor and balance tests were entirely consistent, percentiles were used to represent the variables' distribution. Our approach overcame the limitations of previous studies [14] by examining all components of balance systematically to obtain a complete profile of postural control in individuals with ASD.

Within our study, the presence of intellectual disability could not be ruled out to justify the different performances between TD subjects and participants with ASD. Therefore, the lower scores on the PPA items may be a consequence of an underlying intellectual disability or a combination with the presence of ASD. However, our sample was representative of a large subset of individuals with ASD. Notably, Newschaffer et al. [43] estimated that 70–75% of children with ASD have an intellectual disability.

4.1. Vision

According to a narrative review of literature by Bakroon and Lakshminarayanan [44], 29 to 44% of children and adolescents with ASD reported the presence of refractive errors. Here, half of our sample of children and adolescents with ASD performed poorly in the tests of visual acuity, particularly when the lighting conditions were poor (low-contrast). This result contrasts with the postulated superior visual acuity (eagle vision) of ASD subjects reported by some authors [45–47]. In fact, in our study only five ASD participants performed below the 10th percentile, which demonstrated a very high visual acuity performance. For static contrast sensitivity, our findings seemed to corroborate those presented in Simmons' review [48] whereby there were no differences between ASD and TD performances. As also noted by Simmons et al. [48], depth perception or stereopsis was apparently preserved but has been scarcely studied; here, we found poor depth perception in more than a third of ASD participants. The reasons for the disagreement between the findings reported in the literature and ours may include different modalities of data collection (e.g., different tools to assess vision such as the Freiburg Acuity and Contrast Test) [45]; some authors also outlined the role of visual attention and its importance in visual integration [49].

4.2. Peripheral Sensation

Tactile sensitivity was inferior in our ASD population with three-quarters of participants scoring above the 90th percentile and one performing below the 10th percentile. Our results are in agreement with the literature [50,51] although a recent review questioned the high prevalence of tactile processing dysfunction in ASD [52]. It pointed out the difficulty to assess tactile sensitivity due to the subjectivity of clinical assessments, the heterogeneity of ASD cohorts and the diversity of tactile sensitivity measures;

although it mostly concerns pain stimulation, another potential confounder to consider relates to emotional-affective conditioning in sensitivity tests [53]. Here, we used an aesthesiometer to be more accurate. One-quarter of ASD participants performed poorly in the test of proprioception. Similar to other sensory systems such as vision, the literature on the integrity of proprioception in ASD is conflicting. Some studies have reported altered proprioception [54] while others do not [55]; such discrepancies can be partly attributed to the variety of the test modality used. Notably, we tested proprioception in the leg, which has more relevance to standing postural control but is not as commonly investigated as in the upper limbs. In synthesis, the peripheral sensation was impaired in the ASD participants with most participants showing clear deficits in tactile sensitivity at the ankle and fewer underperforming in the proprioception assessment.

4.3. Reaction Time

We assessed simple reaction time with both the lower and upper limbs in individuals with ASD. More than half of our participants performed above the 90th percentile in the tests of simple reaction time at the finger and the foot, confirming previous reports of slow processing speed in ASD individuals [56]. Some studies [57–59] have also shown an increased response time variability in ASD but these works considered ASD subjects with Attention Deficit Hyperactivity Disorder. We might conclude that children and adolescents with ASD are slower compared with age-matched TD peers.

4.4. Lower Limb Muscle Strength

Over a quarter of the children and adolescents with ASD presented muscle weakness in at least one of the three lower limb muscle groups we investigated. Such deficits in muscle strength are likely to contribute to the altered gait patterns reported in ASD [60]. Interestingly, all of the adolescents with ASD aged 13 years and above presented evident knee flexor muscle weakness compared with age-matched TD peers. These older participants also included individuals with higher levels of intellectual disability and increased ASD severity. Interestingly, Kern et al. [61] reported that handgrip strength in children with ASD was related to the severity of the disorder.

4.5. Balance Tests

Our results for the sway tests with eyes closed are in line with most studies that showed increased postural sway of ASD subjects under these conditions [16,62,63]. Poor performance in the tests of coordinated stability and maximum balance range reflects the difficulty individuals with ASD have to control their center of mass at the limits of their stability [64]. Although the prevalence of balance problems in ASD is well acknowledged, explanations regarding the causes of the postural stability deficits diverge. For example, some authors outline the role of anxiety on postural instability [65] while others attribute the problem to poor cognition [66]. Nevertheless, most of the debate lies in whether postural deficits are related to sensorimotor or integrational problems. In fact, a body of literature suggests that rather than poor perceptive ability, failure in the integration of visual, somatosensory and vestibular information could be the primary contributors to poor balance [28]. While we agree that sensory integration needs to be considered, our findings demonstrate that poor performances in the single sensorimotor tests administered clearly impact on postural control in ASD.

4.6. Correlation with Age

The second aim of this work was to determine if the correlation between age and physiological parameters was similar for TD and ASD children and adolescents. Spearman correlation coefficients calculated for all variables showed a marked difference between the groups. In fact, TD participants' performances improved with increasing age in most components of the PPA (except for edge contrast sensitivity, proprioception and sway on floor eyes open and closed) while for ASD participants, only the coordinated stability test performance was significantly correlated with age. Our findings support previous reports that tactile sensitivity [67], visual acuity [68] and reaction time [69] improve with increasing age in children and adolescents but disagree with those regarding contrast sensitivity [68] and proprioception [70,71]. In these latter studies, proprioception was assessed in the forearm while here proprioception was evaluated in the leg. To this end, our findings suggest that most balance-influencing parameters mature with age but not in ASD.

4.7. Limitations

We acknowledge that our work has some limitations. The first is that we did not collect the intelligence quotient for all participants in this study. We therefore cannot make firm conclusions regarding the potential contribution of cognition on sensorimotor integration and balance in the ASD sample. The second limitation involves the significant amount of interpersonal interactions between the participant and the examiner required to conduct the PPA, which might have affected the testing given communication issues are inherent to ASD. Third, the duration of the PPA could also deter individuals from participating. Finally, the reduced sample sizes of the age-matched individuals with ASD may affect the generalizability of the postural findings to the ASD population. Moreover, we recommend that future studies should investigate postural capacity in individuals with ASD compared with different populations matched on the degree of intellectual disability.

5. Conclusions

In conclusion, our findings support the applicability of the PPA in TD children and adolescents. Moreover, the PPA was successfully administered to a subgroup of age-matched individuals with ASD.

The normative data provided for the TD children and adolescents can be used in clinical and research settings for assessing postural capacity. Although preliminary, the subset data from participants with ASD may contribute to the understanding of postural impairments in developmental disorders. Interestingly, we found a reduced balance performance and age-related development progress decreased in individuals with ASD. Further studies in a larger sample size should investigate sensorimotor integration for postural control using the PPA in individuals with ASD as well as study each postural domain across age groups and ASD severity.

Supplementary Materials: The following are available online at http://www.mdpi.com/2076-3425/10/10/681/s1. Table S1: percentiles for typically developed children and adolescents.

Author Contributions: Conceptualization, C.P., C.G.C. and D.P.; methodology, C.P., C.G.C., J.M. and D.P.; software, C.G.C.; formal analysis, R.M. and C.G.C.; investigation, G.V., M.M., V.G., E.G. and C.P.; data curation, C.P., M.M., V.G. and C.G.C.; writing—original draft preparation, C.P., C.G.C. and D.P.; writing—review and editing, C.P., M.M., J.M. and D.P.; supervision, C.M.C.; project administration, C.G.C. All authors have read and agreed to the published version of the manuscript.

Funding: This research received no external funding.

Acknowledgments: The authors are grateful to Stephen R. Lord for the valuable suggestions relating to the management of the data of the Physiological Profile Assessment. The authors thank the children and the families who participated in this study.

Conflicts of Interest: The authors declare no conflict of interest.

Data Availability Statement:: The data that support the findings of the current study are available from the corresponding author [CP] upon reasonable request.

References

1. Baio, J.; Wiggins, L.; Christensen, D.L.; Maenner, M.J.; Daniels, J.; Warren, Z.; Kurzius-Spencer, M.; Zahorodny, W.; Robinson Rosenberg, C.; White, T.; et al. Prevalence of Autism Spectrum Disorder Among Children Aged 8 Years—Autism and Developmental Disabilities Monitoring Network, 11 Sites, United States, 2014. *MMWR Surveill. Summ.* **2018**, *67*, 1–23. [CrossRef]
2. Narzisi, A.; Posada, M.; Barbieri, F.; Chericoni, N.; Ciuffolini, D.; Pinzino, M.; Romano, R.; Scattoni, M.L.; Tancredi, R.; Calderoni, S.; et al. Prevalence of Autism Spectrum Disorder in a large Italian catchment area: A school-based population study within the ASDEU project. *Epidemiol. Psychiatr. Sci.* **2018**, *29*, e5. [CrossRef]

3. Association, A.P. Diagnostic and statistical manual of mental disorders. *BMC Med.* **2013**, *17*, 133–137.
4. Provost, B.; Lopez, B.R.; Heimerl, S. A comparison of motor delays in young children: Autism spectrum disorder, developmental delay, and developmental concerns. *J. Autism Dev. Disord.* **2007**, *37*, 321–328. [CrossRef]
5. Teitelbaum, P.; Teitelbaum, O.; Nye, J.; Fryman, J.; Maurer, R.G. Movement analysis in infancy may be useful for early diagnosis of autism. *Proc. Natl. Acad. Sci. USA* **1998**, *95*, 13982–13987. [CrossRef]
6. Ghaziuddin, M.; Butler, E. Clumsiness in autism and Asperger syndrome: A further report. *J. Intellect. Disabil. Res.* **1998**, *42 Pt 1*, 43–48. [CrossRef]
7. Mari, M.; Castiello, U.; Marks, D.; Marraffa, C.; Prior, M. The reach-to-grasp movement in children with autism spectrum disorder. *Philos. Trans. R. Soc. Lond. B Biol. Sci.* **2003**, *358*, 393–403. [CrossRef]
8. Miyahara, M.; Tsujii, M.; Hori, M.; Nakanishi, K.; Kageyama, H.; Sugiyama, T. Brief report: Motor incoordination in children with Asperger syndrome and learning disabilities. *J. Autism Dev. Disord.* **1997**, *27*, 595–603. [CrossRef]
9. Noterdaeme, M.; Mildenberger, K.; Minow, F.; Amorosa, H. Evaluation of neuromotor deficits in children with autism and children with a specific speech and language disorder. *Eur. Child Adolesc. Psychiatry* **2002**, *11*, 219–225. [CrossRef]
10. Kindregan, D.; Gallagher, L.; Gormley, J. Gait deviations in children with autism spectrum disorders: A review. *Autism Res. Treat.* **2015**, *2015*, 741480. [CrossRef]
11. Valagussa, G.; Balatti, V.; Trentin, L.; Piscitelli, D.; Yamagata, M.; Grossi, E. Relationship between tip-toe behavior and soleus—gastrocnemius muscle lengths in individuals with autism spectrum disorders. *J. Orthop.* **2020**, *21*, 444–448. [CrossRef]
12. Ament, K.; Mejia, A.; Buhlman, R.; Erklin, S.; Caffo, B.; Mostofsky, S.; Wodka, E. Evidence for specificity of motor impairments in catching and balance in children with autism. *J. Autism. Dev. Disord.* **2015**, *45*, 742–751. [CrossRef]
13. Fournier, K.A.; Kimberg, C.I.; Radonovich, K.J.; Tillman, M.D.; Chow, J.W.; Lewis, M.H.; Bodfish, J.W.; Hass, C.J. Decreased static and dynamic postural control in children with autism spectrum disorders. *Gait Posture* **2010**, *32*, 6–9. [CrossRef]
14. Memari, A.H.; Ghanouni, P.; Shayestehfar, M.; Ghaheri, B. Postural control impairments in individuals with autism spectrum disorder: A critical review of current literature. *Asian J. Sports Med.* **2014**, *5*, e22963. [CrossRef]
15. Ming, X.; Brimacombe, M.; Wagner, G.C. Prevalence of motor impairment in autism spectrum disorders. *Brain Dev.* **2007**, *29*, 565–570. [CrossRef]
16. Minshew, N.J.; Sung, K.; Jones, B.L.; Furman, J.M. Underdevelopment of the postural control system in autism. *Neurology* **2004**, *63*, 2056–2061. [CrossRef]
17. Vernazza-Martin, S.; Martin, N.; Vernazza, A.; Lepellec-Muller, A.; Rufo, M.; Massion, J.; Assaiante, C. Goal directed locomotion and balance control in autistic children. *J. Autism Dev. Disord.* **2005**, *35*, 91–102. [CrossRef]
18. Horak, F.B. Postural orientation and equilibrium: What do we need to know about neural control of balance to prevent falls? *Age Ageing* **2006**, *35* (Suppl. 2), ii7–ii11. [CrossRef]
19. Peterka, R.J. Sensorimotor integration in human postural control. *J. Neurophysiol.* **2002**, *88*, 1097–1118. [CrossRef]
20. Brockevelt, B.L.; Nissen, R.; Schweinle, W.E.; Kurtz, E.; Larson, K.J. A comparison of the Sensory Profile scores of children with autism and an age- and gender-matched sample. *S. D. Med.* **2013**, *66*, 463–465.
21. Cascio, C.J. Somatosensory processing in neurodevelopmental disorders. *J. Neurodev. Disord.* **2010**, *2*, 62–69. [CrossRef]
22. Lloyd, M.; MacDonald, M.; Lord, C. Motor skills of toddlers with autism spectrum disorders. *Autism* **2013**, *17*, 133–146. [CrossRef]
23. Henderson, S.E.; Sugden, D.A.; Barnett, A.L. *Movement Assessment Battery for Children-2 Second Edition [Movement ABC-2]*; The Psychological Corporation: London, UK, 2007.
24. Emck, C.; Bosscher, R.J.; Van Wieringen, P.C.; Doreleijers, T.; Beek, P.J. Gross motor performance and physical fitness in children with psychiatric disorders. *Dev. Med. Child Neurol.* **2011**, *53*, 150–155. [CrossRef]
25. Largo, R.H.; Fischer, J.E.; Rousson, V. Neuromotor development from kindergarten age to adolescence: Developmental course and variability. *Swiss Med. Wkly.* **2003**, *133*, 193–199. [CrossRef] [PubMed]

26. Denckla, M.B. Revised Neurological Examination for Subtle Signs (1985). *Psychopharmacol. Bull.* **1985**, *21*, 773–800. [PubMed]
27. Chen, F.C.; Tsai, C.L. A light fingertip touch reduces postural sway in children with autism spectrum disorders. *Gait Posture* **2016**, *43*, 137–140. [CrossRef] [PubMed]
28. Lim, Y.H.; Partridge, K.; Girdler, S.; Morris, S.L. Standing Postural Control in Individuals with Autism Spectrum Disorder: Systematic Review and Meta-analysis. *J. Autism Dev. Disord.* **2017**, *47*, 2238–2253. [CrossRef]
29. Wang, Z.; Hallac, R.R.; Conroy, K.C.; White, S.P.; Kane, A.A.; Collinsworth, A.L.; Sweeney, J.A.; Mosconi, M.W. Postural orientation and equilibrium processes associated with increased postural sway in autism spectrum disorder (ASD). *J. Neurodev. Disord.* **2016**, *8*, 43. [CrossRef]
30. Lord, S.R.; Menz, H.B.; Tiedemann, A. A physiological profile approach to falls risk assessment and prevention. *Phys. Ther.* **2003**, *83*, 237–252. [CrossRef]
31. Phirom, K.; Kamnardsiri, T.; Sungkarat, S. Beneficial Effects of Interactive Physical-Cognitive Game-Based Training on Fall Risk and Cognitive Performance of Older Adults. *Int. J. Environ. Res. Public Health* **2020**, *17*, 6079. [CrossRef]
32. Gunn, H.; Cameron, M.; Hoang, P.; Lord, S.; Shaw, S.; Freeman, J. Relationship Between Physiological and Perceived Fall Risk in People With Multiple Sclerosis: Implications for Assessment and Management. *Arch. Phys. Med. Rehabil.* **2018**, *99*, 2022–2029. [CrossRef] [PubMed]
33. Lord, S.R.; Delbaere, K.; Gandevia, S.C. Use of a physiological profile to document motor impairment in ageing and in clinical groups. *J. Physiol.* **2016**, *594*, 4513–4523. [CrossRef] [PubMed]
34. Hoang, P.D.; Baysan, M.; Gunn, H.; Cameron, M.; Freeman, J.; Nitz, J.; Low Choy, N.L.; Lord, S.R. Fall risk in people with MS: A Physiological Profile Assessment study. *Mult. Scler. J. Exp. Transl. Clin.* **2016**, *2*. [CrossRef] [PubMed]
35. Rosa, N.M.; Queiroz, B.Z.; Lopes, R.A.; Sampaio, N.R.; Pereira, D.S.; Pereira, L.S. Risk of falls in Brazilian elders with and without low back pain assessed using the Physiological Profile Assessment: BACE study. *Braz. J. Phys. Ther.* **2016**, *20*, 502–509. [CrossRef]
36. Piscitelli, D.; Pellicciari, L. Responsiveness: Is it time to move beyond ordinal scores and approach interval measurements? *Clin. Rehabil.* **2018**, *32*, 1426–1427. [CrossRef]
37. Valagussa, G.; Trentin, L.; Terragni, E.; Cerri, C.; Gariboldi, V.; Perin, C.; Mauri, D.; Grossi, E. 164.188 Postural Control Assessment in Autism Using the Pediatric Balance Scale and the Fall Screen Assessment System: Results from a Pilot Study. In Proceedings of the International Meeting for Autism Research—IMFAR San Francisco, San Francisco, CA, USA, 10 May 2010.
38. Lord, C.; Rutter, M.; DiLavore, P.C.; Risi, S.; Gotham, K.; Bishop, S.L.; Schedule, A.A.D.O. ADOS-2. In *Manual (Part I): Modules 1-4*; Western Psychological Services: Torrance, CA, USA, 2012.
39. World Health Organization. *WHO Child Growth Standards: Length/Height-for-Age, Weight-for-Age, Weight-for-Length, Weight-for-Height and Body Mass Index-For-Age: Methods and Development*; World Health Organization: Geneva, Switzerland, 2006.
40. Mergner, T. A neurological view on reactive human stance control. *Annu. Rev. Control* **2010**, *34*, 177–198. [CrossRef]
41. Chan-Viquez, D.; Hasanbarani, F.; Zhang, L.; Anaby, D.; Turpin, N.A.; Lamontagne, A.; Feldman, A.G.; Levin, M.F. Development of vertical and forward jumping skills in typically developing children in the context of referent control of motor actions. *Dev. Psychobiol.* **2020**, *62*, 1–12. [CrossRef]
42. Assaiante, C. Development of locomotor balance control in healthy children. *Neurosci. Biobehav. Rev.* **1998**, *22*, 527–532. [CrossRef]
43. Newschaffer, C.J.; Croen, L.A.; Daniels, J.; Giarelli, E.; Grether, J.K.; Levy, S.E.; Mandell, D.S.; Miller, L.A.; Pinto-Martin, J.; Reaven, J.; et al. The epidemiology of autism spectrum disorders. *Annu. Rev. Public Health* **2007**, *28*, 235–258. [CrossRef]
44. Bakroon, A.; Lakshminarayanan, V. Visual function in autism spectrum disorders: A critical review. *Clin. Exp. Optom.* **2016**, *99*, 297–308. [CrossRef]
45. Bach, M.; Dakin, S.C. Regarding "Eagle-eyed visual acuity: An experimental investigation of enhanced perception in autism". *Biol. Psychiatry* **2009**, *66*, e19–e20. [CrossRef] [PubMed]
46. Dakin, S.; Frith, U. Vagaries of visual perception in autism. *Neuron* **2005**, *48*, 497–507. [CrossRef]

47. Joseph, R.M.; Keehn, B.; Connolly, C.; Wolfe, J.M.; Horowitz, T.S. Why is visual search superior in autism spectrum disorder? *Dev. Sci.* **2009**, *12*, 1083–1096. [CrossRef] [PubMed]
48. Simmons, D.R.; Robertson, A.E.; McKay, L.S.; Toal, E.; McAleer, P.; Pollick, F.E. Vision in autism spectrum disorders. *Vis. Res.* **2009**, *49*, 2705–2739. [CrossRef] [PubMed]
49. Robertson, C.E.; Kravitz, D.J.; Freyberg, J.; Baron-Cohen, S.; Baker, C.I. Tunnel vision: Sharper gradient of spatial attention in autism. *J. Neurosci.* **2013**, *33*, 6776–6781. [CrossRef] [PubMed]
50. Puts, N.A.; Wodka, E.L.; Tommerdahl, M.; Mostofsky, S.H.; Edden, R.A. Impaired tactile processing in children with autism spectrum disorder. *J. Neurophysiol.* **2014**, *111*, 1803–1811. [CrossRef] [PubMed]
51. Tavassoli, T.; Bellesheim, K.; Tommerdahl, M.; Holden, J.M.; Kolevzon, A.; Buxbaum, J.D. Altered tactile processing in children with autism spectrum disorder. *Autism Res.* **2016**, *9*, 616–620. [CrossRef] [PubMed]
52. Mikkelsen, M.; Wodka, E.L.; Mostofsky, S.H.; Puts, N.A.J. Autism spectrum disorder in the scope of tactile processing. *Dev. Cogn. Neurosci.* **2018**, *29*, 140–150. [CrossRef] [PubMed]
53. Riquelme, I.; Hatem, S.M.; Montoya, P. Abnormal Pressure Pain, Touch Sensitivity, Proprioception, and Manual Dexterity in Children with Autism Spectrum Disorders. *Neural Plast.* **2016**, *2016*, 1723401. [CrossRef]
54. Blanche, E.I.; Reinoso, G.; Chang, M.C.; Bodison, S. Proprioceptive processing difficulties among children with autism spectrum disorders and developmental disabilities. *Am. J. Occup. Ther.* **2012**, *66*, 621–624. [CrossRef]
55. Fuentes, C.T.; Mostofsky, S.H.; Bastian, A.J. No proprioceptive deficits in autism despite movement-related sensory and execution impairments. *J. Autism Dev. Disord.* **2011**, *41*, 1352–1361. [CrossRef] [PubMed]
56. Schmitz, N.; Daly, E.; Murphy, D. Frontal anatomy and reaction time in Autism. *Neurosci. Lett.* **2007**, *412*, 12–17. [CrossRef] [PubMed]
57. Karalunas, S.L.; Geurts, H.M.; Konrad, K.; Bender, S.; Nigg, J.T. Annual research review: Reaction time variability in ADHD and autism spectrum disorders: Measurement and mechanisms of a proposed trans-diagnostic phenotype. *J. Child Psychol. Psychiatry* **2014**, *55*, 685–710. [CrossRef] [PubMed]
58. Truedsson, E.; Bohlin, G.; Wahlstedt, C. The Specificity and Independent Contribution of Inhibition, Working Memory, and Reaction Time Variability in Relation to Symptoms of ADHD and ASD. *J. Atten. Disord.* **2020**, *24*, 1266–1275. [CrossRef] [PubMed]
59. Tye, C.; Johnson, K.A.; Kelly, S.P.; Asherson, P.; Kuntsi, J.; Ashwood, K.L.; Azadi, B.; Bolton, P.; McLoughlin, G. Response time variability under slow and fast-incentive conditions in children with ASD, ADHD and ASD+ADHD. *J. Child Psychol. Psychiatry* **2016**, *57*, 1414–1423. [CrossRef]
60. Eggleston, J.D.; Harry, J.R.; Hickman, R.A.; Dufek, J.S. Analysis of gait symmetry during over-ground walking in children with autism spectrum disorder. *Gait Posture* **2017**, *55*, 162–166. [CrossRef]
61. Kern, J.K.; Geier, D.A.; Adams, J.B.; Troutman, M.R.; Davis, G.; King, P.G.; Young, J.L.; Geier, M.R. Autism severity and muscle strength: A correlation analysis. *Res. Autism Spectr. Disord.* **2011**, *5*, 1011–1015. [CrossRef]
62. Doumas, M.; McKenna, R.; Murphy, B. Postural Control Deficits in Autism Spectrum Disorder: The Role of Sensory Integration. *J. Autism Dev. Disord.* **2016**, *46*, 853–861. [CrossRef]
63. Molloy, C.A.; Dietrich, K.N.; Bhattacharya, A. Postural stability in children with autism spectrum disorder. *J. Autism Dev. Disord.* **2003**, *33*, 643–652. [CrossRef]
64. Graham, S.A.; Abbott, A.E.; Nair, A.; Lincoln, A.J.; Muller, R.A.; Goble, D.J. The Influence of Task Difficulty and Participant Age on Balance Control in ASD. *J. Autism Dev. Disord.* **2015**, *45*, 1419–1427. [CrossRef]
65. Stins, J.F.; Emck, C. Balance Performance in Autism: A Brief Overview. *Front. Psychol.* **2018**, *9*, 901. [CrossRef] [PubMed]
66. Travers, B.G.; Mason, A.; Gruben, K.G.; Dean, D.C., 3rd; McLaughlin, K. Standing Balance on Unsteady Surfaces in Children on the Autism Spectrum: The Effects of IQ. *Res. Autism Spectr. Disord.* **2018**, *51*, 9–17. [CrossRef] [PubMed]
67. Taylor, S.; McLean, B.; Falkmer, T.; Carey, L.; Girdler, S.; Elliott, C.; Blair, E. Does somatosensation change with age in children and adolescents? A systematic review. *Child Care Health Dev.* **2016**, *42*, 809–824. [CrossRef]
68. Leat, S.J.; Yadav, N.K.; Irving, E.L. Development of visual acuity and contrast sensitivity in children. *J. Optom.* **2009**, *2*, 19–26. [CrossRef]
69. Kail, R. Processing time decreases globally at an exponential rate during childhood and adolescence. *J. Exp. Child Psychol.* **1993**, *56*, 254–265. [CrossRef] [PubMed]

70. Goble, D.J.; Lewis, C.A.; Hurvitz, E.A.; Brown, S.H. Development of upper limb proprioceptive accuracy in children and adolescents. *Hum. Mov. Sci.* **2005**, *24*, 155–170. [CrossRef] [PubMed]
71. Holst-Wolf, J.M.; Yeh, I.L.; Konczak, J. Development of Proprioceptive Acuity in Typically Developing Children: Normative Data on Forearm Position Sense. *Front. Hum. Neurosci.* **2016**, *10*, 436. [CrossRef] [PubMed]

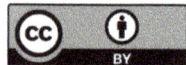

© 2020 by the authors. Licensee MDPI, Basel, Switzerland. This article is an open access article distributed under the terms and conditions of the Creative Commons Attribution (CC BY) license (http://creativecommons.org/licenses/by/4.0/).

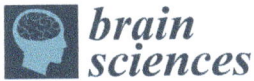 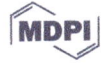

Article

Participatory Art Activities Increase Salivary Oxytocin Secretion of ASD Children

Sanae Tanaka [1,†], Aiko Komagome [2,†], Aya Iguchi-Sherry [3,†], Akiko Nagasaka [4], Teruko Yuhi [5], Haruhiro Higashida [5], Maki Rooksby [6,7], Mitsuru Kikuchi [8], Oko Arai [2], Kana Minami [5,9], Takahiro Tsuji [5,10] and Chiharu Tsuji [5,*]

1. Division of Integrated Art and Sciences and Local Community Support, Research Center for Child Mental Development, Kanazawa University, Kanazawa 920-8640, Japan; tanakast@staff.kanazawa-u.ac.jp
2. The COI Site, Tokyo University of the Arts Tokyo 110-8714, Japan; komagome.aiko@ms.geidai.ac.jp (A.K.); tanaka.oko@ms.geidai.ac.jp (O.A.)
3. Artlink Central, Scotland FK8 1EA, UK; ayaiguchi@icloud.com
4. Department of Childhood Care and Education, Faculty of Social Work, Kinjo University, Hakusan 924-8511, Japan; ngsk-a4@kinjo.ac.jp
5. Department of Basic Research on Social Recognition, Research Center for Child Mental Development, Kanazawa University, Kanazawa 920-8640, Japan; y-teruko@med.kanazawa-u.ac.jp (T.Y.); haruhiro@med.kanazawa-u.ac.jp (H.H.); minami-k@staff.kanazawa-u.ac.jp (K.M.); tsuji-t@u-fukui.ac.jp (T.T.)
6. Adverse Childhood Experiences (ACE) Lab, Institute of Health and Wellbeing, University of Glasgow, Glasgow G12 8RZ, UK; Maki.Rooksby@glasgow.ac.uk
7. Social Brain in Action Lab, Institute of Neuroscience and Psychology, University of Glasgow, Glasgow G12 8QB, UK
8. Department of Psychiatry and Neurobiology, Graduate School of Medical Science, Kanazawa University, Kanazawa 920-8640, Japan; mitsuruk@med.kanazawa-u.ac.jp
9. Department of Health Development Nursing, Institute of Medical, Pharmaceutical and Health Sciences, Kanazawa University, Kanazawa 920-0942, Japan
10. Department of Ophthalmology, Faculty of Medical Sciences, University of Fukui, Fukui 910-1193, Japan
* Correspondence: ctsuji@med.kanazawa-u.ac.jp or higashida.c@gmail.com
† These authors contributed equally to this work.

Received: 15 August 2020; Accepted: 25 September 2020; Published: 27 September 2020

Abstract: Autism spectrum disorder (ASD) occurs in 1 in 160 children worldwide. Individuals with ASD tend to be unique in the way that they comprehend themselves and others, as well as in the way that they interact and socialize, which can lead to challenges with social adaptation. There is currently no medication to improve the social deficit of children with ASD, and consequently, behavioral and complementary/alternative intervention plays an important role. In the present pilot study, we focused on the neuroendocrinological response to participatory art activities, which are known to have a positive effect on emotion, self-expression, sociability, and physical wellbeing. We collected saliva from 12 children with ASD and eight typically developed (TD) children before and after a visual art-based participatory art workshop to measure the levels of oxytocin, a neuropeptide involved in a wide range of social behaviors. We demonstrated that the rate of increase in salivary oxytocin following art activities in ASD children was significantly higher than that in TD children. In contrast, the change rate of salivary cortisol after participatory art activities was similar between the two groups. These results suggest that the beneficial effects of participatory art activities may be partially mediated by oxytocin release, and may have therapeutic potential for disorders involving social dysfunction.

Keywords: autism spectrum disorder; oxytocin; cortisol; group activity; stress; art

1. Introduction

Autism spectrum disorder (ASD) is estimated to occur in 1 in 160 children worldwide [1]; ASD tends to begin in childhood and tends to persist for life. Deficits in social skills are the defining symptoms of ASD [2], which greatly impede the ability of individuals to function in community settings throughout their lives. Effective social interaction is essential for building friendships and avoiding unnecessary aversive interactions with peers during the early years, while communication with coworkers and customers is necessary for successful work performance in adults. Thus, social deficits are likely to lead ASD individuals to socially withdraw or isolate. Despite these serious consequences of social deficits in ASD, there is currently no medication to attenuate the impairment of social behaviors.

Moreover, in many cases, depression and anxiety accompany social deficits and other core symptoms of ASD such as repetitive behaviors and a narrow range of interests [2,3]. Therefore, numerous studies have focused on the hypothalamic–pituitary–adrenal (HPA) axis with regard to level of cortisol (CORT), which is frequently used as a stress biomarker [4]. The HPA axis is a highly regulated system that enables stress adaptation and diurnal rhythm, and CORT is secreted when the HPA axis is activated [5,6]. Previous studies have shown that in children with ASD, diurnal rhythm of CORT differs from that in typically developed (TD) children; in addition, children with ASD exhibit hyperresponsive CORT secretions in the social evaluative context or social situations [7]. Dysfunction of the HPA axis has been shown to negatively affect mental health in TD children and children with ASD [3,8]. Thus, management of stress in children with ASD may help decrease the risk of a concurrent mental disorder.

Recently, the therapeutic use of oxytocin (OT), which has a diverse role in mammalian social behaviors, has gained increasing attention. OT is a nonapeptide produced by the hypothalamic neurons in the brain. It is released to the bloodstream to reach peripheral organs or within the hypothalamic and other limbic regions of the brain [9]. The involvement of OT in social recognition, selective social bonding, attachment, anxiety, and stress coping has been demonstrated in a considerable amount of animal studies [9,10]. Indeed, mice that have a deficiency in OT release, such as OT null mice or CD38 knockout mice, are unable to recognize previously encountered conspecifics [11,12]. Furthermore, OT has been shown to be important for mate-bonding in monogamous prairie voles [13], as well as in parent-infant bonding in prairie voles, sheep, and primates [14,15]. The OT system is activated in stressful, challenging, and threatening conditions, and functions to facilitate stress coping [9]. OT has also been implicated in human emotions and social behaviors [14]; for instance, physical interaction between parents and infants increase endogenous OT in both the mother and father, and the increase in OT correlates with the level of affectionate behavior of the mother [15].

Exogenously administered OT has been shown to modulate social behaviors, stress, and anxiety both in healthy individuals and in patients with neuropsychiatric disorders [16]. Moreover, intranasal administration of OT affects social perception, in that it improves discrimination of facial expressions [17,18] and increases the gaze to the eye region [19]. In addition, OT application has been previously shown to enhance feelings of trust [20] and generosity [21]. Thus, the peripheral application of OT has been considered a potentially effective therapeutic treatment for autism and schizophrenia; however, recent clinical trials have shown conflicting results [22]. Although this is in part due to the underpowered design of the trials, the use of exogenous OT as a therapeutic agent is questionable given it has low blood brain barrier permeability and metabolic stability in plasma [23]. Therefore, nonpharmacological interventions that increase endogenous OT are needed to ameliorate the social deficit of patients with ASD, especially those that can effectively stimulate the release of OT in the brain.

The World Health Organization (WHO) recently summarized how art-based interventions can help improve health and well-being, as well as contribute to the prevention of, and recovery from mental and physical illness [24]. Participatory art, in which participants engage in creative activities during social interaction, is known for its beneficial effects on physical health and emotional well-being [25,26]. In fact, the experience of participating in the creative process itself improves mental health conditions, thereby building resilience, boosting social and communicative skills, and improving self-confidence [26–28]. More broadly, such activities are included in social prescribing, an emerging intervention modality that has garnered interest and attention in the academic and clinical communities [29]. With participatory art, as well as social prescribing, the approach to treating various health ailments is holistic and practical, whereby activities such as art, exercising, and gardening are supervised by trained specialists, many of whom are nonclinicians [30]. Because ASD is a neurodevelopmental disorder for which no specific intervention has been established, such activities may provide valuable coping mechanisms across the life span for those affected and their families.

In the present study, we conducted the preliminary study to investigate whether the salivary OT level changes following participation in visual art-based activities in ASD and typically developed (TD) children. Because ASD individuals often struggle to adapt to changes or a new environment, we also measured the salivary CORT level, which is often used as a psychological stress biomarker. To the best of our knowledge, this is the first study to assess the neuroendocrinological changes in individuals who have taken part in participatory art activities.

2. Materials and Methods

2.1. Participants

For this study, 10 TD children (aged 8–9 years) and 13 children (8–13 years) with ASD were recruited. All the children were volunteers; however, all children did not participate in all five sessions of visual art-based participatory workshops, and the data from children who participated less than twice were not used for analysis. Four boys and 4 girls, aged 8–9 years, who were TD and 11 boys and 1 girl, aged 8–13 years, who had ASD were analyzed (Table 1). ASD was diagnosed by children's psychiatrists or pediatricians, who used criteria from the American Psychiatric Association's Diagnostic and Statistical Manual of Mental Disorders, Fourth Edition, Text Revision (DSM-IV-TR) or Fifth Edition (DSM-V) or from the International Statistical Classification of Diseases and Related Health Problems, 10th edition (ICD-10). The evaluations included IQ testing, behavioral observation, and questionnaires; depending on the child, the Childhood Autism Rating Scale (CARS), Autism Diagnostic Observation Schedule (ADOS), Diagnostic Interview for Social and Communication Disorders (DISCO), or Pervasive Developmental Disorders Autism Society Japan Rating Scale (PARS) was used.

Table 1. Age, mean scores of Early Symptomatic Syndromes Eliciting Neurodevelopmental Clinical Examinations-Questionnaire (ESSENCE-Q) and education for each group of children.

	TD	ASD
Numbers	8 (male: 4, female: 4)	12 (male: 11, female: 1)
Age	96–119 months mean: 107, SD: 6.9	113–162 months mean: 135, SD: 16.7
ESSENCE-Q	Yes: 0.4, Maybe/A Little: 0.1/0.3	Yes: 2.83, Maybe/A Little: 1.58/2.83
Education	regular class	regular or special needs classes or special education support classes

The participants' parents were asked to respond to the Early Symptomatic Syndromes Eliciting Neurodevelopmental Clinical Examinations-Questionnaire (ESSENCE-Q) in order to screen the current status of TD children and children with ASD. The ESSENCE-Q is a brief screening questionnaire established specifically for the purpose of shortening the identification process of a wide variety of neurodevelopmental problems [31].

Among the children with ASD, 10 were enrolled in either regular or special needs classes at local schools in Japan. The other 2 children in this group were students at special support education schools.

2.2. Ethics Statement

The study was approved as a noninvasive medical study by Kanazawa University Graduate School of Medicine in 2018 (approval number #2790-2). The study was performed according to the Declaration of Helsinki and the Ethical Guidelines for Clinical Studies of the Ministry of Health, Labor and Welfare of Japan. After the children and their parents had been given a complete explanation of the study, they provided written informed consent. The participants were informed that they could choose not to supply their saliva on each occasion, even after agreeing to participate in the study.

2.3. Visual Art-Based Participatory Art Workshop

During the visual art-based participatory art workshops, participants created their own original stories and made characters and props with different kind of materials. Then participants used the Smoovie application on an iPad (Apple, Inc., Cupertino, CA, USA) to make their own movies with short stop-motion animation. The subjects of their stories varied from their everyday life to the objects that surrounded them; the theme of the project was fully participant led. The aim of this workshop was to let the participants express themselves as freely as possible and not to make them feel as if they were working on a school task or a job. We provided arts and crafts materials that stimulated different senses—paper (colored, textured, plain; different weights of paper), fabric (patterned, textured), tape (washi tape, colored tape), soft clay (colored, neutral), soft construction material (bubble wrap, wrapping material, cardboard), glue (hot glue gun, glue stick), paint, colored pens, and decorative material (sequins, gems, buttons).

The facilitators and supporters of the art workshop set up a comfortable venue, prepared the tools, explained how to use them, and provided a variety of materials. The art workshops conducted in this study were facilitated by a visual artist and supported by the art faculty, students from the University of the Arts, and a staff member who is licensed in special education. During the activity, the organizers interacted with the participants as and when appropriate and encouraged them throughout the creative processes of generating ideas and producing animations.

2.4. Assessment

The visual art-based participatory art workshops were held five times between 22 July–10 August in 2018 and 2019. The workshops in 2018 were held from 14:30–16:30, while those in 2019 were held from 14:00–15:30. Sessions for TD children and ASD children were organized separately. The saliva samples were collected within 10 min of arrival, and just after the participatory art was finished. The percentage of salivary OT or CORT for each session was determined as (concentration after session/concentration before session) × 100. The total number of sessions analyzed before and after the art workshop and the percentage after the workshops for TD and ASD group were 33 and 42, respectively. The personal average percentage after the workshops was calculated as a mean percentage of all the sessions that each child participated (8 subjects for TD group and 12 subjects for ASD group).

2.5. Saliva Collection and Analysis

The saliva samples (0.3–1.0 mL) were collected in a sterile 50 mL polypropylene tube (Greiner Bio-one Co. Ltd., Tokyo, Japan), and were immediately placed in ice for storage at −20 °C. Three to 5 days later, the samples were thawed and centrifuged twice at 4 °C at 1500× g for 10 min. The samples were divided into 1.5-mL microtubes, each containing 100 µL, and kept again at −80 °C until required for the assay. The salivary OT level was measured using a 96-plate commercial OT-ELISA kit (Enzo Life Sciences, Farmingdale, NY, USA), as described previously [32–34]. The measurements were performed in duplicate. Samples (100 µL) without fractionation were treated according to the manufacturer's instructions. The optical density of the samples and standards was measured at wavelengths of 405 nm by a microplate reader (Bio-Rad, Richmond, CA, USA). The salivary CORT level was measured using a cortisol enzyme immunoassay kit (Salimetrics, State College, PA, USA) as previously described [35].

Samples (25 µL) were treated according to the manufacturer's instructions. The optical density of the samples and standards were measured at wavelengths of 450 nm by a microplate reader (Bio-Rad, Richmond, CA, USA). Measurements were performed in duplicate. Sample concentrations were calculated according to the relevant standard curve. The intraassay and interassay coefficients were <12.4% and <12.1%, respectively.

2.6. Statistical Analysis

Statistical analysis was performed using Prism 8 software (GraphPad Software Inc., San Diego, CA, USA). Wilcoxon rank-sum tests were used to compare the levels of salivary OT or CORT of TD children with children with ASD before and after each visual art-based workshop session. The Mann–Whitney U test was used to compare the average percentage of OT or CORT of TD children with children with ASD after each session. Two-tailed student's t test was used to assess the personal average percentage of salivary OT or CORT after each session in which a child participated. All data were calculated as means ± standard errors of the means. In all analyses, $p < 0.05$ was considered statistically significant.

3. Results

The salivary OT level after each session of visual art-based participatory art workshop showed a significant decrease in the TD group (before, 161.5 ± 19.4 pg/mL, after 136.6 ± 16.0 pg/mL; $p = 0.015$) (Figure 1a), whereas there was no significant difference in the ASD group (before 167.9 ± 17.9 pg/mL, after 175.5 ± 16.4 pg/mL; $p = 0.880$) (Figure 1a). However, the average percentage of salivary OT after each session of the ASD group was significantly higher than that of the TD group (TD, 90.8% ± 6.9%; ASD, 127.9% ± 11.8%; $p = 0.024$) (Figure 1b). Also, the personal average percentage of salivary OT after each participated session of the ASD group was significantly higher than that of the TD group (TD, 88.4% ± 4.8%; ASD, 134.5% ± 15.6%; $p = 0.03$) (Figure 1c).

The concentrations of salivary cortisol were not significantly different before and after the participatory art workshop in either the TD or ASD group (Figure 2a). No significant difference was observed between the TD and ASD groups with regards to the average percentage after each session, and/or in the average percentage of personal salivary CORT after each session (Figure 2b,c).

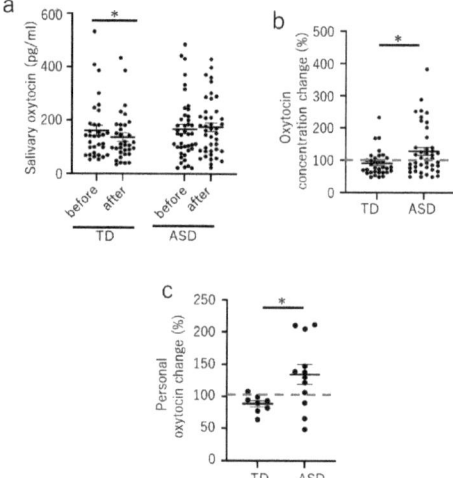

Figure 1. The salivary oxytocin levels before and after participatory art workshops. (**a**). Salivary oxytocin level before and after each session in the typically developed (TD) children and those with autism spectrum disorder (ASD). Note that not all children attended all five sessions of the art workshop (total number of sessions analyzed: 33 for the TD children and 42 for the children with ASD). (**b**). Percentage of salivary oxytocin in the TD children and those with ASD after each session. Note that not all children attended all five sessions of the art workshop (total number of sessions analyzed—33 for the TD children and 42 for the children with ASD). (**c**). Personal average percentage of salivary oxytocin level after each session in the TD and ASD groups (number of children assessed: TD, $n = 8$; ASD, $n = 12$). Data are mean ± sem. * $p < 0.05$.

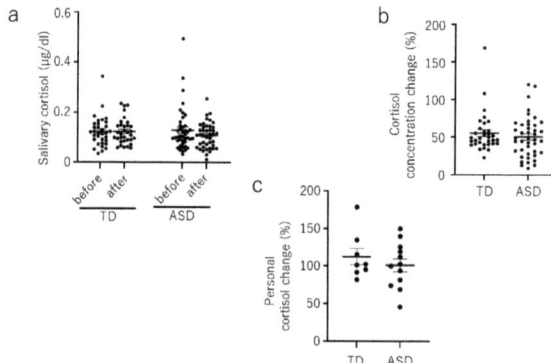

Figure 2. The salivary cortisol level before and after participatory art workshop. (**a**). Salivary cortisol level before and after each session in the TD and ASD groups. Note that not all children attended all five sessions of the art workshop (total number of sessions analyzed—33 for the TD children and 42 for the children with ASD). (**b**). Percentage of salivary cortisol after each session in the TD and ASD groups. Note that not all children attended all five sessions of the art workshop (total number of sessions analyzed—33 for the TD children and 42 for the children with ASD). (**c**). Personal average percentage of salivary cortisol level after each session in the TD and ASD groups (number of children assessed: TD, $n = 8$; ASD, $n = 12$). Data are mean ± sem.

4. Discussion

The current trial was a pioneering study to assess salivary OT and CORT concentrations in ASD and TD children in response to a positive social activity, participatory arts. Although we could not detect a statistical difference in OT levels after each session in the ASD group, the average percentage of salivary OT after each session, and the personal average percentage of salivary OT after each session were increased in ASD children. However, no significant difference in the cortisol level was detected before and after participatory art activities in either the ASD or TD group. Since the cortisol level did not change significantly during the participatory art activities, we suggest that OT is released as a result of positive social activities, rather than a response to stress.

Because all the children participated voluntarily in the visual art-based participatory art workshop, the TD children were expected not to feel anxious or stressed about their participation, and we initially assumed that their OT levels would increase after participatory art activities. However, the OT level decreased instead. As the CORT level in TD children did not change significantly, the decrease in the OT level may not be a result of the stress response. Because both groups of children enjoyed the art activities, the results suggest that the TD children may have felt driven to complete their artwork, which corresponded with a decrease in the OT level afterwards. A decrease in OT levels has been suggested to reflect a reduction in social qualities of attention or, more broadly, in social interaction [36]. In our case, the decrease in the TD group may correspond to a shift in attention upon completion of their work. The children with ASD, on the other hand, required the experience to form a part of their routine over the course of the workshop attendance and may have gained more pleasure out of the process of creativity. It has been reported that attention systems are disrupted and atypical in children with ASD [37]. It is possible that our participants with ASD required more sessions than the TD children in order to understand the structure of the workshops and to focus on their creative activities. Alternatively, there might have been an increase in the OT level in TD children during the activities, but the time course may have differed from that observed in the children with ASD. Larger sample sizes and further follow up will allow a better understanding of the process.

Our preliminary study had several limitations. First, the study was designed to examine the immediate OT response of participatory art activity. Although the percentage change of OT level was increased in ASD children, we failed to show a statistical difference in the salivary OT level before and after each of the workshop due to the modest sample size and the large variance in the OT concentration. Therefore, it is necessary to conduct a further trial with a larger sample size of ASD children to obtain reliable data. Second, we did not include any psychological, emotional, or behavioral measurement that may be relevant to the OT response. As shown in Figure 1c, there is a diverse variability in the personal percentage change in ASD children compared to the TD children; as a result, we need to conduct a further study to elucidate the correlation between the traits of children and the OT responsiveness to participatory art activities. Third, it is worth pointing out that our study did not include a control condition in order to disentangle the potential effect of participatory art from other more generic activities involving crafting or animation making. Such a control could have simply involved being in the premise for the workshop sessions, as in a wait-list group. However, each workshop typically required the entire duration of the children's visit in terms of staff cover and their families who need to fit in taking and collecting their children. Staffs and participants were all volunteers and we faced several practical difficulties which prevented from adding this important aspect to our design this time. We will be mindful for exploring options for adding the control in our future work.

The WHO recently summarized how art interventions can help improve health and well-being, and can help to prevent both mental and physical illness [24]. They also stated that while art is conceptually difficult to define, it is important to verify the effectiveness of art. Indeed, although a wide variety of studies use diverse methodologies, these are often based on psychological tests or subjective feedback. Our study aimed to capture the fluctuations in the neuroendocrine response to participatory art activities. In the future study, we will investigate the association of the neuroendocrine response and the traits of children in order to elucidate for whom and in what aspect participatory art activities can be effective. We will also evaluate the effectiveness of participatory arts activities in the long term. Further, experience in multi-sensory processing has been showing some promising results in children with autism spectrum disorders [38]. Given that crafting and creative activities are familiar and popular in typical as well as atypical development, it would be an important agenda to study the therapeutic role of multi-sensory experiences involved in activities such as participatory art. Ultimately, we would like to utilize our research findings related to the use of neuroendocrine responses in combination with psychological, emotional, or behavioral measurement to establish a method to verify the effectiveness of participatory art activities.

In the current study, ELISA was used to measure the saliva OT concentrations; however, with this technique, there remains the issue of antibody specificity. The antibody may not only detect the free form of the target analyte, but different forms, such as precursors and metabolites, or a form within other protein complexes. These phenomena may partially explain the differences in values observed between different ELISA kits, as well as between ELISA and HPLC-MS or radio immunoassay. Indeed, our detected OT concentration range is one digit higher than that reported by other studies [15,39,40]. However, since we have detected the relative change in salivary OT in the context of physical interaction and/or in social interaction [32,34,41], although the values may not be reflecting the absolute physiological value of free OT, the relative change in monitored values are likely to be comparable.

In conclusion, the current experiment was designed to assess salivary OT and CORT concentrations in ASD and TD children in response to participation in visual art-based activities, since art is known to improve mental and physical health and overall quality of life. We demonstrated increased OT release after participatory art activities that was unrelated to the stress response. Thus, our case study is the first to show the biological link between the social experience of participatory art and its positive psychosocial effects.

Author Contributions: S.T., A.K., A.I.-S. have contributed equally to this work. S.T. and C.T. recruited the participants; S.T., A.K., A.I.-S., M.R. and C.T. conceived and designed the experiments; S.T., A.K., A.I.-S., M.R., A.N., K.M., M.K., and O.A. performed and organized art workshop; T.Y. performed saliva assay; T.T., C.T., H.H. analyzed the data and data interpretation; H.H. contributed to provide analytical tools; C.T. prepared the initial draft and M.R. and C.T. revised the manuscript. All authors have read and agreed to the published version of the manuscript.

Funding: This research is supported by grants from The Great Britain Sasakawa Foundation Grant and JST COI Grant No. JPMJCE1310, the Center of Innovation Program from Japan Science and Technology Agency, JST.

Conflicts of Interest: The authors declare no conflict of interest.

References

1. Elsabbagh, M.; Divan, G.; Koh, Y.J.; Kim, Y.S.; Kauchali, S.; Marcin, C.; Montiel-Nava, C.; Patel, V.; Paula, C.S.; Wang, C.; et al. Global prevalence of autism and other pervasive developmental disorders. *Autism Res.* **2012**, *5*, 160–179. [CrossRef]
2. Geschwind, D.H. Advances in autism. *Annu. Rev. Med.* **2009**, *60*, 367–380. [CrossRef]
3. Simonoff, E.; Pickles, A.; Charman, T.; Chandler, S.; Loucas, T.; Baird, G. Psychiatric disorders in children with autism spectrum disorders: Prevalence, comorbidity, and associated factors in a population-derived sample. *J. Am. Acad. Child. Adolesc. Psychiatry* **2008**, *47*, 921–929. [CrossRef]
4. Hellhammer, D.H.; Wust, S.; Kudielka, B.M. Salivary cortisol as a biomarker in stress research. *Psychoneuroendocrinology* **2009**, *34*, 163–171. [CrossRef]
5. Chrousos, G.P. Stress and disorders of the stress system. *Nat. Rev. Endocrinol.* **2009**, *5*, 374–381. [CrossRef]
6. de Kloet, E.R.; Joels, M.; Holsboer, F. Stress and the brain: From adaptation to disease. *Nat. Rev. Neurosci.* **2005**, *6*, 463–475. [CrossRef]
7. Taylor, J.L.; Corbett, B.A. A review of rhythm and responsiveness of cortisol in individuals with autism spectrum disorders. *Psychoneuroendocrinology* **2014**, *49*, 207–228. [CrossRef]
8. Shirtcliff, E.A.; Essex, M.J. Concurrent and Longitudinal Associations of Basal and Diurnal Cortisol with Mental Health Symptoms in Early Adolescence. *Dev. Psychobiol.* **2008**, *50*, 690–703. [CrossRef]

9. Jurek, B.; Neumann, I.D. The Oxytocin Receptor: From Intracellular Signaling to Behavior. *Physiol. Rev.* **2018**, *98*, 1805–1908. [CrossRef]
10. Modi, M.E.; Young, L.J. The oxytocin system in drug discovery for autism: Animal models and novel therapeutic strategies. *Horm. Behav.* **2012**, *61*, 340–350. [CrossRef]
11. Ferguson, J.N.; Young, L.J.; Hearn, E.F.; Matzuk, M.M.; Insel, T.R.; Winslow, J.T. Social amnesia in mice lacking the oxytocin gene. *Nat. Genet.* **2000**, *25*, 284–288. [CrossRef]
12. Jin, D.; Liu, H.X.; Hirai, H.; Torashima, T.; Nagai, T.; Lopatina, O.; Shnayder, N.A.; Yamada, K.; Noda, M.; Seike, T.; et al. CD38 is critical for social behaviour by regulating oxytocin secretion. *Nature* **2007**, *446*, 41–45. [CrossRef]
13. Tabbaa, M.; Paedae, B.; Liu, Y.; Wang, Z. Neuropeptide Regulation of Social Attachment: The Prairie Vole Model. *Compr. Physiol.* **2016**, *7*, 81–104. [CrossRef]
14. Feldman, R. Oxytocin and social affiliation in humans. *Horm. Behav.* **2012**, *61*, 380–391. [CrossRef]
15. Feldman, R.; Gordon, I.; Schneiderman, I.; Weisman, O.; Zagoory-Sharon, O. Natural variations in maternal and paternal care are associated with systematic changes in oxytocin following parent-infant contact. *Psychoneuroendocrinology* **2010**, *35*, 1133–1141. [CrossRef]
16. Andari, E.; Hurlemann, R.; Young, L.J. A Precision Medicine Approach to Oxytocin Trials. *Curr. Top. Behav. Neurosci.* **2018**, *35*, 559–590. [CrossRef]
17. Domes, G.; Heinrichs, M.; Michel, A.; Berger, C.; Herpertz, S.C. Oxytocin improves "mind-reading" in humans. *Biol. Psychiatry* **2007**, *61*, 731–733. [CrossRef]
18. Savaskan, E.; Ehrhardt, R.; Schulz, A.; Walter, M.; Schachinger, H. Post-learning intranasal oxytocin modulates human memory for facial identity. *Psychoneuroendocrinology* **2008**, *33*, 368–374. [CrossRef]
19. Yamasue, H.; Domes, G. Oxytocin and Autism Spectrum Disorders. *Curr. Top. Behav. Neurosci.* **2018**, *35*, 449–465. [CrossRef]
20. Kosfeld, M.; Heinrichs, M.; Zak, P.J.; Fischbacher, U.; Fehr, E. Oxytocin increases trust in humans. *Nature* **2005**, *435*, 673–676. [CrossRef]
21. Zak, P.J.; Stanton, A.A.; Ahmadi, S. Oxytocin increases generosity in humans. *PLoS ONE* **2007**, *2*, e1128. [CrossRef]
22. Young, L.J.; Barrett, C.E. Neuroscience. Can oxytocin treat autism? *Science* **2015**, *347*, 825–826. [CrossRef]
23. Gulliver, D.; Werry, E.; Reekie, T.A.; Katte, T.A.; Jorgensen, W.; Kassiou, M. Targeting the Oxytocin System: New Pharmacotherapeutic Approaches. *Trends Pharmacol. Sci.* **2019**, *40*, 22–37. [CrossRef]
24. Fancourt, D.; Finn, S. *What is the Evidence on the Role of the Arts in Improving Health and Well-Being? A Scoping Review*; (Health Evidence Network (HEN) Synthesis Report 67); WHO Regional Office for Europe: Copenhagen, Denmark, 2019.
25. Hacking, S.; Secker, J.; Kent, L.; Shenton, J.; Spandler, H. Mental health and arts participation: The state of the art in England. *J. R Soc. Promot. Health* **2006**, *126*, 121–127. [CrossRef]
26. Bone, T.A. Art and Mental Health Recovery: Evaluating the Impact of a Community-Based Participatory Arts Program through Artist Voices. *Community Ment Health J.* **2018**, *54*, 1180–1188. [CrossRef]
27. Hacking, S.; Secker, J.; Spandler, H.; Kent, L.; Shenton, J. Evaluating the impact of participatory art projects for people with mental health needs. *Health Soc. Care Community* **2008**, *16*, 638–648. [CrossRef]
28. Stickley, T.; Wright, N.; Slade, M. The art of recovery: Outcomes from participatory arts activities for people using mental health services. *J. Ment. Health* **2018**, *27*, 367–373. [CrossRef]
29. Bickerdike, L.; Booth, A.; Wilson, P.M.; Farley, K.; Wright, K. Social prescribing: Less rhetoric and more reality. A systematic review of the evidence. *BMJ Open* **2017**, *7*, e013384. [CrossRef]
30. Toma, M.; Morris, J.; Kelly, C.; Jinal-Snape, D. *The Impact of Art Attendance and Participation on Health and Wellbeing: Systematic Literature Review (Work Package 1)*; Glasgow Centre for Population Health: Glasgow, UK, 2014.
31. Hatakenaka, Y.; Fernell, E.; Sakaguchi, M.; Ninomiya, H.; Fukunaga, I.; Gillberg, C. ESSENCE-Q-a first clinical validation study of a new screening questionnaire for young children with suspected neurodevelopmental problems in south Japan. *Neuropsychiatr. Dis. Treat.* **2016**, *12*, 1739–1746. [CrossRef]
32. Tsuji, S.; Yuhi, T.; Furuhara, K.; Ohta, S.; Shimizu, Y.; Higashida, H. Salivary oxytocin concentrations in seven boys with autism spectrum disorder received massage from their mothers: A pilot study. *Front. Psychiatry* **2015**, *6*, 58. [CrossRef]
33. MacLean, E.L.; Gesquiere, L.R.; Gee, N.; Levy, K.; Martin, W.L.; Carter, C.S. Validation of salivary oxytocin and vasopressin as biomarkers in domestic dogs. *J. Neurosci. Methods* **2018**, *293*, 67–76. [CrossRef]

34. Yuhi, T.; Ise, K.; Iwashina, K.; Terao, N.; Yoshioka, S.; Shomura, K.; Maehara, T.; Yazaki, A.; Koichi, K.; Furuhara, K.; et al. Sex Differences in Salivary Oxytocin and Cortisol Concentration Changes during Cooking in a Small Group. *Behav. Sci.* **2018**, *8*, 101. [CrossRef]
35. Kumazaki, H.; Warren, Z.; Corbett, B.A.; Yoshikawa, Y.; Matsumoto, Y.; Higashida, H.; Yuhi, T.; Ikeda, T.; Ishiguro, H.; Kikuchi, M. Android Robot-Mediated Mock Job Interview Sessions for Young Adults with Autism Spectrum Disorder: A Pilot Study. *Front. Psychiatry* **2017**, *8*. [CrossRef]
36. Nishizato, M.; Fujisawa, T.X.; Kosaka, H.; Tomoda, A. Developmental changes in social attention and oxytocin levels in infants and children. *Sci. Rep. UK* **2017**, *7*. [CrossRef]
37. Guillon, Q.; Hadjikhani, N.; Baduel, S.; Roge, B. Visual social attention in autism spectrum disorder: Insights from eye tracking studies. *Neurosci. Biobehav. Rev.* **2014**, *42*, 279–297. [CrossRef]
38. Case-Smith, J.; Weaver, L.L.; Fristad, M.A. A systematic review of sensory processing interventions for children with autism spectrum disorders. *Autism* **2015**, *19*, 133–148. [CrossRef]
39. Schladt, T.M.; Nordmann, G.C.; Emilius, R.; Kudielka, B.M.; de Jong, T.R.; Neumann, I.D. Choir versus Solo Singing: Effects on Mood, and Salivary Oxytocin and Cortisol Concentrations. *Front. Hum. Neurosci.* **2017**, *11*, 430. [CrossRef]
40. Jong, T.R.; Menon, R.; Bludau, A.; Grund, T.; Biermeier, V.; Klampfl, S.M.; Jurek, B.; Bosch, O.J.; Hellhammer, J.; Neumann, I.D. Salivary oxytocin concentrations in response to running, sexual self-stimulation, breastfeeding and the TSST: The Regensburg Oxytocin Challenge (ROC) study. *Psychoneuroendocrinology* **2015**, *62*, 381–388. [CrossRef]
41. Yuhi, T.; Kyuta, H.; Mori, H.A.; Murakami, C.; Furuhara, K.; Okuno, M.; Takahashi, M.; Fuji, D.; Higashida, H. Salivary Oxytocin Concentration Changes during a Group Drumming Intervention for Maltreated School Children. *Brain Sci.* **2017**, *7*, 152. [CrossRef]

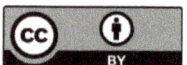

© 2020 by the authors. Licensee MDPI, Basel, Switzerland. This article is an open access article distributed under the terms and conditions of the Creative Commons Attribution (CC BY) license (http://creativecommons.org/licenses/by/4.0/).

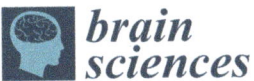 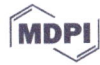

Article

Tele-Assisted Behavioral Intervention for Families with Children with Autism Spectrum Disorders: A Randomized Control Trial

Flavia Marino, Paola Chilà, Chiara Failla, Ilaria Crimi, Roberta Minutoli, Alfio Puglisi, Antonino Andrea Arnao, Gennaro Tartarisco, Liliana Ruta, David Vagni [†] and Giovanni Pioggia *,[†]

Institute for Biomedical Research and Innovation (IRIB), National Research Council of Italy (CNR), 98164 Messina, Italy; flavia.marino@cnr.it (F.M.); paola.chila@irib.cnr.it (P.C.); chiara.failla@irib.cnr.it (C.F.); ilaria.crimi@irib.cnr.it (I.C.); roberta.minutoli@irib.cnr.it (R.M.); alfio.puglisi@irib.cnr.it (A.P.); antoninoandrea.arnao@cnr.it (A.A.A.); gennaro.tartarisco@cnr.it (G.T.); liliana.ruta@irib.cnr.it (L.R.); david.vagni@cnr.it (D.V.)
* Correspondence: giovanni.pioggia@cnr.it
† These authors contributed equally to the study.

Received: 24 August 2020; Accepted: 16 September 2020; Published: 18 September 2020

Abstract: Background: Telehealth is useful for both autism spectrum disorder (ASD) diagnosis and treatment, but studies with a direct comparison between teletherapy and traditional in-person therapy are limited. Methods: This randomized control trial—ISRCTN (International Standard Randomised Controlled Trial Number) primary clinical trial registry ID ISRCTN15312724—was aimed at comparing the effect of a tele-assisted and in-person intervention based on a behavioral intervention protocol for families with children affected by ASDs. Forty-two parents with children with autism (30 months to 10 years old) were randomly assigned to 12 sessions of an applied behavioral analysis (ABA) intervention implemented in an individual and group setting, either with or without the inclusion of tele-assistance. Pre- and postintervention assessments were conducted using the Home Situation Questionnaire (HSQ-ASD) and the Parental Stress Index (PSI/SF). Results: Substantial improvements in the perception and management of children's behavior by parents, as well as in the influence of a reduction in parent stress levels on said children's behavior through the use of a tele-assisted intervention, were obtained. Conclusions: This randomized controlled trial demonstrates the evidence-based potential for telehealth to improve treatment of ASDs.

Keywords: telehealth; ASD; ABA; behavioral intervention; RCT

1. Introduction

Social communication deficits and restricted and repetitive interests and behaviors are the core symptom domains of autism spectrum disorders (ASDs) [1,2]. In addition, language, perceptual and sensory processing abnormalities, as well as delays in ASD detection and access to care during the crucial toddler years, remain unique challenges [3,4]. Nevertheless, intensive evidence-based treatments supported by parent-mediated interventions are crucial to obtain improvements in the developmental trajectories and functional outcomes of children with ASDs [5]. Telehealth represents a new technology able to emphasize the strengths of current treatment methods [4,6], mainly because it offers: (i) possible remote diagnostic methods with a consequent reduction in the delay in ASD detection; (ii) a continuous and ubiquitary access to care for families with children with autism; (iii) the chance to directly involve family members in the child's development by actively applying effective parent-mediated interventions.

Telehealth is defined by the Global Health Observatory (GHO) of the WHO as the delivery of healthcare services, where patients and providers are separated by distance [7]. Information and communication technologies are used to interact directly with both clinicians and algorithms. Telehealth is also used for exchanging information to enable the diagnosis and treatment of diseases and injuries, as well as for improving patient access to quality, cost-effective, health services, wherever they may be. It is especially relevant for vulnerable groups [7].

Telehealth is a delivery model demonstrating the potential to deliver early intervention services effectively and efficiently, thereby improving access and reducing the impact of resources shortages in underserved areas. The use of a telehealth delivery model facilitates interdisciplinarity and services coordination, and it also makes possible the consultation with specialists not available within a local community [8].

Despite the undeniable advantages of telehealth and the interest in exploring the feasibility of implementing telehealth-supported behavioral interventions, the number of papers suggesting its effectiveness with children or adults with ASDs are extremely limited in the literature [3,6,9–12]. Recent findings of a scoping review [3] show the potential for telehealth to improve access for the assessment and diagnosis of ASDs, even in the very early diagnostic stages. A recent systematic literature review analyzed 28 studies reporting how telehealth is useful for both diagnosis and treatment in the case of ASDs [9], and the authors concluded that more research is needed before considering telehealth as an efficacious evidence-based treatment model. This seems mainly due to the shortage of direct comparisons between on-site and online teletherapy with ASDs [6]. The most widely used implementation is parent training programs for families with children with ASDs in order to increase their knowledge about the condition, to suggest behavioral intervention strategies to manage the children's inadequate behaviors in everyday life, and to recommend psychotherapy for parents to ameliorate their emotional burden and to reduce their stress levels. In various studies, the objective of telehealth has been to make parents competent, as well as to ensure that they are able to perform a functional analysis of their children's behavior and to learn functional communication techniques. Such objectives are usually achieved through dedicated remote training with the support of educational videos, web-based programs, and weekly videoconferencing coaching sessions with an operator [3,9–12]. The results show that, in the case of direct training with a behavioral analyst, parents become competent and increase their ability to perform a functional analysis and to use functional communication techniques. Thus, telematic tools become effective, acceptable, and usable for the parents [3,6,9,12–17]. The application of these techniques by parents makes it possible to reduce the inadequate behavior of children, with a peak reduction greater than 90%, and to improve the children's social communication skills.

2. Materials and Methods

To contribute to the growing research of telehealth applied to ASDs, in this paper, we aimed to investigate the feasibility and efficacy of a tele-assisted parent-mediated intervention for children with ASD in the context of an applied behavior analysis (ABA)-based treatment [9,18]. We compared, in a randomized controlled trial (RCT), the efficacy of the parent-mediated intervention that was delivered via telehealth or in-person approaches. The RCT is registered with ID ISRCTN15312724 at the ISRCTN (International Standard Randomised Controlled Trial Number) primary clinical trial registry—http://www.isrctn.com/ISRCTN15312724. Using tele-interventions, we aim at reducing parental distress due to commute time, strict schedules and unfamiliar environments. Furthermore, we aim to create a higher family engagement in the therapy and foster skills generalization in the home context.

We hypothesize that the parents of children on the autism spectrum randomly assigned to the tele-assisted intervention will perceive (1) a decrease in the severity of disruptive and noncompliant behavior in their children after the intervention and (2) that their children become easier to manage compared to children on the autism spectrum who undergo the intervention without telehealth assistance, and that he/she will show (3) lower parental distress and (4) improvements in the parent–child functional interaction.

The tele-assisted intervention was designed and implemented through a web platform, providing video conference tools and ABA assignments for parents that included cues, prompts, and reinforcements. The tele-assisted intervention was planned by chartered ABA psychotherapists, well-experienced in parent coaching and treatment, who delivered the intervention to both groups. The psychotherapists were teamed with bioengineers who implemented the intervention protocol via a web platform. The web platform was developed within the G Suite, a suite of cloud computing, productivity, and collaboration tools, software, and products developed by Google (https://gsuite.google.com).

2.1. Applied Behavior Analysis Therapy for Autism Spectrum Disorders

The ABA method studies particular dynamic interactions between the organism and its environment, and this method has been adapted to improve challenging behaviors in children with ASDs [18,19]. ABA therapy for autism is usually administered with a high intensity and used to achieve specific, measurable goals [19]. In this field, ABA is based on behaviorist theories that state that simple and complex behavior can be taught through a system of rewards and consequences. Most of the time, this therapy is intended to "extinguish" undesirable behaviors and to teach desired behaviors and skills.

ABA focuses on a behavioral approach, making it possible to simultaneously improve behavioral, cognitive, social, and communicative skills [19,20]. This system uses "reinforcement" (i.e., rewards) to motivate children with autism to learn new skills, as well as multiple trials that start with a prompt (i.e., antecedent) to execute the desired behavior. ABA therapy starts with an evaluation to determine a child's challenges and strengths in the areas of behavior, cognition, communication, and social interactions. Then, the ABA therapist sets appropriate goals for the child and recommends a particular number of hours of therapy per week.

The basic structure of an ABA intervention is a set of repeated behavioral trials consisting of an antecedent, behavior, and consequence in discrete trial training (DTT) implementation, while in natural environment teaching (NET), the motivators are selected by the preferences of the children during natural social interactions, while any attempt at compliance is rewarded [21].

Overall, systematic reviews [18,19,21,22] have demonstrated that ABA interventions show promising evidence in terms of efficacy and are a viable intervention for individuals on the autism spectrum, both in telehealth and in-person [9,23], although the variability of the study designs, the heterogeneity of the participants' clinical presentation, and the methodological limitations reduce the generalizability of study findings.

ABA protocols in children and adults on the autism spectrum are individually delivered, with the involvement of family members or in a group-based format. While individual ABA protocols ensure a better personalization of the therapy objectives and strategies to the specific needs and skills of the single subject, group-based ABA interventions take advantage of the influence of social interaction, promoting experience-sharing, improving self-acceptance, and supporting insights of both personal strengths and impairments.

2.2. Inclusion Criteria

The inclusion criteria were as follows: (1) parents of children aged between 30 months and 10 years; (2) a clinical diagnosis of an ASD for the children of the recruited families based on the Diagnostic and Statistical Manual of Mental Disorders-Fifth Edition (DSM-5) criteria from a licensed clinical child neuropsychiatrist; (3) DSM-5 severity scores from moderate (level 2) to severe (level 3) in both the social communication and the restricted interests and repetitive behaviors domains; (4) not being on psychiatric medication; (5) not receiving any other intervention directly related to behavioral skills during the trial.

All children had a previous diagnosis that was further confirmed through the assessment and the consensus of the experienced professionals on the research team (i.e., a child neuropsychiatrist and a clinical psychologist).

2.3. Participants

Families were recruited as part of an ongoing research program and were tested at our clinical facilities. We enrolled $N = 88$ parents of 44 children with ASDs, aged 30 months–10 years. A first screening based on inclusion criteria was implemented, and $n = 74$ parents of children with ASDs were eligible; $n = 36$ (30:6 male/female) children fully met the entry criteria and their parents were enrolled in the present study (Figure 1).

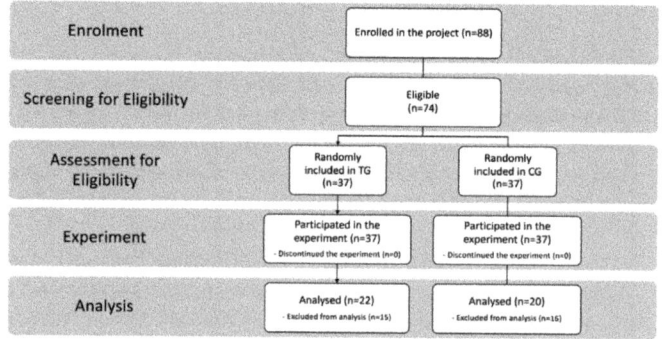

Figure 1. Subject recruitment, assignment, and assessment procedures.

Parents were randomly assigned to the tele-assisted group (TG) or to the control group (CG), applying exactly the same protocol without telehealth assistance. A randomized block design was used to ensure that intervention groups were balanced with respect to gender, age, and developmental quotient (DQ). Finally, another 30 parents were excluded due to missing data. There were no dropouts during the interventions. Data were complete for $N = 20$ parents (9:11 males/females) of $N = 11$ children (9:2 males/females; mean age in months = 69.6; standard deviation (SD) = 32.9; mean DQ = 68.8; SD = 21.4) in the CG and for $N = 22$ parents (10:12 males/females) of $N = 12$ children (10:2 males/females; mean age in months = 69.1; SD = 22.5; mean DQ = 63.8; SD = 16.9) in the experimental group (Table 1).

Table 1. Demographic and clinical characteristics of the sample.

Preintervention Variables			CG (n = 20)		TG (n = 22)		Comparison between Groups				
			M	SD	M	SD	M	SE	t	d.f. *	p-Value
Child Demographic	Age in months		69.6	32.9	69.1	22.5	0.509	8.79	0.058	33.1	0.945
	DQ		68.8	21.4	63.8	16.9	4.93	5.99	0.822	36.1	0.416
Outcome Variables	PSI/SF	PD	30.1	9.31	31.8	10.5	−1.77	3.05	−579	40.0	0.566
		P–CDI	28.6	9.41	29.4	7.09	−0.809	2.59	−0.312	35.2	0.757
		DC	38.2	6.79	40.0	8.50	0.245	2.36	0.104	39.4	0.918
		Total	96.9	13.8	99.2	11.7	−2.33	3.97	−0.588	37.6	0.560
	HSQ-ASD	SI	3.10	1.69	3.68	1.50	−0.577	0.495	−1.17	40.0	0.251
		DS	2.48	1.41	2.46	1.60	0.026	0.465	0.056	40.0	0.956
		Total	2.67	1.34	2.92	1.42	−0.258	0.427	−0.604	40.0	0.549

Developmental Quotient (DQ); Mean (M); Standard Deviation (SD); Standard Error (SE); Parental Stress Index/Short Form (PSI/SF); Home Situation Questionnaire-ASD Version (HSQ-ASD); Parental Distress (PD); Parent–Child Dysfunctional Interaction (P–CDI); Difficult Child (DC); * equal variance not assumed.

All of the above-mentioned children were attending mainstream public schools for 27 h a week, with a special teacher for 10–12 h. All children were Italian.

All children were scored at or above the clinical cut-off on the Autism Diagnostic Observation Schedule, Second Edition (ADOS-2), module three. The child psychologist collected information from parents concerning developmental milestones (including joint attention, social interaction, pretend play, and repetitive behaviors, with an onset prior to 3 years of age) and current behaviors.

2.4. Intervention Protocols

The protocol consisted of three consecutive phases. In phase I, all of the enrolled parents received 12 2 h-long plenary sessions of informative parent training about ASD characteristics and ABA/behavioral principles. The intervention protocol then consisted of two consecutive sections of 12 weeks each, i.e., phases II and III. The present study reports the results of the phase III comparison between CG and TG groups.

Phase II lasted 12 weeks. In phase II, all of the enrolled parents received 2 h/week of group behavioral therapy administered in homogeneous groups (based on the developmental age, target behaviors, and ASD level of their children). In this phase, all of the children of the enrolled parents received 1 h/week of one-to-one ABA therapy, where parents were allowed and invited to observe the therapists during treatment sessions.

Phase III lasted 12 weeks. In phase III, the intervention protocol consisted of the administration of 2 h/week of tele-assisted one-to-one behavioral parent training and coaching to participants belonging to the TG, while 2 h/week of in-person one-to-one behavioral parent training and couching was administered to participants belonging to the CG.

All of the therapies were administered by a clinical psychologist with a postmaster's degree in behavioral modification and analysis. Considering the usual ABA protocols last 25–40 h/week, our protocol can be considered to be low intensity. Testing the efficacy of low-intensity protocols, mediated by parents in natural environments, is of the utmost importance to develop more efficient implementations.

2.5. Ethics

All subjects gave their informed consent for inclusion before they participated in the study. The study was conducted in accordance with the Declaration of Helsinki, and the protocol was approved by the Ethic Committee of the Research Ethics and Bioethics Committee (http://www.cnr.it/ethics) of the National Research Council of Italy (CNR) (Prot. N. CNR-AMMCEN 54444/2018 01/08/2018). All of the parents of the children who took part in the study gave their consent to participate in this study, signing a written consent form.

2.6. Outcome Measures

The outcome measures for all of the TG and CG participants were assessed during the weeks before and after the intervention sessions (week 1 and week 12 of phase III, respectively). The general measures were assessed by direct observations of the parents. The primary outcome measurement tools were the Home Situation Questionnaire (HSQ-ASD) [24] and the Parental Stress Index (PSI/SF) [25,26], both of which are objective measures of the perception and influence of children's behavior on the psychological state of their parents. The investigators who assessed the outcome measures were blinded to intervention allocation. There were no significant differences between the prephase III outcome measures of either group (Table 1).

2.6.1. Home Situation Questionnaire (HSQ-ASD)

The HSQ-ASD is a caregiver-rated scale designed to assess the severity of disruptive and noncompliant behavior in children. Its modified and revised version for ASD consists of 27 items describing different situations or settings that are common for children on the spectrum. Parents are asked to indicate whether their children have problems with compliance in these situations and, if so, to rate the severity on a 0–9 Likert scale, with higher scores indicating greater non-compliance. Factor analysis of the questionnaire yielded two distinctive 12-items subscales: (1) Social Inflexibility (SI) ($\alpha = 0.84$) and (2) Demand-Specific (DS) ($\alpha = 0.89$) [24]. The first subscale comprises items regarding compliance with changes in daily social routines, while the second one is related to demand avoidance for daily living tasks. The two subscales are moderately correlated ($r = 0.51$). The subscale totals' test–retest reliability were all significant with $r = 0.57$ for socially inflexible, $r = 0.58$ for demand specific, and $r = 0.57$ for the combined total. Convergent validity was assessed with previously known scales. HSQ-ASD was correlated with scales measuring problem behaviors and daily living skills, while was not correlated with IQ or communication skills.

2.6.2. Parental Stress Index/Short Form (PSI/SF)

The PSI/SF is a self-assessment questionnaire designed for the early identification of factors that can compromise the normal development of a child. The Italian validation of the test affects only the short form (PSI/SF), which derives directly from the extended form, since it contains all entries with identical words. The test is based on the hypothesis that the stress that a parent experiences is the joint result of certain characteristics of their children, the parents themselves, and a series of situations closely related to their parental role. Data relating to the mother have been added to the short form, including age, marital status, education, and profession. This test investigates three main domains of stressors, namely, those associated with the characteristics of the children, those of the parents, and those of situational-demographic events. The short form is composed of 36 items, divided into three subscales: (1) Parental Distress (PD), which taps into parental feelings; (2) Parent–Child Dysfunctional Interaction (P–CDI), which focuses on the perception of the child as not responding to parental expectations; (3) Difficult Child (DC), which is centered on some of the characteristics of the child that make it easy or difficult to manage. The expected time to complete the questionnaire was between 10 and 15 min [25]. Raw total scores above 90 or 33 on the PD and DC subscales and above 27 on the PCDI subscale are considered clinically elevated. Test–retest reliability coefficients of the total stress score have been reported to be $r = 0.84$, for the PD subscale $r = 0.85$, for the PCDI subscale $r = 0.68$ and for the DC subscale $r = 0.78$. For the internal consistency of the PSI/SF, reports for total stress have been $\alpha = 0.91$, for PD $\alpha = 0.87$, for PCDI $\alpha = 0.80$ and for the DC subscale $\alpha = 0.85$. A subsequent study on parents of ASD children [26] found a similar internal consistency: PD $\alpha = 0.91$, for PCDI $\alpha = 0.85$ and for the DC subscale $\alpha = 0.82$ and $\alpha = 0.91$ for the total score.

2.7. Statistical Analysis

After having controlled for multivariate analysis of covariance (MANCOVA) assumptions of normality using the Shapiro–Wilk test and homogeneity using Box's M test of the equality of covariance matrices, parametric statistics were applied in order to analyze the group effects on the intervention. Levene's test of equality of error variances was performed post hoc.

Total HSQ-ASD and PSI/SF scores were used as primary outcome measures, while the single subscales were used as secondary measures. Group and parental gender were used as factors, while child age and DQ, together with the preintervention variables, were used as covariates. A two-sided test with an alpha level of 0.05 was used, after adjustment using the Šidák correction for multiple comparisons. Sensitivity analysis was performed using G*Power 3.1 for MANOVA with 2 groups and 2 factors and 4 covariates. With a total sample size of 42, we can identify large effects with sizes with $f^2(U) > 0.631$. To increase the confidence in the results, we computed 95% bias-corrected confidence intervals for our data using a bias-corrected and accelerated (BCa) bootstrap ($n = 1000$).

Finally, to further explore the intervention effects, as an ancillary analysis we also used a paired t-test between pre- and postintervention variables for each group separately.

The raw data for each participant comprising the demographics and assessment, HSQ-ASD and PSI/SF preintervention and postintervention scores (Table S1), as well as the complete statistics for the assumptions (Tables S2–S5), are provided in the Supplementary Materials, together with the complete analysis of covariance (ANCOVA) for the secondary outcomes variables (Tables S6 and S7), in order to provide an analytical picture of the sample distribution and to allow replicability.

SPSS software (v. 26, IBM Corporation, Armonk, NY, USA) was used to run statistical analyses.

3. Results

The demographic and clinical characteristics of the sample are reported in Table 1. No significant differences between the TG and the CG were found with respect to any demographic or clinical variable (Table 1).

The multivariate test found no effect of age, DQ, or parental gender on the outcome variables. There was a statistically significant effect in the outcome variables PSI/SF, $F(2, 33) = 39.9$, $p < 0.001$ (Wilk's $\Lambda = 0.293$, $\eta_p^2 = 0.707$) and HSQ-ASD, $F(2, 33) = 3.59$, $p = 0.039$ (Wilk's $\Lambda = 0.821$, $\eta_p^2 = 0.179$). There was also a significant effect of the experimental group, $F(2, 33) = 11.7$, $p < 0.001$ (Wilk's $\Lambda = 0.586$, $\eta_p^2 = 0.414$) (Table 2). Univariate analyses led to a significant effect of the group on both outcome variables: PSI/SF ($M = 8.28$, standard error (SE) = 1.91; $F(1, 34) = 18.7$, $p < 0.001$, $\eta_p^2 = 0.355$) and HSQ-ASD ($M = 0.742$, $SE = 0.358$; $F(1, 34) = 4.30$, $p = 0.046$, $\eta_p^2 = 0.112$) with a larger decrease in the TG (Table 3).

Table 2. Multivariate tests for primary outcome variables.

Effect	Wilks' Λ	$F(2, 33)$	p-Value	η_p^2	Obs. Power
PSI/SF	0.293	39.9	<0.001 *	0.707	1.00
HSQ-ASD	0.821	3.59	0.039 *	0.179	0.624
Group	0.586	11.7	<0.001 *	0.414	0.990
Parental Gender (PG)	0.976	0.406	0.669	0.024	0.110
Group × PG	0.978	0.378	0.688	0.022	0.106
Intercept	0.830	3.37	0.046 *	0.170	0.596
Age	0.955	0.785	0.464	0.045	0.172
DQ	0.994	0.103	0.902	0.006	0.064

Developmental Quotient (DQ) i.e., Griffiths Mental Development Scales III total score; Parental Stress Index/Short Form (PSI/SF); Home Situation Questionnaire-ASD Version (HSQ-ASD); Design: Intercept + Age + DQ +PSI + HSQ + Group + PG + Group × PG. * $p < 0.001$.

Table 3. Univariate Analysis for primary outcome variables.

Source	Dependent Variable	Hyp. df	df Errors	MS	F	p-Value	η_p^2	Obs. Power
Group	PSI/SF	1	34	686	18.7	<0.001 *	0.355	0.988
	HSQ-ASD	1	34	5.50	4.30	0.046 *	0.112	0.522
Parental Gender	PSI/SF	1	34	30.2	0.824	0.370	0.024	0.143
	HSQ-ASD	1	34	0.010	0.005	0.946	0.000	0.051
Group × PG	PSI/SF	1	34	11.1	0.305	0.586	0.009	0.083
	HSQ-ASD	1	34	0.660	0.517	0.477	0.015	0.108

Mean Square (MS). Design: Intercept + Age + DQ +PSI + HSQ + Group + Parental Gender + Group. * Parental Gender.

Extending the analyses to the subscales, we found no interaction among the secondary outcome variables and age, DQ, or parental gender. All subscales had a significant multivariate effect (Table S6). Univariate effects for group differences were significant for PD ($M = 4.93$, $SE = 2.16$; $F(1, 31) = 5.23$, $p = 0.029$, $\eta_p^2 = 0.145$), SI ($M = 4.92$, $SE = 0.386$; $F(1, 31) = 5.69$, $p = 0.023$, $\eta_p^2 = 0.155$), and DS ($M = 1.16$, $SE = 0.383$; $F(1, 31) = 9.23$, $p = 0.005$, $\eta_p^2 = 0.229$), while barely significant for P–CDI ($M = 3.82$, $SE = 1.92$; $F(1, 31) = 3.94$, $p = 0.056$, $\eta_p^2 = 0.113$) and not significant for DC ($M = 0.173$, $SE = 2.63$; $F(1, 31) = 0.004$, $p = 0.948$, $\eta_p^2 < 0.001$).

Finally, we analyzed the two groups separately; as shown in Figure 2 (and Table 4), the TG displayed a significant improvement in PSI/SF, $t(21) = 5.10$, $p = 0.001$, with a decrease in stress of 7%. Conversely, the CG showed no significant change—$t(19) = -1.19$, $p = 0.241$. Likewise, the postintervention total scores of the HSQ-ASD decreased by 20% in the TG (Figure 3). The paired t-test indicated a significant improvement in the TG, $t(21) = 2.32$, $p = 0.035$, but not in the CG, $t(19) = 0.145$, $p = 0.890$. All children in the TG improved. Complete descriptive statistics of outcome variables are reported in the Supplementary Materials (Tables S8 and S9).

The complete raw data (Table S1) and pre- and postphase III results for each participant are reported in the Supplementary Materials (Tables S2–S9).

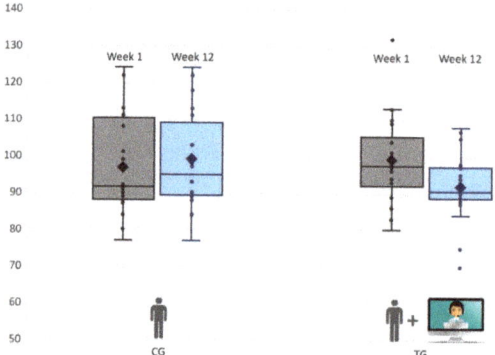

Figure 2. Box-plot of postphase III gains for Control Group (CG) and Tele-assisted Group (TG) in the Parental Stress Index/Short Form (PSI/SF) Test.

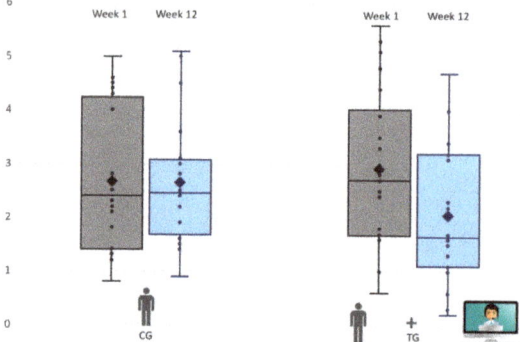

Figure 3. Box-plot of postphase III gains for gains for control group (CG) and tele-assisted group (TG) in the Home Situation Questionnaire-ASD Version (HSQ-ASD) Test.

Table 4. Pre- and postphase III comparison of outcome measures for control group (CG) and tele-assisted group (TG) separately.

Group	Test	Factor	MD	SE	t	df	BCa 95% Difference C.I.			p-Value
CG	PSI/SF	PD	−0.450	2.03	−0.225	19	−4.46	-	3.26	0.844
		P–CDI	1.65	2.13	0.777	19	−3.27	-	5.89	0.464
		DC	−3.00	2.34	−1.30	19	−7.45	-	1.79	0.225
		Total	−1.80	1.44	−1.19	19	−4.53	-	0.797	0.241
	HSQ-ASD	SI	0.050	0.172	0.288	19	−0.230	-	0.422	0.778
		DS	0.140	0.227	0.596	19	−0.250	-	0.573	0.542
		Total	0.020	0.133	0.145	19	−0.208	-	0.275	0.890
TG	PSI/SF	PD	3.13	1.75	1.80	21	−0.176	-	6.16	0.090
		P–CDI	3.68	1.22	3.02	21	1.17	-	6.32	0.010 *
		DC	0.227	2.50	0.091	21	−5.39	-	5.26	0.919
		Total	6.95	1.34	5.10	21	4.57	-	9.67	0.001 *
	HSQ-ASD	SI	0.823	0.393	2.06	21	0.036	-	1.53	0.052
		DS	1.03	0.351	2.90	21	0.378	-	1.69	0.012 *
		Total	0.863	0.367	2.32	21	0.137	-	1.57	0.035 *

Mean Difference (MD) between pre- and postintervention for each scale; Standard Deviation (SD); Standard Error (SE); Parental Stress Index/Short Form (PSI/SF); Home Situation Questionnaire-ASD Version (HSQ-ASD); Parental Distress (PD); Parent–Child Dysfunctional Interaction (P–CDI); Difficult Child (DC); Bias Corrected Accelerated Bootstrap (BCa). * $p < 0.05$.

4. Discussion

In this study, the feasibility and efficacy of a tele-assisted ABA intervention program for families with children with ASDs was described and evaluated in a randomized controlled trial. To the best of our knowledge, this study is one of the first to focus on a tele-assisted ABA intervention program [9]. The intervention consisted of informative group parent training, behavioral group therapy, and individual therapy, engaging parents in behavioral interactive play activities with their young children, aged 3–10, with or without the addition of tele-assistance.

We found an effect of the tele-assisted intervention group on the parents' stress levels and perception of the disruptive and noncompliant behavior of their children. This can be inferred by a significant change in the PSI/SF scores in the TG with a mean decrease of 8.28 points (−8.39%), in comparison to the CG and HSQ-ASD scores by the TG with a mean decrease of 0.742 points (−28.1%).

We found an increased ability of parents belonging to the TG to face stress, as highlighted by the PD subscale (−4.93 points; −16.1%), in comparison to the CG, and to cope with their children's inadequate behaviors, as pointed out by a significant decrease in the SI (−0.920 points; −30.1%) and DS (−1.16 points; −49.5%) subscales and as suggested by the barely significant effect of the P–CDI subscale (−3.82 points; −14.2%).

Interestingly, we found no change in the judgment of the difficulties associated with a specific child (DC subscale, as well as if both the parental stress was reduced and the children's behaviors were perceived as improved). This result is not surprising, given that our experimental intervention focused on teaching parents coping and interactional skills to manage challenging behaviors, rather than to change their perception regarding their children's temperament. The strength of this study is also its limitation. Focusing on parental perception allowed us to better understand it, but in order to generalize the results and to assess the therapeutic efficacy of the protocol, future replication should also assess behavioral changes through direct and independent measures.

We had no parents drop out during the trial. All of the parents in the TG demonstrated high interest in the web-based platform and sustained motivation throughout each experimental session. Unfortunately, 40% of the parents did not complete all of the pre- and post-tests and were therefore excluded; thus, increasing the parents' collaboration not only for the therapy sessions, but also to complete the tests would be important for future replications. Participants identified several benefits associated with telehealth including its flexibility, reduction in commute time, access to providers, and more family engagement. Parents and children experiencing the tele-assisted sessions showed the usually demonstrated parent–child interactions at home, especially initiating and sharing play activities. This is in line with the previous literature reporting how effective, acceptable, and usable ubiquitous communication technology is for the parents [27–29]. Moreover, as reported by themselves, all parents in the TG spontaneously practiced the learned lessons at home subsequent to the tele-assisted intervention, just as is usually reported by parents following in-person parent coaching sessions.

Parent–child interactions were not influenced by computer, tablet, or general technology concerns, e.g., internet connection, digital divide, or anxiety regarding their performance when using technology. These qualitative results are in contrast with those reported by Cole et al. who identified access to high speed internet and the opinion that telehealth was not as effective as in-person treatment as their primary barriers [30]. Our hypothesis is that given the specificity of our center, which is highly focused on technology, recruited parents could had a more favorable propensity toward technology, and future study should replicate the results with a more diverse population and aim to validate structured interviews or questionnaires to assess parental propensity to initiate a tele-intervention in an easily replicable fashion.

Furthermore, while ABA interventions are usually time-intensive, we administered a low-dose intervention, suggesting that the additional hour of tele-assistance could be pivotal for the success of the implementation. From informal exchanges with the participants, many parents reported challenges in generalizing and personalizing the techniques learned during the courses and in generalizing the daily life situations the skills learned through observations in the laboratory. The addition of tele-assistance helped the therapists fill the gap, reaching families of children with ASDs in their homes.

This evidence encourages further experimental studies regarding the long-term application of tele-assisted interventions in ASD therapy.

5. Conclusions

The obtained results support the idea that an ABA tele-assistive intervention can be an effective treatment for families with children on the autism spectrum following initial parent training. In line with our hypothesis, we found a significant positive effect of the ABA tele-assistive intervention in terms of parents' stress levels, perception of the disruptive and noncompliant behavior of their children, coping with their children in cases of inadequate behaviors, as well as in the influence on their children's behavior. We expect that further studies with larger samples may replicate these findings. All of the raw data gathered, and the analysis described in this study, are reported in the Supplementary Materials for future comparisons.

Supplementary Materials: The following are available online at http://www.mdpi.com/2076-3425/10/9/649/s1, Table S1. Raw Data of Analyzed Participants, Tables S2–S9: Pre- and postintervention results for each participant.

Author Contributions: Conceptualization, F.M., D.V. and G.P.; methodology, F.M., L.R., D.V. and G.P.; software, A.P., G.T. and G.P.; validation, F.M., L.R., P.C., C.F., I.C., and R.M.; formal analysis, G.T., A.A.A., D.V. and G.P.; investigation, F.M., P.C., C.F., I.C. and R.M.; resources, F.M., P.C., L.R., D.V. and G.P.; data curation, F.M., P.C., C.F., I.C., R.M. and A.A.A.; writing—original draft preparation, F.M., D.V. and G.P.; writing—review and editing, F.M., D.V. and G.P.; visualization, F.M., D.V. and G.P.; supervision, F.M., D.V. and G.P.; project administration, G.P.; funding acquisition, G.P. All authors have read and agreed to the published version of the manuscript.

Funding: This research was funded by Project SIRENA—Sistemi Innovativi di Ricerca E-health per la Neuro-Abilitazione, Prot. CNR-IRIB n. 2346/2019-20/12/2019-CUP B44D19000210007 by Soc. Coop. Soc. Occupazione e Solidarietà, Bari, Italy.

Acknowledgments: We acknowledge all the children and their parents for their help and participation. A special thank you to the Soc. Coop. Soc. Occupazione e Solidarietà for its constant support.

Conflicts of Interest: The authors declare no conflict of interest.

References

1. American Psychiatric Association. *The Diagnostic and Statistical Manual of Mental Disorders: DSM-5*; American Psychiatric Publishing: Washington, DC, USA, 2013.
2. Styles, M.; Alsharshani, D.; Samara, M.; Alsharshani, M.; Khattab, A.; Qoronfleh, M.W.; Al-Dewik, N.I. Risk factors, diagnosis, prognosis and treatment of autism. *Front. Biosci. (Landmark. Ed.)* **2020**, *25*, 1682–1717. [PubMed]
3. Alfuraydan, M.; Croxall, J.; Hurt, L.; Kerr, M.; Brophy, S. Use of telehealth for facilitating the diagnostic assessment of Autism Spectrum Disorder (ASD): A scoping review. *PLoS ONE* **2020**, *15*, e0236415. [CrossRef] [PubMed]
4. Solomon, D.; Soares, N. Telehealth Approaches to Care Coordination in Autism Spectrum Disorder. In *Interprofessional Care Coordination for Pediatric. Autism Spectrum Disorder*; McClain, M.B., Shahidullah, J., Mezher, K., Eds.; Springer Nature: Cham, Switzerland, 2020; pp. 289–306.
5. Reichow, B.; Hume, K.; Barton, E.E.; Boyd, B.A. Early intensive behavioral intervention (EIBI) for young children with autism spectrum disorders (ASD). *Cochrane Database Syst. Rev.* **2018**, *5*, CD009260. [CrossRef] [PubMed]
6. Hao, Y.; Franco, J.H.; Sundarrajan, M.; Chen, Y. A Pilot Study Comparing Tele-therapy and In-Person Therapy: Perspectives from Parent-Mediated Intervention for Children with Autism Spectrum Disorders. *J. Autism Dev. Disord.* **2020**. [CrossRef] [PubMed]
7. World Health Organization. *Global Diffusion of eHealth: Making Universal Health Coverage Achievable*; Report of the Third Global Survey on eHealth; World Health Organization: Geneva, Switzerland, 2016.

8. Juárez, A.P.; Weitlauf, A.S.; Nicholson, A.; Pasternak, A.; Broderick, N.; Hine, J.; Stainbrook, A.; Warren, Z. Early identification of ASD through telemedicine: Potential value for underserved populations. *J. Autism Dev. Disord.* **2018**, *48*, 2601–2610. [CrossRef] [PubMed]
9. Ferguson, J.; Craig, E.A.; Dounavi, K. Telehealth as a Model for Providing Behaviour Analytic Interventions to Individuals with Autism Spectrum Disorder: A Systematic Review. *J. Autism Dev. Disord.* **2019**, *49*, 582–616. [CrossRef]
10. Knutsen, J.; Wolfe, A.; Burke, B.L.; Hepburn, S.; Lindgren, S.; Coury, D. A systematic review of telemedicine in autism spectrum disorders. *Rev. J. Autism Dev. Disord.* **2016**, *3*, 330–344. [CrossRef]
11. Lindgren, S.; Wacker, D.P.; Suess, A.; Schieltz, K.; Pelzel, K.; Kopelman, T.; Lee, J.; Romani, P.; Waldron, D. Telehealth and autism: Treating challenging behavior at a lower cost. *Pediatrics* **2016**, *137*, S167–S175. [CrossRef]
12. Parsons, D.; Cordier, R.; Vaz, S.; Lee, H.C. Parent-mediated intervention training delivered remotely for children with autism spectrum disorder living outside of urban areas: Systematic review. *J. Med. Int. Res.* **2017**, *19*, e198. [CrossRef]
13. Machalicek, W.; Lequia, J.; Pinkelman, S.; Knowles, C.; Raulston, T.; Davis, T.; Alresheed, F. Behavioral telehealth consultation with families of children with autism spectrum disorder. *Behav. Interv.* **2016**, *31*, 223–250. [CrossRef]
14. Simacek, J.; Dimian, A.F.; McComas, J.J. Communication intervention for young children with severe neurodevelopmental disabilities via telehealth. *J. Autism Dev. Disord.* **2017**, *477*, 44–67.
15. Suess, A.N.; Wacker, D.P.; Schwartz, J.E.; Lustig, N.; Detrick, J. Preliminary evidence on the use of telehealth in an outpatient behavior clinic. *J. Appl. Behav. Anal.* **2016**, *49*, 686–692. [CrossRef] [PubMed]
16. Salomone, E.; Arduino, G.M. Parental attitudes to a telehealth parent coaching intervention for autism spectrum disorder. *J. Telemed. Telecare* **2017**, *23*, 416–420. [CrossRef] [PubMed]
17. Ingersoll, B.; Wainer, A.L.; Berger, N.I.; Pickard, K.E.; Bonter, N. Comparison of a Self-Directed and Therapist-Assisted Telehealth Parent-Mediated Intervention for Children with ASD: A Pilot RCT. *J. Autism Dev. Disord.* **2016**, *46*, 2275–2284. [CrossRef] [PubMed]
18. Mazza, M.; Pino, M.C.; Vagnetti, R.; Filocamo, A.; Attanasio, M.; Calvarese, A.; Valenti, M. Intensive intervention for adolescents with autism spectrum disorder: Comparison of three rehabilitation treatments. *Int. J. Psychiatry Clin. Pract.* **2020**, 1–9. [CrossRef] [PubMed]
19. Yu, Q.; Li, E.; Li, L.; Liang, W. Efficacy of Interventions Based on Applied Behavior Analysis for Autism Spectrum Disorder: A Meta-Analysis. *Psychiatry Investig.* **2020**, *17*, 432–443. [CrossRef]
20. Leaf, J.B.; Leaf, R.; McEachin, J.; Cihon, J.H.; Ferguson, J.L. Advantages and Challenges of a Home- and Clinic-Based Model of Behavioral Intervention for Individuals Diagnosed with Autism Spectrum Disorder. *J. Autism Dev. Disord.* **2018**, *48*, 2258–2266. [CrossRef]
21. Booth, N.; Keenan, M. Discrete Trial Teaching: A study on the comparison of three training strategies. *Interdiscip. Educ. Psychol.* **2018**, *2*, 3. [CrossRef]
22. Leaf, J.B.; Cihon, J.H.; Ferguson, J.L.; Milne, C.M.; Leaf, R.; McEachin, J. Advances in Our Understanding of Behavioral Intervention: 1980 to 2020 for Individuals Diagnosed with Autism Spectrum Disorder. *J. Autism Dev. Disord.* **2020**. [CrossRef]
23. Tang, J.S.Y.; Falkmer, M.; Chen, N.T.M.; Bölte, S.; Girdler, S. Development and Feasibility of MindChip™: A Social Emotional Telehealth Intervention for Autistic Adults. *J. Autism Dev. Disord.* **2020**. [CrossRef]
24. Chowdhury, M.; Aman, M.G.; Lecavalier, L.; Smith, T.; Johnson, C.; Swiezy, N.; McCracken, J.T.; King, B.; McDougle, C.J.; Bearss, K.; et al. Factor structure and psychometric properties of the revised Home Situations Questionnaire for autism spectrum disorder: The Home Situations Questionnaire-Autism Spectrum Disorder. *Autism* **2016**, *20*, 528–537. [CrossRef] [PubMed]
25. Abidin, R.R. *Parenting Stress Index*, 3rd ed.; Psychological Assessment Resource: Odessa, FL, USA, 1995.
26. Dardas, L.A.; Ahmad, M.M. Psychometric properties of the Parenting Stress Index with parents of children with autistic disorder. *J. Intellect. Disabil. Res.* **2014**, *58*, 560–571. [CrossRef] [PubMed]
27. Baharav, E.; Reiser, C. Using telepractice in parent training in early autism. *Telemed. e-Health* **2010**, *16*, 727–731. [CrossRef] [PubMed]
28. Cason, J.; Behl, D.; Ringwalt, S. Overview of states' use of telehealth for the delivery of early intervention (IDEA Part C) services. *Int. J. Telerehabil.* **2012**, *4*, 39. [CrossRef]

29. Owen, N. Feasibility and acceptability of using telehealth for early intervention parent counselling. *Adv. Ment. Health* **2020**, *18*, 39–49. [CrossRef]
30. Cole, B.; Pickard, K.; Stredler-Brown, A. Report on the use of telehealth in early intervention in Colorado: Strengths and challenges with telehealth as a service delivery method. *Int. J. Telerehabil.* **2019**, *11*, 33. [CrossRef]

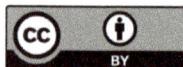 © 2020 by the authors. Licensee MDPI, Basel, Switzerland. This article is an open access article distributed under the terms and conditions of the Creative Commons Attribution (CC BY) license (http://creativecommons.org/licenses/by/4.0/).

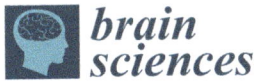 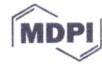

Article

Developing Employment Environments Where Individuals with ASD Thrive: Using Machine Learning to Explore Employer Policies and Practices

Amy Jane Griffiths [1,*], Amy Hurley Hanson [2], Cristina M. Giannantonio [2], Sneha Kohli Mathur [1], Kayleigh Hyde [3] and Erik Linstead [4]

1. Attallah College of Educational Studies, Chapman University, One University Drive, Orange, CA 92866, USA; mathu109@mail.chapman.edu
2. Argyros School of Business and Economics, Chapman University, One University Drive, Orange, CA 92866, USA; ahurley@chapman.edu (A.H.H.); giannant@chapman.edu (C.M.G.)
3. Schmid College of Science and Technology, Chapman University, One University Drive, Orange, CA 92866, USA; khyde@chapman.edu
4. Fowler School of Engineering, Chapman University, One University Drive, Orange, CA 92866, USA; linstead@chapman.edu
* Correspondence: agriffit@chapman.edu

Received: 27 June 2020; Accepted: 9 September 2020; Published: 11 September 2020

Abstract: An online survey instrument was developed to assess employers' perspectives on hiring job candidates with Autism Spectrum Disorder (ASD). The investigators used K-means clustering to categorize companies in clusters based on their hiring practices related to individuals with ASD. This methodology allowed the investigators to assess and compare the various factors of businesses that successfully hire employees with ASD versus those that do not. The cluster analysis indicated that company structures, policies and practices, and perceptions, as well as the needs of employers and employees, were important in determining who would successfully hire individuals with ASD. Key areas that require focused policies and practices include recruitment and hiring, training, accessibility and accommodations, and retention and advancement.

Keywords: autism spectrum disorder; machine learning; employment

1. Introduction

Research suggests that competitive employment may be difficult to attain for individuals with Autism Spectrum Disorder (ASD). Although companies are beginning to recognize the value of hiring employees with ASD, the academic literature on the benefits and current practices of recruiting people with ASD is limited [1,2]. Providing supportive employment services for adults with ASD is seen as a positive investment. Individuals with ASD can typically gain employment with the right support [3]. Research indicates that employees with ASD have many skills that can contribute a great deal to the workforce. Despite the skill sets of individuals with ASD, the unemployment and underemployment rates for these individuals, as compared to the general population, remains staggeringly low [4–10]. This discrepancy suggests that it is critical to understand employers' perspectives and experiences, so that hiring practices and outcomes may be improved for both organizations and employees with ASD.

2. Background

Organizations' interest in hiring neurodiverse individuals, including those with ASD, has increased [2]. This interest is due in part to companies recognizing the value of hiring employees with ASD. Research indicates that employees with ASD typically pay close attention to detail, enjoy certain job tasks that other employees may find repetitive or socially isolating, and bring a different perspective to issues, allowing for innovative solutions to common problems [3,11]. Research also suggests that employees with ASD have high levels of trustworthiness, integrity, and honesty. They are reliable, precise, efficient, and consistent [4,7,12,13].

Additionally, employees with ASD may demonstrate "above standard" workplace performance compared to their counterparts related to increased attention to detail, work ethic, and quality of work [9]. Employees with ASD have been found to have fewer absences and are more likely to arrive at work on time than other employees [12,14,15]). Research has also found that employees with autism have dramatically lower turnover rates than neurotypical employees. Turnover is a large expense for organizations. In some industries, such as software, the turnover rate is close to fifteen percent nationally. Employees with autism have a seven percent turnover rate. The costs of replacing a worker earning less than $50,000 are estimated to be twenty percent of their annual salary [16]. As salaries rise, so do the costs of replacing those employees.

Moreover, an increase in the employment of people with ASD can lead to significant economic benefits to society [3,17–19]. A study in Australia found that reducing the unemployment of people with ASD by one-third would lead to a $43 billion increase in the Australian Gross Domestic Product [20]. The Dandelion Employment Program in Australia calculates that every 100 individuals with ASD who were previously unemployed, and who participate in the program for three years, save the Australian government over six million dollars in the form of tax gains, savings in welfare benefits, and savings in unemployment services costs.

Despite these individual positive qualities, and benefits to organizations and society, many individuals with ASD remain unemployed, underemployed, and underpaid. Recent unemployment statistics for adults with ASD reveal that 85% are unemployed (National Autistic Society, 2016). Research has shown that many individuals with ASD have never been members of the labor force [21]. The authors of [10] found that thirty-five percent of young adults with autism have never held a job, been members of the labor force, or attended educational programs after high school [10,21]. A study of 200 transition-age young adults with ASD found that 81% were unemployed [22].

Understanding the factors that contribute to unemployment is critical. The number of people affected by Autism Spectrum Disorder (ASD) is estimated in the tens of millions worldwide and 3.5 million in the United States [2]. Moreover, it is predicted that over the next decade, close to half a million children with ASD will reach adulthood (https://www.cdc.gov/ncbddd/autism/index.html). If they cannot be employed and live independently, the services they will require will place a financial toll on families and society [3]. Supporting an individual with ASD may exceed two million dollars throughout their lifetime [17]. The total cost of ASD support services in the U.S. exceeds 236 billion dollars annually [17]. This number is expected to rise to one trillion dollars by 2025 [4]. There are additional financial and non-financial costs that are difficult to measure, such as income losses for individuals with ASD and their families, as well as the emotional and psychological costs associated with long term unemployment [1].

Research must examine why organizations hire individuals with ASD and the barriers to their employment [2]. The literature on the employment of people with disabilities has found that, although many employers say they are willing to hire those with disabilities, their actual hiring practices do not show efforts in this area [23–25]. Employer's attitudes and perceptions towards people with disabilities, and organizational practices and policies, are two significant barriers to employment success [23]. This paper examines the role of employers' attitudes, perceptions, organizational practices, and policies on the hiring and retention of employees with ASD.

2.1. Research on Employer Attitudes and Perceptions

The literature on employer attitudes and perceptions towards employees with ASD is limited. However, there are studies in the disabilities literature that may lend insight into employers' attitudes and perceptions of individuals with ASD. Investigators at Cornell University surveyed over 800 private sector employers and over 400 federal sector employers in regard to actual hiring and retention processes for employees with disabilities [26,27].

When considering hiring individuals with disabilities, employers have several concerns. These concerns include potential legal risks, the time and effort to supervise and train, safety issues, the financial burden of accommodations, and the belief that they would never be able to terminate the disabled employee once hired [24,28–31]. Specifically looking at ASD, the authors of [32] found that employers who do not hire employees with ASD tend to have the following concerns; focusing on the employee's ability to adapt to work situations, a concern for adverse outcomes, and a lower interest in receiving new information and training. A study focusing on employees with Asperger's Syndrome (now categorized as ASD), found that employers' resistance and negative attitudes about the (perceived) need to provide accommodations, concerns about high costs, low productivity, and high turnover, as well as the need to provide outside supports, were associated with lower rates of hiring and higher rates of termination of individuals with ASD [7].

However, research has contradicted employer attitudes and perceptions that hiring adults with ASD may result in a loss of productivity and increased costs associated with workplace modifications and additional training and supervision. A few studies have compared the job performance ratings of employees with and without ASD [3]. Managers tended to rate the job performance of the employee with ASD as average or above average [11,14,33]. The authors of [34] compared employees with and without ASD on the extent to which they met standard requirements for good workplace performance. They found that employees with ASD performed at an "above standard level" regarding attention to detail, work ethic, and quality of work. This study found that employers do not incur additional costs when employing an adult with ASD over and above that of any new employee. They also found that while they may require some workplace modifications, supervision, and training, there is no significant difference between them and their colleagues concerning weekly employment, supervision, and training costs. Twaronite found that those with ASD were able to identify process improvements that cut training time in half (https://wwTw.ey.com/en_us/diversity-inclusiveness/six-ways-to-advance-disability-inclusion-in-your-organization). They also found that quality of work, efficiency, and productivity was equal to their other employees. JP Morgan & Chase Company has employed over 70 individuals with ASD over the past three years (https://www.forbes.com/sites/jpmorganchase/2017/06/05/how-jpmorgan-chases-autism-at-work-program-is-helping-to-win-top-tech-talent/#660a965830bb). Representatives of JP Morgan & Chase Company report that their employees with ASD are producing forty-eight to one-hundred-and-forty percent more work than their neurotypical colleagues (https://fortune.com/2018/06/24/where-autistic-workers-thrive/). They anticipate hiring hundreds more individuals with ASD globally in the coming years. A survey of employers who had hired individuals with ASD found that fifty-seven percent of employers reported no additional costs from hiring an individual with ASD and did not require assistance from tax incentives to hire them (https://askjan.org/topics/costs.cfm). Consequently, at the organizational level, these results contradict employers' attitudes and perceptions that hiring adults with ASD may result in a loss of productivity and increased costs associated with workplace modifications and additional training and supervision.

2.2. Research on Employer Practices and Policies

Research on employers' practices and policies to support employees with ASD is in its infancy. Although many organizations have created hiring initiatives to hire individuals with disabilities, some are beginning to focus on explicitly hiring individuals with ASD [27]. Organizational practices and policies may influence all stages of employment. A holistic approach to hiring for employees with ASD should be encouraged [35]. To better assist organizations in improving their employment practices, the barriers and facilitators to hiring individuals with ASD must be understood [2].

Much attention has focused on how the traditional selection interview may operate as a barrier to employment for individuals with ASD. The authors of [36] note that one of the obstacles to hiring neurodiverse employees is the traditional interview process. Current recruitment interview processes have not been found to provide adequate accommodations for neurodiverse individuals [37,38]. The authors of [36,39] found that the employment interview poses a unique barrier for individuals with ASD. Their research found that it is difficult for individuals with autism to navigate the social cues present during an interview. Research has found that individuals with ASD experience high anxiety during employment interviews [4,40]. A study of adults with ASD participating in an interview process found that 100% of the participants found that their high levels of anxiety negatively influenced their experience with the interview process. The participants also reported that their anxiety negatively affected their communication and performance in the interview (https://search.proquest.com/openview/b2bf39c3621955296526edd36f51dde6/1?pq-origsite=gscholar&cbl=18750&diss=y). The study also found that all participants viewed the interview as a negative experience due to issues of verbal and nonverbal communication, the process of the interview, and anxiety. For example, when companies use online applications, candidates may not be able to complete the application without adaptive technology, such as talk-to-text software. This can prevent a potential employee from even being eligible for an interview. Some organizations replace traditional interviews with opportunities for applicants with ASD to engage in a job trial or to demonstrate their skills with alternative methods [27].

The work in [35] found that, in Australia and Sweden, employers reported that knowledge and understanding of ASD, work environment, and job match led to successful employment of individuals with ASD. The authors of [35] noted that, when employees had a working knowledge of the needs of individuals with ASD, they fostered successful workplace relationships, minimized misunderstandings, and increased communication. The authors of [41], who interviewed employment support service providers, found that accommodations need to begin during the hiring process, not after the person has been hired. Some organizations may benefit from using support specialists in the hiring process. Support specialists help employers to see how the organization can successfully hire individuals with disabilities, including ASD. They will also assist them with training other employees and needed accommodations [42–48]. When education comes directly from employment support specialists during the hiring process, employers feel more confident about hiring employees with ASD. Employers reported that having an employment support specialist allows them to have someone to rely on. Employers can then ask disability-related questions, understand accommodation needs, and ease legal concerns [31,42,48–50]. Research is needed that examines organizational policies and practices that lead to successful employment outcomes for individuals with ASD [2].

2.3. Current Study

The literature explores employer perspectives and practices in regard to hiring employees with disabilities. There is limited research on employer factors that contribute to successful hiring and retention practices of employees with ASD, specifically. In this study, we used K-means clustering, a form of unsupervised machine learning, to categorize companies in different clusters based on their response to an online survey. This analysis allowed us to assess and compare aspects of businesses that successfully hire employees with ASD versus those that do not. Clustering algorithms aim to partition the dataset into groups (clusters) in which members of each group are similar to those in their cluster and dissimilar to those in other clusters. This type of analysis allows for a better understanding of the characteristics of those companies that are more successful in hiring employees with ASD.

3. Data

An online survey instrument was developed to assess employers' perspectives on hiring candidates with "High Functioning" Autism Spectrum Disorder (HFASD). This term was used to provide a brief descriptor of a particular group of individuals with ASD (i.e., those with average to above-average cognitive skills). However, the term HFASD can be problematic, as the term suggests those with average or above cognitive skills perform well in other functional areas, while the evidence indicates this is a poor predictor of functional skills [51]. To ameliorate some of these concerns, while still maintaining a "short descriptor", investigators clearly defined what was meant by HFASD as it related to the survey. Example behaviors based on the Diagnostic and Statistical Manual of mental disorders, 5th edition [52] were described in the survey and included areas of difficulty in functional domains. Specifically, for the purposes of this study, a person with HFASD is defined as someone who has identified themselves as having Autism, Aspergers, or HFASD has approximately average intellectual ability (when compared to peers) but may have marked difficulties in social interactions, including communication. The employee may have difficulty initiating or responding to social interactions, or may not seem interested in interacting with colleagues or customers. The person may be able to have a conversation when necessary, but may have difficulty keeping the conversation going or knowing how and when to end the conversation. The person may require a structured environment and/or schedule and may not deal well with change. The person may have difficulty with organization and planning.

A review of the literature was conducted to identify related studies across various stakeholders [53,54] to develop a basic framework and a list of questions. Questions used to assess these perspectives were organized into several categories including employer background and characteristics of employees; policies and practices related to recruitment and hiring; training, accessibility, and accommodations; and retention and advancement; barriers and facilitators to hiring individuals with ASD; and finally, the employer needs to improve hiring outcomes for individuals with ASD.

Employers from five local businesses agreed to participate as early reviewers and provided feedback about content as well as readability. A staff member from one local business volunteered to take the survey, along with the authors, and read aloud and answered each question on the computer and verbally. The volunteer asked questions for clarification and provided feedback during the process. In addition, the research team completed the survey multiple times, taking on varying respondent perspectives (e.g., employers with experience in hiring individuals with ASD, employers who had no experience) to assess whether the survey branching logic was appropriate; also discussed were potential answers, the survey flow, and whether the questions were sequenced in a logical order based on earlier responses. All pretest feedback was considered and resulted in multiple revisions. After obtaining Institutional Review Board approval, the survey instrument was finalized and placed in an electronic survey platform (Qualtrics), and a unique resource locator (URL) was created.

To access a broad range of employers across a larger geographical region, the team utilized the Qualtrics research services to recruit survey respondents. An invitation was sent out through their platform. The request to complete the survey included a statement regarding the researchers' interest in the employer's opinions on organizational practices, policies, and needs, related to employing people with ASD. However, it was made clear that the employer did not have to have experience hiring an individual with ASD to participate. Respondents were selected if they had a significant role in hiring decisions for their company. The survey link was active and open for three weeks. Participants were able to direct any questions or concerns to the authors; however, no questions or concerns were received.

The survey research methodology involved a traditional analytical process. The researchers had knowledge only about the demographic categories that the respondents provided, and no other identifying information was provided. Quantitative and qualitative data were collected via the survey. Quantitative data were obtained primarily through forced-choice or ranking questions. For most items, standard survey nomenclature (e.g., Likert scales) was used. Specifically, for the policy- and practices-related questions, respondents were asked if a particular policy or practice was not in place, being considered, in place but not effective, in place and somewhat effective, or in place and very effective. When asked about barriers and facilitators, employers were given a range of options to choose from, and an "other" or short text box was available for many questions so that respondents could provide a more detailed response [55]. For example, when asked, "Do any of the following pose a barrier to employment or advancement for people with ASD in your organization?" Respondents could select all that apply from a range of options including (but not limited to) cost of accommodations, cost of training/additional supervision, attitudes/stereotypes, lack of requisite skills among individuals with ASD, productive and performance of an individual, etc. All of the response options are based on previous research described above. When explicitly asked about employer needs related to hiring individuals with ASD, employers were asked a variety of questions about training, tax incentives and support, and experience with incentive and support programs. For example, employers were asked, "If an agency were to provide training and support for employing people with ASD, what would make it worthwhile for your organization to utilize the training?" Employers were able to select all applicable response options including the training would be free of cost, the training would be in partnership with a well-respected community organization concerning HFASD, and the training would be tailored to my company's needs. They were also asked if they would be willing to pay for training to assist their company in hiring individuals with ASD. The results of the quantitative data analysis are reported in this paper.

The instrument consisted of 50 to 80 questions, depending on the participant's hiring experience. Specifically, the number of items offered to each respondent varied based on his or her experience with hiring individuals with High Functioning ASD (HFASD). It took approximately 20 min to complete the survey online, and a total of 285 respondents completed the online survey. Of the 285 respondents, 166 (58%) indicated they had hired at least one individual with HFASD in the past five years. Of the 285 respondents, 120 possessed a high school diploma, 36 held an associates degree, 107 held a bachelors degree or higher, and the remainder indicated "other" as their highest level of education. Of the respondents, 14 worked for organizations with 15 or less employees, 7 at organizations with 16–49 employees, 26 at organizations with 50–99 employees, 26 at organizations with 100–499 employees, 13 at organizations with 500–999 employees, and the remainder at organizations with 1000 or more employees.

To create the data matrix, 41 questions and sub-questions from the survey were used to create a binary variable for each item. For each variable, a 1 indicated a favorable response in relation to HFASD. The variables were then broken into five categories: (1) Hiring ($n = 15$), (2) Training ($n = 8$), (3) Accommodations ($n = 8$), (4) Retention ($n = 10$), and (5) Perceptions ($n = 18$). To reduce the dimensions of the dataset, the average score for each respondent in each of the four categories was calculated. Creating an average score for each category also helped to normalize the data. Because the number of variables differed among the categories, using a count (as opposed to an average score) would put more weight on the categories with more variables. For example, if a respondent had a favorable response for seven of the Hiring variables, he or she would have a Hiring score of $7/15 = 0.47$. After assessing the cluster model, all clusters had virtually the same Perception score, which led to overlapping clusters. Thus, the Perception scores from the final data matrix were excluded. Having a dataset with large dimensions often leads to a sparse dataspace (all objects may seem dissimilar in this space) and analysis results that may be true with higher dimensionality but that will not necessarily hold in a lower dimensional space. Thus, the final data matrix was a 285×4 dimensional matrix that represents the average scores of 285 employers' responses to the 41 questions mapped to 4 categories. The variable descriptions and survey averages for each category can be found in Tables 1–4.

Table 1. Accommodation.

Description	Survey Average
Regularly reviews the accessibility of its online application system to people with visual, hearing, finger dexterity, and cognitive impairments	61.0%
Analyzes our job descriptions to determine whether the responsibilities could be broken down into discrete tasks that could be performed by an individual with ASD	61.0%
Provides advance notice to job applicants that reasonable accommodations are provided during the job application process	68.0%
Evaluates pre-employment occupational screenings to ensure they are unbiased	71.0%
Has company-wide fund to provide accommodations for people with disabilities	61.0%
Has a designated office or person to address accommodation questions	69.0%
Has an established grievance procedure to address reasonable accommodation issues	70.0%

Table 2. Hiring.

Description	Survey Average
Hired someone with ASD in the last 5 years	58.0%
Actively recruits people with ASD	53.0%
Works with community organizations that promote hiring of people with ASD	57.0%
Includes people with ASD explicitly in its diversity and inclusion plan	58.0%
Has explicit organizational goals related to the recruitment or hiring of people with ASD	54.0%
Includes progress toward hiring goals for people with ASD in the performance appraisals of senior management	52.0%
Participates in internships that target people with ASD	53.0%
Has senior management that demonstrates a strong commitment to ASD hiring	56.0%
Utilizes tax incentives for hiring people with disabilities	54.0%
Requires subcontractors/suppliers to adhere to disability nondiscrimination requirements	56.0%
Does not automatically exclude job applicants with a history of unemployment	79.0%
Does not automatically exclude job applicants with a large gap in employment	76.0%
Has company initiative to hire people with HFASD	53.0%
Works with universities to hire people with HFASD	49.0%
Uses social media ads to recruit people with HFASD	45.0%

Table 3. Retention.

Description	Survey Average
Has a formal mentoring program to support employees with ASD	53.0%
Encourages flexible work arrangements for all employees with ASD (e.g., flextime, part-time, telecommuting)	62.0%
Offers special career planning and development tools for employees with ASD	55.0%
Has an ASD-focused employee network (e.g., employee resource group or affinity group)	52.0%
Invites employees to confidentially disclose whether they have a disability (e.g., staff surveys)	73.0%
Has explicit organizational goals related to retention or advancement of employees with ASD	54.0%
Includes progress toward retention of advancement goals for employees with ASD in the performance appraisals of senior management	54.0%
Allows an employee to exceed the maximum duration of medical leave as an accommodation	54.0%
Has defined career paths at our company for all employees	75.0%
Opportunities for advancement of employees with HFASD	61.0%

Table 4. Training.

Description	Survey Average
Offers ASD awareness and sensitivity training (internal)	60.0%
Offers ASD awareness and sensitivity training (external)	51.0%
Trains HR staff and supervisors on effective interviewing of people with ASD	62.0%
Trains HR staff and supervisors on inclusion practices of people with ASD in the workplace	62.0%
Requires training for supervisors on legal requirements of disability and non-discrimination and accommodation	68.0%
Includes ASD awareness and sensitivity as a topic in training for managers/ supervisors	58.0%
In contract with an agency that can help our business provide the support needed for working with employees with ASD now and in the future	52.0%

4. Methods

K-means is an unsupervised learning algorithm that is capable of discerning latent clusters in data [56]. We chose this algorithm for our analysis based on data visualizations which showed no irregular shapes or non-homogeneous behavior which would require a more sophisticated technique. Unlike supervised learning (classification), which requires labeled data to measure the accuracy of prediction, unsupervised learning methods are instead assessed on the "goodness" of the clusters identified using one or more common quantitative metrics, such as silhouette score. K-means requires a single parameter, k, as input, which represents the number of clusters to be fit to the data. The algorithm then proceeds as follows.

1. A centroid (mean) for each of the k clusters is assigned by randomly selecting a data point from the data.
2. Every other data point is assigned to the cluster whose centroid is closest. Distance can be calculated using any valid distance metric, with Euclidean and Cosine distance being popular choices.
3. The centroids are reevaluated by averaging each data point assigned to a specific cluster.
4. Steps 2 and 3 are repeated, alternating between assigning data points to their nearest centroids, and then reevaluating the value of the centroids based on the new assignments. When the centroids no longer change, or the cluster assignments for the data points become static, the algorithm terminates.

For the work presented here, we found the most likely number of clusters to be five. This was calculated by using the gap statistic [57], a common technique for assessing the number of latent clusters in unsupervised machine learning. This was further validated using the Hopkins statistic, which denotes the overall likelihood that the data can be partitioned into clusters. For the data presented here, the Hopkins score was 0.72, indicating that the dataset exhibits strong clustering tendency.

With clustering, the lack of labeled data means there is not an independent data set to validate accuracy. Instead, silhouette scores [58] were used to measure how well the clusters explained the latent structure of the data. Silhouette scores quantify how similar a data point is to the other points in its cluster compared to those represented in other nearby clusters. The silhouette scores vary from -1 to $+1$, with values close to 1 suggesting that the point is well clustered and a negative silhouette as suggesting that the data point likely should not belong to its assigned cluster. The mean silhouette score for our model was 0.54.

5. Model Results

The data from the complete set of respondents were partitioned into five clusters and visualized in Figure 1, with average category scores listed in Table 5. The remaining figures (presented according to cluster) provide a visualization of the individual cluster average category scores, with the last (presented at the end of this section) that shows all graphs on the same axis for comparison.

Table 5. Cluster average scores.

Cluster	Size	Accommodation	Hiring	Retention	Training
1	41	0.67	0.21	0.28	0.11
2	32	0.84	0.56	0.78	0.70
3	62	0.10	0.12	0.06	0.04
4	24	0.30	0.34	0.25	0.61
5	126	0.97	0.95	0.97	0.98

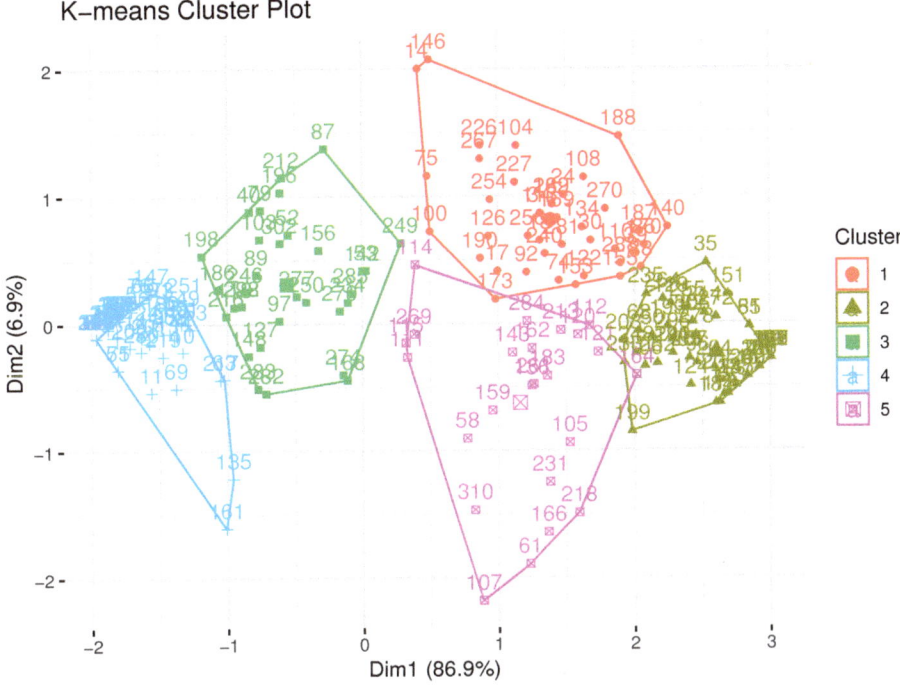

Figure 1. Employer K-means cluster plot.

5.1. Cluster 1

The 41 employer respondents in Cluster 1 (14.0% of sample) had only 29.0% in a management/owner role, while 54.0% were in a human resource/recruiting position. Although employers in Cluster 1 had the lowest five-year hiring rates (24.0% vs. survey average 58.0%) for individuals with high functioning ASD, they are able to offer full-time employment to those they do hire. Almost all, 98.0%, of the employers in Cluster 1 have high functioning ASD employees employed full time. In the past two years, 63.0% of employers in Cluster 1 have hired more than 11 employees.

This cluster had employers in 19 out of the 24 different industries listed and a company size of 218 employees on average (survey average 285 employees). Most respondents in all clusters and the survey were representing health care/social assistance employers. Only the health care/social assistance and construction industries represented at least 10.0% of Cluster 1. A college degree is required by 32.0% of employers in Cluster 1, and 63.0% require a high school diploma for employment. Employers in this cluster had 5.0% in the Southwest, 12.0% in the Northeast, 22.0% in the Southeast, 24.0% in the Midwest, and 34.0% located in the West.

Employers in this cluster do not have policies and practices to foster hiring, retaining, or training employees with high functioning ASD (significantly lower than survey averages for all variables). No employers in Cluster 1 had a hiring initiative for high functioning ASD or a job-related training program for employees with high functioning ASD (compared to 53.0% and 56% of survey respondents, respectively).

Employers in this cluster have most accommodations in place for high functioning ASD comparable to the survey averages. Only the following four accommodation variables were significantly higher than the average for the survey. More than 80.0% of employers in Cluster 1 allow an employee to exceed the maximum duration of medical leave as an accommodation, have an established grievance procedure to address reasonable accommodation issues, have a designated office to address accommodation questions, and provide advance notice to job applicants that reasonable accommodations are provided during the job application process (Figure 2).

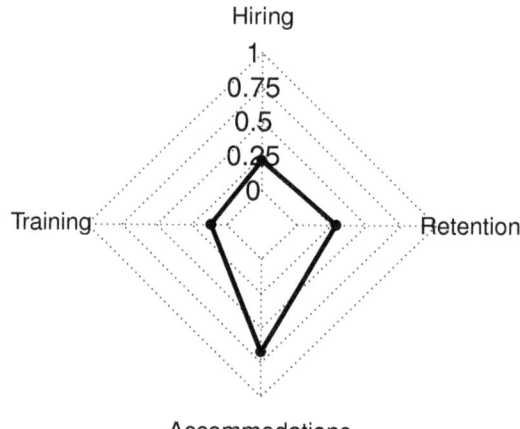

Figure 2. Cluster 1 radar graph.

5.2. Cluster 2

The 32 employer respondents in Cluster 2 (11.0% of sample) had 44.0% in a management/owner role, while 53.0% were in a human resource/recruiting position. Respondents in Cluster 2 had a five-year high functioning ASD hiring rate above the survey average (66.0% vs. survey average 58.0%). Cluster 2 had 72.0% of respondents who were involved in the hiring process for less than 10 years (survey average 64.0%). In this cluster, 72.0% of employers have hired over 11 employees in the last 2 years.

This cluster had employers in 18 out of the 24 different industries listed and had a company size of 400 employees on average (40.0% higher than the survey average of 285 employees). Cluster 2 had the highest number, 24.0%, of employers having over 1000 employees compared to the other clusters. Only the insurance/finance (12.0%) and health care/social assistance (16.0%) industries represented at least 10.0% of Cluster 2. A high school diploma is required by 47.0% of employers in Cluster 2, and a college degree is needed for 50.0% of employers in this cluster. Employers in Cluster 2 had

3.0% in the Southwest, 16.0% in the Midwest, 25.0% in the West, 28.0% in the Northeast, and 28.0% in the Southeast.

Cluster 2 employers had most hiring practices similar to the survey averages. Of these employers, 75.0% had senior management that exhibited a strong commitment to high functioning ASD hiring and recruitment (survey average of 56.0%); however, only 25.0% of employers in this cluster require suppliers/subcontractors to follow disability non-discrimination requirements (survey average of 56.0%). Cluster 2 have employers who have human resource staff and supervisors training on high functioning ASD sensitivity and awareness approximately 20.0% more than the survey average. However, only 19.0% do the training internally (survey average of 60.0%). Employers in Cluster 2 also impart training on effective inclusion and interviewing practices for employees with high functioning ASD approximately 20.0% more than the average for survey. In addition, this cluster had about 20.0% higher instances of favorable policies and procedures regarding accommodations and accessibility than the averages for the survey. More than 90.0% of Cluster 2 employers have a defined career path for every employee, have opportunities for advancement for employees with high functioning ASD, and invite employees to confidentially disclose whether they have a disability (Figure 3).

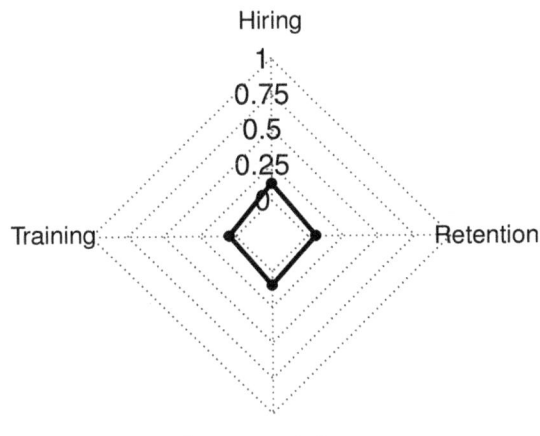

Figure 3. Cluster 2 radar graph.

5.3. Cluster 3

The 62 employer respondents in Cluster 3 (22.0% of sample) had 45.0% in a management/owner role, while 42.0% were in a human resource/recruiting position. Employers in Cluster 3 had a five-year high functioning ASD hiring rate below the survey average (42.0% vs. survey average 58.0%). Cluster 3 had 52.0% of respondents who were involved in the hiring process for less than 10 years (survey average 64.0%). In this cluster, only 42.0% of employers have hired over 11 employees in the last 2 years.

Cluster 3 had employers in 15 out of the 24 different industries listed and had a company size of 108 employees on average (62.0% lower than the survey average of 285 employees). Only the construction (11.0%), Other (13.0%), and health care/social assistance (19.0%) industries represented at least 10.0% of Cluster 3. A high school diploma is required by 55.0% of employers in Cluster 3, and a college degree is needed for only 29.0% of employers in this cluster. Over half of the employers in Cluster 3 were located in the eastern United States. This cluster had 6.0% in the Southwest, 15.0% in the Midwest, 18.0% in the West, 29.0% in the Northeast, and 35.0% in the Southeast.

Cluster 3 only had two policies and procedures, in any category, that were within 40% of the average for the survey: 47.0% do not automatically exclude applicants with a large gap in employment (76.0% survey average), and 45.0% do not automatically exclude applicants with a history of unemployment (79.0% survey average).

Employers in this cluster had very few favorable hiring policies and procedures in place for individuals with high functioning ASD. Only the following three hiring variables were in place for more than 10.0% of employers in Cluster 3: 11.0% actively recruit individuals with high functioning ASD, 13.0% require suppliers/subcontractors to follow disability non-discrimination requirements, and 46.0% do not automatically exclude applicants with a gap in employment or a history of unemployment. The single training variable present in more than 10.0% of Cluster 3 employers was the 23.0% that train supervisors on the legal requirements related to disability, non-discrimination, and accommodation.

Cluster 3 employers also had few favorable accommodations and accessibility policies and procedures in place for individuals with high functioning ASD. Only the following two accommodations variables were in place for more than 10.0% of employers in Cluster 3: 23.0% allow employees to exceed the maximum medical leave duration, and 19.0% evaluate pre-employment occupational screenings to verify they are unbiased.

This cluster only had two favorable policies related to retention of employees with high functioning ASD present in more than 10.0% of employers: 25.0% invite employees to confidentially disclose whether they have a disability, and have a defined career path for all employees (Figure 4).

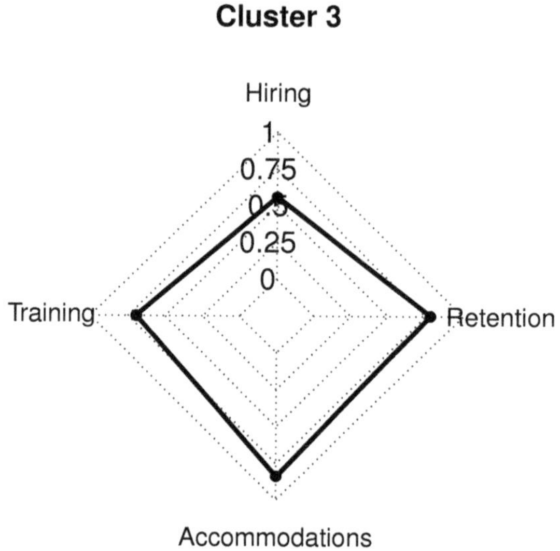

Figure 4. Cluster 3 radar graph.

5.4. Cluster 4

The 28 employer respondents in Cluster 4 (8.0% of sample) had 33.0% in a management/owner role, while 67.0% were in a human resource/recruiting position. Employers in Cluster 4 had a five-year high functioning ASD hiring rate below the survey average (46.0% vs. survey average 58.0%). Cluster 4 had 67.0% of respondents who were involved in the hiring process for less than 10 years (survey average 64.0%). In this cluster, 54.0% of employers have hired less than 11 employees in the last 2 years.

Cluster 4 had employers in 13 out of the 24 different industries listed and had a company size of 250 employees on average (survey average of 285 employees). Only the retail trade (12.0%) and health care/social assistance (29.0%) industries represented at least 10.0% of Cluster 4. A high school diploma is required by only 38.0% of employers in Cluster 4, and a college degree is needed for 63.0% of employers in this cluster. Over half of the employers in Cluster 4 were located in the eastern United States. This cluster had 8.0% in the Midwest, 13.0% in the Southwest, 21.0% in the West, 29.0% in the Northeast, and 29.0% in the Southeast.

Most employers in in Cluster 4 had training policies and procedures in place within 10.0% of the survey averages. There were four training policies in place in ~20.0% more employers than the survey averages: work with an agency to provide the support needed for working with individuals with high functioning ASD, train human resource supervisors and staff on effective inclusion and inclusion practices, and offer sensitivity and awareness training internally.

The majority of employers in Cluster 4 did not have policies in place to stimulate accommodating, hiring, or retaining individuals with high functioning ASD. Nearly all hiring procedures related to employees with high functioning ASD were approximately 20.0–40.0% below the average for the survey. Only one hiring variable had an average comparable to to the survey average: 50.0% actively recruit employees with high functioning ASD (53.0% survey average)

All accommodations and accessibility variables were approximately 30.0–44.0% below the survey average for employers in Cluster 4. All but one retention policies were 30.0–45.0% below the survey average: 54.0% of employers provide a defined career path for all employees (Figure 5).

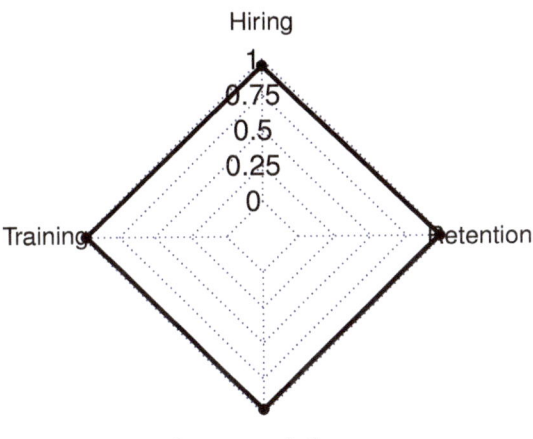

Figure 5. Cluster 4 radar graph.

5.5. Cluster 5

Cluster 5 is the largest cluster of the model. The 126 employer respondents in Cluster 5 (44.0% of sample) had 40.0% in a management/owner role, while 56.0% were in a human resource/recruiting position. Employers in Cluster 5 had a five-year high functioning ASD hiring rate far above the survey average (86.0% vs. survey average 58.0%). Cluster 5 had 75.0% of respondents who were involved in the hiring process for less than 10 years. This is consistent with the work in [59], which found employers newer to the hiring process were more likely to hire an individual with high functioning ASD. In this cluster, 71.0% of employers have hired over 11 employees in the last 2 years.

This cluster had employers in all 24 different industries listed and had a company size of 375 employees on average. The average company size is higher than the survey average of 285 employees, but comparable to the that of Cluster 2 (400 employees). Cluster 5 had 19.0% of employers with over 1000 employees compared to the other clusters. Only the educational services (12.0%) and health care/social assistance (20.0%) industries represented at least 10.0% of Cluster 5. A high school diploma is required by 29.0% of employers in Cluster 5, and a college degree is needed for 64.0% of employers in this cluster. Most employers in this cluster were located in the eastern United States. Employers in Cluster 5 had 7.0% in the Southwest, 15.0% in the West, 18.0% in the Midwest, 22.0% in the Northeast, and 40.0% in the Southeast.

Cluster 5 employers had very high rates of favorable policies and practices in place for individuals with high functioning ASD. The following three polices were in place for *all* employers in this cluster; have a company-wide initiative to higher employees with high functioning ASD, offer a job-related training program for individuals with high functioning ASD, and include individuals with high functioning ASD explicitly in their diversity and inclusion plan.

All but two hiring policies and procedures in place for more than 90% of the Cluster 5 employers: 82.0% have relationships with community organizations that promote the employment of individuals with high functioning ASD, and 88.0% actively recruit individuals with high functioning ASD. Every accommodation, retention, and training policies included in the survey were in place for almost all, 94.0%, of Cluster 5 employers (Figure 6).

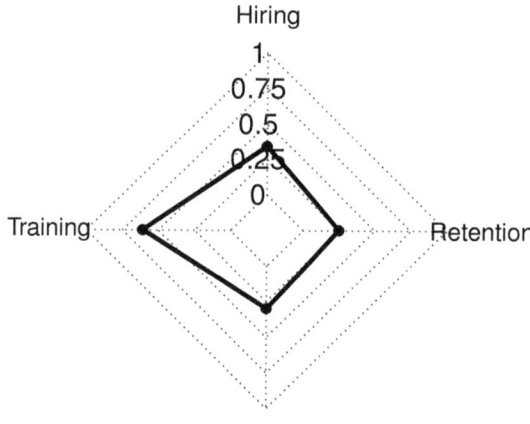

Figure 6. Cluster 5 radar graph.

5.6. Summary of Cluster Comparisons

Most of the respondents were employed in Human Resources and/or Recruiting, which was consistent across all clusters. Cluster 5 had the highest high functioning ASD hiring rate for the past five years, at 86.0%, and, surprisingly also had the most cluster members. The two largest clusters (3 and 5) also had the most extreme average scores for each category. This could indicate that employers tend to have either extremely favorable policies and practices in place or none at all. The most prevalent industry in the survey and all clusters was health care/social assistance, but the cluster with the highest rate of high functioning ASD employment (Cluster 5) did not have the highest rate of health care/social assistance.

Only two clusters (2 and 5) have employment rates above the survey average of 58.0%. These also are the only two clusters with an average company size above the survey average. Although large companies hire more employees, over 50.0% of employers in both of these clusters require a college degree for entry-level jobs. Clusters 1 and 3 had the lowest rates of hiring high function ASD (24.0% and 26.0%, respectively) and are the only two clusters with rates for requiring a college degree below 50.0% (32.0% and 29.0%, respectively). Figure 7 shows all graphs on the same axis.

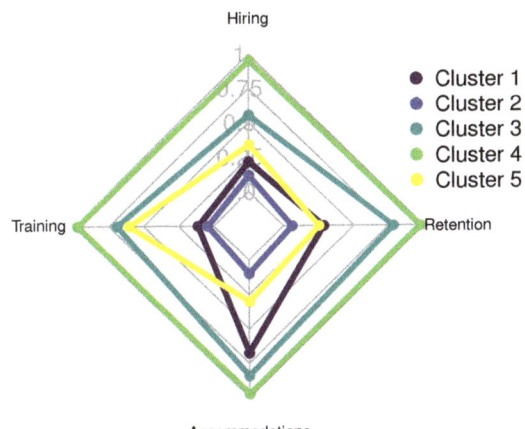

Figure 7. Radar graph for all clusters.

6. Discussion

Although Cluster 3 had the lowest overall score across four categories (hiring, training, accommodation, and retention), Cluster 1 had the lowest hiring rate for individuals with ASD. For this reason, Cluster 1 was compared to Cluster 5, which had the highest hiring rate for individuals with ASD. Cluster 5 also offered a sharp contrast to Cluster 1 in the number of policies in place in support of employees with ASD. Comparing the company structures, policies and practices, perceptions, and needs of employers and employees within these two clusters allows a determination of best practices for companies that are looking to improve their employment rates of individuals with ASD.

6.1. Company Structure, Policies, and Practices

Given that company size and job structures affect hiring practices, company data across the two clusters are included. For size, 58.5% of companies in Cluster 1 had more than 50 employees, compared to 75.3% of Cluster 5 companies. This is important to note, as larger companies may have more opportunities to hire employees with ASD. There also was a difference between job availability and skill sets needed for the different clusters. In Cluster 5, over half of the entry-level jobs require a bachelor's degree (53.2%), whereas, for Cluster 1, only 24.4% require a bachelor's degree, and most require a high school diploma (63.4%). This may be affected by the fact that 70.7% of employers in Cluster 5 work directly with universities to hire employees with HFASD.

In comparison to Cluster 1, companies in Cluster 5 provide their employees with ASD more opportunities for professional growth. For example, 73.0% of Cluster 5 employees with HFASD are paid more now than when they started, and 65.0% of Cluster 5 employees with HFASD have been promoted or had an increase in job responsibilities, versus just 7% in Cluster 1. Further, 50.0% of respondents in Cluster 5 reported that their employees disclosed their HFASD during the application or interview process, rather than after being hired (37.5%) or not at all (12.5%) This could reflect a tendency of the companies in Cluster 5 to be responsive and supportive to a disability disclosure during the interview process.

In Cluster 5, 65.1% of companies created incentives to work at their companies by offering credit-based internships for employees with high functioning ASD, compared to 7.3% in Cluster 1. In addition, about half of the organizations in Cluster 5 show purposeful initiatives to hire employees with high functioning ASD. In contrast, every company in Cluster 1 responded that they did *not* have any purposeful initiatives to hire individuals with high functioning ASD. This indicates that there are no current or future plans for initiatives related to hiring people with high functioning ASD, in contrast to Cluster 5, which included positive responses to many of the initiatives to specifically hire, support, and retain employees with high functioning ASD. One of the few initiatives that 58.6% of Cluster 1 organizations did have was advance notice to job applicants that reasonable accommodations are provided during the job application process. Cluster 1 responses, however, indicated that employers did not offer much beyond this, whereas 81.0% of organizations in Cluster 5 had the accommodations in place. Although none of the companies in Cluster 1 reported having hiring initiatives for employees with high functioning ASD, Cluster 5 reported having specific initiatives to hire employees with high functioning ASD to create a more inclusive workplace (21.0%), because they recognize the skills of employees with high functioning ASD (21.0%), to increase the company's reputation benefits (7.0%), and to decrease employee turnover (2.0%).

Employers in Cluster 1 provide far fewer accommodations than do those in Cluster 5. For example, 81.7% of Cluster 5 employees state that they have a centralized accommodations fund to specifically provide accommodations for employees with disabilities, compared to 39.1% in Cluster 1. Further, just 2.4% of employers in Cluster 5 reported *not* having a designated office or person to address accommodation questions compared to 17.1% in Cluster 1 who do not have a designated accommodation office or person. These data indicate that it may be necessary for employers to provide a menu of accommodation options for their employees, rather than using a one-size-fits-all approach.

Because all respondents in Cluster 1 indicated that they did not have initiatives to specifically hire employees with high functioning ASD, their survey was auto-formatted to skip questions regarding these specific hiring practices. Although this does not allow for comparisons of specific high functioning ASD hiring practices between Clusters 1 and 5, the difference in responses indicates that Cluster 1 companies did not have any initiatives to specifically hire employees with high functioning ASD, while Cluster 5 companies did.

Many employers in Cluster 5 said that they have relationships with community organizations that promote the employment of people with high functioning ASD, with 81.8% that reported that such a program was already in place, and 17.5%, that such a program was being considered. Approximately, 70.7% of Cluster 5 also reported having relationships with universities, with 23.0% that noted that such a program was being considered, and 4.0%, that such a program was not currently in place.

6.2. Perceptions and Attitudes

Questions related to employer attitudes demonstrated, in Cluster 5, a company belief in the high competency of their employees with high functioning ASD. For example, 74.6% of employers in Cluster 5 reported being likely to hire employees with high functioning ASD versus 17.1% of Cluster 1. In Cluster 5, 65.1% of employees with high functioning ASD have been promoted or taken on additional job responsibilities, whereas only 7.3% of Cluster 1 had. Generally, employers in Cluster 5 reported having supportive coworkers, reflecting a positive work environment as well as an overall positive experience in working with employees with high functioning ASD, with 20.6% rating their experience as positive and 53.2% as very positive. The majority (78.0%) of respondents in Cluster 1 did not have experience with working with high functioning ASD; thus, comparison data were not available.

The data from Cluster 5 demonstrate an inclusive culture in which high functioning ASD training is offered to employees. Employers offer HR and staff training on inclusive practices (80.2%) and legal requirements (77.8%), high functioning ASD sensitivity and awareness training (72.9%), and training related to effective interviewing of potential employees with high functioning ASD (83.4%). In Cluster 1, 87.8% do not offer high functioning ASD sensitivity and awareness training, 87.8% do not have training in effective interviewing of potential employees with high functioning ASD, 63.4% do not require training related to legal requirements and nondiscrimination accommodation, and 90.2% do not train staff on inclusive workplace practices of people with high functioning ASD.

The biggest fears of hiring someone with high functioning ASD were the same for both clusters: high functioning ASD employees would have behaviors that put themselves or others at risk (Cluster 1: 24.0%; Cluster 5: 29.0%) and employees with high functioning ASD would not perform well (Cluster 1: 24.0%; Cluster 5: 23.0%). Despite having the same fears, Cluster 5 businesses responded positively to hiring employees with high functioning ASD.

6.3. Needs of Employers and Employees

When asked about obtaining additional training in hiring practices, respondents in Clusters 1 and 5 stated that they would prefer that training in hiring employees with high functioning ASD be free, but only 43.9% of Cluster 1 were willing to pay, whereas 80.0% of Cluster 5 were willing to pay.

Having a supportive environment helps to alleviate stress and boost productivity [35]. In Cluster 5, the majority of high functioning ASD employees seem to need some form of support, but these companies appear to be prepared to provide that support. Cluster 1 has a far lower perceived need of support for high functioning ASD employees, but perhaps employers are simply unaware of the support needed or less open to offering extra support. For the level of support that their employees with high functioning ASD need, 75.6% of Cluster 1 companies did not respond, indicating a lack of experience with high functioning ASD employees. Of those who did respond, their answers were that their employees with high functioning ASD required: no support (7.3%), some support (12.2%), substantial support (2.4%), or very substantial support (2.4%). In Cluster 5, 12.1% did not respond, but the remaining responded: no support (6.3%), some support (30.2%), substantial support (28.6%), or very substantial support (19.8%). In Cluster 5, 47.6% reported that high functioning ASD employees are in a job-related training program, whereas, in Cluster 1, employers responded that none of their employees with high functioning ASD is in a job-related training program. After considering the notable factors in the in-depth cluster comparisons and reviewing the literature in the field, the researchers identified best practices in employment that would likely lead to the successful hiring of individuals with ASD. These components were organized under a summary of best practices for improving employment, to assist with applying the study outcomes to the field and presented in Table 6.

Table 6. Practices for improving employment of individuals with high functioning ASD.

Category	Practice	Supporting Citations
Recruitment and Hiring	Foster relationships with community organizations for recruitment of employees with ASD. Encourage relationships with universities and employment agencies to help bridge the gap between college and employment and allow for a smoother transition. Have a supportive interview process. It is not enough to simply note that accommodations will be provided during interview (e.g., Cluster 1); more is needed Have specific hiring and retention practices and policies related to ASD employees, along with training for managers, hiring personnel (specify who)	Culler et al. (2011); Fraser et al. (2010); Fraser et al. (2011); Gewurtz et al. (2018); Graffam et al. (2002); Peck & Kirkbride (2001); Wiggett-Barnard and Swarts (2012)
Training	Make hiring personnel, managers, and employees aware of the many positive professional traits that employees with ASD have; foster an inclusive workplace that reflects a belief in the high competency of employees. Provide training about the myths of ASD employment "challenges".	Fraser et al. (2011); Lengnick-Hall et al. (2008); Lopez & Keenan (2014); Luecking (2011); Nesbitt (2000); Peck & Kirkbride (2001); Richards (2012)
Accessibility & Accommodations	Provide a menu of options, rather than just a few, that the employer believes are effective, for individuals to hire and retain employees with ASD. Offer for-credit internships; this creates more of an incentive to work there and can provide a transition opportunity for employees with ASD to adjust to the work environment. Provide the same professional growth opportunities for ASD as for neurotypical colleagues.	Project SEARCH [60]; Taube (2014) [61]
Retention & Advancement	Create and monitor a professional growth plan. Support employers (encourage ride-sharing, peer mentor/support, relationships of open communication and trust). Partner with or provide an on-site job training program.	Lindsay et al. (2019); Wiggett-Barnard and Swarts (2012)

7. Conclusions

This study supports some of the findings of the research on employer perspectives on hiring employees with ASD [7,25,32], but also expands upon Lindsay et al.'s study by using machine learning to analyze trends in businesses that have successfully hired and retained employees with ASD [27]. To foster such diversity and inclusion, it is critical to understand the needs of both the employees and employers. The results of this analysis may be utilized to make suggestions for stakeholders who are working to make improvements to the employment of individuals with high functioning ASD.

The comparison of clusters of employers with the highest and lowest rates of employing individuals with ASD revealed company policies and practices that can be effective for hiring, training, and retaining employees with ASD. The results show that purposeful diversity initiatives and relationships with community organizations that promote ASD are likely effective in increasing employment for those with ASD. Offering disability and diversity training is also helpful for understanding the needs of employees with ASD. These steps may affect perceptions and attitudes as well, as shown through the belief in high competency of employees with ASD; promotions; and supportive, positive coworker experiences. These results are promising for developing recommendations that can be implemented to increase employment opportunities for individuals with ASD on a large scale. More research, however, needs to be conducted to continue to identify best practices for supporting employees with ASD. As these recommendations are further researched and refined, employers will need training and support to translate these concepts into practice.

Author Contributions: Conceptualization, A.J.G., A.H.H., and C.M.G.; data curation, A.J.G., A.H.H., and C.M.G.; methodology, K.H. and E.L.; software, K.H. and E.L.; writing—original draft preparation, A.J.G., A.H.H., C.M.G., S.K.M., and K.H.; writing—review and editing, A.J.G., A.H.H., C.M.G., S.M., K.H., and E.L. All authors have read and agreed to the published version of the manuscript.

Funding: The APC was funded by the Machine Learning and Assistive Technology Lab at Chapman University.

Conflicts of Interest: The authors declare no conflicts of interest.

Abbreviations

The following abbreviations are used in this manuscript.

ASD	Autism Spectrum Disorder
HFASD	High Functioning Autism Spectrum Disorder
HR	Human Resources

References

1. Hurley-Hanson, A.E.; Giannantonio, C.M.; Griffiths, A.J. *Autism in the Workplace: Creating Positive Employment and Career Outcomes for Generation A*; Palgrave Macmillan: Basingstoke, UK, 2020.
2. Hedley, D.; Uljarević, M.; Cameron, L.; Halder, S.; Richdale, A.; Dissanayake, C. Employment programmes and interventions targeting adults with autism spectrum disorder: A systematic review of the literature. *Autism* **2017**, *21*, 929–941. [CrossRef]
3. Jacob, A.; Scott, M.; Falkmer, M.; Falkmer, T. The costs and benefits of employing an adult with autism spectrum disorder: A systematic review. *PLoS ONE* **2015**, *10*, e0139896. [CrossRef] [PubMed]
4. Baldwin, S.; Costley, D.; Warren, A. Employment activities and experiences of adults with high-functioning Autism and Asperger's disorder. *J. Autism Dev. Disord.* **2014**, *44*, 2440–2449. [CrossRef] [PubMed]
5. Kreiger, B.; Kinebanian, A.; Prodinger, B.; Heigl, F. Becoming a member of the workforce: Perceptions of adults with Asperger syndrome. *Work* **2012**, *43*, 141–157. [CrossRef] [PubMed]
6. Nord, D.K.; Stancliffe, R.J.; Nye-Legerman, K.; Hewitt, A.S. Employment in the community for people with and without autism: A comparative analysis. *Res. Autism Spectr. Disord.* **2016**, *24*, 11–16. [CrossRef]
7. Richards, J. Examining the exclusion of employees with Asperger syndrome from the workplace. *Pers. Rev.* **2012**, *41*, 630–646. [CrossRef]

8. Roux, A.M.; Shattuck, P.T.; Cooper, B.P.; Anderson, K.A.; Wagner, M.; Narendorf, S.C. Postsecondary employment experiences among young adults with an Autism Spectrum Disorder RH: Employment in young adults with autism. *J. Am. Acad. Child Adolesc. Psychiatry* **2013**, *52*, 931–939. [CrossRef]
9. Scott, M.; Falkmer, M.; Girdler, S.; Falkmer, T. Viewpoints on factors for successful employment for adults with autism spectrum disorder. *PLoS ONE* **2015**, *10*, e0139281.
10. Shattuck, P.T.; Narendorf, S.C.; Cooper, B.; Sterzing, P.R.; Wagner, M.; Taylor, J.L. Postsecondary education and employment among youth with an autism spectrum disorder. *Pediatrics* **2012**, *129*, 1042–1049. [CrossRef]
11. Hagner, D.; Cooney, B.F. "I do that for everybody": Supervising employees with autism. *Focus Autism Other Dev. Disabil.* **2005**, *20*, 91–97. [CrossRef]
12. Hendricks, D. Employment and adults with autism spectrum disorders: Challenges and strategies for success. *J. Vocat. Rehabil.* **2010**, *32*, 125–134. [CrossRef]
13. de Schipper, E.; Mahdi, S.; de Vries, P.; Granlund, M.; Holmann, M.; Karande, S.; Almodayfer, O.; Shulman, C.; Tonge, B.; Wong, V.; et al. Functioning and disability in Autism Spectrum Disorder: A worldwide survey of experts. *Autism Res.* **2016**, *9*, 959–969. [CrossRef] [PubMed]
14. Hillier, A.; Campbell, H.; Mastriani, K.; Izzo, M.V.; Kool-Tucker, A.K.; Cherry, L.; Beversdorf, D.Q. Two-Year Evaluation of a Vocational Support Program for Adults on the Autism Spectrum. *Career Dev. Except. Individ.* **2007**, *30*, 35–47. [CrossRef]
15. Howlin, P.; Alcock, J.; Burkin, C. An 8 year follow-up of a specialist supported employment service for high-ability adults with autism or Asperger syndrome. *Autism* **2005**, *9*, 533–549. [CrossRef] [PubMed]
16. Boushey, H.; Glynn, S.J. There are significant business costs to replacing employees. *Cent. Am. Prog.* **2012**, *16*, 1–9.
17. Buescher, A.V.; Cidav, Z.; Knapp, M.; Mandell, D.S. Costs of autism spectrum disorders in the United Kingdom and the United States. *JAMA Pediatr.* **2014**, *168*, 721–728. [CrossRef]
18. Kemper, A.; Stolarick, K.; Milway, J.B.; Treviranus, J. *Releasing Constraints: Projecting the Economic Impacts of Increased Accessibility in Ontario*; Martin Prosperity Institute: Toronto, ON, Canada, 2009.
19. Knapp, M.; Romeo, R.; Beecham, J. Economic cost of autism in the UK. *Autism* **2009**, *13*, 317–336. [CrossRef]
20. Lee, E.A.; Black, M.H.; Tan, T.; Falkmer, T.; Girdler, S. "I'm destined to ace this": Work experience placement during high school for individuals with autism spectrum disorder. *J. Autism Dev. Disord.* **2019**, *49*, 3089–3101. [CrossRef]
21. Cidav, Z.; Marcus, S.C.; Mandell, D.S. Implications of childhood autism for parental employment and earnings. *Pediatrics* **2012**, *129*, 617–623. [CrossRef]
22. Gewurtz, R.E.; Langan, S.; Shand, D. Hiring people with disabilities: A scoping review. *Work* **2016**, *54*, 135–148. [CrossRef]
23. Chen, J.L.; Leader, G.; Sung, C.; Leahy, M. Trends in Employment for Individuals with Autism Spectrum Disorder: A Review of the Research Literature. *Rev. J. Autism Dev. Disord.* **2015**, *2*, 115–127. [CrossRef]
24. Hernandez, B.; Keys, C.; Balcazar, F. Employer attitudes toward workers with disabilities and their ADA employment rights: A literature review. *J. Rehabil.* **2000**, *66*, 4–16.
25. López, B.; Keenan, L. Barriers to employment in autism: Future challenges to implementing the Adult Autism Strategy. In *Autism Research Network*; University of Portsmouth: Portsmouth, UK, 2014.
26. Bruyere, S.M. *Disability Employment Policies and Practices in Private and Federal Sector Organizations*; Cornell University: Ithaca, NY, USA, 2000.
27. Lindsay, S.; Cagliostro, E.; Leck, J.; Shen, W.; Stinson, J. Employers' perspectives of including young people with disabilities in the workforce, disability disclosure and providing accommodations. *J. Vocat. Rehabil.* **2019**, *50*, 141–156. [CrossRef]
28. Kaye, H.S.; Jans, L.H.; Jones, E.C. Why don't employers hire and retain workers with disabilities? *J. Occup. Rehabil.* **2011**, *21*, 526–536. [CrossRef] [PubMed]
29. Loprest, P.; Maag, E. Issues in Job Search and Work, Accommodation. *Res. Soc. Sci. Disabil.* **2003**, *3*, 87–108.
30. Morgan, R.L.; Alexander, M. The employer's perception: Employment of individuals with developmental disabilities. *J. Vocat. Rehabil.* **2005**, *23*, 39–49.
31. Peck, B.; Kirkbride, L.T. Why businesses don't employ people with disabilities. *J. Vocat. Rehabil.* **2001**, *16*, 71–75.
32. Nesbitt, S. Why and why not? Factors influencing employment for individuals with Asperger syndrome. *Autism* **2000**, *4*, 357–369. [CrossRef]

33. Unger, D.D. Employers' attitudes toward persons with disabilities in the workforce: Myths or realities? *Focus Autism Other Dev. Disabil.* **2002**, *17*, 2–10. [CrossRef]
34. Scott, M.; Jacob, A.; Hendrie, D.; Parsons, R.; Girdler, S.; Falkmer, T. Employers' perception of the costs and the benefits of hiring individuals with autism spectrum disorder in open employment in Australia. *PLoS ONE* **2017**, *12*, e0177607. [CrossRef]
35. Dreaver, J.; Thompson, C.; Girdler, S.; Adolfsson, M.; Black, M.H.; Falkmer, M. Success Factors Enabling Employment for Adults on the Autism Spectrum from Employers' Perspective. *J. Autism Dev. Disord.* **2019**, *50*, 1657–1667. [CrossRef] [PubMed]
36. Austin, R.D.; Pisano, G.P. Neurodiversity as a competitive advantage. *Harv. Bus. Rev.* **2017**, *95*, 96–103.
37. Demer, L. The Autism Spectrum: Human Rights Perspectives. *Pediatrics* **2018**, *141*, 369–374. [CrossRef]
38. Hensel, W.F. People with Autism spectrum disorder in the workplace: An expanding legal frontier. *Harv. Civ.-Rights-Civ. Lib. Law Rev.* **2017**, *52*, 74–103.
39. Vogus, T.J.; Lounds-Taylor, J. Flipping the script: Bringing an organizational perspective to the study of autism at work. *Autism* **2018**, *22*, 514–516. [CrossRef] [PubMed]
40. Hara, K.; Bigham, J.P. Introducing people with ASD to crowd work. In Proceedings of the 19th International ACM SIGACCESS Conference on Computers and Accessibility, Baltimore, MD, USA, 29 October–1 November 2017; pp. 42–51.
41. Gerhardt, P.F.; Lainer, I. Addressing the needs of adolescents and adults with autism: A crisis on the horizon. *J. Contemp. Psychother.* **2011**, *41*, 37–45. [CrossRef]
42. Fraser, R.; Ajzen, I.; Johnson, K.; Hebert, J.; Chan, F. Understanding employers' hiring intention in relation to qualified workers with disabilities. *J. Vocat. Rehabil.* **2011**, *35*, 1–11. [CrossRef]
43. Bricout, J.C.; Bentley, K.J. Disability status and perceptions of employability by employers. *Soc. Work. Res.* **2000**, *24*, 87–95. [CrossRef]
44. Chan, F.; Strauser, D.; Maher, P.; Lee, E.J.; Jones, R.; Johnson, E.T. Demand-side factors related to employment of people with disabilities: A survey of employers in the Midwest region of the United States. *J. Occup. Rehabil.* **2010**, *20*, 412–419. [CrossRef]
45. Hand, C.; Tryssenaar, J. Small business employers' views on hiring individuals with mental illness. *Psychiatr. Rehabil. J.* **2006**, *29*, 166. [CrossRef]
46. Hazer, J.T.; Bedell, K.V. Effects of seeking accommodation and disability on preemployment evaluations. *J. Appl. Soc. Psychol.* **2000**, *30*, 1201–1223. [CrossRef]
47. Jasper, C.R.; Waldhart, P. Employer attitudes on hiring employees with disabilities in the leisure and hospitality industry. *Int. J. Contemp. Hosp. Manag.* **2013**, *25*, 577–594. [CrossRef]
48. Wiggett-Barnard, C.; Swartz, L. What facilitates the entry of persons with disabilities into South African companies? *Disabil. Rehabil.* **2012**, *34*, 1016–1023. [CrossRef]
49. Culler, K.H.; Wang, Y.C.; Byers, K.; Trierweiler, R. Barriers and facilitators of return to work for individuals with strokes: perspectives of the stroke survivor, vocational specialist, and employer. *Top. Stroke Rehabil.* **2011**, *18*, 325–340. [CrossRef]
50. Graffam, J.; Shinkfield, A.; Smith, K.; Polzin, U. Factors that influence employer decisions in hiring and retaining an employee with a disability. *J. Vocat. Rehabil.* **2002**, *17*, 175–181.
51. Alvares, G.A.; Bebbington, K.; Cleary, D.; Evans, K.; Glasson, E.J.; Maybery, M.T.; Pillar, S.; Uljarevic, M.; Varcin, K.; Wray, J.; Whitehouse, A.J. The misnomer of 'high functioning autism': Intelligence is an imprecise predictor of functional abilities at diagnosis. *Autism* **2020**, *24*, 221–232. [CrossRef]
52. American Psychiatric Association. *Diagnostic and Statistical Manual of Mental Disorders*, 5th ed.; American Psychiatric Publishing: Washington, DC, USA, 2013.
53. Erickson, W.A.; von Schrader, S.; Bruyère, S.M.; VanLooy, S.A. The employment environment: Employer perspectives, policies, and practices regarding the employment of persons with disabilities. *Rehabil. Couns. Bull.* **2014**, *57*, 195–208. [CrossRef]
54. Newman, L.; Wagner, M.; Knokey, A.M.; Marder, C.; Nagle, K.; Shaver, D.; Wei, X. *The Post-High School Outcomes of Young Adults with Disabilities up to 8 Years after High School: A Report from the National Longitudinal Transition Study-2 (NLTS2). NCSER 2011–3005*; National Center for Special Education Research: Washington, DC, USA, 2011.
55. Dillman, D.A.; Smyth, J.D.; Christian, L.M. *Internet, Phone, Mail, and Mixed-Mode Surveys: The Tailored Design Method*; John Wiley & Sons: Hoboken, NJ, USA, 2014.

56. MacQueen, J. Some methods for classification and analysis of multivariate observations. In Proceedings of the Fifth Berkeley Symposium on Mathematical Statistics and Probability, Berkeley, CA, USA, 21 June–18 July 1965; University of California: Oakland, CA, USA, 1967; Volume 1, pp. 281–297.
57. Tibshirani, R.; Walther, G.; Hastie, T. Estimating the number of clusters in a data set via the gap statistic. *J. R. Stat. Soc. Ser. (Stat. Methodol.)* **2001**, *63*, 411–423. [CrossRef]
58. Rousseeuw, P.J. Silhouettes: A graphical aid to the interpretation and validation of cluster analysis. *J. Comput. Appl. Math.* **1987**, *20*, 53–65. [CrossRef]
59. Hyde, K.; Griffiths, A.J.; Giannantonio, C.; Hurley-Hanson, A.; Linstead, E. Predicting employer recruitment of individuals with autism spectrum disorders with decision trees. In Proceedings of the 2018 17th IEEE International Conference on Machine Learning and Applications (ICMLA), Orlando, FL, USA, 17–20 December 2018; pp. 1366–1370.
60. Wehman, P.; Schall, C.; McDonough, J.; Molinelli, A.; Riehle, E.; Ham, W.; Thiss, W.R. Project SEARCH for youth with autism spectrum disorders: Increasing competitive employment on transition from high school. *J. Posit. Behav. Interv.* **2013**, *15*, 144–155. [CrossRef]
61. Taube, A. *Two MIT Grads Founded A Startup That Almost Exclusively Employs People On The Autism Spectrum*; Organization for Autism Research: Arlington County, VA, USA, 2014.

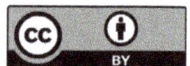

© 2019 by the authors. Licensee MDPI, Basel, Switzerland. This article is an open access article distributed under the terms and conditions of the Creative Commons Attribution (CC BY) license (http://creativecommons.org/licenses/by/4.0/).

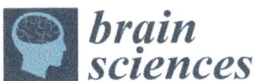 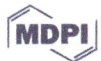

Article

An Assessment of the Motor Performance Skills of Children with Autism Spectrum Disorder in the Gulf Region

Rehab H. Alsaedi [1,2]

1. Faculty of Education, Queensland University of Technology (QUT), Brisbane 4059, Australia; r-alsaidi@hotmail.com
2. Department of Special Education, Taibah University, Madinah 41477, Saudi Arabia

Received: 29 June 2020; Accepted: 29 August 2020; Published: 3 September 2020

Abstract: This study aims to determine the prevalence, severity, and nature of the motor abnormalities seen in children with autism spectrum disorder (ASD) as well as to elucidate the associated developmental profiles. The short-form of the Bruininks-Oseretsky Test of Motor Proficiency, Second Edition (BOT-2) was used to assess various aspects of the motor performance of 119 children with ASD and 30 typically developing children (age range: 6–12 years) from three Gulf states. The results revealed the high prevalence of motor abnormalities among the ASD group when compared with the normative data derived from the BOT-2 manual as well as with the data concerning the typically developing group. The results also indicated that the motor performance of the children with ASD fell within the below-average range according to the BOT-2 cut-off score. Further, the results suggested that the age variable may influence the overall motor performance of children with ASD, since the children's motor abnormalities may decrease with maturation. The results concerning the specific motor dysfunction profiles seen in individuals with ASD could help practitioners, parents, and educators to better understand the nature of the motor deficits exhibited by children with ASD, which could assist with the design and implementation of treatment and rehabilitation programs for such children. Overall, motor performance represents an important aspect that should be considered during the clinical evaluation of ASD and that should not be ignored during early interventions.

Keywords: motor performance skills; autism spectrum disorder; Gulf; BOT-2

1. Introduction

Motor skills are associated with "activities that require a chain of sensory (vision, hearing, touch, and smell), central (brain and nervous systems), and motor mechanisms whereby the performer is able to maintain constant control of the sensory input and in accordance with the goal of the movement" [1]. The child development literature tends to assume that motor ability is an important indicator of overall development, particularly if it is compromised [2]. Indeed, early motor disturbances and delays are likely to have far-reaching consequences for later development, and they may be predictive of developmental disorders in later life [3,4]. Children with autism spectrum disorder (ASD) represent a population likely to experience motor impairments [5].

ASD affects every domain of human existence. An impairment in the motor domain can have profound effects on a child's development in areas such as schooling, socialisation, and communication [6,7]. It has been estimated that "80–90% of children with ASD show some degree of motor abnormality" [8]. However, it should be noted that previous results regarding prevalence rates vary depending on the utilised cut-off scores, diagnoses, and instruments [9].

Motor dysfunction represents an important neurological symptom in those with ASD. A growing body of evidence illustrates the motor difficulties experienced by children with ASD when compared with their typically developing peers [10–13]. However, such difficulties have traditionally been considered secondary aspects of ASD [14].

The only motor abnormalities currently included in the diagnostic criteria for ASD are stereotypical and repetitive behaviours [15]. However, the relevant motor abnormalities are not limited to such behaviours, as individuals with ASD, including children [16], often display motor issues consisting of both delays and deficits. Delays occur in the gross and fine motor skills [12], while deficits manifest in praxis [17], coordination and gait [18], postural control [19], and motor planning [20]).

Little is currently known about the underlying neurobiology of ASD-related motor problems, although the disruptions observed in those with ASD may stem from abnormal brain connectivity [10,21]. Some studies report reduced cerebellar activation in individuals with ASD during motor tasks when compared with neurotypical controls [22,23]. Dysfunctions in the frontostriatal pathways of children with ASD have also been demonstrated [24,25]. Further, the aberrant neural connectivity patterns observed between the cerebellar and frontostriatal pathways indicate the role of the cortical and subcortical structures and the pathways connecting them in controlling the accuracy of motor outputs [21].

Considerable ambiguity persists regarding the nature of such motor abnormalities and whether they are universal and specific to ASD. Some findings indicate that motor impairments constitute a cardinal feature of ASD [10,26–28]. The identified impairments remain consistent across ages and levels of functioning [11,29,30]. Additionally, evidence from prospective studies of at-risk infants indicates motor deficits to have been documented in infants later diagnosed with ASD [31–34]. Therefore, motor symptoms could serve as diagnostic markers and guide the early identification of ASD [26,35,36]. However, other evidence suggests that motor delays can be attributed to developmental disorders in general, meaning that they are not specific to ASD [37].

Some preliminary evidence indicates that motor impairments represent an essential part of a broader autistic phenotype [38], although other studies have not found such impairments to represent an essential aspect [8,37]. It is important to recognise that motor impairments are not limited to one disorder (e.g., ASD), as they are also present in other developmental disorders [9,39–41]. The debate regarding the prevalence and importance of motor deficits is not surprising given that ASD is a spectrum disorder, meaning that every child exhibits a wide variety of symptoms with different degrees of severity. This variability can offer a unique opportunity to identify disorder subtypes [42].

Jeste (2011) offers a number of justifications for investigating motor dysfunction in individuals with ASD [20]. First, motor symptoms are easily quantifiable and so can be objectively measured. Second, motor impairments may elucidate the heterogeneity within the autistic spectrum. Third, the investigation of motor abnormalities may yield insights into the aberrant neural mechanisms underlying ASD and the defining characteristics of the disorder. Fourth, motor performance is critical to the development of a wide variety of skills, which would all benefit from the early identification of deficits and the implementation of appropriate interventions. Lastly, determining when motor deficits manifest in individuals with ASD may assist with the early diagnosis of the disorder [20].

Age might be a critical factor in determining the nature of the motor dysfunction seen in individuals with ASD. However, the available research concerning the developmental acquisition of motor skills by children with ASD is limited. Evidence suggests that the different subsystems supporting motor development mature at different times and rates, which results in nonlinear development [43]; thereby, indicating the dynamic development of motor skills. Thus, Darrah et al. (2003) suggest the adoption of a developmental change perspective rather than one that emphasises the stability of motor development [44].

No firm conclusions regarding the stability or instability of motor performance can yet be drawn in relation to ASD. Some longitudinal studies indicate the persistent and constant nature of impaired motor performance in children with ASD [45]. Further, other longitudinal research confirms that motor problems among preschool children are not always stable, although they do appear to be so in most children with ASD [46]. However, some cross-sectional studies note the changing nature of motor problems in children with ASD, with the prevalence of motor deficits being lower in older children than younger children [16]. In contrast, other studies indicate that motor difficulties become increasingly problematic over time [34]. A number of factors could contribute to this decline in motor performance, including a lack of early intervention programs targeting motor skills and a lack of parental involvement in children's treatment [34].

A growing body of evidence gathered in Western contexts suggests motor abnormalities to be a marker of clinical severity and an important therapeutic target in children with ASD [26,36,47]. However, despite this increasing recognition, the evaluation and intervention processes related to motor abnormalities are still not seen as priorities, meaning that they are unlikely to attract the attention of professionals in our research context (the Gulf region). Indeed, motor dysfunctions arguably represent one of the most commonly overlooked comorbidities associated with ASD in the Gulf context. It is important to conduct research regarding motor performance in individuals with ASD in different cultures so as to achieve a clearer understanding of ASD and its phenotypes in different socio-cultural contexts.

The present study had three main aims. First, to determine the ratio of motor impairments seen in children with ASD, as identified using the short form of the Bruininks-Oseretsky Test of Motor Proficiency, Second Edition (BOT-2) [48]. It was expected that children with ASD would surpass the cut-off point for being "motor impaired". Second, to examine the extent of the differences in the motor performance of children with ASD and typically developing children. It was hypothesised that the motor performance of children with ASD would be significantly worse than that of typically developing children. Third, to investigate the effect of chronological age on the motor performance of children with ASD. Due to the lack of relevant evidence, no predictions were made regarding the relation between motor performance and age.

2. Materials and Methods

2.1. Study Design

This observational study applied a quantitative research approach that entailed the use of a cross-sectional design to characterize the motor proficiency levels of the participants at a given point in time. There were a number of reasons why this particular research approach was chosen. First, the study relied on a quantitative measurement instrument (i.e., the BOT-2) that provided a numerical evaluation of various aspects of the participants' motor performance, which meant that it was possible to objectively assess the performance of the study sample. Second, due to the nature of the research aims, outcomes in the form of numerical values were required to allow for comparisons between the ASD population and the corresponding BOT-2 norms and/or those children without ASD, as well as to reflect the relationship between the participants' age and their test outcomes.

2.2. Participants

Data for the present study were collected in Bahrain, Saudi Arabia, and the United Arab Emirates (UAE). The participants comprised children who were participating in an ongoing large-scale study evaluating neurobehavioral problems in children with ASD. They were recruited through purposive sampling on a voluntary basis.

The initial sample consisted of 235 children, who were divided into the ASD ($n = 180$) and typically developing (TD) ($n = 55$) groups. Among them, 61 children with ASD and 25 TD children were excluded from the final sample. The recruitment process is illustrated in Figure 1.

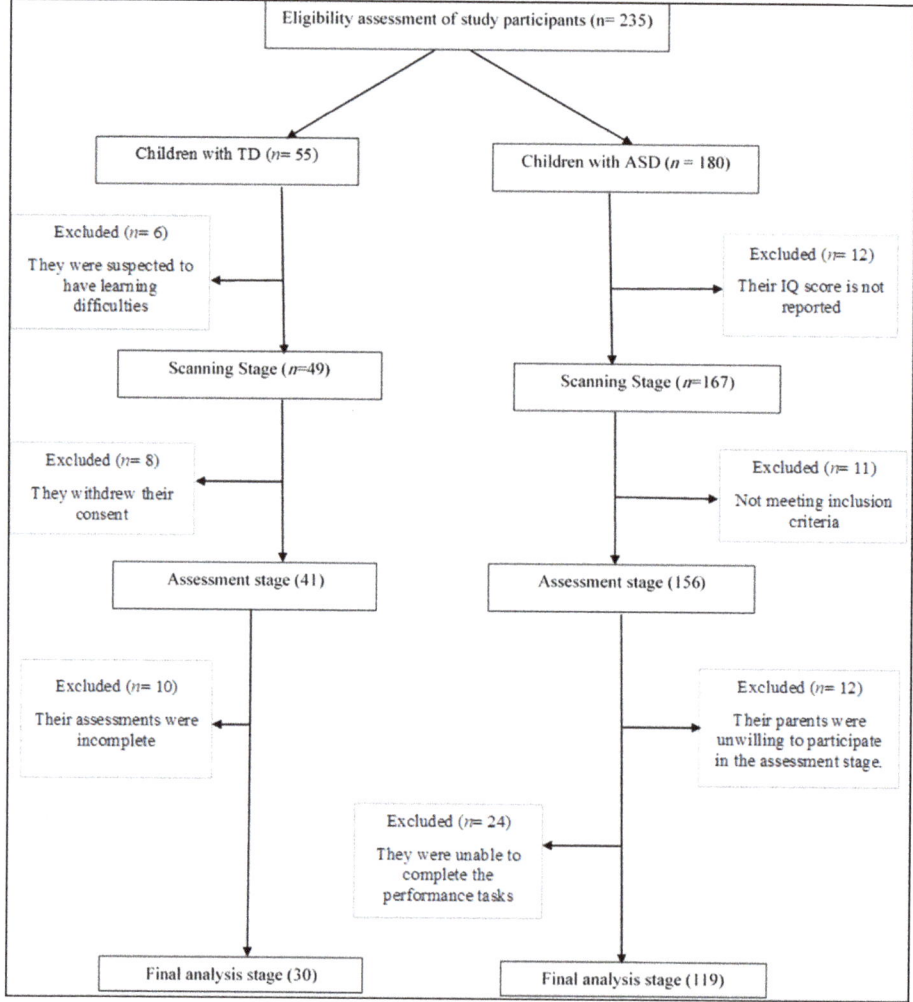

Figure 1. Recruitment of the Participants.

All the children with ASD (age range: 6–12 years; mean age = 8.75 years) had received a formal diagnosis prior to their recruitment for the present study. They attended three different types of educational settings, namely a fully inclusive school ($N = 26$; 21.8%), a partially inclusive school ($N = 19$; 15.9%), or a specialised ASD school or centre ($N = 74$; 62.18%).

The inclusion criteria for the ASD group were as follows. First, all the children with ASD had an IQ score of 70 or above. This IQ-related criterion was required to ensure that they could understand the test items and instructions and so that any identified differences in performance reflected autistic symptomatology rather than general intellectual functioning. The intelligence test scores were obtained from the children's school records. In the three countries of interest, a child's IQ is normally determined by a clinical psychologist or school psychologist using the Arabic version of the Wechsler Intelligence Scale for Children, Third Edition (WISC-III; 1991). Second, they all met the diagnostic criteria for level 1 of the ASD severity scale included within the DSM-5, indicating that they had mild symptoms and required support [49]. Third, all their scores on the Michigan Autism Spectrum Questionnaire

(MASQ) [50] were 22 or above, indicating high-functioning performance. Moreover, they all scored ≥ 71 on the Gilliam Autism Rating Scale—Third Edition (GARS-3) [51], indicating that an ASD diagnosis is very likely.

The exclusion criterion for the ASD group was the presence of comorbid affective and/or behavioural symptoms (e.g., intractable epilepsy, severe self-injury, aggression, uncorrected hearing loss, or visual impairment precluding participation). The absence of such comorbidities was verified by the researcher through interviewing the parents and reviewing the children's medical records.

The comparison (non-ASD or TD) group comprised 30 TD children (age range: 6–12 years; mean age = 9.06 years) recruited from mainstream primary schools. The exclusion criteria were (i) a history of any psychiatric, neurological, or developmental disorder, (ii) a family history of ASD, (iii) a need to regularly use any psychotropic medication, (iv) a physical disability that hinders motor performance, and/or (v) undergoing physical therapy to address motor issues. One obstacle to recruiting a sufficient number of TD participants concerns parents' reluctance to permit their children to participate in research. This reluctance could indicate that parents are concerned about their children's assessment results. Data collection can prove particularly challenging in the Arab context due to recognised delays in certain developmental skills and the potential for stigmatisation.

All the participants (i.e., with and without ASD) were group-wise matched according to their gender, chronological age, handedness (rated using the Edinburgh Handedness Inventory (EHI) [52], non-verbal IQ (assessed using Raven's Coloured Progressive Matrices (RCPM) [53]), and parental education level (see Table 1). The results of the group-wise analyses revealed no significant between-group differences ($p < 0.05$) with regard to any factor relevant to the comparison outcome variables.

Table 1. Demographic and Clinical Characteristics of the Participants.

Comparison Characteristics		Target Group (N = 119) Children with ASD	Control Group (N = 30) TD Children	t/χ^2	p	ES
Continuous variables						
Age (years)		8.72 (1.96) *	9.06 (1.42) *	1.05	0.71	0.21
Non-verbal IQ		29.76 (1.92) *	29.80 (2.64) *	0.69	0.060	0.17
Categorical variables						
Gender	Male	95 (79.8%)	24 (80.0%)	0.00	0.98	-
	Female	24 (20.2%)	6 (20.0%)			
Handedness	Right	104 (87.4%)	23 (76.7%)	2.191	0.14	-
	Lift	15 (12.6%)	7 (23.3%)			
Father's education level	Secondary	67 (56.3%)	16 (53.3%)	0.09	0.77	-
	College degree	52 (43.7%)	14 (46.7%)			
Mother's education level	Secondary	78 (65.5%)	20 (66.7%)	0.01	0.91	-
	College degree	41 (34.5%)	10 (33.3%)			

Note: * Mean (SD) non-verbal IQ (Raven's raw score range 0–36). The continuous variables are summarised as the mean and standard deviation using t-tests, while the categorical variables are summarised as the count and percentage using the chi-square χ^2. ES = effect size, which is calculated using Cohen's d.

2.3. Instruments

This study relied on two types of instruments, namely screening questionnaires, and assessment measures.

2.3.1. Screening Questionnaires

The following three screening questionnaires were used to verify the participant's clinical diagnosis and to determine the severity of their autistic symptoms. The first two measures were completed by at least one parent of each participant with ASD, while the third measure was used by the researcher to independently assess the severity of the ASD symptoms.

1. Gilliam Autism Rating Scale—Third Edition (GARS-3) [51]: After obtaining written permission from the publisher (Pro-Ed), the researcher had previously translated the GARS-3 and made certain cultural adaptations to facilitate its use in the Gulf region. The GARS-3 is a norm-referenced, standardised informant rating scale designed to identify and rate the severity of autism symptomatology in individuals. The GARS-3 items correspond to the diagnostic criteria for ASD set out in the DSM-5 [54]. It consists of 56 Likert-type items that comprise six subtests: restricted/repetitive behaviours (RB; 13 items), social interaction (SI; 14 items), social communication (SC; nine items), emotional responses (ER; eight items), cognitive style (CS; seven items), and maladaptive speech (MS; seven items). The summation of the subscales' scaled scores yields the composite autism index, which is also reported in terms of the standard score, percentile rank, severity level, and probability of ASD. Two autism indices (four or six) can be formed, depending on whether or not the individual is mute. Higher scaled scores indicate increasingly severe autistic symptoms. Caregivers require approximately 5–10 min to complete the measure.

2. Michigan Autism Spectrum Questionnaire (MASQ) [50]: The MASQ is based on the clinical characteristics that may be suggestive of Asperger's syndrome (AS) or high-functioning ASD (HFA). It includes ten items representing two main functional areas: the quality of the social interaction patterns and the style of both the content and form of communication. The items are rated on a four-point (0–3) scale, with their sum yielding the total score (maximum 30). A cut-off score ≥ 22 is recommended to screen for individuals with HFA or AS. Cut-off scores between 14 and 21 are predictive of ASD or pervasive developmental disorder-not otherwise specified (PDD-NOS), while scores < 14 are predictive of other psychiatric disorders.

3. The Clinician-Rated Severity of Autism Spectrum and Social Communication Disorders (CRSASSC) [49]: This two-item scale is used to assess the severity of an individual's autistic symptoms and his/her level of functioning based on the amount of support required due to challenges associated with the social and communication (SC) domain and the restricted interests and repetitive behaviours (RRB) domain, respectively. Each domain is rated on a four-point Likert scale consistent with the DSM-5 diagnostic criteria: 0 (none), 1 (requiring support), 2 (requiring substantial support), or 3 (requiring very substantial support). The clinical criteria may also help to assign a specific functional level to an individual: mild (level 1), moderate (level 2), or severe (level 3). The level of severity for each item should be independently reported, and a combined overall severity score should not be calculated.

2.3.2. Assessment Measures

There are a number of different tools available to assist clinicians and researchers with the evaluation and measurement of different aspects of motor skills development and their contribution to motor performance [55,56]. This study used the following measure.

Bruininks-Oseretsky Test of Motor Proficiency, Second Edition (BOT-2; [48]): The BOT-2 is a standardised, norm-referenced test of motor proficiency used to assess the gross and fine motor skills involved in engaging, goal-directed activities among children aged 4–21 years. It includes eight subtests: fine motor precision, fine motor integration, manual dexterity, bilateral coordination, balance, running speed and agility, and upper-limb coordination and strength. The BOT-2 results in four composite scores and one comprehensive measure of overall motor proficiency. The different administration options include the complete form, the short form, selected composites, and selected subtests. The short form (14 items), which was used in this study, takes 15–20 min to administer, with another five minutes being required to tape off the running course. Liu et al. (2015) noted that it is most efficient for practitioners to evaluate a child using the short form first [56]. The short-form BOT-2 consists of 14 items covering eight subtests and including the widest possible range of abilities to produce sufficiently reliable scores (see Table 2). It is a quick and user-friendly screening tool that provides a single overall motor proficiency score. The total composite score is reported as the standardised score (mean = 50.0, standard deviation = 10.0).

Table 2. Short-Form Items.

The BOT-2 Subtest	Item	Assessment
Subtest 1 *Fine Motor Precision*	Drawing Lines Through Paths Folding Paper	# of Errors # of Errors
Subtest 2 *Fine Motor Integration*	Copying a Square Copying a Star	# of Errors # of Errors
Subtest 3 *Manual Dexterity*	Transferring Pennies	# of Pennies in 15 s
Subtest 4 *Bilateral Coordination*	Jumping in Place-Same Sides Synchronized Tapping Feet and Fingers-Same Sides Synchronized	Repetitions Repetitions
Subtest 5 *Balance*	walking Forward on a Line Standing on One Leg on a Balance Beam-Eyes Open	Steps Time
Subtest 6 *Running Speed Agility*	One-Legged Stationary Hop	# of Hops in 15 s
Subtest 7 *Upper-Limb Coordination*	Dropping and Catching a Ball-Both Hands Dropping a Ball-Alternating Hands	Catches Dribbles
Subtest 8 *Strength*	Full Push-Ups Sit-Ups	# Performed in 30 s # Performed in 30 s

Note: (#) The hash symbol expresses the number of errors made during task completion and the number of tasks completed.

The BOT-2 SF exhibited strong psychometric properties. Its high internal consistency was determined using the stratified alpha method with regard to each composite and the split-half method with regard to each subtest [48]. The alpha value for the total motor composites was found to equal 0.93, while the test-retest correlations were found to be >0.80. Further, the interrater reliability correlations were noted to range between 0.92 and 0.98 [48].

In terms of the validity of the measure, the internal structure of the BOT-2 has been examined using the correlations among the subtest scale scores and the composite scores [57]. The validity of the BOT-2 was also established using a confirmatory factor analysis [58]. The BOT-2 was further determined to be correlated with other measures of motor performance (Bruininks and Bruininks, 2005 [48]). Moreover, the BOT-2 SF was reported to exhibit high sensitivity (84%) but poor specificity (42.9%) with 76.5% accuracy among 153 neurotypical children aged 8–11 years [59]. As per the test manual, the BOT-2 is noted to be able to differentiate between children in different clinical groups, including an ASD group, and children in the normative group.

2.4. Procedures

All the involved procedures were carried out in accordance with the ethical standards of the Queensland University of Technology, the research ethics committee of which approved the study protocol. The children involved in this project participated with the full written informed consent of their parents and legal guardians after the study procedures were explained; however, it was also important that the child participants were asked to give their verbal assent to participate. The parents of children with ASD provided information about the severity of their child's autism by answering the questions on the GARS-3 and MASQ. In addition, the children with ASD underwent an assessment based on the CRSASSC scale that was conducted by the researcher in order to determine the level of severity. Each child was individually evaluated according to the BOT-2 by the researcher in a noise- and distraction-free room at their school. The verbal instructions given were adapted to fit each child's level of language ability. The instructions for the test were also accompanied by photos of a child performing the main components of the test. All scores were recorded and converted into standardised scores according to the procedure described in the test manual. The assessment sessions were scheduled according to the times suggested by the children's parents and teachers. The children were all given adequate praise throughout the test. At the start of the testing session, the children were informed that they could cease to participate at any time and for any reason.

2.5. Analysis

All the data analyses in the present study were performed using the Statistical Package for the Social Sciences (SPSS) version 23.0 (IBM, Chicago, IL, USA). A one-sample z-test was performed to determine whether the mean of the motor scores of the ASD group statistically differed from the corresponding normative mean derived from the standardisation sample, as available in the BOT-2 manual. Further, the BOT-2 cut-off score (40 or less) was used to calculate the proportions of the actual clinical scores (i.e., the proportion of participants who scored below the clinical cut-off point).

Descriptive statistics were calculated concerning the raw scores for all the BOT-2 subtests. The overall differences between the raw scores of the children with ASD on the BOT-2 and those of the typically developing children were analysed by means of an independent samples *t*-test.

Generally speaking, when performing multiple comparisons using the same data set, the risk of a type I error occurring increases. To overcome this problem, the probabilities were not maintained at the chosen level (0.05), while a Bonferroni adjustment was made to control the overall type I error rate. When performing a Bonferroni adjustment, the alpha is estimated by taking the desired alpha level (0.05) and then dividing it by the number of comparisons being conducted. In the present study, for the multiple comparison analysis of the eight BOT-2 subtests, the significance level was set at $p = 0.006$.

The effect sizes were expressed using Cohen's d [60]. According to Cohen (1988), the magnitude of the effect size can be categorised into one of three graded levels, namely small (0.2–0.5), medium (0.5–0.8) or large (>0.8) [60].

Further, the effect of the age variable on the participants' motor performance was investigated using a regression analysis, with age being considered the predictor variable and the total raw score for each child's motor performance being considered the outcome of interest. The level of statistical significance was set as $p < 0.01$ in order to avoid type I errors.

For linear regression, the effect size was calculated using Cohen's $f2$. According to Cohen's guidelines (1988) concerning the interpretation of the magnitude of the R-squared value, the values of Cohen's $f2 = 0.02$, 0.13 and 0.26 are considered to be small, medium, and large effect size, respectively. The equation to compute Cohen's effect size is ($f2 = R2/1 - R2$) [60].

3. Results

The results of this study are presented in three stages according to the sequence of the research objectives:

3.1. The Proportion of Children with ASD Who Exhibit Motor Impairments

The BOT-2 standardized test was used in this study in order to evaluate motor proficiency in the child participants. Lower scores on the BOT-2 items are considered to be indicative of lower motor performance. On the short form of the BOT-2, the subtests are administered to find the raw scores. Each raw score for the subtests was then converted into a point score using the graded scale provided. The point scores are summed to give the total point score (max = 88), which is in turn converted into the standard score considering age and sex (ranging from 20 to 80), with a mean of 50 (SD = 10). A total composite standard score of 40 or less (one standard deviation below) is classified as indicative of motor impairment. This total motor composite can be reported as a categorical variable with five descriptive categories: well above average "≥70", above average "60–69", average "41–59", below average "31–40", and well below average "≤30". Based on this process, the overall score, which is the sum of the eight subscales, was compared with the BOT-2 norms. Table 3 presents descriptive statistics concerning the total BOT-2 motor composite scores of the children with ASD as well as the results of the z-test comparing their overall motor performance to the performance of the normative test sample.

Table 3. Descriptive Statistics and Z-Test Results Concerning the Total Motor Composite.

BOT-2	ASD Sample (N = 119)					95% Confidence Interval for the Mean		One-Sample Z-Test		
	Min	Max	M	SD	SE	Lower	Upper	Z	p	d
Standard score for the total motor composite *	47.0	85.0	31.90	5.03	0.46	30.98	32.81	−19.74	<0.001	1.81

Note: * A standard score less than 40 is regarded as the cut-off point for an abnormal motor performance.

As shown in Table 3, the mean BOT-2 score of the ASD group for the total motor composite (M = 31.90, SD = 5.03, $p < 0.001$) statistically deviated from the norm with a large effect size; thereby, indicating the presence of motor impairment within the overall level of motor proficiency. In light of the cut-off score set out in the BOT-2 guidelines, 88% of participants with ASD scored below the normal threshold when compared with the normative BOT-2 data. Based on the descriptive standard scoring categories detailed in the BOT-2 guidelines, the children with ASD were classified as displaying a motor performance deficit that fell within the below-average range.

3.2. Comparing the ASD and TD Children Based on the BOT-2 Test Raw Scores

Table 4 shows the participants' mean raw scores and standard deviations on the eight BOT-2 subtests, namely fine motor precision, fine motor integration, manual dexterity, upper-limb coordination, bilateral coordination, balance, running speed and agility, and strength, as well as the total motor composite. It therefore indicates the differences identified between the children in the ASD group and the typically developing children. The highest point score for the test is 88. Higher scores on the BOT-2 items are indicative of higher motor performance, and vice versa.

Table 4. Comparison of the autism spectrum disorder and typically developing groups based on the BOT-2 raw scores and total motor composite.

The BOT-2 Test Scores	ASD Sample (N = 119)		TDC Group (N = 30)		t-Statistic	p	D
	M	SD	M	SD			
Fine Motor Precision	5.38	2.66	10.17	2.10	9.171 ***	<0.001 ***	1.99
Fine Motor Integration	7.43	2.17	9.53	1.36	6.623 ***	<0.001 ***	1.16
Manual Dexterity	3.28	1.62	6.33	1.56	9.322 ***	<0.001 ***	1.92
Bilateral Coordination	4.60	1.68	6.67	0.85	9.489 ***	<0.001 ***	1.55
Balance	5.69	1.10	7.30	0.75	7.563 ***	<0.001 ***	1.71
Running Speed and Agility	3.08	2.03	6.97	1.40	12.267 ***	<0.001 ***	2.23
Upper-Limb Coordination	5.13	2.80	10.20	1.73	12.472 ***	<0.001 ***	2.18
Strength	3.21	2.08	8.97	2.24	13.352 ***	<0.001 ***	2.66
Total Motor Composite	37.79	12.25	66.13	8.24	15.097 ***	<0.001 ***	2.71

Note: *** $p < 0.001$ by independent samples t-test. ADS: Autism spectrum disorder without intellectual disability; TDC: typically developing children; BOT-2: Bruininks-Oseretsky Test of Motor Proficiency, Second Edition; d values are effect sizes (ESs) of ASD versus TDC. Bonferroni correction: α = 0.05/8 = 0.006.

The independent samples t-test found significant differences in terms of all the BOT-2 short-form subtests and the total score when comparing the children with ASD and the typically developing children. All the differences are significant at the $p < 0.001$ level, with the size effects on the eight BOT-2 subtests ranging from 1.16 to 2.66 and the total motor composite equalling 2.71 (Cohen's d). This indicates that the children with ASD performed more poorly on the BOT-2 items than the TD controls. The performance on the eight motor subtests was variable. The children with ASD scored their lowest point scores on the strength element of all the subtests (Cohen's $d = 2.66$), while Fine Motor Integration was associated with their highest point scores (Cohen's $d = 1.16$).

3.3. Relationship between Motor Performance and Age

The relationship between the ASD participants' age and their overall motor performance was examined using linear regression analyses. The results indicated the significant main effect of age, which suggested that the children with ASD exhibited age-related gains in terms of their overall motor performance. Indeed, positive correlation was noted between their overall motor performance and their age ($\beta = 0.52$, $p \leq 0.001$, $R^2 = 0.26$, Cohen's $f^2 = 0.36$). This correlation pattern indicated that the children with ASD exhibited fewer deficits during the performance of motor tasks as they aged.

4. Discussion

The results relevant to each aim of the study will be discussed separately in the following subsections

4.1. Prevalence of Children with ASD Who Exhibited Clinically Significant Motor Abnormalities

Our first objective was to identify the prevalence of children with ASD who exhibited clinically significant motor abnormalities. The results indicated that the majority of the ASD sample fell outside the normal range in terms of motor performance. Indeed, the prevalence of children with ASD who exhibited clinically significant motor performance problems was found to be 88%. These children had a score of 40 or less on the total composite, which indicates deficits in their motor skills.

These results regarding the motor impairments seen in children with ASD are consistent with our expectations, since they reflect the motor abnormalities seen in those with autism. Additionally, such findings regarding deficient motor functioning in children with ASD are in line with the findings of several prior studies that relied on a similar measure to the BOT-2 [8,17,29,61–63]. The mean standard score for the overall motor composite in these previous studies ranged from 33.0 to 39.6, indicating the existence of motor impairments among children with ASD. A similar pattern of results was also found in the clinical sample of 45 individuals with autism aged 4–21 years described in the BOT-2 manual (M = 37.0; SD = 8.4) [48]. The present results are also in line with those of other studies that used different measures [6,11]. However, our results contrast with those found in a study by Hilton et al. (2014) that used the BOT-2 but did not identify a significant deficit in the motor skills of individuals with ASD [64]. However, the small sample size involved in Hilton et al.'s (2014) study should be considered, since they only investigated seven children with ASD.

The motor disruptions seen in children with ASD may be attributed to the increase in the total brain volume seen in such children, as well as to certain affected brain regions that are regularly suspected to be involved in the neural underpinnings of autism, including the cerebellum, basal ganglia, brain stem functions, and alterations in the frontostriatal and frontocerebellar pathways [10,65]. However, the brain mechanisms underlying the motor disruptions observed in those with autism are not conclusive, meaning that they warrant further investigation.

Environmental factors may also contribute to the poor motor skills performance exhibited by those with ASD. An individual's motor skills development stems from the dynamic relationship that exists between organismic and environmental factors; hence, any changes in such properties will influence the acquisition of motor skills [66]. A study by Maksoud (2016) indicated that certain environmental factors might explain the poor performance exhibited by Egyptian children with Down's syndrome in relation to the BOT-2 instrument [67]. These factors included low enhancement and poor support from the parent(s), as well as limited opportunities to practice during the early years of their lives [67].

A proposition drawn from these findings is that these factors may also be applicable to children with ASD.

It is important to note, however, that the prevalence of motor performance abnormalities identified in the context of our research was high when compared to the prevalence reported in other studies [17,61–63]. It is possible that the high frequency of motor performance abnormalities seen in the children with ASD in the present study could be attributed to several factors largely related to the local cultural context.

First, low levels of physical activity can contribute to reducing the motor proficiency of children with ASD. The relationship between an individual's motor proficiency level and his/her level of physical activity was confirmed by Wrotniak, Epstein, Dorn, Jones, and Kondilis (2006) [68]. The majority of families in the Gulf region depend on domestic servants to help care for their children and to do the housework [69]. These domestic servants also typically assist the children with numerous tasks associated with daily living, especially in the case of children who have been diagnosed with a disability. This assistance could involve, for example, buttoning up clothes, zipping up zippers, tying shoes, bathing, feeding, cleaning teeth, and combing hair. Hence, it is possible that the children might come to overly rely on the domestic servants to help them perform everyday activities. This could in turn have a negative impact on the physical activity levels of the children, and therefore adversely affect their motor development.

Second, a lack of opportunities to engage in physical activity/practice responding to physical stimuli could stem from various familial factors. The negative relationship between motor development and insufficient physical activity has been confirmed in the literature [70,71]. The parents of children with ASD in the Arab Gulf region tend toward an overprotective parenting style, and they often exhibit excessive concern about their children's safety when outdoors. This parenting style is likely to have contributed to the children with ASD being less physically active than is ideal and, relatedly, to their insufficient motor skills proficiency [72].

Additionally, children living in the Gulf region tend to only rarely engage in physical activities out in the natural environment. Prior research evidence has suggested that the physical environment that we inhabit can offer both opportunities and barriers in terms of engaging in physical activities [70]. For example, countries in the Gulf region frequently experience very high temperatures during the daytime [73]. Therefore, it is rarely considered safe or appropriate for children to engage in outdoor activities during that time/in such conditions. Children with ASD are particularly prone to being prevented for participating in outdoor activities due to both the perceived inconvenience of them doing so and the associated security concerns. This lack of participation may affect the development of the children's gross motor skills.

Finally, children with ASD typically lack exercise partners of the same age and are frequently isolated from their peers, which means that they generally lack opportunities to engage in social interactions. Unfortunately, children with ASD are particularly susceptible to social exclusion due to both the stigma experienced by their families (i.e., feelings of shame about their child's condition) and the rejection and lack of acceptance shown by their peers (i.e., evasion and discrimination). Some families attempt to keep their children's condition a secret, and hence prevent their children from attending social events and engaging in social interactions with their peers. It has been reported that the lack of a peer exercise partner represents one of the key barriers to physical activity experienced by children with ASD [74]. Such non-participation in peer activities may limit children's opportunities to develop their motor proficiency.

4.2. Distinct Nature of Motor Performance Exhibited by Children with ASD and Typically Developing Children

This study also sought to examine the differences between the motor performance, as assessed using the BOT-2, of children with ASD and typically developing children. The results demonstrated that the children with ASD exhibited weaker motor skills performance than the typically developing children, which indicated deficits in their motor proficiency. The results, therefore, support the findings of prior studies concerning motor behaviours, which indicated a general impairment of motor functioning in individuals with ASD [10,11]. The results contribute to our understanding of definitive areas of motor dysfunction among children with ASD and their long-term developmental consequences. Further, the results add weight to previous insights intended to assist caregivers and therapists in addressing such issues. Overall, the results provide further evidence of the need to reconceptualise ASD to include motor delays and deficits.

When considering all eight subscales used to evaluate the overall motor proficiency of the children with ASD, it appears that the identified motor deficits manifested with different degrees of severity. For instance, fine motor precision tasks require precise control over finger and hand movements. Our results indicated that the children with ASD experienced difficulties drawing lines through paths and folding paper. This finding is in accordance with the notion that individuals with ASD experience difficulties completing tasks that require the planning and sequencing of movement [75]. As some children with ASD also exhibit hypotonia, it is likely that the hypotonia in their hands results in severe fine-motor and graph-motor delays due to an inability to manipulate objects and control a pencil [76]. Such difficulties may lead to problems during many activities associated with daily living, including buttoning clothes and writing.

Fine motor integration skills require the capacity to integrate visual stimuli with motor control. This kind of integration is commonly referred to as "visual motor integration". Our results indicated that the children with ASD were generally unable to perform the hand-eye coordination tasks. This finding is in line with prior evidence that some individuals with ASD exhibit underlying deficits in visual-motor integration [77]. Such deficits may stem from sensory problems since hand-eye coordination requires the assimilation of several types of sensory inputs to direct movement toward the target [78]. Moreover, children with ASD demonstrate delayed manipulation skills, which are also important for activities such as writing and fastening clothing [79]. These fine motor integration skills tend to be affected when an individual with ASD experiences a tactile perception problem, especially when tactile defensiveness is present. Ayres noted that hyper-responsivity to tactile stimuli may render it difficult for younger children to develop in-hand manipulation, fine motor skills, and hand-eye coordination [80]. It has been established that children with ASD often exhibit difficulties with tactile awareness, which may impede their fine motor skills. Thus, it has a bearing on their ability to develop fine motor skills.

Our findings also revealed the impaired performance of the children with ASD on the manual dexterity subtest, which is in line with the results of prior studies [11,14,81,82]. Deficits in manual coordination may occur due to the poor hand-eye coordination typically seen in children with ASD, since good hand-eye coordination allows individuals to pick up small objects and precisely manipulate them. Further, perception-action coupling is crucial to the production of purposeful, coherent movements [14]. However, prior evidence has suggested that such manual coordination deficits may be related to the use of a dual-scored task that involves both spatial accuracy and age-related temporal parameters [14]. Interestingly, a recent study indicated that the worst results for children with ASD were seen in relation to the fine motor skills component, while the gross motor skills component gave rise to the best results [83]. During the indicative qualitative evaluation, the researchers found more children with ASD to be able to manage the manual tasks when provided with unlimited time and support [83]. In contrast, the majority of children with ASD could not manage the gross motor tasks at all [83].

The bilateral coordination subtest concerns the capacity to use both sides of the body in a controlled and organized manner to accomplish a functional task [79]. The results indicated that the children with ASD experienced problems when attempting movements involving both sides of the body. This finding is consistent with the fact that individuals with ASD are typically characterised by poor bilateral coordination [84]. Further, Staples and Reid found that children with ASD experienced difficulty coordinating both sides of their body, or both arms and legs, while performing motor tasks [82]. Bilateral coordination problems may be associated with vestibular dysfunction, as when the vestibular system is unable to adequately integrate information, it can contribute to poor bilateral coordination.

Moreover, the vestibular system allows the two sides of the body to communicate with each other at the level of the brain stem via the vestibular nuclei [85].

The balance subtest evaluates the motor control skills integral to an individual's posture when standing. Balance is necessary for both movement and stillness, which is why it is sometimes referred to as postural control [86,87]. The balance subtest consists of movement activities that measure the stability of the trunk support as well as stasis and movement. Our results suggested that the balance skills of the children with ASD were significantly impaired when compared with the typically developing children, which is in line with the findings of previous studies [10,11,14,81]. However, Ament et al. found that deficits in the balance skills of children with ASD were only demonstrated during static balance tasks and not during dynamic balance tasks [88]. Further, the presence of balance deficits in children with ASD is often interpreted as indicating a deficit in the integration of information obtained from the visual, proprioception and vestibular afferent systems [10,89]. The maintenance of successful postural stability during static balance postures is thought to require the integration of vestibular, somatosensory, and visual inputs. If one of these inputs is impaired or disrupted, then both simple and complex motor tasks prove more difficult [19].

The running speed and agility subtest includes activities that require both speed and agility. Hopping is defined as the elevation of the body off the ground and the subsequent landing on a single foot [90]. It appears to be an extension of the ability to balance while standing on one leg. This type of balance is referred to as "dynamic balance". Our results indicated that the children with ASD experienced difficulty in hopping on one foot when compared with the typically developing children. This is in accordance with prior clinical observations that many autistic children experience great difficulty when hopping [91,92]. For instance, Noterdaeme et al. found that children with ASD experienced difficulties performing motor skills that require standing and hopping on one foot for a predetermined period of time when compared with typically developing children [93]. A similar result was found by Pusponegoro et al., who noted that only five out of 40 (12.5%) children with ASD could hop on one foot without falling over [92]. Comparable to the situation with balance and bilateral coordination, a possible contributing factor to the impairment seen in children with ASD is the vestibular problems they experience. Hopping requires the ability to balance on either foot, which relies heavily on a sensitive vestibular system and motor coordination [94]. The vestibular system also plays an important role in controlling the mutual interaction of sensory inputs and motor outputs [95]. As the ASD population typically exhibits an impairment in vestibular processing that results in poor balance, this impairment may impact the ability of a child with ASD to hop.

The upper-limb coordination (ULC) subtest consists of activities designed to measure visual tracking with coordinated arm and hand movements. Our results revealed that the children with ASD exhibited ULC difficulties, which is consistent with prior evidence that individuals with ASD exhibit poor ULC during visuomotor activities [96]. The results also indicated that the use of both hands to drop and catch a ball proved difficult for the children with ASD [14]. It appears, therefore, that children with ASD experience difficulty completing tasks involving both hands. When attempting to catch a ball with two hands, their arm movements are often poorly coordinated [97,98]. These deficits may be attributed to insufficient information processing [99]. As activities involving ball skills are often social in nature, such motor impairments may result in the exclusion of children with ASD from games, which may disrupt their psychosocial development [98,100].

The strength subtest is intended to assess the trunk flexor muscles and the upper and lower extremity strength. It involves activities such as push-ups and sit-ups. Our results indicated that the children with ASD showed an insufficient level of strength during such activities. They were able to complete fewer push-up and sit-up repetitions than the typically developing children. This is in line with the results obtained by Pan (2014), who found individuals with ASD to be able to complete fewer push-ups and sit-ups than age-matched peers without ASD [29]. The inability to master the push-up skill may indicate weakness in an individual's general upper body condition. Further, difficulty performing sit-ups may result from relatively low middle-body strength [101]. One explanation for the poor performance of the children with ASD in relation to strength skills could be their limited general body strength. Such activities require a great deal of muscle strength, which is also necessary for many aspects of movement and motor control, including postural control, balance, and coordination [102].

4.3. The Relationship between Age and Motor Performance

The final aim of this study was to determine whether the chronological age of the children with ASD affected their overall motor performance. Ultimately, it was determined that age did impact the motor performance of the children with ASD. The total score for motor performance was positively related to the age of the children with ASD. In general, the present results indicate that children with ASD demonstrated fewer deficits during motor tasks with age. This finding is consistent with the general pattern of the developmental acquisition of motor skills with age [43,48]. Relatively few studies have examined age differences in terms of motor performance in those with ASD, although the current results are in line with those of a study by Ming et al. (2007), who found that older children with ASD tend to perform better in relation to the motor skills than younger children with ASD [16]. However, the present results stand in contrast to the results of longitudinal work indicating that these motor deficits remain relatively stable over time in children with ASD [46]. The identified age-related gains could be due to the natural maturity of motor skills or the result of therapeutic interventions [16]. Structural environmental changes may promote motor development in children with ASD. However, the children with ASD in the context in which this study was conducted, whether they exhibited motor deficits or not, were not expected to receive any services to assist with their motor development. Hence, the results of the present study support the hypothesis that the development of fine and gross motor skills is characterized by change rather than stability.

5. Conclusions

The present study outlined the prevalence of motor impairments in children with ASD, as well as the nature of the motor abnormalities seen in school-aged children with ASD when compared to typically developing children, through the use of a standardized test so as to facilitate a better understanding of the motor profiles associated with ASD. An additional focus of the study was the exploration of the relationship between motor performance ability and age. Based on the impairment cut-off detailed in the BOT-2 guidelines, the majority of children with ASD in our sample showed mild to extremely negative deviation from population norms, and therefore were classified as exhibiting a motor performance deficit. This study also found evidence that the children with ASD performed significantly poorer than the typically developing children in relation to all the items of the BOT-2. In addition, the study demonstrated the existence of a positive relationship between age and motor performance ability, which indicated that motor skills may improve as children grow older.

The overall findings of this study served to reinforce and extend the results of prior studies concerning motor abnormalities in those with ASD. In particular, the present findings contributed significantly to our understanding of such motor characteristics in non-Western individuals diagnosed with ASD.

A strength of this study is related to the use of a standardised assessment of motor impairment (i.e., the BOT-2), which is one of the most commonly applied means of evaluating and discriminating motor function in children. However, only the short form of the chosen motor proficiency test (SFBOT-2) was used in this study, which limited our interpretation of the subcategories. However, the use of the SFBOT-2 can be justified based on the findings of our unpublished pilot study, which revealed both the difficulty and the high time requirements associated with applying the full version of the test. Additionally, a number of comorbid psychiatric disorders, including anxiety, could potentially impact children's performance during a motor task [103,104]. However, the results of this study do not contribute to the ongoing discussion regarding the effect of anxiety on test performance. Thus, future studies could examine the possible relationship between anxiety levels and performance levels during motor tasks. Although the severity of the ASD symptoms has been found to be related to the severity of the experienced motor problems [8,105–107], examining this relationship in more detail is beyond the scope of the present study. It does, however, represent an interesting avenue for future studies to explore.

Another limitation of the present study is related to the cross-sectional methodological approach chosen to explore the impact of chronological age on the motor difficulties exhibited by children with ASD, which limited our ability to interpret the findings from a developmental perspective. Future studies should employ a longitudinal design so as to be better able to investigate the developmental trajectories of motor impairments in children with ASD and to provide us with further insights into the mechanisms that underlie such motor disruptions. The final limitation of this study concerned the study sample. Only children with ASD who exhibited an average or above-average IQ were included in the study. Therefore, the findings are limited to that group, and hence are not representative of individuals with ASD who exhibit lower cognitive function. Additionally, the fact that the sample of typically developing children included in the study was relatively small should be considered. Indeed, the typically developing participants in this study may not be representative of the population as a whole.

Despite the above-mentioned limitations, the findings of the present study have a number of important implications for practice. First, the results reported here suggested that motor abnormalities represent a prevalent feature of ASD. However, such problems do not typically form part of the assessments for ASD nor are they typically included in intervention programs. Therefore, the inclusion of a motor assessment in the evaluation protocols associated with ASD should prove highly useful. Second, although motor deficits are present from very early on in the development of children with ASD and may actually reflect an underlying brain deficit, they do not generally represent a key focus for either parents or professionals. It is recommended that motor functioning should be considered during the clinical assessment and management of ASD, and it should not be ignored during early interventions. Further, it is recommended that additional research be undertaken in this regard so as to ensure greater clinical recognition of motor dysfunctions among children with ASD.

Moreover, the wide-ranging implications of poor motor performance on the part of individuals with ASD can extend beyond the motor domain and into the educational, social, cognitive, and behavioural domains. Hence, motor functioning represents another area that we should be mindful of in the clinical context. The identification of motor abnormalities could be a potentially valuable marker of the degree and the nature of the other defining clinical features of ASD. Finally, the results of the present study highlighted the need for increased efforts to improve the clinical surveillance process in order to better identify potential developmental delays or deficits in terms of motor performance, as well as to implement intervention strategies intended to address motor problems, in children with ASD. Early identification and proper intervention with regard to motor problems in children with ASD may lead to such children experiencing improved self-confidence and self-esteem, increased performance quality, and enhanced occupational engagement and social participation.

Funding: This study was partly funded by Taibah University, Saudi Arabia. More specifically, Taibah University funded the study instruments used during the large-scale evaluation project intended to identify neurobehavioral problems in children with ASD that was conducted by the author as part of her Ph.D. thesis.

Acknowledgments: The author would like to thank the parents and staff members from the autism centers and mainstream primary schools in Bahrain, Saudi Arabia, and the UAE. for their assistance with the data collection. This study was conducted as part of the author's PhD thesis.

Conflicts of Interest: The author declares that there are no financial interests or potential conflicts of interest regarding the publication of this article.

References

1. Haibach, P.; Reid, G.; Collier, D. *Motor Learning and Development*, 2nd ed.; Human Kineticsl: Champaign, IL, USA, 2017.

2. Piek, J.P.; Hands, B.; Licari, M.K. Assessment of motor functioning in the preschool period. *Neuropsychol. Rev.* **2012**, *22*, 402–413. [CrossRef] [PubMed]
3. Catama Bryan, V.; Calalang Wielm Mae, S.; Cada Renz Karlo, D.; Ballog Angelica, C.; Batton Kaylee, B.; Bigay Ma Lourdes, R.; Borje Denice Jan, J. Motor intervention activities for children with autism spectrum disorders. *Int. J. Res. Stud. Psychol.* **2017**, *6*, 27–42. [CrossRef]
4. Libertus, K.; Hauf, P. Motor skills and their foundational role for perceptual, social, and cognitive development. *Front. Psychol.* **2017**, *8*, 301. [CrossRef] [PubMed]
5. Gowen, E.; Hamilton, A. Motor abilities in autism: A review using a computational context. *J. Autism Dev. Disord.* **2013**, *43*, 323–344. [CrossRef]
6. Abu-Dahab, S.M.N.; Skidmore, E.R.; Holm, M.B.; Rogers, J.C.; Minshew, N.J. Motor and tactile-perceptual skill differences between individuals with high-functioning autism and typically developing individuals ages 5–21. *J. Autism Dev. Disord.* **2013**, *43*, 2241–2248. [CrossRef]
7. Dowd, A.; Rinehart, N.; McGinley, J. Motor function in children with autism: Why is this relevant to psychologists? *Clin. Psychol.* **2010**, *14*, 90–96. [CrossRef]
8. Hilton, C.L.; Zhang, Y.; Whilte, M.R.; Klohr, C.L.; Constantino, J. Motor impairment in sibling pairs concordant and discordant for autism spectrum disorders. *Autism* **2012**, *16*, 430–441. [CrossRef]
9. Van Damme, T.; Simons, J.; Sabbe, B.; Van West, D. Motor abilities of children and adolescents with a psychiatric condition: A systematic literature review. *World J. Psychiatry* **2015**, *5*, 315. [CrossRef]
10. Fournier, K.A.; Hass, C.J.; Naik, S.K.; Lodha, N.; Cauraugh, J.H. Motor coordination in autism spectrum disorders: A synthesis and meta-analysis. *J. Autism Dev. Disord.* **2010**, *40*, 1227–1240. [CrossRef]
11. Green, D.; Charman, T.; Pickles, A.; Chandler, S.; Loucas, T.; Simonoff, E.; Baird, G. Impairment in movement skills of children with autistic spectrum disorders. *Dev. Med. Child Neurol.* **2009**, *51*, 311–316. [CrossRef]
12. Liu, T.; Breslin, C.M. Fine and gross motor performance of the MABC-2 by children with autism spectrum disorder and typically developing children. *Res. Autism Spectr. Disord.* **2013**, *7*, 1244–1249. [CrossRef]
13. Moseley, R.L.; Pulvermueller, F. What can autism teach us about the role of sensorimotor systems in higher cognition? New clues from studies on language, action semantics, and abstract emotional concept processing. *Cortex* **2018**, *100*, 149–190. [CrossRef] [PubMed]
14. Whyatt, C.P.; Craig, C.M. Motor skills in children aged 7–10 years, diagnosed with autism spectrum disorder. *J. Autism Dev. Disord.* **2012**, *42*, 1799–1809. [CrossRef] [PubMed]
15. McCleery, J.P.; Elliott, N.A.; Sampanis, D.S.; Stefanidou, C.A. Motor development and motor resonance difficulties in autism: Relevance to early intervention for language and communication skills. *Front. Integr. Neurosci.* **2013**, *7*, 30. [CrossRef]
16. Ming, X.; Brimacombe, M.; Wagner, G.C. Prevalence of motor impairment in autism spectrum disorders. *Brain Dev.* **2007**, *29*, 565–570. [CrossRef]
17. Dewey, D.; Cantell, M.; Crawford, S.G. Motor and gestural performance in children with autism spectrum disorders, developmental coordination disorder, and/or attention deficit hyperactivity disorder. *J. Int. Neuropsychol. Soc.* **2007**, *13*, 246–256. [CrossRef]
18. Nobile, M.; Perego, P.; Piccinini, L.; Mani, E.; Rossi, A.; Bellina, M.; Molteni, M. Further evidence of complex motor dysfunction in drug naive children with autism using automatic motion analysis of gait. *Autism* **2011**, *15*, 263–283. [CrossRef]
19. Travers, B.G.; Powell, P.S.; Klinger, L.G.; Klinger, M.R. Motor difficulties in autism spectrum disorder: Linking symptom severity and postural stability. *J. Autism Dev. Disord.* **2013**, *43*, 1568–1583. [CrossRef]
20. Jeste, S.S. The neurology of autism spectrum disorders. *Curr. Opin. Neurol.* **2011**, *24*, 132–139. [CrossRef]
21. Stefanatos, G.A. Autism Spectrum Disorders. In *The Neuropsychology of Psychopathology*; Noggle, C., Dean, R., Eds.; Springer Publishing Company: New York, NY, USA, 2013; pp. 97–170.
22. Mostofsky, S.H.; Powell, S.K.; Simmonds, D.J.; Goldberg, M.C.; Caffo, B.; Pekar, J.J. Decreased connectivity and cerebellar activity in autism during motor task performance. *Brain* **2009**, *132*, 2413–2425. [CrossRef]
23. Takarae, Y.; Minshew, N.J.; Luna, B.; Sweeney, J.A. Atypical involvement of frontostriatal systems during sensorimotor control in autism. *Psychiatry Res. Neuroimaging* **2007**, *156*, 117–127. [CrossRef] [PubMed]
24. McAlonan, G.M.; Suckling, J.; Wong, N.; Cheung, V.; Lienenkaemper, N.; Cheung, C.; Chua, S.E. Distinct patterns of grey matter abnormality in high-functioning autism and Asperger's syndrome. *J. Child Psychol. Psychiatry* **2008**, *49*, 1287–1295. [CrossRef] [PubMed]

25. Rinehart, N.J.; Tonge, B.J.; Iansek, R.; McGinley, J.; Brereton, A.V.; Enticott, P.G.; Bradshaw, J.L. Gait function in newly diagnosed children with autism: Cerebellar and basal ganglia related motor disorder. *Dev. Med. Child Neurol.* **2006**, *48*, 819–824. [CrossRef]
26. Cairney, J.; King-Dowling, S. Developmental coordination disorder. In *Comorbid Conditions among Children with Autism Spectrum Disorders*; Matson, J.L., Ed.; Springer: Berlin, Germany, 2016; pp. 303–322.
27. Mosconi, M.W.; Sweeney, J.A. Sensorimotor dysfunctions as primary features of autism spectrum disorders. *Sci. China Life Sci.* **2015**, *58*, 1016–1023. [CrossRef] [PubMed]
28. Pluta, M. Parental perceptions of the effect of child participation in hippotherapy programme on overall improvement of child mental and physical wellbeing. *Ann. UMCS Zootech.* **2011**, *29*, 74–84. [CrossRef]
29. Pan, C.Y. Motor proficiency and physical fitness in adolescent males with and without autism spectrum disorders. *Autism* **2014**, *18*, 156–165. [CrossRef]
30. Travers, B.G.; Kana, R.K.; Klinger, L.G.; Klein, C.L.; Klinger, M.R. Motor learning in individuals with autism spectrum disorder: Activation in superior parietal lobule related to learning and repetitive behaviors. *Autism Res.* **2015**, *8*, 38–51. [CrossRef]
31. Choi, B.; Leech, K.A.; Tager-Flusberg, H.; Nelson, C.A. Development of fine motor skills is associated with expressive language outcomes in infants at high and low risk for autism spectrum disorder. *J. Neurodev. Disord.* **2018**, *10*, 14. [CrossRef]
32. Flanagan, J.E.; Landa, R.; Bhat, A.; Bauman, M. Head lag in infants at risk for autism: A preliminary study. *Am. J. Occup. Ther.* **2012**, *66*, 577–585. [CrossRef]
33. Landa, R.; Garrett-Mayer, E. Development in infants with autism spectrum disorders: A prospective study. *J. Child Psychol. Psychiatry* **2006**, *47*, 629–638. [CrossRef]
34. Lloyd, M.; MacDonald, M.; Lord, C. Motor skills of toddlers with autism spectrum disorders. *Autism* **2013**, *17*, 133–146. [CrossRef] [PubMed]
35. Esposito, G.; Pasca, S. Motor abnormalities as a putative endophenotype for Autism Spectrum Disorders. *Front. Integr. Neurosci.* **2013**, *7*, 43. [CrossRef] [PubMed]
36. Marrus, N.; Eggebrecht, A.T.; Todorov, A.; Elison, J.T.; Wolff, J.J.; Cole, L.; Emerson, R.W. Walking, gross motor development, and brain functional connectivity in infants and toddlers. *Cereb. Cortex* **2017**, *28*, 750–763. [CrossRef] [PubMed]
37. Ozonoff, S.; Young, G.S.; Goldring, S.; Greiss-Hess, L.; Herrera, A.M.; Steele, J.; Rogers, S.J. Gross motor development, movement abnormalities, and early identification of autism. *J. Autism Dev. Disord.* **2008**, *38*, 644–656. [CrossRef] [PubMed]
38. Bhat, A.N.; Galloway, J.C.; Landa, R.J. Relation between early motor delay and later communication delay in infants at risk for autism. *Infant Behav. Dev.* **2012**, *35*, 838–846. [CrossRef]
39. Baranek, G.T.; Parham, L.D.; Bodfish, J.W. Sensory and motor features in autism: Assessment and intervention. In *Handbook of Autism and Pervasive Developmental Disorders*; Volkmar, F., Ed.; John Wiley & Sons: Hoboken, NJ, USA, 2017; pp. 831–857.
40. Setoh, P.; Marschik, P.B.; Einspieler, C.; Esposito, G. Autism spectrum disorder and early motor abnormalities: Connected or coincidental companions? *Res. Dev. Disabil.* **2005**, *60*, 13–15. [CrossRef]
41. Williams JH, G.; Whiten, A.; Singh, T. A systematic review of action imitation in autistic spectrum disorder. *J. Autism Dev. Disord.* **2004**, *34*, 285–299. [CrossRef]
42. Chinello, A.; Di Gangi, V.; Valenza, E. Persistent primary reflexes affect motor acts: Potential implications for autism spectrum disorder. *Res. Dev. Disabil.* **2018**, *83*, 287–295. [CrossRef]
43. Piek, J. *Infant Motor Development*; Human Kinetics: Champaign, IL, USA, 2006.
44. Darrah, J.; Hodge, M.; Magill-Evans, J.; Kembhavi, G. Stability of serial assessments of motor and communication abilities in typically developing infants—Implications for screening. *Early Hum. Dev.* **2003**, *72*, 97–110. [CrossRef]
45. Pless, M.; Carlsson, M.; Sundelin, C.; Persson, K. Preschool children with developmental coordination disorder: A short-term follow-up of motor status at seven to eight years of age. *Acta Paediatr.* **2002**, *91*, 521–528. [CrossRef]
46. Van Waelvelde, H.; Oostra, A.; Dewitte, G.; Van Den Broeck, C.; Jongmans, M.J. Stability of motor problems in young children with or at risk of autism spectrum disorders, ADHD, and/or developmental coordination disorder. *Dev. Med. Child Neurol.* **2010**, *52*, e174–e178. [CrossRef] [PubMed]

47. Baumer, F.; Sahin, M. Neurological comorbidities in autism spectrum disorder. In *Autism Spectrum Disorder*; McDougle, C.J., Ed.; Oxford University Press: Oxford, UK, 2016; pp. 99–116.
48. Bruininks, R.H.; Bruininks, B.D. *Bruininks-Oseretsky Test of Motor Proficiency*, 2nd ed.; Pearson Assessments: Minneapolis, MN, USA, 2005.
49. American Psychiatric Association. DSM-5 Task Force. The Clinician-Rated Severity of Autism Spectrum and Social Communication Disorders. 2013. Available online: http://www.psychiatry.org/dsm5 (accessed on 29 February 2020).
50. Ghaziuddin, M.; Welch, K. The Michigan Autism Spectrum Questionnaire: A Rating Scale for High-Functioning Autism Spectrum Disorders. *Autism Res. Treat.* **2013**, *2013*, 1–5. [CrossRef] [PubMed]
51. Gilliam, J.E. *Gilliam Autism Rating Scale*, 3rd ed.; Pro-Ed: Austin, TX, USA, 2013.
52. Oldfield, R. The assessment and analysis of handedness: The Edinburgh inventory. *Neuropsychologia* **1971**, *9*, 97–113. [CrossRef]
53. Raven, J.; Raven, J.; Court, J. *Manual for Raven's Progressive Matrices and Vocabulary Scales*; Oxford Psychologists Press: Oxford, UK, 1998.
54. American Psychiatric Association. DSM-5 Task Force, & American Psychiatric Association. In *Diagnostic and Statistical Manual of Mental Disorders: DSM-5*, 5th ed.; American Psychiatric Association: Arlington, VA, USA, 2013.
55. Holloway, J.M.; Long, T.M.; Biasini, F. Relationships between gross motor skills and social function in young boys with autism spectrum disorder. *Pediatric Phys. Ther.* **2018**, *30*, 184–190. [CrossRef] [PubMed]
56. Liu, T.; Breslin, C.M.; ElGarhy, S. Methods and Procedures for Measuring Comorbid Disorders: Motor Movement and Activity. In *Comorbid Conditions among Children with Autism Spectrum Disorders*; Matson, J.L., Ed.; Springer: Berlin, Germany, 2015; pp. 91–134.
57. Deitz, J.C.; Kartin, D.; Kopp, K. Review of the Bruininks-Oseretsky test of motor proficiency, (BOT-2). *Phys. Occup. Ther. Pediatr.* **2007**, *27*, 87–102. [CrossRef]
58. Okuda, P.; Pangelinan, M.; Capellini, S.; Cogo-Moreira, H. Motor skills assessments: Support for a general motor factor for the Movement Assessment Battery for Children-2 and the Bruininks-Oseretsky Test of Motor Proficiency-2. *Trends Psychiatry Psychother.* **2019**, *41*, 51–59. [CrossRef]
59. Jírovec, J.; Musálek, M.; Mess, F. Test of motor proficiency second edition (bot-2): Compatibility of the complete and short form and its usefulness for middle-age school children. *Front. Pediatr.* **2019**, *7*, 153. [CrossRef]
60. Cohen, J. *Statistical Power Analysis for the Behavioral Sciences*, 2nd ed.; L. Erlbaum Associates: Hillsdale, NJ, USA, 1988.
61. Hilton, C.L.; Attal, A.; Best, J.R.; Reistetter, T.; Trapani, P.; Collins, D. Exergaming to improve physical and mental fitness in children and adolescents with autism spectrum disorders: Pilot study. *Int. J. Sports Exerc. Med.* **2015**, *1*, 1–6. [CrossRef]
62. Mattard-Labrecque, C.; Amor, L.B.; Couture, M.M. Children with autism and attention difficulties: A pilot study of the association between sensory, motor, and adaptive behaviors. *J. Can. Acad. Child Adolesc. Psychiatry* **2013**, *22*, 139.
63. Olzenak, D.L. Adding Motor Assessment to the Disability Determination Process in School-Aged Children with ASD: Implications for Participation. 2015. Available online: https://ddp.policyresearchinc.org/wp-content/uploads/2015/09/Olzenak_Final-Report.pdf (accessed on 5 December 2019).
64. Hilton, C.L.; Cumpata, K.; Klohr, C.; Gaetke, S.; Artner, A.; Johnson, H.; Dobbs, S. Effects of exergaming on executive function and motor skills in children with autism spectrum disorder: A pilot study. *Am. J. Occup. Ther. Off. Publ. Am. Occup. Ther. Assoc.* **2014**, *68*, 57–65. [CrossRef]
65. Mosconi, M.W.; Takarae, Y.; Sweeney, J.A. Motor functioning and dyspraxia in autism spectrum disorders. In *Autism Spectrum Disorder*; Amaral, D.G., Dawson, G., Geschwind, H.D., Eds.; Oxford University Press: New York, NY, USA, 2011; pp. 355–380.
66. Gaul, D.; Issartel, J. Fine motor skill proficiency in typically developing children: On or off the maturation track? *Hum. Mov. Sci.* **2016**, *46*, 78–85. [CrossRef] [PubMed]
67. Maksoud, G. Fine motor skill proficiency in children with and without down syndrome. *J. Phys. Ther. Health Promot.* **2016**, *4*, 43–50. [CrossRef]
68. Wrotniak, B.H.; Epstein, L.H.; Dorn, J.M.; Jones, K.E.; Kondilis, V.A. The relationship between motor proficiency and physical activity in children. *Pediatrics* **2006**, *118*, e1758–e1765. [CrossRef] [PubMed]

69. Khalifa, B.; Nasser, R. The closeness of the child to the domestic servant and its mediation by negative parenting behaviors in an Arab Gulf country. In Proceedings of the Australasian Conference on Business and Social Sciences, Sydney, Australia, 6 December 2015; pp. 258–269.
70. Duncan, M.J.; Spence, J.C.; Mummery, W.K. Perceived environment and physical activity: A meta-analysis of selected environmental characteristics. *Int. J. Behav. Nutr. Phys. Act.* **2005**, *2*, 11. [CrossRef]
71. Zeng, N.; Ayyub, M.; Sun, H.; Wen, X.; Xiang, P.; Gao, Z. Effects of physical activity on motor skills and cognitive development in early childhood: A systematic review. *Biomed. Res. Int.* **2017**, *2017*, 1–13. [CrossRef]
72. Al-Heizan, M.O.; Al-Abdulwahab, S.S.; Kachanathu, S.J.; Natho, M. Sensory processing dysfunction among Saudi children with and without autism. *J. Phys. Ther. Sci.* **2015**, *27*, 1313–1316. [CrossRef]
73. Alkhalifah, S. Psychometric properties of the Sensory Processing Measure Preschool-Home among Saudi children with autism spectrum disorder: Pilot study. *J. Occup. Ther. Sch. Early Interv.* **2019**, *12*, 401–416. [CrossRef]
74. Must, A.; Phillips, S.; Curtin, C.; Bandini, L.G. Barriers to physical activity in children with autism spectrum disorders: Relationship to physical activity and screen time. *J. Phys. Act. Health* **2015**, *12*, 529–534. [CrossRef]
75. Patz, J.A.; Messina, R.M. Fine motor, oral motor, and self-care development. In *Young Children with Special Needs*, 5th ed.; Hooper, S.R., Umansky, W., Eds.; Pearson: Upper Saddle River, NJ, USA, 2009; pp. 168–235.
76. McCarton, C. Assessment and diagnosis of pervasive developmental disorder. In *Autism Spectrum Disorders*; Hollander, E., Ed.; Dekker: New York, NY, USA, 2003; pp. 101–132.
77. Coffin, A.B.; Myles, B.S.; Rogers, J.; Szakacs, W. Supporting the Writing Skills of Individuals with Autism Spectrum Disorder through Assistive Technologies. In *Technology and the Treatment of Children with Autism Spectrum Disorder*; Cardon, T.A., Ed.; Springer: Berlin, Germany, 2016; pp. 59–73.
78. Abdel Karim, A.E.; Mohammed, A.H. Effectiveness of sensory integration program in motor skills in children with autism. *Egypt. J. Med Hum. Genet.* **2015**, *16*, 375–380. [CrossRef]
79. Betts, D.; Jacobs, D. *Everyday Activities to Help Your Young Child with Autism Live Life to the Full: Simple Exercises to Boost Functional Skills, Sensory Processing, Coordination and Self-Care*; Jessica Kingsley Publishers: London, UK, 2011.
80. Semel, E.; Rosner, S. *Understanding Williams Syndrome: Behavioral Patterns and Interventions*; L. Erlbaum: Mahwah, NJ, USA, 2003.
81. Hilton, C.; Wente, L.; LaVesser, P.; Ito, M.; Reed, C.; Herzberg, G. Relationship between motor skill impairment and severity in children with Asperger syndrome. *Res. Autism Spectr. Disord.* **2007**, *1*, 339–349. [CrossRef]
82. Staples, K.L.; Reid, G. Fundamental movement skills and autism spectrum disorders. *J. Autism Dev. Disord.* **2010**, *40*, 209–217. [CrossRef] [PubMed]
83. Zikl, P.; Petrů, D.; Daňková, A.; Doležalová, H.; Šafaříková, K. Motor skills of children with autistic spectrum disorder. In *SHS Web of Conferences*; EDP Sciences: Les Ulis, France, 2016; Volume 26, p. 1076.
84. Paris, B. Characteristics of autism. In *Exploring the Spectrum of Autism and Pervasive Developmental Disorders*; Murray-Slutsky, C., Paris, B., Eds.; Therapy Skill Builders (Harcourt Health Sciences): San Antonio, TX, USA, 2000; pp. 7–23.
85. Dejean, V.M. *Vestibular Re Integration of the Autistic Child: Developmental Model for Autism*; iUniverse, Inc.: New York, NY, USA, 2008.
86. Coetzee, D. Strength, running speed, agility and balance profiles of 9-to 10-year-old learners: NW-child study. *S. Afr. J. Res. Sport Phys. Educ. Recreat.* **2016**, *38*, 13–30.
87. Deponio, P.; Macintyre, C. *Identifying and Supporting Children with Specific Learning Difficulties: Looking Beyond the Label to Support the Whole Child*; Routledge: London, UK, 2003.
88. Ament, K.; Mejia, A.; Buhlman, R.; Erklin, S.; Caffo, B.; Mostofsky, S.; Wodka, E. Evidence for specificity of motor impairments in catching and balance in children with autism. *J. Autism Dev. Disord.* **2015**, *45*, 742–751. [CrossRef]
89. Molloy, C.A.; Dietrich, K.N.; Bhattacharya, A. Postural stability in children with autism spectrum disorder. *J. Autism Dev. Disord.* **2003**, *33*, 643–652. [CrossRef] [PubMed]
90. Van Sant, A.; Goldberg, C. Normal motor development. In *Pediatric Physical Therapy*; Tecklin, J.S., Ed.; Lippincott Williams & Wilkins: New York, NY, USA, 1999; pp. 22–25.
91. DeLong, G.R. The cerebellum in autism. In *The Neurology of Autism*; Coleman, M., Ed.; Oxford University Press: Oxford, UK, 2005; pp. 75–90.

92. Pusponegoro, H.D.; Efar, P.; Soebadi, A.; Firmansyah, A.; Chen, H.J.; Hung, K.L. Gross motor profile and its association with socialization skills in children with autism spectrum disorders. *Pediatr. Neonatol.* **2016**, *57*, 501–507. [CrossRef] [PubMed]
93. Noterdaeme, M.; Mildenberger, K.; Minow, F.; Amorosa, H. Evaluation of neuromotor deficits in children with autism and children with a specific speech and language disorder. *Eur. Child Adolesc. Psychiatry* **2002**, *11*, 219–225. [CrossRef]
94. Dixon, G.; Addy, L. *Making Inclusion work for Children with Dyspraxia: Practical Strategies for Teachers*; Routledge Falmer: London, UK, 2004.
95. Memari, A.H.; Ghanouni, P.; Shayestehfar, M.; Ghaheri, B. Postural control impairments in individuals with autism spectrum disorder: A critical review of current literature. *Asian J. Sports Med.* **2014**, *5*, e22963. [CrossRef]
96. Bhat, A.N.; Landa, R.J.; Galloway, J.C. Current perspectives on motor functioning in infants, children, and adults with autism spectrum disorders. *Phys. Ther.* **2011**, *91*, 1116–1129. [CrossRef]
97. Attwood, T. *The Complete Guide to Asperger's Syndrome*; Jessica Kingsley Publishers: London, UK, 2006.
98. Baetti, S. Argentinian ambulatory integral model to treat autism spectrum disorders. In *Autism: The Movement Sensing Perspective*; Torres, E.B., Whyatt, C., Eds.; CRC Press; Taylor & Francis Group: Boca Raton, FL, USA, 2017; pp. 253–269.
99. Dirksen, T.; Lussanet, D.; Marc, H.E.; Zentgraf, K.; Slupinski, L.; Wagner, H. Increased Throwing Accuracy Improves Children's Catching Performance in a Ball-Catching Task from the Movement Assessment Battery (MABC-2). *Front. Psychol.* **2016**, *7*, 1122. [CrossRef]
100. Emck, C.; Bosscher, R.; Beek, P.; Doreleijers, T. Gross motor performance and self-perceived motor competence in children with emotional, behavioural, and pervasive developmental disorders: A review. *Dev. Med. Child Neurol.* **2009**, *51*, 501–517. [CrossRef]
101. Neporent, L. *Fitness Walking for Dummies*; John Wiley & Sons: New York, NY, USA, 2011.
102. Siri, K.; Lyons, T. *Cutting-Edge Therapies for Autism*; Skyhorse Publishing Inc.: New York, NY, USA, 2014.
103. Mayall, L.A.; D'Souza, H.; Hill, E.L.; Karmiloff-Smith, A.; Tolmie, A.; Farran, E.K. Motor Abilities and the Motor Profile in Individuals with Williams Syndrome. *Adv. Neurodev. Disord.* **2020**, *8*, 1–15. [CrossRef]
104. Wilson, R.B.; Enticott, P.G.; Rinehart, N.J. Motor development and delay: Advances in assessment of motor skills in autism spectrum disorders. *Curr. Opin. Neurol.* **2018**, *31*, 134–139. [CrossRef] [PubMed]
105. Jasmin, E.; Couture, M.; McKinley, P.; Reid, G.; Fombonne, E.; Gisel, E. Sensori-motor and daily living skills of preschool children with autism spectrum disorders. *J. Autism Dev. Disord.* **2009**, *39*, 231–241. [CrossRef]
106. MacDonald, M.; Lord, C.; Ulrich, D.A. The relationship of motor skills and social communicative skills in school-aged children with autism spectrum disorder. *Adapt. Phys. Act. Q.* **2013**, *30*, 271–282. [CrossRef]
107. Purpura, G.; Fulceri, F.; Puglisi, V.; Masoni, P.; Contaldo, A. Motor coordination impairment in children with autism spectrum disorder: A pilot study using Movement Assessment Battery for Children-2 Checklist. *Minerva Pediatrica* **2016**, *72*. [CrossRef] [PubMed]

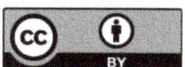

© 2020 by the author. Licensee MDPI, Basel, Switzerland. This article is an open access article distributed under the terms and conditions of the Creative Commons Attribution (CC BY) license (http://creativecommons.org/licenses/by/4.0/).

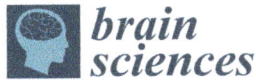

Article

Grammatical Comprehension in Italian Children with Autism Spectrum Disorder

Jessica Barsotti [1], Gloria Mangani [1], Roberta Nencioli [1], Lucia Pfanner [1], Raffaella Tancredi [1], Angela Cosenza [1], Gianluca Sesso [1], Antonio Narzisi [1], Filippo Muratori [1,2,*], Paola Cipriani [1] and Anna Maria Chilosi [1]

[1] IRCCS Stella Maris Foundation, Calambrone, 56018 Pisa, Italy; jessica.barsotti@fsm.unipi.it (J.B.); gloria.man96@hotmail.it (G.M.); roberta.nencioli@fsm.unipi.it (R.N.); lucia.pfanner@fsm.unipi.it (L.P.); raffaella.tancredi@fsm.unipi.it (R.T.); angela.cosenza@fsm.unipi.it (A.C.); gianluca.sesso@fsm.unipi.it (G.S.); antonio.narzisi@fsm.unipi.it (A.N.); paola.cipriani@fsm.unipi.it (P.C.); anna.chilosi@fsm.unipi.it (A.M.C.)
[2] Department of Clinical and Experimental Medicine, University of Pisa, Via Savi, 10, 56126 Pisa, Italy
* Correspondence: filippo.muratori@fsm.unipi.it

Received: 26 June 2020; Accepted: 30 July 2020; Published: 2 August 2020

Abstract: Language deficits represent one of the most relevant factors that determine the clinical phenotype of children with autism spectrum disorder (ASD). The main aim of the research was to study the grammatical comprehension of children with ASD. A sample of 70 well-diagnosed children (60 boys and 10 girls; aged 4.9–8 years) were prospectively recruited. The results showed that language comprehension is the most impaired language domain in ASD. These findings have important clinical implications, since the persistence of grammatical receptive deficits may have a negative impact on social, adaptive and learning achievements. As for the grammatical profiles, persistent difficulties were found during the school-age years in morphological and syntactic decoding in children with relatively preserved cognitive and expressive language skills. These data and the lack of a statistically significant correlation between the severity of ASD symptoms and language skills are in line with the DSM-5 (Diagnostic and Statistical Manual of Mental Disorders, Fifth Edition) perspective that considers the socio-communication disorder as a nuclear feature of ASD and the language disorder as a specifier of the diagnosis and not as a secondary symptom anymore. The presence of receptive difficulties in school-age ASD children with relatively preserved non-verbal cognitive abilities provides important hints to establish rehabilitative treatments.

Keywords: autism spectrum disorder; language profiles; grammatical comprehension

1. Introduction

Children with autism spectrum disorder (ASD) show heterogeneous functional profiles and outcomes [1,2]. Language deficits represent one of the most relevant factors that determine the clinical phenotype of children with ASD. Language deficits in ASD children can be described as a continuum, as on one hand there are non-verbal or minimally verbal children or those who do not acquire verbal language (in variable percentages up to 50% according to different studies) [3–8], and on the other hand there are children with formally appropriate but pragmatically inadequate language [9,10]. Within this continuum, highly variable language profiles can be found, with children exhibiting language delay, children with language disorders, and those who, despite reaching their first language milestones (i.e., speaking their first words between 12 and 18 months), later experience an arrest or a regression in language development.

Though communication and language in children with ASD have been extensively investigated [4,9–13], the nature of the language deficit still remains an open issue. According to the DSM-5 [14], social communication disorder is considered a nuclear feature of ASD, while language disorder is only defined as a "specifier" of the condition. Some authors consider language disorders and ASD as potentially comorbid conditions [10,15] and use the term ASD-LI to refer to individuals with ASD who have impairments in structural language, regardless of their overall cognitive functioning.

The majority of published studies report that, in ASD, receptive language is more impaired than expressive language [5,11,16–21], but this finding has not been completely confirmed [22,23]. Moreover, the issue of the discrepancy between receptive and expressive competences is still unclear in terms of whether it should be considered as a possible marker of ASD, or whether both receptive and expressive language difficulties are comorbid to ASD.

Receptive language disorders in children with ASD are part of a wide and more complex phenotype characterized by pragmatic and neuropsychological deficits that may impair the acquisition of verbal comprehension. According to Tager-Flusberg and colleagues [24], the ASD's problems of language comprehension are especially present in everyday situations, rather than during single-word comprehension testing. Children with ASD exhibit impairments in the ability to decode relevant contextual cues and deficits in social attention [25–28], whereas typically developing (TD) children are able from an early age to identify and select salient sensory stimuli and crucial social cues that are relevant both for comprehension and communication [29,30].

Grammatical comprehension, as a specific language skill that is required for decoding verbal messages in interactions, would represent a crucial matter of research in the field of ASD. However, it is worth noticing that relatively few studies are available which assess the comprehension of someone with ASD by means of specific tasks that differentially evaluate their lexical and grammatical skills. The evaluation of receptive abilities in children with ASD is of crucial importance in the clinical context in order to more clearly define the language profile, which has always been considered a paramount prognostic marker of development. Indeed, minimally verbal children with ASD exhibit a greater severity of autistic symptoms and globally worse clinical outcomes [31] than those with normal or mildly delayed language development, for whom an outcome could be more satisfactory [32]. Considering the above mentioned prognostic significance of language skills on the developmental perspective of children with ASD, the aims of the present study were:

1. To assess grammatical receptive skills in relation to other language abilities;
2. To investigate the relative contributions of non-verbal cognitive abilities and the severity of autistic symptoms on the language profile of children with ASD;
3. To examine the qualitative and quantitative differences in grammatical comprehension between ASD and TD children.

2. Materials and Methods

2.1. Sample

The present study was conducted on a sample of 70 children (60 boys) aged 4.9–8 years (mean age: 6.3 years; SD: 11 months; age range: 4.9–8 years) prospectively recruited at IRCCS Stella Maris Foundation (Calambrone, Pisa, Italy) from February 2009 to May 2018.

Inclusion criteria were as follows:

- A diagnosis of either autistic disorder according to DSM-IV-TR criteria or autism spectrum disorder according to DSM-5 criteria;
- Average or borderline non-verbal intellectual or developmental functioning level assessed through standardized psychometric tests;
- Expressive language at the level of multiword productions.

In order to qualitatively analyze grammatical comprehension, a subsample of 54 children with ASD and performance IQ $\geq$ 85 was selected and compared to 54 age- and sex-matched typically developing (TD) children. TD children were recruited from kindergarten and elementary schools in the area of Pisa, excluding subjects exposed to bilingualism.

Both groups were subdivided into four age groups at 12 months intervals, from 4.10 to 8 years. Informed written consent was obtained from the parents of all participants. This study was approved by the Pediatric Ethical Committee of the Tuscany Region (approval number: 178/2016) and was conducted according to the Helsinki Declaration.

2.2. Tests and Procedures

Grammatical comprehension was assessed using the Grammatical Comprehension Test for Children (Test Comprensione Grammaticale per Bambini; TCGB) [33] standardized on Italian children aged 3.6–8 years. The TCGB is a picture multiple-choice language test composed of 76 sentences pertaining to eight main blocks of grammatical structures: locatives, inflectionals, both affirmative and negative actives and passives, relatives and datives. Within each block of structures, the clauses differ not only in grammatical complexity, but also in semantic complexity (i.e., irreversible vs. reversible and probable vs. improbable clauses).

Children with ASD also underwent a comprehensive assessment of language skills by means of a receptive vocabulary test (PPVT-R: Peabody Picture Vocabulary Test—Revised) [34], an expressive picture naming test (One-Word Picture Vocabulary Test) [35] and the analysis of spontaneous language performed according to a six level rating system (Grid of Analysis of Spontaneous speech—GASS) [36,37]. For a detailed description of the TCGB and GASS, see Tables S1 and S2 in the Supplementary Materials. For all language tests, z-scores below —1.5 SD of the mean were considered as deficient.

Wechsler Preschool and Primary Scale of Intelligence, 3rd Ed (WPPSI-III, [38]) performance IQ, the Perceptual Reasoning Index at WISC-IV [39] or Griffiths [40] developmental quotient of the performance scale were used as measures of the non-verbal intellectual functioning level.

Finally, the Autism Diagnostic Observation Schedule-Generic (ADOS-G) [41] and Autism Diagnostic Observation Schedule-Second Edition (ADOS-2) [42] semi-structured observations were performed in ASD children for the evaluation of the autistic symptomatology severity.

2.3. Statistical Analysis

Skewness and Kurtosis statistics did not demonstrate a normal distribution for language-related variables, thus non-parametric tests were utilized. On the whole sample of 70 children with ASD, Spearman's rank correlation coefficients between the grammatical comprehension non-verbal cognitive scores and ADOS severity scores were calculated. The Mann–Whitney U test was used to compare: (1) the non-verbal cognitive scores between children who performed averagely in the TCGB and children whose performances were classed as deficient; (2) the TCGB scores between the 54 ASD and the 54 TD children. The Kruskal–Wallis test for independent samples was also used to assess significant differences between the four age groups (5, 6, 7 and 8-year-old groups) of 54 children with ASD and 54 TD controls. Statistical analyses were performed using SPSS 21 software (IBM SPSS Statistics, Chicago, IL, USA).

3. Results

3.1. Language Profiles

Considering the mean z scores of the whole sample (see Table 1), grammatical comprehension appeared the most impaired domain compared to the other language measures. The TGCB mean total z score and the mean z score of the different structures (with the exception of active negative sentences) fell below −1.5 SD of the mean. Sixty-three percent of children with ASD had impaired grammatical comprehension. As for the vocabulary measures, the mean receptive lexical quotient at the PPVT was in the borderline range, with 56% of children showing an impaired performance. The expressive vocabulary scores were in the average range both for high and low frequency words (only 18% of children exhibited an impaired performance). According to the GASS, expressive language was at level 4, which corresponds to a deficient control of complex grammar, and only 14% of children had a more severe deficit.

Table 1. Sample characteristics ($n = 70$).

Children's Language, Cognitive and ADS Profiles	Mean	SD	Mean z Score
Age	76.43	11.80	-
Grammatical Comprehension (TCGB)	20.33	11.27	−3.25
Locative	2.55	2.14	−1.66
Inflectional	3.29	2.47	−2.55
Affirmative Active	1.99	1.98	−2.59
Negative Active	1.90	1.68	−0.86
Affirmative Passive	3.31	2.29	−2.58
Negative Passive	2.74	1.79	−2.61
Relative	2.59	1.85	−2.97
Dative	1.96	1.33	−4.73
Receptive Vocabulary (QL PPVT-R)	80.72	11.12	−1.22
Grammatical production level (GASS)	4.18	0.62	-
Expressive Vocabulary for high-frequency words (Brizzolara)	13.58	5.27	−0.38
Expressive Vocabulary for low-frequency words (Brizzolara)	32.32	6.09	−0.77
NVIQ	100.62	14.66	-
ADOS Comparison Score	5.30	1.42	-

Abbreviations: SD: standard deviation; NVIQ: non-verbal intelligence quotient.

3.2. Correlations between Language Measures, Non-Verbal Cognitive Skills and Autistic Symptoms Severity

Statistically significant correlations were found between the non-verbal IQ and total TCGB scores ($p = 0.020$). Non-verbal IQ was also correlated with active negative and passive negative clauses ($p = 0.000$ and $p = 0.023$, respectively). However, it is worth noting that non-verbal cognitive abilities did not differ significantly between ASD children with average and impaired comprehensions ($p = 0.073$).

The severity of the autistic symptoms assessed through the ADOS was low/moderate and did not correlate significantly with any expressive and receptive language measure.

3.3. Grammatical Comprehension Profiles of ASD and TD Children

The subsample of 54 children with ASD with a non-verbal IQ ≥ 85, was subdivided into four age groups (i.e., 5, 6, 7 and 8-year-old groups). These subgroups did not differ significantly in terms of non-verbal cognitive abilities ($p = 0.296$) or the severity of autistic symptoms ($p = 0.212$).

As displayed in Table 2 and Figure 1, the comparison between ASD and TD children showed that ASD children had significantly lower scores than TD children for most types of grammatical clauses at different ages. As expected, performances of both ASD and TD children changed with age; however, the ASD children's performances changed at a significantly slower rate compared to the TD children. In the 5-year-old subgroup, statistically significant differences emerged for affirmative active, negative passive and dative clauses, whereas, in the 6- and 7-year-old subgroup, ASD children scored significantly lower than TD children in all types of clauses (with the exception of negative active clauses). The 8-year-old subgroup showed a significant reduction in their error scores, compared to 5- and 6-year-old children ($p = 0.030$ and $p = 0.010$, respectively). Nonetheless, significant differences between ASD and TD children were still evident for locative, affirmative passive, relative and dative clauses. Considering the semantic and grammatical complexity of the different clause types (for details see Table 3), markedly significant differences between ASD and TD children were observed for the more complex but not for the simpler sentences (i.e., verbal vs. nominal inflexions, projective vs. topological locatives, semantically improbable vs. probable and neutral active affirmative clauses, reversible vs. irreversible clauses) [33]. The comparison between the reversible and irreversible clauses total scores showed a highly significant difference between TD and ASD children in the comprehension of reversible clauses ($p = 0.000$), but not in irreversible clauses ($p = 0.834$).

Table 2. Comparison between typically developing (TD) and autism spectrum disorder (ASD) children in the different age ranges.

Grammatical Comprehension	5 Years			6 Years			7 Years			8 Years		
	TD (n = 21)	ASD (n = 21)	p	TD (n = 14)	ASD (n = 14)	p	TD (n = 12)	ASD (n = 12)	p	TD (n = 7)	ASD (n = 7)	p
TCGB Total score	14.00 (6.51)	21.38 (8.95)	0.004	6.86 (2.64)	20.68 (3.27)	0.000	2.79 (1.12)	14.00 (7.48)	0.000	2.21 (2.02)	9.14 (4.92)	0.005
Locative	1.79 (1.52)	2.38 (1.84)	ns	1.00 (0.70)	2.11 (1.36)	0.012	0.38 (0.57)	2.17 (1.70)	0.002	0.14 (0.24)	1.14 (0.85)	0.011
Inflectional	3.21 (2.22)	3.60 (2.40)	ns	1.04 (1.15)	2.33 (0.62)	0.002	0.29 (0.33)	2.42 (1.04)	0.000	0.29 (0.39)	0.57 (0.45)	ns
Affirmative Active	0.88 (0.74)	2.29 (1.55)	0.001	0.61 (0.56)	1.61 (1.66)	0.043	0.25 (0.50)	1.08 (1.28)	0.047	0.21 (0.57)	0.64 (0.80)	ns
Negative Active	1.71 (1.27)	2.07 (1.54)	ns	1.25 (1.03)	1.64 (1.26)	ns	0.46 (0.58)	1.00 (1.19)	ns	0.50 (0.58)	0.79 (0.99)	ns
Affirmative Pass.	2.45 (2.64)	3.19 (2.11)	ns	1.07 (1.47)	3.71 (2.55)	0.003	0.38 (0.38)	3.00 (2.13)	0.000	0.29 (0.57)	2.00 (1.68)	0.025
Negative Passive	1.64 (1.43)	2.71 (1.51)	0.023	0.71 (0.80)	3.07 (1.20)	0.000	0.42 (0.51)	1.79 (1.47)	0.006	0.43 (0.53)	1.21 (1.55)	ns
Relative	1.74 (1.34)	2.74 (1.86)	ns	0.93 (0.92)	3.11 (1.91)	0.001	0.50 (0.56)	1.50 (1.46)	0.038	0.29 (0.39)	1.71 (0.81)	0.001
Dative	0.57 (0.81)	2.38 (1.22)	0.000	0.25 (0.38)	2.04 (1.42)	0.000	0.13 (0.31)	0.92 (0.63)	0.001	0.07 (0.19)	1.07 (0.67)	0.003

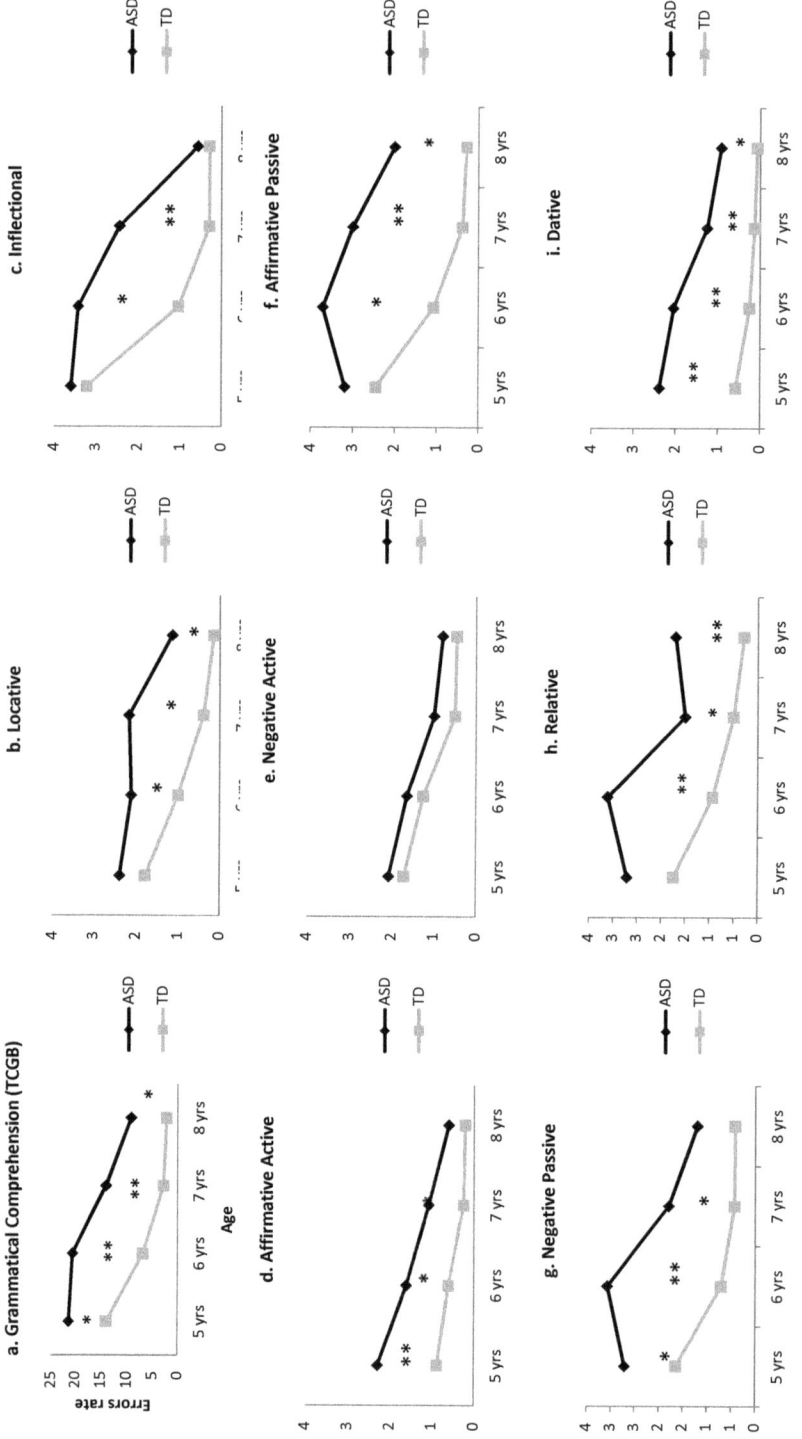

Figure 1. ASD and TD children's total (a) and single clause type (b–i) error scores (* $p \leq 0.05$; ** $p \leq 0.001$). Abbreviation: yrs: years.

Table 3. Comparison between ASD and TD children: qualitative assessment of the clause type related subcategories.

Structure	Sub-Categories	TD (n = 54)	ASD (n = 54)	Mann–Whitney Test
Locative	topological	0.12 (0.34)	0.42 (0.88)	0.021
	projective	0.94 (1.07)	1.57 (1.31)	0.009
Inflectional	nominal	0.07 (0.20)	0.16 (0.50)	ns
	verbal	0.84 (1.14)	1.80 (1.46)	0.000
	possessive	0.70 (1.16)	0.89 (0.92)	0.027
Affirmative Active	SV (reflexive)	0.08 (0.30)	0.41 (0.46)	0.000
	reversible probable	0.11 (0.21)	0.05 (0.18)	0.048
	reversible neutral	0.13 (0.28)	0.28 (0.50)	ns
	reversible improbable	0.07 (0.26)	0.54 (0.66)	0.000
	reversible with subject object inanimate-animate	0.19 (0.37)	0.30 (0.65)	ns
Negative Active	SV	0.01 (0.07)	0.13 (0.48)	0.041
	SVO irreversible	0.50 (0.67)	0.43 (0.65)	ns
	SVO reversible	0.65 (0.84)	1.00 (0.92)	0.023
Affirmative Passive	irreversible	0.53 (1.08)	0.40 (0.53)	ns
	reversible probable	0.22 (0.49)	0.94 (1.06)	0.000
	reversible improbable	0.35 (0.55)	0.95 (0.84)	0.000
	reversible neutral	0.25 (0.59)	0.78 (1.02)	0.000
Negative Passive	SV	0.10 (0.36)	0.77 (0.72)	0.000
	SVA irreversible	0.34 (0.53)	0.55 (0.68)	ns
	SVA reversible	0.53 (0.88)	1.05 (0.96)	0.002
Relative	embedded	0.61 (0.70)	1.44 (1.09)	0.000
	right branching	0.45 (0.75)	0.92 (1.12)	0.022
Dative	AAA	0.26 (0.56)	0.92 (0.85)	0.000
	AIA	0.07 (0.24)	0.86 (0.88)	0.000

Abbreviations: SV: subject verb; SVO: subject verb object; SVA: subject verb agent; AAA: animate animate animate; AIA: animate inanimate animate.

4. Discussion

The present research is the first Italian study aimed at assessing grammatical comprehension in children with ASD. Our results support the hypothesis proposed by some authors [9,11,17,20,43] that language comprehension would be the most impaired language domain in autism, in spite of its highly heterogeneous linguistic phenotype [1]. Around two thirds of our patients exhibited an impaired grammatical comprehension, whereas grammatical production was impaired in only 14% of children. Additionally, in the lexical domain, receptive skills were more impaired than expressive ones. However, the deficit of language comprehension was not homogeneous, since receptive grammar was more impaired than receptive vocabulary. The above language profile differs from the one usually observed in children with a primary developmental language disorder, which is generally characterized by better receptive abilities as opposed to expressive language abilities [16,44–46]. The discrepancy between receptive and expressive skills in children with ASD is, however, still a debated issue, because it is not clear whether it could be considered a specific marker of ASD.

As for the relationship between language and non-verbal cognitive abilities, a positive correlation between non-verbal intellectual functioning and grammatical comprehension was found, but non-verbal cognitive abilities did not differ statistically between children with a normal comprehension and those with an impaired comprehension. These apparently conflicting findings suggest that the grammar comprehension deficit is quite specific in children with ASD, and, thus, is relatively independent from non-verbal cognitive skills. This evidence is in line with the results of a study conducted on a sample of ASD children with average or borderline intellectual functioning [43] in which non-verbal IQ explained a limited amount of the variance of language scores.

The lack of statistically significant correlations between the severity of ASD symptoms and language skills seems to confirm the DSM-5's choice to let language deficits outside the nuclear symptoms of autism. In this way, the DSM-5 avoids the risk of automatically establishing an overlap between communication and structural language skills.

4.1. Grammatical Comprehension Profiles in Children with ASD and TD

To date, the qualitative assessment of grammatical decoding strategies in children with ASD has generally been carried out on English-speaking subjects [47–49], with few reports in the recent literature [50]. In the present Italian study, the qualitative assessment of language comprehension showed significant differences between TD and ASD children. The latter showed both delayed and atypical receptive grammatical skills.

Data on the development of grammatical comprehension in TD children show a significant change between 5 and 6 years of age, a period characterized by an increasing integration of the different decoding strategies, and by a sharp reduction in the inter-individual variability. By 7 or 8 years old, TD children show a further increase in their capacity to generalize the use of linguistic principles and rules for decoding more complex grammatical structures [33]. In children with ASD, improvements in grammatical comprehension occurred around 7 or 8 years of age, but their receptive skills remained significantly impaired in comparison to TD children. This result has important clinical implications, since the persistence of grammatical receptive deficits may have a negative impact on social, adaptive and learning achievements during the school-age years [43,51,52].

As for the grammatical profiles, persistent difficulties were found in morphological (i.e., inflectional clauses) and syntactic decoding (i.e., locative, passive, relative and dative clauses). Similar to what was observed in TD children, the comprehension of active negative sentences was more difficult than the comprehension of active affirmative sentences. This might be due to the poor representability of negative actions and to the fact that decoding of such structures requires inferential reasoning (e.g., the correct answer for the sentence "the child does not eat the soup" is represented by a picture in which the child is eating an ice-cream).

Relative, passive and dative clauses were more difficult for children with ASD than for TD children. In the case of relative clauses, the persistence of difficulties up to 8 years of age probably depends on their length and structural complexity. For passive and dative clauses, the crucial factor may be the reversibility of actions. The significant difficulty in decoding reversible, but not irreversible sentences, which characterizes the profiles of children with ASD, is an important result because it suggests the presence of a specific linguistic deficit. In fact, in reversible sentences the roles of the agent or patient of the action are interchangeable, as they are both animate referents (e.g., "the girl pushes the boy" or vice versa). Therefore, decoding these sentences is crucially based on the word order, that is, on syntactic strategies. Conversely, in irreversible sentences, the agent and patient roles are not interchangeable, because of semantic restrictions linked to the animate/inanimate nature of referents (e.g., "the car is washed by the boy"). In this case, lexical factors can drive the sentence decoding. Difficulties in processing reversible sentences have also been described [47] in a study reporting that impairments in reversible sentence comprehension was greater than expected from the global level of receptive skills. We would suggest that ASD children with average or borderline intellectual functioning may be able to process lexical information, while showing difficulties to acquire an integrate system for decoding morpho-syntactic information.

4.2. Limitations

This study presents several limitations. A first limitation is that the non-verbal IQ tests we chose to administer require verbal comprehension skills to follow the instructions, which might have contributed to the positive correlation between the non-verbal IQ scores and the grammatical comprehension scores. Another limit is the typology of our structured picture-based comprehension test, which does not tap into ecologically natural and contextual-based comprehension abilities, thus not providing a comprehensive profile of ASD children's receptive skills.

Finally, although there was no a priori restriction on patient selection according to the severity of autistic symptomatology applied in the present study, the children with ASD showed a low to moderate severity of autistic symptomatology. This may be due to the fact that only patients who were able to complete the structured language evaluation were included, creating a bias in the selection of the sample. Patients on the autism spectrum exhibit quite heterogeneous clinical pictures, while the present study focuses on the language comprehension of intellectually unimpaired verbal children with a low/moderate severity of autistic symptoms. Hence, our results may not be generalizable to the whole population of patients with ASD.

5. Conclusions

Our results are in line with the DSM-5 perspective according which emphasizes that the socio-communication disorder is a nuclear feature of ASD, whereas the language disorder should be considered as a specifier of the diagnosis, not a nuclear deficit or a secondary symptom. Among the language abilities we have described, a specific receptive grammatical deficit was found, whilst cognitive and expressive language are relatively preserved. It would be important in the future to evaluate the relationship between language comprehension and some neuropsychological abilities, such as working memory and executive functions to shed some light on the nature of the comprehension deficits in children with ASD.

The presence of receptive difficulties in school-age ASD children with relatively preserved non-verbal cognitive abilities provides important hints about treatment. Receptive language difficulties, when not associated with expressive deficits, may go unnoticed [43] and may be neglected despite their relevance in everyday life functioning, communication and social interaction. Early support to aid in the acquisition of adequate receptive language skills is crucial for further development. Moreover, as grammatical comprehension difficulties tend to persist in ASD children up to school-age (when generally speech therapy gradually diminishes), a specific intervention on both oral and written receptive skills is mandatory.

Supplementary Materials: The following are available online at http://www.mdpi.com/2076-3425/10/8/510/s1, Table S1: The Test of grammatical Comprehension for Children TCGB, [33], Table S2: Grid of Analysis of Spontaneous Speech GASS.

Author Contributions: Conceptualization, J.B., R.N., L.P., R.T., A.N., F.M. and A.M.C.; Data curation, J.B., G.M., R.N., L.P., R.T., A.C. and A.N.; Methodology, J.B., G.M. and A.M.C.; Supervision, A.N., F.M., P.C. and A.M.C.; Writing—original draft, J.B., G.M., R.N., L.P., G.S. and A.M.C.; Writing—review and editing, J.B., R.N., L.P., G.S., A.N., F.M., P.C. and A.M.C. All authors have read and agreed to the published version of the manuscript.

Funding: This research was funded by the Italian Ministry of the Health RC2019 and 5 ×1000 founds.

Acknowledgments: We would like to acknowledge the children and families who participated in this study, we also thank Linda Tieu for English editing.

Conflicts of Interest: The authors declare no conflict of interest.

References

1. Lombardo, M.V.; Pierce, K.; Eyler, L.; Carter Barnes, C.; Ahrebs-Barbeau, C.; Solso, S.; Campbell, K.; Courchesne, E. Different functional neural substrates for good and poor language outcome in autism. *Neuron* **2015**, *86*, 567–577. [CrossRef]
2. Lombardo, M.V.; Lai, M.; Baron-Cohen, S. Big data approaches to decomposing heterogeneity across the autism spectrum. *Mol. Psychiatry* **2019**, *24*, 1435–1450. [CrossRef]
3. Rapin, I. *Preschool Children with Inadequate Communication: Developmental Language Disorder, Autism, Low IQ*; Mac Keith: London, UK, 1996.
4. Wetherby, A.M.; Prizant, B.M.; Schuler, A.L. Understanding the nature of communication and language impairments. In *Autism Spectrum Disorders: A Transactional Developmental Perspective*; Wetherby, A., Prizant, B.M., Eds.; Paul H. Brookes Publishing: Baltimore, MD, USA, 2000; pp. 109–142.
5. Boucher, J. Research Review: Structural language in autistic spectrum disorder—characteristics and causes. *J. Child Psychol. Psychiatry* **2012**, *53*, 219–233. [CrossRef]
6. Anderson, D.K.; Lord, C.; Risi, S.; Di Lavore, P.S.; Shulman, C.; Thurm, A.; Welch, K.; Pickles, A. Patterns of growth in verbal abilities among children with autism spectrum disorder. *J. Consult. Clin. Psychol.* **2007**, *75*, 594–604. [CrossRef] [PubMed]
7. Gotham, K.; Pickles, A.; Lord, C. Trajectories of autism severity in children using standardized ADOS scores. *Pediatrics* **2012**, *130*, 1278–1284. [CrossRef] [PubMed]
8. Pickles, A.; Anderson, D.K.; Lord, C. Heterogeneity and plasticity in the development of language: A 17-year follow-up of children referred early for possible autism. *J. Child Psychol. Psychiatry* **2014**, *5*, 1354–1362. [CrossRef] [PubMed]
9. Tager-Flusberg, H.; Caronna, E. Language disorders: Autism and other pervasive developmental disorders. *Pediatr. Clin. N. Am.* **2007**, *54*, 469–481. [CrossRef] [PubMed]
10. Tager-Flusberg, H. Defining language impairments in a subgroup of children with autism spectrum disorder. *Sci. China Life Sci.* **2015**, *58*, 1044–1052. [CrossRef]
11. Mitchell, S.; Brian, J.; Zwaigenbaum, L.; Roberts, W.; Szatmari, P.; Smith, I.; Bryson, S. Early language and communication development of infants later diagnosed with autism spectrum disorder. *J. Dev. Behav. Pediatr.* **2006**, *27*, 69–78. [CrossRef]
12. Kjellmer, L.; Hedvall, A.; Fernell, E.; Gillberg, C.; Norrelgen, F. Language and communication skills in preschool children with autism spectrum disorders: Contribution of cognition, severity of autism symptoms, and adaptive functioning to the variability. *Res. Dev. Disabil.* **2012**, *33*, 172–180. [CrossRef]
13. Tager-Flusberg, H. On the nature of linguistic functioning in early infantile autism. *J. Autism Dev. Disord.* **1981**, *54*, 469–481. [CrossRef] [PubMed]
14. American Psychiatric Association (APA). *Diagnostic and Statistical Manual of Mental Disorders*, 5th ed.; American Psychiatry Association: Washington, DC, USA, 2013.
15. Williams, D.; Botting, N.; Boucher, J. Language in autism and specific language impairment: Where are the links? *Psychol. Bull.* **2008**, *134*, 944–963. [CrossRef] [PubMed]
16. Davidson, M.M.; Ellis Weismer, S. A discrepancy in comprehension and production in early language development in ASD: Is it clinically relevant? *J. Autism Dev. Disord.* **2017**, *47*, 2163–2175. [CrossRef] [PubMed]

17. Hudry, K.; Leadbitter, K.; Temple, K.; Slonims, V.; McConachie, H.; Aldre, C.; Howlin, P.; Charman, T. Preschoolers with autism show greater impairment in receptive compared with expressive language abilities. *Int. J. Lang. Commun. Disord.* **2010**, *45*, 681–690. [CrossRef]
18. Seol, K.I.; Song, S.H.; Kim, K.L.; Oh, S.T.; Kim, Y.T.; Im, W.Y.; Song, D.H.; Cheon, K.A. A comparison of receptive-expressive language profiles between toddlers with autism spectrum disorder and developmental language delay. *Yonsei Med. J.* **2014**, *55*, 1721–1728. [CrossRef]
19. Woynarosky, T.; Yoder, P.; Watson, L.R. Atypical cross-modal profiles and longitudinal associations between vocabulary scores in initially minimally verbal children with ASD. *Autism Res.* **2016**, *9*, 301–310. [CrossRef]
20. Charman, T.; Drew, A.; Baird, C.; Baird, G. Measuring early language development in preschool children with autism spectrum disorder using the MacArthur Communicative Development Inventory (Infant Form). *J. Child Lang.* **2003**, *30*, 213–236. [CrossRef]
21. Ellis Weismer, S.; Lord, C.; Esler, A. Early language patterns of toddlers on the autism spectrum compared to toddlers with developmental delay. *J. Autism Dev. Disord.* **2010**, *40*, 1259–1273. [CrossRef]
22. Kwok, E.Y.L.; Brown, H.M.; Smyth, R.E.; Cardy, J.O. Meta-analysis of receptive and expressive language skills in autism spectrum disorder. *Res. Autism Spectr. Disord.* **2015**, *9*, 202–222. [CrossRef]
23. Reinhartsen, D.B.; Tapia, A.L.; Watson, L.; Crais, E.; Bradley, C.; Fairchild, J.; Herring, A.H.; Daniels, J. Expressive Dominant Versus Receptive Dominant Language Patterns in Young Children: Findings from the Study to Explore Early Development. *J. Autism Dev. Disord.* **2019**, *49*, 2447–2460. [CrossRef]
24. Tager-Flusberg, H.; Paul, R.; Lord, C. Language and Communication in Autism. In *Handbook of Autism and Pervasive Developmental Disorders: Diagnosis, Development, Neurobiology, and Behavior*; Volkmar, F.R., Paul, R., Klin, A., Cohen, D., Eds.; John Wiley & Sons Inc.: Hoboken, NJ, USA, 2005; pp. 335–364.
25. Young, N.; Hudry, K.; Trembath, D.; Vivanti, G. Children With Autism Show Reduced Information Seeking When Learning New Tasks. *Am. J. Intellect. Dev. Disabil.* **2016**, *121*, 65–73. [CrossRef] [PubMed]
26. Cornew, L.; Dobkins, K.R.; Akshoomoff, N.; McCleery, J.P.; Carver, I.J. Atypical social referencing in infant siblings of children with Autism Spectrum Disorders. *J. Autism Dev. Disord.* **2012**, *42*, 2611–2621. [CrossRef] [PubMed]
27. Scambler, D.; Hepburn, S.; Rutherford, M.; Wehner, E.; Rogers, S. Emotional responsivity in children with autism, children with other developmental disabilities, and children with typical development. *J. Autism Dev. Disord.* **2007**, *37*, 553–563. [CrossRef] [PubMed]
28. Volkmar, F.R. Understanding the social brain in autism. *Dev. Psychobiol.* **2011**, *53*, 428–434. [CrossRef]
29. Menyuk, P. *Language Development: Knowledge and Use*; Addison-Wesley Longman: Chicago, IL, USA, 1988.
30. Menyuk, P.; Liebergott, J.W.; Schultz, M.C. *Early Language Development in Full-Term and Premature Infants*; Psychology Press: New York, NY, USA, 2014.
31. Tager-Flusberg, H.; Kasari, C. Minimally verbal school-aged children with autism spectrum disorder: The Neglected End of the Spectrum. *Autism Res.* **2013**, *6*, 468–478. [CrossRef]
32. Fein, D.; Barton, M.; Eigsti, I.M.; Kelley, E.; Naigles, L.; Schultz, R.T. Optimal outcome in individuals with a history of autism. *J. Child Psychol. Psychiatry* **2013**, *54*, 195–205. [CrossRef]
33. Chilosi, A.M.; Cipriani, P. *TCGB Test di Comprensione Grammaticale Per Bambini*; Edizioni Del Cerro: Tirrenia, Pisa, Italy, 2006.
34. Dunn, L.M.; Dunn, L.M. *Peabody Picture Vocabulary Test*; Guidance Associates: Wilmingston, DE, USA, 1981.
35. Brizzolara, D. *Test di Vocabolario Figurato*; Technical Report of the Research Project 500.4/62.1/1134; Italian Department of Health to IRCCS Stella Maris: Calambrone, Pisa, Italy, 1989.
36. Cipriani, P.; Chilosi, A.M.; Bottari, P.; Pfanner, L. *L'acquisizione Della Morfosintassi Dell'italiano: Fasi e Processi*; Uipress: Padova, Italy, 1993.
37. Cipriani, P.; Chilosi, A.M.; Pfanner, L.; Villani, S.; Bottari, P. Il ritardo di linguaggio in età precoce: Profili evolutivi e indici di rischio. In *Indici di Rischio Nel Primo Sviluppo Del Linguaggio*; Caselli, C., Capirci, O., Eds.; Franco Angeli: Milano, Italy, 2002; pp. 95–108.
38. Wechsler, D. *Wechsler Preschool and Primary Scale of Intelligence*, 3rd ed.; Harcourt Assessment: San Antonio, TX, USA, 2002.
39. Wechsler, D. *Wechsler Intelligence Scale for Children*, 4th ed.; Psychological Corporation: San Antonio, TX, USA, 2003.
40. Griffiths, R. *The Abilities of Young Children: A Comprehensive System of Mental Measurement for the First Eight Years of Life (Revised Edition)*; Bucks: A.R.I.C.D. Test Agency Limited: London, UK, 1984.

41. Lord, C.; Risi, S.; Lambrecht, L.; Cook, E.H.; Leventhal, B.L.; DiLavore, P.C.; Pickles, A.; Rutter, M. The Autism Diagnostic Observation Schedule-Generic: A Standard Measure of Social and Communication Deficits Associated with the Spectrum of Autism. *J. Autism Dev. Disord.* **2000**, *30*, 205–223. [CrossRef]
42. Lord, C.; Rutter, M.; DiLavore, P.C.; Risi, S.; Luyster, R.J.; Gotham, K.; Bishop, S.L.; Guthrie, W. *ADOS-2—Autism Diagnostic Observation Schedule-Second Edition*; Colombi, C., Tancredi, R., Persico, A., Faggioli, R., Eds.; Hogrefe: Göttingen, Germany, 2013.
43. Kjellmer, L.; Fernell, E.; Gillberg, C.; Norrelgen, F. Speech and language profiles in 4- to 6-year-old children with early diagnosis of autism spectrum disorder without intellectual disability. *Neuropsychiatr. Dis. Treat.* **2018**, *14*, 2415–2427. [CrossRef]
44. Rapin, I. Language and its development in the autism spectrum disorders. In *Language: Normal and Pathological Development*; Riva, D., Rapin, I., Zardini, G., Eds.; John Libbey Eurotext: Montrange, France, 2006; pp. 121–137.
45. Rapin, I.; Allen, D.A.; Aram, D.M.; Dunn, M.A.; Fein, D.; Morris, R.; Waterhouse, L. Classification issues, in Rapin, I. In *Preschool Children with Inadequate Communication*; MacKeith: London, UK, 1996; pp. 190–201.
46. Chilosi, A.M.; Pfanner, L.; Pecini, C.; Salvadorini, R.; Casalini, C.; Brizzolara, D.; Cipriani, P. Which linguistic measures distinguish transient from persistent language problems in Late Talkers from 2 to 4 years? A study on Italian speaking children. *Res. Dev. Disabil.* **2019**, *89*, 59–68. [CrossRef]
47. Paul, R.; Fischer, M.L.; Cohen, D.J. Brief Report: Sentence comprehension strategies in children with autism and specific language disorders. *J. Autism Dev. Disord.* **1988**, *18*, 669–679. [CrossRef]
48. Prior, M.R.; Hall, L.C. Comprehension of transitive and intransitive phrases by autistic, retarded, and normal children. *J. Commun. Disord.* **1979**, *12*, 103–111. [CrossRef]
49. Tager-Flusberg, H. Sentence comprehension in autistic children. *Appl. Psycholinguist.* **1981**, *2*, 5–24. [CrossRef]
50. Kover, S.T.; Haebig, E.; Oakes, A.; McDuffie, A.; Hagerman, R.J.; Abbeduto, L. Sentence comprehension in boys with autism spectrum disorder. *Am. J. Speech Lang. Pathol.* **2014**, *23*, 385–394. [CrossRef] [PubMed]
51. Catts, H.W.; Fey, M.E.; Tomblin, J.B.; Zhang, X. A longitudinal investigation of reading outcomes in children with language impairments. *J. Speech Lang. Hear. Res.* **2002**, *45*, 1142–1157. [CrossRef]
52. Stothard, S.E.; Snowling, M.J.; Bishop, D.V.; Chipchase, B.B.; Kaplan, C.A. Language-impaired preschoolers: A follow-up into adolescence. *J. Speech Lang. Hear. Res.* **1998**, *41*, 407–418. [CrossRef]

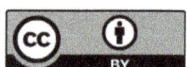

© 2020 by the authors. Licensee MDPI, Basel, Switzerland. This article is an open access article distributed under the terms and conditions of the Creative Commons Attribution (CC BY) license (http://creativecommons.org/licenses/by/4.0/).

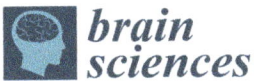 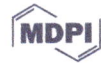

Article

Alexithymia Profile in Relation to Negative Affect in Parents of Autistic and Typically Developing Young Children

Elisa Leonardi [1], Antonio Cerasa [1,2], Francesca Isabella Famà [1], Cristina Carrozza [1], Letteria Spadaro [1], Renato Scifo [3], Sabrina Baieli [3], Flavia Marino [1], Gennaro Tartarisco [1], David Vagni [1], Giovanni Pioggia [1,†] and Liliana Ruta [1,*,†]

1. Institute for Biomedical Research and Innovation (IRIB), National Research Council of Italy, 98164 Messina, Italy; elisa.leonardi@istitutomarino.it (E.L.); antonio.cerasa@irib.cnr.it (A.C.); francescaisabella.fama@istitutomarino.it (F.I.F.); cristina.carrozza@istitutomarino.it (C.C.); spadarolia@gmail.com (L.S.); flavia.marino@irib.cnr.it (F.M.); gennaro.tartarisco@irib.cnr.it (G.T.); david.vagni@irib.cnr.it (D.V.); giovanni.pioggia@irib.cnr.it (G.P.)
2. S. Anna Institute and Research in Advanced Neurorehabilitation (RAN), 88900 Crotone, Italy
3. Centre for Autism Spectrum Disorders, Child Psychiatry Unit, Provincial Health Service of Catania (ASP CT), 95100 Catania, Italy; renato.scifo@aspct.it (R.S.); sabrina.baieli@aspct.it (S.B.)
* Correspondence: liliana.ruta@irib.cnr.it
† These Authors contributed equally to the study.

Received: 25 May 2020; Accepted: 27 July 2020; Published: 29 July 2020

Abstract: In our study, we explored the construct of alexithymia in parents of children with and without ASD using a multi-method approach based on self-rated and external rater assessment. We also assessed the level of self-report measures of negative affect states such as trait anxiety and depression, and investigated the correlation between the alexithymia construct, trait anxiety, and depression within the broader autism phenotype (BAP). A total sample of 100 parents (25 mothers and 25 fathers in each group) were administered the TAS-20 and the TSIA to measure self-reported and observer-rated alexithymia traits, as well as self-report measures of anxiety and depression. Study results showed that the TSIA but not the TAS-20 was able to detect significant group differences in alexithymia traits among parents of children with and without ASD, with parents of ASD children displaying significantly higher levels of alexithymia. Furthermore, differently from the TAS-20, no significant correlations between the TSIA and measures of anxiety and depression were detected. Taken together, our results suggest the importance of using multi-method approaches to control for potential measurement bias and to detect psychological constructs such as alexithymia in subclinical samples such as parents of children with ASD.

Keywords: autism; alexithymia; anxiety; depression; TAS-20; TSIA; parents; broader autism phenotype

1. Introduction

Alexithymia literally means "absence of words for emotions". It is a personality construct, normally distributed in the general population [1,2], characterized by deficits identifying and describing one's own emotions and feelings, problems distinguishing between feelings and bodily sensations of emotional arousal, lack of fantasy, externally oriented cognitive style, and impairment in cognitively mapping their feeling states onto internal bodily responses [3–6]. Difficulties in emotional awareness may have a negative impact on subjective emotion regulation [7] and, in turn, may compromise the understanding of others' emotions, giving rise to problems in social interaction. It has been reported, indeed, that individuals with alexithymia show difficulties distinguishing and appreciating emotions expressed by others, and consequently, they are likely to show nonempathic and idiosyncratic socio-emotional responses [8]. Deficits in empathy, specifically in the cognitive component of recognizing and understanding others emotions, have also been reported as one of the distinctive features of autism spectrum disorders (ASD) [9–13], a neurodevelopmental condition characterized by socio-communicative impairments and restricted and repetitive patterns of behaviors and interests [14]. A significant association between ASD and alexithymia has been reported, with at least half of individuals with ASD experiencing co-occurring alexithymia [15–19]. The interrelationship between the two conditions is complex, and it is still debated whether alexithymia and ASD share common etiological roots or if, instead, alexithymia is a symptomatological manifestation within the ASD neuropsychological functioning [20]. Some broad genetic and neurobiological overlapping between the two conditions have been reported, including the involvement of the serotonin and oxytocin systems, and brain areas related to emotion processing, specifically the amygdala, cingulate, and prefrontal cortex [21]. It has been suggested that a common genetic vulnerability between autism and alexithymia could lead to atypical brain networks, associated in turn with different behavioral patterns that manifest themselves mainly with symptoms of alexithymia, autism, or both [22,23]. At the behavioral level, the intersection between alexithymia and ASD is equally controversial and questions the role of alexithymia in relation to emotion recognition and interoception (the ability to interpret the internal state of the body). Indeed, the abilities to perceive one's own emotions and bodily signals are closely interrelated in social-emotional development [24]. Some studies, comparing individuals with and without ASD on alexithymia, have found that alexithymia, rather than autism per se, predicts difficulties in facial emotion recognition [17], while other evidence in nonclinical samples reported that autism traits more than alexithymia were a stronger predictor of atypical empathy [25]. In relation to interoception, across clinical and nonclinical samples, alexithymia, but not autism, has been associated with impaired interoception [23,24]. Furthermore, alexithymia associated traits have also been reported in relatives of individuals with ASD [26] who show subclinical autism traits, reported as the broader autism phenotype (BAP) [27–31]. The BAP is characterized by below the diagnostic threshold social and cognitive deficits, restricted behavior patterns, ASD-like personality characteristics, and psychiatric difficulties in relatives of autistic individuals [28–37]. Furthermore, higher levels of alexithymia in fathers of children with ASD were related to higher severity on the repetitive behavior domain in their children [38]. The most widely used questionnaire to evaluate alexithymia is the Toronto Alexithymia Scale (TAS-20) [39]. The TAS-20 is a self-report measure consisting of 20 items rated on a five-point Likert scale. The higher the score on the TAS-20, the greater the alexithymia traits. Although consistent empirical evidence over the past 25 year period has confirmed the reliability and validity of the TAS-20 to tap into the alexithymia construct [40], some concerns about applying a self-report measure to individuals who have difficulties identifying their own emotional states and lack the appropriate insight on this impairment, have been raised. Self-assessment of the interoceptive deficit in alexithymia would, in fact, imply a self-reliance bias being that the main characteristic of alexithymia is exactly the absence of recognition of one's feelings and bodily sensations [19,41–43]. Another shortcoming of the TAS-20 is that the measure does not include the dimension of the imaginative processes, which represents one of the facets of the complex alexithymia construct. Furthermore, scores at the TAS-20 have been correlated with negative affect states, particularly depression and anxiety. This association may be partially explained by a neuropsychological overlap between these dimensions, being that impairment in interoception is frequently associated with negative affect [44], but might also be related to a negativity response bias due to the self- report nature of the TAS-20 [45–47]. To overcome this limitation, in 2006, Bagby, Taylor, and Parker developed the Toronto structured interview for Alexithymia (TSIA) [48], a structured interview consisting of 24 questions and carried out by an external examiner who scores the items based on the individual responses across four core domains such as difficulty identifying feelings (DIF), difficulty describing feelings (DDF), externally oriented thinking (EOT), and imaginal processes (IMP). Several studies have confirmed the internal and convergent validity as well as cultural stability of the TAS-20 and the TSIA in nonclinical populations, as well as clinical patients, and have suggested that the TSIA is able to more reliably assess the "fantasy" facet of the alexithymia construct and to better disentangle negative affect states such as depression and anxiety that may partially overlap with the alexithymia construct [48–53].

To the best of our knowledge, the only study assessing alexithymia in family members using the TSIA was conducted in parents of anorexic daughters [54], reported significantly higher levels of alexithymia using the observer-rated measure as compared to the self-report measure in parents of the clinical group. Also, as far as we are aware, no studies assessing the alexithymia profile through both self-report and interviewer-administered measures in relatives of ASD individuals have been conducted. Hence, in our study, we used both the TAS-20 and the TSIA to investigate alexithymia in parents of children with and without ASD. Furthermore, since it has been demonstrated an association between alexithymia as measured by the TAS-20 and negative affect states, a secondary goal of the study is to explore the association between both self-report and rater-assessed alexithymia scores and measures of depression and trait anxiety. Previous findings have reported, in fact, significantly higher self-reported levels of trait anxiety and depression symptoms in parents of children with ASD [55–60] and it may be relevant to investigate the overlapping alexithymia construct in relation to these dimensions within the BAP trying to disentangle potential biases related to the administration method.

We expect that parents of ASD children, compared to parents of typically developing children, present higher levels of alexithymia at both the TAS-20 and the TSIA, and that the TSIA, in particular, will be able to keep aside co-occurrent traits of depression and anxiety.

2. Methods

2.1. Participants

Parents were enrolled and tested in the context of an ongoing study on young children with and without ASD, aged between 3 and 6 years of age, both males and females (30% females in the ASD group and 48% females in the TD group). Parents of children with ASD were recruited and tested at the clinical facilities of the Institute for Research and Innovation in Biomedicine of the National Research Council of Italy (IRIB-CNR) in Messina and at the Centre for Autism Spectrum Disorders, Child Psychiatry Unit, Provincial Health Service (ASP-CT) in Catania, Italy. Parents of typically developing children (TD) were recruited and tested in three different mainstream nursery schools and primary schools in Messina. Inclusion criteria in both the ASD and TD parent groups were: (1) biological parents; (2) native Italian speakers; (3) between the age of 25 and 55 years. Specific inclusion criterion in the ASD parent group was having a child with a confirmed clinical diagnosis of ASD according to the Diagnostic and Statistical Manual of Mental Disorders, Fifth Edition [14], while exclusion criteria in the TD parents group were having a child with a clinical diagnosis of neurodevelopmental conditions (such as language and/or motor delay, ADHD, etc.) and a family history of intellectual disabilities, language delay and ASD. A total sample of 112 parents were recruited. According to the inclusion and exclusion criteria, 12 parents (8 parents in the TD group and 5 parents in the ASD group) were excluded for the following reasons: four couples of parents (2 couples in each group) were adoptive parents; two couples of parents of TD children had a first degree relative with ASD; one parent (mother) in the TD group presented a mild intellectual disability; one parent (mother) in the ASD group was a foreigner and had significant difficulties with understanding written and spoken Italian language and finally 4 couples of parents (3 couples in the TD group and 1 couple in the ASD group) who initially agreed to participate, subsequently refused to contribute to the study. A final sample of 50 parents (25 mothers and 25 fathers) of ASD children and 50 parents of TD children (25 mothers and 25 fathers) were fully tested and analyzed in the study.

The study received ethical clearance by the Ethics Committees of CNR (ethical clearance, 01.08.2018) and ASP-CT (Prot. N. 498), respectively, and all the caregivers signed an informed consent to participate in the study.

2.2. Measures and Procedures

All enrolled subjects completed the following neuropsychological assessment battery: (1) the State Trait Anxiety Inventory-Form Y (STAI-Y), a self-report questionnaire which consists of 20 questions scored on a 4-point Likert-type scale, ranging from 1 to 4 (from "almost never" to "almost always"). The total score at the STAI-Y ranges from 20 to 80, with scores >40 indicating above-average levels of anxiety. (2) The Beck Depression Inventory (BDI-II) is a self-report questionnaire with 21 items, rated on a 4-point scale from 0 to 3, based on the diagnostic criteria for depressive disorders. Inventory cutoffs are: 0–13: minimal depression, 14–19: mild depression, 20–28: moderate depression, and 29–63: severe depression [61,62]; (3) The Toronto Alexithymia Scale (TAS-20) [39] is a self-report scale comprised of 20 items. Each item is rated on a five-point Likert scale ranging from 1 ("strongly disagree") to 5 ("strongly agree"). The TAS-20 is a reliable and valid measure of emotion processing in adults and includes a total score and three subscales: Difficulty Identifying Feelings (DIF), Difficulty Describing Feelings (DDF), and Externally-Oriented Thinking (EOT). The empirically derived cutoff score of 61 is used for identifying individuals with "high" versus "low" alexithymia. (4) The Toronto Structured Interview for Alexithymia (TSIA) is a structured interview with prompts and probes which incorporates the same three subscales included in the TAS-20 (DIF, DDF, and EOT, respectively), and an extra subscale investigating Imaginal Processes (IMP). The TSIA consists of 24 items, six items for each of the four salient facets of the alexithymia construct; (5) the "Reading the Mind in the Eyes" Test Revised (Eyes Test) [63]. In the Eyes Test, the participant is presented with a series of 36 black and white photographs of the eye-region of different actors and actresses and is asked to choose which of four words best describes what the person in the photograph is thinking or feeling. We implemented the test on an iPad tablet 9.7 in and collected both accuracy (number of correct answers) and reaction time (RT = length of time taken to answer in seconds); (6) the Wechsler Abbreviated Scale of Intelligence Second Edition (WASI-II) [64] to assess the intelligent quotient (IQ) in all the participants. All questionnaires were administered in a standardized way and in the same sequence to all participants. Assessment administration took about 2 h and was split into two sessions over two consecutive days. In the first session, participants filled in the TAS-20, the STAI-Y and the BDI-II, while during the second visit, the TSIA and the WASI-II were administered by an experienced clinical neuropsychologist (E.L.), specially trained on the administration procedures and scoring of the measures.

2.3. Statistical Analysis

Statistical analyses were performed using SPSS Version 23.0. Kolmogorov–Smirnov test was carried out and confirmed the assumptions of normality for all variables. A chi-square test was used for categorical variables, while the Mann–Whitney U-test was run for ordinal variables. An independent two-sample t-test was used to analyze between-group differences for continuous, normally distributed variables. The t-test's effect size was calculated using Cohen d, where an effect size value of 0.2 is considered a small effect, of 0.5 is considered a medium effect, and values of 0.8 and above are considered large effects. Pearson's correlations between TAS-20 and TSIA total scores and their dimensions, correlations between TAS-20 and TSIA and correlations of TSIA and TAS-20 with BDI-II and STAI-Y2 respectively, were performed.

All statistical analyses were 2-tailed; α levels were corrected for multiple comparisons using hierarchical Sidak correction. We used two primary measures (TAS-20 and TSIA) for fathers' and mothers' questionnaires respectively, therefore, we had 4 primary variables, and we set $\alpha_c < 0.013$. Only if the total score is significant, we analyzed the sub-scales for each measure. TAS-20 has 3 sub-scales and TSIA has 6 sub-scales, therefore $\alpha_c < 0.017$ for the first sub-scales analysis and $\alpha_c < 0.009$ for the second one. The Eyes Test accuracy and reaction Time were added as secondary measures of the BAP and $\alpha_c < 0.01$ was set. In the ancillary correlation analyses, we used a similar procedure setting $\alpha_c < 0.003$ for the correlation among Eyes Test, STAI-Y and BDI-II with TAS-20 and TSIA total scores, $\alpha_c < 0.009$ and $\alpha_c < 0.004$ for the correlation among Eyes Test, STAI-Y and BDI-II with TAS-20 and TSIA sub-scales.

3. Results

Table 1 shows the demographic and clinical characteristics of the sample. Parents of children with and without ASD did not differ as regards to descriptive variables and IQ. Parents on the ASD group were characterized by significantly higher levels of trait anxiety (both for mothers and fathers) and depression (more evident in the mothers) with respect to TD parents. Furthermore, mothers of ASD children were significantly slower than mothers of TD children in recognizing emotions from the eyes. Inter-correlations among TAS-20 and TSIA with their respective subscales were all statistically significant (all p-values < 0.001) and correlations ranged from moderate to high (from $r = 0.59$ to $r = 0.80$ for the TAS-20 and from $r = 0.65$ to $r = 0.82$ for the TSIA in the ASD parent group and from $r = 0.66$ to $r = 0.77$ for the TAS-20 and from $r = 0.61$ to $r = 0.73$ for the TSIA in the TD parent group). The TAS-20 demonstrated also a modest association with the TSIA ($r = 0.40$; $p = 0.001$ and $r = 0.44$; $p = 0.001$ in the ASD and TD parent group respectively), confirming convergent validity of the two measures. On the TAS-20 total score and subscales, no significant between-group difference has been detected, neither in the mothers nor in the fathers (Table 2). Conversely, using the TSIA, we found a significant group difference on the total score, with parents in the ASD group scoring significantly higher (i.e., demonstrating more alexithymia traits) than parents in the TD group ($p = 0.003$ and $p = 0.0001$ for mothers and fathers respectively). Furthermore, investigating the TSIA subdomains, mothers on the ASD group scored significantly higher in the "operative thinking (OT)" subscale ($p = 0.004$), while fathers on the ASD group, showed significantly higher scores in all the subscales apart from the "difficulty identifying feelings (DIF)" subscale (all p's < 0.009). When we analyzed the correlations between the TAS-20 and the TSIA (and their subscales) with the negative effect self-report measures (STAI-Y and the BDI-II) separately in the ASD and TD parent samples, additional significant findings were detected. In the ASD parent group, measures of anxiety and depression were significantly associated to the TAS-20 total scores in both mothers ($r = 0.58$, $p < 0.0001$ and $r = 0.61$, $p < 0.0001$ respectively) and fathers ($r = 0.37$, $p = 0.02$ and $r = 0.36$, $p = 0.03$ respectively). However, in the ASD father group, statistical significance did not survive correction for multiple comparisons. Comparable results were obtained in the TD parent group, with a significant positive association between the TAS-20 total scores and the STAI-Y and BDI-II scores in both mothers ($r = 0.45$, $p = 0.002$ and $r = 0.36$, $p = 0.01$ respectively) and fathers ($r = 0.51$, $p < 0.0001$ and $r = 0.31$, $p = 0.03$ respectively). However, in both mothers and fathers, correlations between the TAS-20 and the BDI-II did not survive the threshold for multiple comparisons. Conversely, we did not observe any significant relationship between the TSIA total scores and measures of anxiety and depression in neither group. Correlations between the alexithymia scales (and subscales) and the anxiety and depression measures, corrected for multiple comparisons, are reported in Tables 3 and 4. As an ancillary analysis, to explore if the group difference on the Eyes Test RT in mothers was driving the group differences found on alexithymia, anxiety, and depression, we analyzed the relationship between these measures in the ASD group. We found no significant correlations between the Eyes Test RT and the other measures (Eyes Test RT vs. TAS-20 total score: $r = -0.13$, $p = 0.3$; vs. TSIA total score: $r = -0.12$, $p = 0.4$; vs. STAI-Y: $r = -0.06$, $p = 0.6$; vs. BDI-II: $r = -0.16$, $p = 0.2$).

Table 1. Descriptive and neuropsychological characteristics in parents of ASD and TD children.

	ASD (n = 50)	TD (n = 50)	p-Level	d's Cohen
Age Mother	38.3 ± 4.8	39.9 ± 5.3	0.31 *	-
Age Father	41.7 ± 8.4	43.2 ± 5.2	0.95 *	-
Education Mother	3 [2–5]	5 [2–6]	0.05 °	-
Education Father	3 [2–6]	3 [2–6]	0.66 °	-
Verbal IQ Mother	97.8 ± 8.9	98.8 ± 9.9	0.67 *	0.11
Performance IQ Mother	102.1 ± 12.5	101.7 ± 13.9	0.91 *	0.02
Total IQ Mother	100.1 ± 10.3	104.7 ± 22.7	0.3 *	0.26
Verbal IQ Father	97.9 ± 8.1	95.6 ± 8.3	0.31 *	0.28
Performance IQ Father	101.7 ± 12.2	105.7 ± 12.2	0.23 *	0.32
Total IQ Father	103.5 ± 23.8	104.4 ± 8.4	0.53 *	0.05
STAI-Y Mother	50.3 ± 10.9	43.9 ± 7.8	0.002 *	0.68
STAI-Y Father	49.5 ± 9.6	44.8 ± 7.9	0.01 *	0.54
BDI-II Mother	11.4 ± 8.8	7.2 ± 5.9	0.01 *	0.56
BDI-II Father	7.6 ± 6.3	4.8 ± 4.6	0.03	0.51
Eyes Test Accuracy Mother	22.6 ± 4.2	22.4 ± 4.4	0.93	0.02
Eyes Test RT Mother	328.3 ± 185.2	230.2 ± 82.7	0.005	0.68
Eyes Test Accuracy Father	20.8 ± 4.1	22.1 ± 3.5	0.23	0.31
Eyes Test RT Father	257.8 ± 88.6	247.3 ± 49.9	0.59	0.14

Data are given as mean values (SD), percentage or median [range] as appropriate. § chi-square test; ° = Mann–Whitney U-test; * = Two sample t-test. ASD, autism spectrum disorders; TD, typical development; education labels, 1 = primary school; 2 = secondary school; 3 = high school; 4 = bachelor degree; 5 = master degree; IQ, intelligent quotient; STAI-Y, State Trait Anxiety Inventory-Form Y; BDI-II, Beck depression inventory; eyes test accuracy, number of correct answers; eyes test RT, length of time taken to answer in seconds.

Table 2. Alexithymia profile in parents of ASD and TD children.

	ASD (Mean ± SD)	TD (Mean ± SD)	p-Level *	d's Cohen
Toronto Alexithymia Scale (TAS-20)				
Total score Mother	39.6 ± 12.3	39.1 ± 9.5	0.79	0.05
DIF Mother	12.1 ± 5.5	11.4 ± 4.8	0.53	0.13
DDF Mother	10.3 ± 4.6	10.3 ± 4.5	0.97	0.01
EOT Mother	17.5 ± 4.2	17.1 ± 4.3	0.65	0.09
Total score Father	42.3 ± 10.8	40.9 ± 9.9	0.53	0.13
DIF Father	11.4 ± 5.2	11.4 ± 4.7	0.99	0.01
DDF Father	11.4 ± 4.4	10.6 ± 9.1	0.38	0.11
EOT Father	19.4 ± 4.7	19.1 ± 3.9	0.68	0.07
Toronto Structured Interview for Alexithymia (TSIA)				
DIF Mother	1.6 ± 1.5	0.9 ± 0.7	0.02	0.6
DDF Mother	2.2 ± 2.3	1.6 ± 1.9	0.22	0.29
EOT Mother	2.9 ± 1.9	2.1 ± 1.7	0.04	0.44
IMP Mother	3.8 ± 1.9	2.7 ± 2.0	0.02	0.56
AA Mother	3.8 ± 3.0	2.5 ± 2.4	0.04	0.48
OT Mother	6.7 ± 2.9	4.8 ± 2.5	**0.004**	0.71
Total score Mother	10.5 ± 4.6	7.3 ± 4.4	**0.003**	0.71
DIF Father	2.3 ± 2.6	1.0 ± 1.6	0.04	0.6
DDF Father	3.8 ± 3.3	1.3 ± 1.5	**0.001**	0.97
EOT Father	4.2 ± 2.8	2.3 ± 1.5	**0.006**	0.85
IMP Father	4.2 ± 2.3	2.1 ± 1.2	**0.001**	1.15
AA Father	5.9 ± 5.3	2.3 ± 2.4	**0.004**	0.87
OT Father	8.5 ± 4.5	4.4 ± 2.1	**0.0001**	1.16
Total score Father	14.9 ± 9.1	6.7 ± 3.7	**0.0001**	1.19

DIF, difficulty identifying feelings; DDF, difficulty describing feelings (DDF); OT, externally-oriented thinking; IMP, imaginal processing; AA, affect awareness; OT, operative thinking. * α levels are corrected for multiple comparisons using hierarchical Sidak correction. An $α_c < 0.01$ was set for the TAS-20 total score and subscales and for the TSIA total score and an $α_c < 0.009$ was set for the TSIA subscales.

Table 3. Correlations between alexithymia scales, trait anxiety, and depression in parents of ASD children.

ASD Parent Group	STAI-Y Mother	STAI-Y Father	BDI-II Mother	BDI-II Father
Toronto Alexithymia Scale (TAS-20)				
Total score Mother	$r = 0.58$ $p < 0.0001$		$r = 0.61$ $p < 0.0001$	
DIF Mother	$r = 0.67$ $p < 0.0001$		$r = 0.73$ $p < 0.0001$	
DDF Mother	$r = 0.46$ $p = 0.002$		$r = 0.54$ $p < 0.0001$	
EOT Mother	$r = 0.09$ $p = 0.54$		$r = 0.21$ $p = 0.19$	
Total score Father		$r = 0.37$ $p = 0.02$		$r = 0.36$ $p = 0.03$
DIF Father		$r = 0.32$ $p = 0.04$		$r = 0.45$ $p = 0.005$
DDF Father		$r = 0.33$ $p = 0.04$		$r = 0.21$ $p = 0.21$
EOT Father		$r = 0.18$ $p = 0.27$		$r = 0.13$ $p = 0.43$
Toronto Structured Interview for Alexithymia (TSIA)				
Total score Mother	$r = 0.11$ $p = 0.51$		$r = 0.15$ $p = 0.35$	
DIF Mother	$r = 0.31$ $p = 0.07$		$r = 0.25$ $p = 0.13$	
DDF Mother	$r = 0.11$ $p = 0.52$		$r = 0.11$ $p = 0.49$	
EOT Mother	$r = 0.15$ $p = 0.39$		$r = 0.21$ $p = 0.22$	
IMP Mother	$r = 0.24$ $p = 0.15$		$r = 0.17$ $p = 0.32$	
AA Mother	$r = 0.23$ $p = 0.16$		$r = 0.22$ $p = 0.19$	
OT Mother	$r = 0.07$ $p = 0.07$		$r = 0.35$ $p = 0.04$	
Total score Father		$r = 0.13$ $p = 0.51$		$r = 0.17$ $p = 0.36$
DIF Father		$r = 0.07$ $p = 0.7$		$r = 0.25$ $p = 0.19$
DDF Father		$r = 0.38$ $p = 0.04$		$r = 0.08$ $p = 0.68$
EOT Father		$r = 0.21$ $p = 0.28$		$r = 0.03$ $p = 0.88$
IMP Father		$r = 0.05$ $p = 0.81$		$R = -0.26$ $p = 0.18$
AA Father		$r = 0.28$ $p = 0.13$		$r = 0.05$ $p = 0.81$
OT Father		$r = 0.11$ $p = 0.59$		$R = -0.17$ $p = 0.41$

DIF, difficulty identifying feelings; DDF, difficulty describing feelings (DDF); OT, externally-oriented thinking; IMP, imaginal processing; AA, affect awareness; OT: operative thinking. * α levels were corrected for multiple comparisons using hierarchical Sidak correction. We set an $\alpha_c < 0.006$ for the correlation among STAI-Y and BDI-II with TAS-20 and TSIA total scores and an $\alpha_c < 0.009$ for the correlation among STAI-Y and BDI-II with TAS-20 and TSIA subscales.

Table 4. Correlations between alexithymia scales, trait anxiety, and depression in parents of TD children.

TD Parent Group	STAI-Y Mother	STAI-Y Father	BDI-II Mother	BDI-II Father
	Toronto Alexithymia Scale (TAS-20)			
Total score Mother	**r = 0.45** **p = 0.002**		r = 0.36 p = 0.01	
DIF Mother	**r = 0.37** **p = 0.008**		r = 0.28 p = 0.06	
DDF Mother	r = 0.35 p = 0.01		r = 0.26 p = 0.07	
EOT Mother	r = 0.11 p = 0.43		r = 0.21 p = 0.15	
Total score Father		r = 0.51 p < 0.0001		r = 0.31 p = 0.03
DIF Father		r = 0.42 p = 0.003		r = 0.4 p = 0.007
DDF Father		r = 0.45 p = 0.002		r = 0.39 p = 0.007
EOT Father		r = 0.41 p = 0.004		r = 0.11 p = 0.47
	Toronto Structured Interview for Alexithymia (TSIA)			
Total score Mother	r = 0.43 p = 0.01		r = 0.45 p = 0.007	
DIF Mother	r = 0.29 p = 0.1		r = 0.43 p = 0.01	
DDF Mother	r = 0.28 p = 0.11		r = 0.39 p = 0.02	
EOT Mother	r = 0.42 p = 0.01		r = 0.41 p = 0.02	
IMP Mother	r = 0.19 p = 0.28		r = 0.005 p = 0.98	
AA Mother	r = 0.32 p = 0.06		r = 0.45 **p = 0.008**	
OT Mother	r = 0.43 p = 0.01		r = 0.35 p = 0.04	
Total score Father		r = 0.42 p = 0.04		r = 0.36 p = 0.09
DIF Father		r = 0.39 p = 0.06		r = 0.43 p = 0.04
DDF Father		r = 0.4 p = 0.05		r = 0.25 p = 0.25
EOT Father		r = 0.03 p = 0.87		r = 0.02 p = 0.92
IMP Father		r = 0.21 p = 0.34		r = 0.19 p = 0.37
AA Father		r = 0.51 p = 0.01		r = 0.44 p = 0.03
OT Father		r = 0.15 p = 0.49		r = 0.13 p = 0.54

DIF, difficulty identifying feelings; DDF, difficulty describing feelings (DDF); OT, externally-oriented thinking; IMP, imaginal processing; AA, affect awareness; OT, operative thinking. * α levels were corrected for multiple comparisons using hierarchical Sidak correction. We set an α_c <0.006 for the correlation among STAI-Y and BDI-II with TAS-20 and TSIA total scores and an α_c <0.009 for the correlation among STAI-Y and BDI-II with TAS-20 and TSIA subscales.

4. Discussion

In our study, we explored the construct of alexithymia in parents of children with and without ASD using a multi-method approach based on self-rated and external rater assessment. Both the TAS-20 and the TSIA were administered to all the participants showing that the TSIA but not the TAS-20 was able to detect significant group differences in alexithymia traits among parents of children with and without ASD, with parents of ASD children displaying significantly higher levels of alexithymia as reflected by the total score and the subscale scores, especially for fathers. This result suggests that the assessment method has an impact on the capacity to detect alexithymic traits in subclinical populations such as parents of ASD children. The TAS-20, in fact, implies that people are aware and able to identify and describe their own feelings and strongly relies on the self-perception of the subject. Individuals with higher alexithymia traits may lack awareness of their own difficulties because of their meta-emotional impairment [65], and a structured interview such as the TSIA may possibly avoid this bias, as the examiner can use probes and examples to more in-depth assess the presence and degree of alexithymia. This result is in line with previous evidence, in a different clinical sample, reporting that parents of anorexic daughters display significantly higher alexithymia traits at the TSIA as compared to the TAS-20 [54]. Furthermore, we explored the dimensions of negative affect and trait anxiety in our sample of parents, and in agreement with previous studies, we found significantly higher levels of self-reported trait anxiety and depression in parents of children with ASD (both in mothers and fathers), compared with parents of TD children. Last but not least, we analyzed the correlation between measures of alexithymia and self-report measures of depression and trait anxiety to investigate if negative affect may influence rater's answers to the TAS-20. We found that the TAS-20 total score and the subscales "difficulty identifying feelings (DIF)" and "difficulty describing feelings (DDF)", but not the TSIA total and subscale scores, were strongly associated with measures of both anxiety and depression in mothers of ASD children. Similar results were observed in the TD parent group, with the TAS-20 being strongly associated with anxiety traits and depression, especially in fathers, and the TSIA showing no significant correlations (apart from the subscale "affect awareness" which was associated with depression in mothers). These findings may suggest that symptoms related to negative emotional states such as reduced cognitive flexibility, emotional awareness, and affective range may influence self-rated responses on the TAS-20. Co-occurring anxiety and depression, in fact, may affect the way one's emotions are self-judged and instead, having a structured interview such as the TSIA, may ensure a more objective and reliable assessment of the facets related to alexithymia reducing the potential misinterpretation of one's emotional state due to self-judgment in relation to negative affect. In line with our results, previous evidence reported that negative affectivity influences the rater's self-report on the TAS-20 items, especially on the DIF and DDF factor subscales, while no association between the TSIA scores and scores at the STAI-Y and the DBI-II was found [46,49,53].

Finally, to explore if aspects of the broader autism phenotype (BAP) in the ASD parent group would account for the results obtained on the alexithymia and negative affect dimensions, we used the Eyes Test to measure emotion recognition and Theory of Mind (ToM) abilities in both groups. Previous evidence, reported impairment in emotion recognition at the Eyes Test in parents of ASD children [66]. We found that mothers of ASD children were significantly slower than mothers of TD children in detecting emotional, mental states from eyes, but no relationship between this measure and measures of alexithymia, anxiety, and depression was found, suggesting that in our ASD parent sample, atypical empathy is not associated to alexithymia traits nor to negative affectivity. Our results, in the light of the mixed findings reported in the literature about the influence of alexithymia on atypical empathy [17,25,67], clearly indicate that measuring these two constructs in relation to autism traits is not simple and generalization from clinical samples to sub-clinical samples such as parents of ASD children to the general population poses complex conceptual and methodological issues that should be taken into account.

Some limitations should be considered with regard to the study and the use of the TSIA. Firstly, the study sample size was relatively small, although rigorously selected according to precise inclusion and exclusion criteria to avoid sampling bias; furthermore, there was no opportunity to conduct a specific psychometric and clinical evaluation on the TD children, to exclude not diagnosed neuropsychiatric conditions, which may have influenced the responses in the TD parent group. Finally, in relation to the use of the TSIA, it should be considered that the time needed to complete the interview, as well as the need for appropriate training in administration procedures and scoring, make the use of the TSIA still limited and more difficult in clinical practice. Further studies are warranted to replicate these results and to generalize these findings from clinical samples to the general population.

5. Conclusions

Our study explored the construct of alexithymia in parents of children with and without ASD using a multi-method approach, and also investigated the correlation between the alexithymia construct, trait anxiety, and depression within the broader autism phenotype (BAP). Based on our findings, in subclinical populations such as parents of children with ASD, the use of an external-rater assessment should be considered to allow a more accurate detection of the presence and degree of alexithymia and to disentangle potential influences of negative affect states and trait anxiety on the alexithymia dimension.

Author Contributions: E.L. participated in the study design, enrolled and tested the participants and contributed to the manuscript draft. L.R. designed and supervised the study and drafted the manuscript. A.C. conducted the statistical analysis and participated in the manuscript draft. F.M., F.I.F., C.C., L.S., S.B., and R.S. helped with participants' enrollment and contributed with data interpretation. D.V. and G.T. contributed with statistical analysis and statistical data interpretations. G.P. contributed in the coordination of the study. All authors read and approved the final manuscript.

Funding: This research was partially supported by the grant from the Sicilian Region of Italy (Assessorato Regionale dell'Istruzione e della Formazione Professionale, Avviso 11/2017 Rafforzare l'occupabilità nel sistema R&S e la nascita di spin off di ricerca in Sicilia—P.O. FSE 2014/2020, project no. 2014.IT.05.SFOP.014/3/10.4/9.2.10/0011—CUP G47B17000100009, entitled SANi) and partially supported by the grant from Azienda Sanitaria Provinciale di Catania (deliberations no. 2005 24/06/2016 and no. 3304 04/10/2017).

Acknowledgments: We acknowledge all the parents who volunteered to participate in the study.

Conflicts of Interest: All authors declare no potential conflicts of interest, including any financial, personal or other relationships with other people or organizations relevant to the subject of their manuscript.

References

1. Eccleston, D. *Disorders of Affect Regulation: Alexithymia in Medical and Psychiatric Illness;* Taylor, G.J., Bagby, R.M., Parker, J.D.A., Eds.; Cambridge University Press: Cambridge, UK, 1998; ISBN 0-521-45610-X.
2. Franz, M.; Popp, K.; Schaefer, R.; Sitte, W.; Schneider, C.; Hardt, J.; Decker, O.; Braehler, E. Alexithymia in the German general population. *Soc. Psychiatry Psychiatr. Epidemiol.* **2008**, *43*, 54–62. [CrossRef] [PubMed]
3. Taylor, G.J.; Michael Bagby, R.; Parker, J.D.A. The Alexithymia Construct: A Potential Paradigm for Psychosomatic Medicine. *Psychosomatics* **1991**, *32*, 153–164. [CrossRef]
4. Parker, J.D.A.; Taylor, G.J.; Bagby, R.M. The 20-Item Toronto Alexithymia Scale. *J. Psychosom. Res.* **2003**, *55*, 269–275. [CrossRef]
5. Picardi, A.; Toni, A.; Caroppo, E. Stability of Alexithymia and Its Relationships with the 'Big Five' Factors, Temperament, Character, and Attachment Style. *Psychother. Psychosom.* **2005**, *74*, 371–378. [CrossRef] [PubMed]
6. Vermeulen, N.; Luminet, O.; Corneille, O. Alexithymia and the automatic processing of affective information: Evidence from the affective priming paradigm. *Cogn. Emot.* **2006**, *20*, 64–91. [CrossRef]
7. Connelly, M.; Denney, D.R. Regulation of emotions during experimental stress in alexithymia. *J. Psychosom. Res.* **2007**, *62*, 649–656. [CrossRef] [PubMed]
8. FeldmanHall, O.; Dalgleish, T.; Mobbs, D. Alexithymia decreases altruism in real social decisions. *Cortex* **2013**, *49*, 899–904. [CrossRef] [PubMed]
9. Baron-Cohen, S.; Wheelwright, S. The Empathy Quotient: An Investigation of Adults with Asperger Syndrome or High Functioning Autism, and Normal Sex Differences. *J. Autism Dev. Disord.* **2004**, *34*, 163–175. [CrossRef]

10. Auyeung, B.; Baron-Cohen, S.; Ashwin, E.; Knickmeyer, R.; Taylor, K.; Hackett, G. Fetal testosterone and autistic traits. *Br. J. Psychol.* **2009**, *100*, 1–22. [CrossRef]
11. Lombardo, M.V.; Barnes, J.L.; Wheelwright, S.J.; Baron-Cohen, S. Self-Referential Cognition and Empathy in Autism. *PLoS ONE* **2007**, *2*, e883. [CrossRef] [PubMed]
12. Sucksmith, E.; Allison, C.; Baron-Cohen, S.; Chakrabarti, B.; Hoekstra, R.A. Empathy and emotion recognition in people with autism, first-degree relatives, and controls. *Neuropsychologia* **2013**, *51*, 98–105. [CrossRef] [PubMed]
13. Aaron, R.V.; Benson, T.L.; Park, S. Investigating the role of alexithymia on the empathic deficits found in schizotypy and autism spectrum traits. *Pers. Individ. Dif.* **2015**, *77*, 215–220. [CrossRef]
14. American Psychiatric Association. DSM-5 Diagnostic Classification. In *Diagnostic and Statistical Manual of Mental Disorders*; American Psychiatric Association: Washington, DC, USA, 2013.
15. Hill, E.; Berthoz, S.; Frith, U. Brief Report: Cognitive Processing of Own Emotions in Individuals with Autistic Spectrum Disorder and in Their Relatives. *J. Autism Dev. Disord.* **2004**, *34*, 229–235. [CrossRef] [PubMed]
16. Berthoz, S.; Hill, E.L. The validity of using self-reports to assess emotion regulation abilities in adults with autism spectrum disorder. *Eur. Psychiatry* **2005**, *20*, 291–298. [CrossRef] [PubMed]
17. Cook, R.; Brewer, R.; Shah, P.; Bird, G. Alexithymia, Not Autism, Predicts Poor Recognition of Emotional Facial Expressions. *Psychol. Sci.* **2013**, *24*, 723–732. [CrossRef]
18. Griffin, C.; Lombardo, M.V.; Auyeung, B. Alexithymia in children with and without autism spectrum disorders. *Autism Res.* **2016**, *9*, 773–780. [CrossRef]
19. Gaigg, S.B.; Cornell, A.S.F.; Bird, G. The psychophysiological mechanisms of alexithymia in autism spectrum disorder. *Autism* **2018**, *22*, 227–231. [CrossRef]
20. Kinnaird, E.; Stewart, C.; Tchanturia, K. Investigating alexithymia in autism: A systematic review and meta-analysis. *Eur. Psychiatry* **2019**, *55*, 80–89. [CrossRef]
21. Poquérusse, J.; Pastore, L.; Dellantonio, S.; Esposito, G. Alexithymia and Autism Spectrum Disorder: A Complex Relationship. *Front. Psychol.* **2018**, *9*, 1–10. [CrossRef]
22. Bird, G.; Cook, R. Mixed emotions: The contribution of alexithymia to the emotional symptoms of autism. *Transl. Psychiatry* **2013**, *3*, e285. [CrossRef]
23. Shah, P.; Hall, R.; Catmur, C.; Bird, G. Alexithymia, not autism, is associated with impaired interoception. *Cortex* **2016**, *81*, 215–220. [CrossRef] [PubMed]
24. Livingston, L.A.; Livingston, L.M. Commentary: Alexithymia, not autism, is associated with impaired interoception. *Front. Psychol.* **2016**, *7*, 7–9. [CrossRef] [PubMed]
25. Shah, P.; Livingston, L.A.; Callan, M.J.; Player, L. Trait Autism is a Better Predictor of Empathy than Alexithymia. *J. Autism Dev. Disord.* **2019**, *49*, 3956–3964. [CrossRef] [PubMed]
26. Berthoz, S.; Lalanne, C.; Crane, L.; Hill, E.L. Investigating emotional impairments in adults with autism spectrum disorders and the broader autism phenotype. *Psychiatry Res.* **2013**, *208*, 257–264. [CrossRef]
27. Bailey, A.; Le Couteur, A.; Gottesman, I.; Bolton, P.; Simonoff, E.; Yuzda, E.; Rutter, M. Autism as a strongly genetic disorder: Evidence from a British twin study. *Psychol. Med.* **1995**, *25*, 63–77. [CrossRef]
28. Bolton, P.; Macdonald, H.; Pickles, A.; Rios, P.; Goode, S.; Crowson, M.; Bailey, A.; Rutter, M. A Case-Control Family History Study of Autism. *J. Child Psychol. Psychiatry* **1994**, *35*, 877–900. [CrossRef]
29. Piven, J.; Palmer, P.; Jacobi, D.; Childress, D.; Arndt, S. Broader autism phenotype: Evidence from a family history study of multiple-incidence autism families. *Am. J. Psychiatry* **1997**, *154*, 185–190. [CrossRef] [PubMed]
30. Piven, J. The broad autism phenotype: A complementary strategy for molecular genetic studies of autism. *Am. J. Med. Genet.* **2001**, *105*, 34–35. [CrossRef]
31. Szatmari, P.; MacLean, J.E.; Jones, M.B.; Bryson, S.E.; Zwaigenbaum, L.; Bartolucci, G.; Mahoney, W.J.; Tuff, L. The Familial Aggregation of the Lesser Variant in Biological and Nonbiological Relatives of PDD Probands: A Family History Study. *J. Child Psychol. Psychiatry* **2000**, *41*, 579–586. [CrossRef]
32. Landa, R.; Piven, J.; Wzorek, M.M.; Gayle, J.O.; Chase, G.A.; Folstein, S.E. Social language use in parents of autistic individuals. *Psychol. Med.* **1992**, *22*, 245–254. [CrossRef]
33. Piven, J.; Wzorek, M.; Landa, R.; Lainhart, J.; Bolton, P.; Chase, G.A.; Folstein, S. Personality characteristics of the parents of autistic individuals. *Psychol. Med.* **1994**, *24*, 783–795. [CrossRef] [PubMed]

34. Hurley, R.S.E.; Losh, M.; Parlier, M.; Reznick, J.S.; Piven, J. The Broad Autism Phenotype Questionnaire. *J. Autism Dev. Disord.* **2007**, *37*, 1679–1690. [CrossRef] [PubMed]
35. Wolff, S.; Narayan, S.; Moyes, B. Personality Characteristics of Parents of Autistic Children: A Controlled Study. *J. Child Psychol. Psychiatry* **1988**, *29*, 143–153. [CrossRef]
36. Murphy, M.; Bolton, P.F.; Pickles, A.; Fombonne, E.; Piven, J.; Rutter, M. Personality traits of the relatives of autistic probands. *Psychol. Med.* **2000**, *30*, 1411–1424. [CrossRef]
37. Yirmiya, N.; Shaked, M. Psychiatric disorders in parents of children with autism: A meta-analysis. *J. Child Psychol. Psychiatry* **2005**, *46*, 69–83. [CrossRef]
38. Papageorgiou, V.; Georgiades, S.; Mavreas, V. Brief report: Cross-cultural evidence for the heterogeneity of the restricted, repetitive behaviours and interests domain of autism: A Greek study. *J. Autism Dev. Disord.* **2008**, *38*, 558–561. [CrossRef]
39. Bagby, R.M.; Parker, J.D.A.; Taylor, G.J. The twenty-item Toronto Alexithymia scale—I. Item selection and cross-validation of the factor structure. *J. Psychosom. Res.* **1994**, *38*, 23–32. [CrossRef]
40. Bagby, R.M.; Parker, J.D.A.; Taylor, G.J. Twenty-five years with the 20-item Toronto Alexithymia Scale. *J. Psychosom. Res.* **2020**, *131*, 109940. [CrossRef] [PubMed]
41. Lane, R.D.; Weihs, K.L.; Herring, A.; Hishaw, A.; Smith, R. Affective agnosia: Expansion of the alexithymia construct and a new opportunity to integrate and extend Freud's legacy. *Neurosci. Biobehav. Rev.* **2015**, *55*, 594–611. [CrossRef]
42. Luminet, O.; Taylor, G.; Bagby, R. Assessment of alexithymia: Self-report and observer-rated measures. In *The Handbook of Emotional Intelligence: Theory, Development, Assessment, and Application at Home, School, and in the Workplace*; Bar-On, R., Parker, J.D.A., Eds.; Jossey-Bass: San Francisco, CA, USA, 2000; pp. 301–319.
43. Meganck, R.; Vanheule, S.; Desmet, M. Factorial Validity and Measurement Invariance of the 20-Item Toronto Alexithymia Scale in Clinical and Nonclinical Samples. *Assessment* **2008**, *15*, 36–47. [CrossRef]
44. Mikhailova, E.S.; Vladimirova, T.V.; Iznak, A.F.; Tsusulkovskaya, E.J.; Sushko, N.V. Abnormal recognition of facial expression of emotions in depressed patients with major depression disorder and schizotypal personality disorder. *Biol. Psychiatry* **1996**, *40*, 697–705. [CrossRef]
45. Leising, D.; Grande, T.; Faber, R. The Toronto Alexithymia Scale (TAS-20): A measure of general psychological distress. *J. Res. Pers.* **2009**, *43*, 707–710. [CrossRef]
46. Lumley, M.A. Alexithymia and negative emotional conditions. *J. Psychosom. Res.* **2000**, *49*, 51–54. [CrossRef]
47. Marchesi, C.; Giaracuni, G.; Paraggio, C.; Ossola, P.; Tonna, M.; De Panfilis, C. Pre-morbid alexithymia in panic disorder: A cohort study. *Psychiatry Res.* **2014**, *215*, 141–145. [CrossRef] [PubMed]
48. Bagby, R.M.; Taylor, G.J.; Parker, J.D.A.; Dickens, S.E. The development of the Toronto structured interview for Alexithymia: Item selection, factor structure, reliability and concurrent validity. *Psychother. Psychosom.* **2006**. [CrossRef]
49. Caretti, V.; Porcelli, P.; Solano, L.; Schimmenti, A.; Bagby, R.M.; Taylor, G.J. Reliability and validity of the Toronto Structured Interview for Alexithymia in a mixed clinical and nonclinical sample from Italy. *Psychiatry Res.* **2011**, *187*, 432–436. [CrossRef]
50. Grabe, H.J.; Löbel, S.; Dittrich, D.; Bagby, R.M.; Taylor, G.J.; Quilty, L.C.; Spitzer, C.; Barnow, S.; Mathier, F.; Jenewein, J.; et al. The German version of the Toronto Structured Interview for Alexithymia: Factor structure, reliability, and concurrent validity in a psychiatric patient sample. *Compr. Psychiatry* **2009**, *50*, 424–430. [CrossRef] [PubMed]
51. Inslegers, R.; Meganck, R.; Ooms, E.; Vanheule, S.; Taylor, G.J.; Bagby, R.M.; De Fruyt, F.; Desmet, M. The Dutch Language Version of the Toronto Structured Interview for Alexithymia: Reliability, Factor Structure and Concurrent Validity. *Psychol. Belg.* **2013**, *53*, 93. [CrossRef]
52. Rosenberg, N.; Rufer, M.; Lichev, V.; Ihme, K.; Grabe, H.J.; Kugel, H.; Kersting, A.; Suslow, T. Observer-Rated Alexithymia and its Relationship with the Five-Factor-Model of Personality. *Psychol. Belg.* **2016**, *56*, 118–134. [CrossRef] [PubMed]
53. Montebarocci, O.; Surcinelli, P. Correlations between TSIA and TAS-20 and their relation to self-reported negative affect: A study using a multi-method approach in the assessment of alexithymia in a nonclinical sample from Italy. *Psychiatry Res.* **2018**, *270*, 187–193. [CrossRef]
54. Mannarini, S.; Nacinovich, R.; Bomba, M.; Balottin, L. Alexithymia in parents and adolescent anorexic daughters: Comparing the responses to TSIA and TAS-20 scales. *Neuropsychiatr. Dis. Treat.* **2014**, *10*, 1941–1951. [CrossRef] [PubMed]

55. Piven, J.; Chase, G.A.; Landa, R.; Wzorek, M.; Gayle, J.; Cloud, D.; Folstein, S. Psychiatric Disorders in the Parents of Autistic Individuals. *J. Am. Acad. Child Adolesc. Psychiatry* **1991**, *30*, 471–478. [CrossRef] [PubMed]
56. Bitsika, V.; Sharpley, C.F. Stress, Anxiety and Depression Among Parents of Children With Autism Spectrum Disorder. *Aust. J. Guid. Couns.* **2004**, *14*, 151–161. [CrossRef]
57. Hamlyn-Wright, S.; Draghi-Lorenz, R.; Ellis, J. Locus of control fails to mediate between stress and anxiety and depression in parents of children with a developmental disorder. *Autism* **2007**, *11*, 489–501. [CrossRef] [PubMed]
58. Kuusikko-Gauffin, S.; Pollock-Wurman, R.; Mattila, M.-L.; Jussila, K.; Ebeling, H.; Pauls, D.; Moilanen, I. Social Anxiety in Parents of High-Functioning Children with Autism and Asperger Syndrome. *J. Autism Dev. Disord.* **2013**, *43*, 521–529. [CrossRef]
59. Al-Farsi, O.; Al-Farsi, Y.; Al-Sharbati, M.; Al-Adawi, S. Stress, anxiety, and depression among parents of children with autism spectrum disorder in Oman: A case-control study. *Neuropsychiatr. Dis. Treat.* **2016**, *12*, 1943–1951. [CrossRef]
60. Schnabel, A.; Youssef, G.J.; Hallford, D.J.; Hartley, E.J.; McGillivray, J.A.; Stewart, M.; Forbes, D.; Austin, D.W. Psychopathology in parents of children with autism spectrum disorder: A systematic review and meta-analysis of prevalence. *Autism* **2020**, *24*, 26–40. [CrossRef]
61. Beck, A.T.; Steer, R.A.; Brown, G.K. *Manual for the Beck Depression Inventory-II*; Psychological Corporation: San Antonio, TX, USA, 1996; ISBN 0158018389.
62. Sica, C.; Ghisi, M. *The Italian versions of the Beck Anxiety Inventory and the Beck Depression Inventory-II: Psychometric Properties and Discriminant Power*; Lange, M.A., Ed.; Nova Science: Hauppauge, NY, USA, 2007; ISBN 1-60021-571-8 (Hardcover), 978-1-60021-571-1 (Hardcover).
63. Baron-Cohen, S.; Wheelwright, S.; Hill, J.; Raste, Y.; Plumb, I. The "Reading the Mind in the Eyes" Test revised version: A study with normal adults, and adults with Asperger syndrome or high-functioning autism. *J. Child Psychol. Psychiatry.* **2001**, *42*, 241–251. [CrossRef]
64. Wechsler, D. *Wechsler Abbreviated Scale of Intelligence–Second Edition (WASI-II)*; NCS Pearson: San Antonio, TX, USA, 2011.
65. Lundh, L.-G.; Johnsson, A.; Sundqvist, K.; Olsson, H. Alexithymia, memory of emotion, emotional awareness, and perfectionism. *Emotion* **2002**, *2*, 361–379. [CrossRef]
66. Baron-Cohen, S.; Hammer, J. Parents of Children with Asperger Syndrome: What is the Cognitive Phenotype? *J. Cogn. Neurosci.* **1997**, *9*, 548–554. [CrossRef]
67. Oakley, B.F.M.; Brewer, R.; Bird, G.; Catmur, C. Theory of mind is not theory of emotion: A cautionary note on the reading the mind in the eyes test. *J. Abnorm. Psychol.* **2016**, *125*, 818–823. [CrossRef] [PubMed]

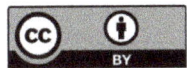 © 2020 by the authors. Licensee MDPI, Basel, Switzerland. This article is an open access article distributed under the terms and conditions of the Creative Commons Attribution (CC BY) license (http://creativecommons.org/licenses/by/4.0/).

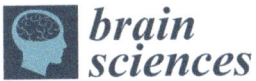 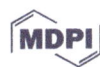

Article

The Role of Executive Functions in the Development of Empathy and Its Association with Externalizing Behaviors in Children with Neurodevelopmental Disorders and Other Psychiatric Comorbidities

Chiara Cristofani [1,†], Gianluca Sesso [1,2,†], Paola Cristofani [1], Pamela Fantozzi [1], Emanuela Inguaggiato [1], Pietro Muratori [1], Antonio Narzisi [1], Chiara Pfanner [1], Simone Pisano [3,4], Lisa Polidori [1], Laura Ruglioni [1], Elena Valente [1], Gabriele Masi [1] and Annarita Milone [1,*]

1. IRCCS Stella Maris Foundation, 56128 Pisa (Calambrone), Italy; ccristofani@fsm.unipi.it (C.C.); gsesso@fsm.unipi.it (G.S.); pcristofani@fsm.unipi.it (P.C.); pfantozzi@fsm.unipi.it (P.F.); einguaggiato@fsm.unipi.it (E.I.); pmuratori@fsm.unipi.it (P.M.); anarzisi@fsm.unipi.it (A.N.); cpfanner@fsm.unipi.it (C.P.); lpolidori@fsm.unipi.it (L.P.); lruglioni@fsm.unipi.it (L.R.); evalente@fsm.unipi.it (E.V.); gmasi@fsm.unipi.it (G.M.)
2. Department of Clinical and Experimental Medicine, University of Pisa, 56126 Pisa, Italy
3. Department of Neuroscience, AORN Santobono-Pausilipon, 80122 Naples, Italy; pisano.simone@gmail.com
4. Department of Translational Medical Sciences, Federico II University, 80138 Naples, Italy
* Correspondence: annarita.milone@fsm.unipi.it
† These authors contributed equally to this work.

Received: 6 July 2020; Accepted: 21 July 2020; Published: 28 July 2020

Abstract: Executive functions have been previously shown to correlate with empathic attitudes and prosocial behaviors. People with higher levels of executive functions, as a whole, may better regulate their emotions and reduce perceived distress during the empathetic processes. Our goal was to explore the relationship between empathy and executive functioning in a sample of children and adolescents diagnosed with Attention Deficit and Hyperactivity Disorder alone or associated with comorbid Disruptive Behavior Disorders and/or Autism Spectrum Disorder. We also aimed to examine the role of empathic dimensions and executive skills in regulating externalizing behaviors. The 151 participants with ADHD were assigned to four groups according to their psychiatric comorbidity (either "pure" or with ASD and/or ODD/CD) and assessed by means of either parent- or self-reported questionnaires, namely the BRIEF-2, the BES, and the IRI. No questionnaire was found to discriminate between the four groups. Affective Empathy was found to positively correlate with Emotional and Behavioral Regulation competences. Furthermore, Aggressiveness and Oppositional Defiant Problems were positively associated with Executive Emotional and Behavioral Regulation competences. On the other hand, Rule-Breaking Behaviors and Conduct Problems were negatively associated with Affective Empathy and with Behavioral skills. Our study provides an additional contribution for a better understanding of the complex relationship between empathic competence and executive functions, showing that executive functioning and empathic attitudes interact with each other to regulate aggressive behaviors. This study further corroborates developmental models of empathy and their clinical implications, for which externalizing behaviors could be attenuated by enhancing executive functioning skills.

Keywords: empathy; executive functions; attention deficit and hyperactivity disorder; autism spectrum disorder; disruptive behavior disorders

1. Introduction

Feeling empathy for someone means understanding his/her emotions and/or personally experiencing the same; it means creating a customized space in one's own inner world to host the world of the other. In other words, it refers to the ability to share and comprehend another person's thoughts and moods [1]. Feeling and understanding the emotions of others are important assumptions to guide one's actions in a prosocial sense and, particularly, to avoid those behaviors that can cause harm and suffering to the other. The cognitive facet of empathy implies the ability to understand the inner situation of the other and to take his/her own perspective [2]. On the other hand, the affective component of empathy is defined as the ability to share the emotional state of others [3]. The latter implies the involvement of limbic and paralimbic structures and develops earlier than the cognitive one, which assumes a fine-tuned maturation of prefrontal and temporal networks [4].

In light of the close association of empathy with contextual factors, early childhood experiences and social behaviors, it is direct to assume that psychopathological conditions are often convoyed by empathy deficits [5,6]. Empathy deficits have been implicated in several neurodevelopmental disorders, among which autism spectrum disorder (ASD) is the most studied [7–9]. ASD have been primarily associated with cognitive empathy deficits [9,10] but the potential role of affective empathy in this framework has been questioned [11].

The reduction or absence of empathy represents the cornerstone of Conduct Disorders (CD) characterized by disruptive and antisocial behaviors [12]. Adults with psychopathic traits show a selective deficit of the affective component of empathy related to impaired emotional responses to facial expressions of feelings of sadness and fear [13–15], which is likely due to dysfunctional neuronal circuits underlying the amygdala [16]. A recent study by our group [17] confirmed these findings in a cohort of young boys with CD, corroborating the association between callous-unemotional (CU) traits and affective empathic attitudes. Interestingly, studies aimed at outlining the differences between children with CD and CU traits and ASD [18] show that, while psychopathy seems to be best characterized by a preserved understanding of what the other thinks, with a deficient capacity to share compassionate feelings towards the others, ASD specifically lacks the ability to take others' perspective. Conversely, a study conducted by Mazza et al., 2014 [11] on a group of adolescents with ASD reported a difficulty in cognitive empathy and a deficit in affective empathy specific for the negative emotional valence, assuming, also for these subjects, the existence of an atypical function and structure of the amygdala [19].

Some evidence has also shown that empathy is compromised in a proportion of children with Attention Deficit and Hyperactivity Disorder (ADHD); in particular, lower levels of social perspective taking are observed [20–22]. Indeed, young people with ADHD may have low cognitive empathic attitudes, as demonstrated for instance by the frequently observed unawareness of other children playing the same game [23]. Further corroborating evidence appeared in a recent study by Maoz et al., 2019 [24], who confirmed the existence of a global deficit in both components of empathy by using the Interpersonal Reactivity Index [25] in its self-report form. In another study conducted by the same research group [26], differences in the empathic profile are identified between the Combined and the Inattentive subtypes of ADHD, identifying a greater impairment in the former for all scales of the IRI questionnaire. According to Uekermann et al., 2010 [27], these deficits might be explained at least in part by the impulsive response modalities typically found in ADHD patients, and thus may be linked to dysfunctions of the fronto-striatal brain networks, functionally related to empathic processing and executive functioning. Interestingly, Barkley, 2006 [28], argues that behavioral inhibition deficits, the core symptoms of ADHD children, might impair social cognition skills, but how much they could affect empathic abilities still remains an unsolved question.

Despite the identification of selective or global impairments of empathy in clinical settings, functional studies, aimed at assessing brain correlates of the experience of feeling the emotions of others, found that empathic attitudes are activated through an emotional processing which is regulated both by bottom-up and top-down circuitry within the prefrontal and limbic cortex [29].

An early influential theory, the Perception-Action Model by Preston and de Waal, 2002 [30], based on an evolutionary perspective, proposed that empathy is considered an uncontrolled response that operates automatically and develops early in life. More recently, the Russian Doll Model by the same authors [31] questioned this simplistic view and posited that bottom-up routes of empathic processing and top-down executive modulators are two interrelated systems that develop sequentially. This model has included executive functions as a regulating factor and considered it as a fundamental ground for the development of cognitive empathy [31–33].

According to the Russian Doll Model, several components of the empathic response, which have been added layer by layer during evolution, remain functionally integrated [34]. At its core is the perception-action mechanism, which induces a similar emotional state in the observer as in the target. Indeed, its basic expressions are motor mimicry and emotional contagion, representing the functional reactions of newborns and infants according to Hoffman's developmental theory of empathy [35]. On the other hand, the external layers of the doll, such as empathic concern and perspective taking, are grounded on the previously described socio-affective basis but require a fine-tuned regulation of emotional responses and a distinct perception between self and cognition. Although the outer layers of the doll depend on prefrontal circuitry, they remain functionally connected to the basic perception-action mechanism [31]. Therefore, cognitive empathic attitudes are supported by the neural regions that underlie working memory, executive functioning, emotional regulation and visuo-spatial processing, overpowering the affective representations of the other in a top-to-bottom fashion [31,36]. In other words, the effective control of empathic responses is thus obtained through the executive functioning regulation system, which allows a fine adaptation and modulation of the sharing experience.

A stepwise transition from immature forms of emotional contagion to more sophisticated expressions of prosocial attitudes, as brilliantly theorized by Hoffman's developmental theory of empathy [37], may be indeed paralleled by the progressive maturation of prefrontal circuitry and executive functions (EF) required to perform a fine-tuned control of such responses. Interestingly, a discrete amount of studies, conducted in community and clinical samples, has repeatedly shown that EF as a whole can modulate empathic attitudes, or in other words people with higher EF competences may better regulate their emotions and reduce perceived distress during the empathic processes [38–46]. Moreover, Gökçen et al. [43,44] found positive correlations between EF and empathic attitudes in individuals with ASD traits, suggesting the role of EF in regulating empathic competences in neurodevelopmental disorders. Similarly, a recent study in ADHD patients versus healthy controls by Abdel-Hamid et al., 2019 [47], found significant positive correlations between theory of mind (ToM) and empathy competences and EF performances in the ADHD group but not in the control group. In a recent review, which analyzed fifteen studies conducted on ADHD samples, with or without comorbidities and included mostly male children, Pineda-Alhucema et al., 2018 [48], found the EF most correlated with ToM were inhibitory control, working memory, cognitive flexibility and attention (for further updated details on the relationship between EF and ToM please refer to Andreou et al. 2020 [49]).

It should be noted, however, that in these studies, EF were variably measured through different neuropsychological tasks, such as the Go/No-Go test and the Wisconsin Card Sorting Test, which assess specific EF such as Cognitive Flexibility and Working Memory in laboratory settings. No study, however, used caregiver-reported measures of behavioral patterns for children and adolescents to evaluate EF in everyday life environments. Given the centrality of EFs in controlling behaviors in everyday life, relying only on laboratory measures of EF performances, detected with clinical tests, may limit the confidence and completeness of the clinical evaluation. The measures based on performances, in fact, depict only limited aspects of the EF system in a narrow time frame and do not fully capture the integrated multidimensional decision-making process based on an analysis of the priority which is often that of real life situations [50].

A recent meta-analysis [29] summarized these results, corroborating the evidence that empathy is strongly related to EF, and interestingly its cognitive facet is more closely related to executive skills than the affective one. Particularly, strong relationships were found between cognitive empathy and specific subcomponents of EF, including Inhibitory Control, Working Memory and Cognitive Flexibility, while affective empathy would only correlate to Inhibitory Control. Despite this, it should be observed that this meta-analysis did not consider further subdivisions of EF in their subgroup analyses, such as emotional regulation abilities and several other metacognitive skills. Moreover, no significant effect of age was demonstrated, though a considerable heterogeneity in the age range of samples of included studies is noticeable. Another potential source of bias was the inclusion of the results of three unpublished dissertations. Finally, many of these studies are made up of heterogeneous samples, while the meta-analysis does not take into account psychiatric comorbidities. The authors emphasized indeed that this field of research is still under open investigation, since the results of single studies are somewhat inconsistent and inadequate to draw definite conclusions.

The present study aims to explore possible relationships between the different facets of empathy and the specific subcomponents of EF in a clinical sample of children and adolescents primarily diagnosed with ADHD, compared to children with comorbid ASD or ODD/CD or both. EF profiles have been evaluated through the Behavior Rating Inventory of Executive Function (BRIEF) [51] questionnaire, which provides a structured assessment of EF behaviors in everyday life environments. Since the EF deficits can strongly affect the cognitive and behavioral manifestations of ADHD and ASD [52,53], our aim was indeed to investigate if and how EF are associated with the dimensions of empathy within these neurodevelopmental disorders.

Moreover, the current study examined the role of empathic dimensions and executive skills in regulating the externalizing behaviors typical of some clinical manifestations of ADHD and ODD/CD, such as for instance aggression, oppositional behaviors and rule transgression. It is believed, in fact, that emotional regulation plays an important role in inhibiting aggressive behaviors by implementing perspective-taking abilities and empathic concern towards the others [54].

2. Methods

2.1. Participants and Diagnostic Procedures

Our study included 151 drug-naïve participants (137 boys, age range 6–18 years old, mean age 9.51 ± 2.64 years) recruited in our third-level Department of Child and Adolescent Psychiatry from March 2019 to December 2019. Subjects underwent a multi-dimensional assessment, through individual clinical evaluations and observations of social interactions within a group of peers, in order to thoroughly investigate ASD symptomatology. The diagnoses were made according to the Diagnostic and Statistical Manual of Mental Disorders–Fifth edition (DSM−5) [55], based on medical history, clinical observations, a structured interview, the Kiddie Schedule for Affective Disorders and Schizophrenia–Present and Lifetime version (K-SADS-PL) [56], and clinical questionnaires, namely the Child Behavior Checklist and the Social Communication Questionnaire, commonly used to assist the diagnostic process.

The Child Behavior Checklist for ages 6 to 18 years (CBCL–6/18) [57,58] is a 118-item scale, completed by parents, with 8 different syndromes scales, a Total Problem Score and two broad-band scores designated as Internalizing Problems and Externalizing Problems. The reliability coefficients (Cronbach's alpha) of the original validation study were 0.82, 0.81 and 0.82, respectively. The Social Communication Questionnaire (SCQ) [59] is a widely used screening measure for ASD. It was designed as a questionnaire version of the Autism Diagnostic Interview–Revised (ADI-R) [60], the gold standard developmental history measure that is widely used in research and often in clinical practice. Caregivers can rate the individual's lifetime and/or current characteristics. Compared to other rating scales, the development research was significantly more robust, including good diagnostic validation on participants, and it has been widely adopted by both the research and clinical community worldwide.

Patients were included if they received a diagnosis of ADHD, with or without comorbid psychiatric conditions, including ODD/CD and ASD. The latter was suspected based on either medical history and clinical observations or a total SCQ score above the cut-off value and later confirmed through the administration of the Autism Diagnostic Observation Schedule–Second Edition (ADOS-2) [61]. The exclusion criteria were as follows: presence of comorbid intellectual disability, as detected through formal psychometric assessment by means of the WISC-IV, i.e., when either the Full-Scale Intelligence Quotient or the General Ability Index were below than 70 points; younger than 6 years old or older than 18 years old; current or previous use of psychoactive medications; neurologic impairments or neurodegenerative conditions.

We identified four clinical groups in our samples: "pure" ADHD group (namely, without comorbid ASD and/or ODD/CD, here-in-after referred as the ADHD alone group), including 64 subjects (12.5% girls, mean age 10.02 ± 2.49 years); comorbid ADHD + ODD/CD group (here-in-after referred as the ADHD+ODD/CD group), including 43 subjects (9.3% girls, mean age 9.37 ± 2.95 years); comorbid ADHD + ASD group (here-in-after referred as the ADHD+ASD group), including 19 subjects (5.26% girls, mean age 9.58 ± 2.69 years); comorbid ADHD + ASD + ODD/CD group (here-in-after referred as the ADHD+ODD/CD+ASD group), including 25 subjects (4% girls, mean age 8.40 ± 2.24 years). All participants and parents were informed about assessment instruments and participated voluntarily in the study after written informed consent was obtained for assessment procedures from parents of all children. The study conformed to the Declaration of Helsinki and the Regional Ethics Committee for Clinical Trials of Tuscany, Pediatric Ethics Committee section, approved the study (ethical approval code: GENCU/03/2019).

2.2. Clinical Assessment

Patients' clinical profiles were also assessed by means of several questionnaires, either through self or parental reports. Particularly, the Italian versions of the following measures were used: the Behavior Rating Inventory of Executive Functions–Second version (BRIEF-2) [51] administered to parents of all included children for the assessment of EF profiles; the Antisocial Process Screening Device (APSD) [62] administered to parents of all included children for the evaluation of CU traits; the Basic Empathy Scale (BES) [12], administered to parents of all children aged 11 years old or less, and the Interpersonal Reactivity Index (IRI) [25], administered in its self-report version to adolescents aged 12 years old or more, for the assessment of empathic competences.

The Behavior Rating Inventory of Executive Function–Second version (BRIEF-2) [51] is the updated version of the BRIEF questionnaire which provides a structured assessment of executive function behaviors in everyday life environments, allowing the identification of helpful clinical manifestations in different contexts, i.e., home and school. In its parent-report version that was used in the present study, this tool has been validated for 5- to 18-year-old children and adolescents. BRIEF-2 is a multi-dimensional measure and items are nearly equally distributed across nine factors, each referring to specific executive functions: Inhibit, Self-Monitor, Shift, Emotional Control, Initiate, Working Memory, Plan/Organize, Task Monitor, Organization of Materials. Three composite scales are also identifiable, each including at least two factors: Behavioral Regulation Index (BRI) (including Inhibit and Self-Monitor), Emotional Regulation Index (ERI) (Shift and Emotional Control) and Cognitive Regulation Index (CRI) (Initiate, Working Memory, Plan/Organize, Task Monitor, Organization of Materials). A Global Executive Composite (GEC) score is also computed as sum of the three aforementioned composite indexes.

The Antisocial Process Screening Device (APSD) [62] is a 20-item clinician-administered rating scale normed on a community sample of pre-adolescent children. The available version of the APSD was designed to be completed by parents and teachers; the former was used in the present study. Items are rated on a three-point Likert scale and the scale consists of three main dimensions, based on factor analysis: Narcissism, Impulsivity and Callous-Unemotional. There is substantial support for the validity of the APSD for distinguishing sub-groups of antisocial youths with more severe and aggressive behavior, with characteristics similar to adults with psychopathy [63] (Cronbach's $\alpha = 0.86$).

The Basic Empathy Scale (BES) [12] is a self- or parent-reported questionnaire, the latter being used in this study, for children and/or adolescents composed of 20 items distributed across two subscales, respectively, referring to the affective and cognitive components of empathy. Both exploratory and confirmatory analyses of the original validation established good internal consistency for each subscale with Cronbach's α ranging from 0.79 to 0.85. The Interpersonal Reactivity Index (IRI) was originally developed by Davis, 1980 [25], as a self-reported questionnaire for adults and subsequently adapted for adolescents by Litvack-Miller and colleagues [64]; it is composed of 28 items distributed across four subscales, respectively referring to Fantasy and Perspective-Taking (combined into the Cognitive Empathy subscale), Empathic Concern and Personal Distress (combined into the Affective Empathy subscale).

2.3. Data Analysis

Statistical analyses were performed by means of MatLab® (MathWorks, Natick, MA, USA) and RStudio® (RStudio Inc., Boston, MA, USA) software. For each clinical variable with continuous distribution, outliers were defined as observations lying outside the range between [first quartile − 1.5 * interquartile range] and [third quartile + 1.5 * interquartile range] and removed. For each BRIEF-2 subscale-related variable, observations were removed whether the corresponding values at either the Infrequency or the Inconsistency scale was higher than 99° percentile of normalized data. As for the BES and the IRI questionnaires, z-scores were computed for each subscales, i.e., the Cognitive and the Affective Empathy scales; thus, z-scores of the two questionnaires were merged together so that a single pair of variables assessing cognitive and affective empathy was available for all subjects irrespectively of the age.

Analyses of Variance (ANOVA) were used to assess significant differences (p-value < 0.05) between clinical variables with continuous distribution. A Tukey post-hoc test was used whenever the ANOVA led to a statistically significant result in order to identify significant comparisons between variables. Spearman's ranks correlation coefficients were estimated to detect significant relationships between rank values of questionnaire variables. Benjamini and Hochberg's False Discovery Rate (FDR) correction method [65] for multiple comparisons was applied after assessing significant differences at a traditional significance level of 5%.

Finally, four linear regression models were applied to identify statistically significant relationships between selected subscales of the administered questionnaires. Namely, four subscales of the CBCL (Aggressive Behavior [AB], Rule-Breaking Behavior [RBB], Oppositional Defiant Problems [ODP], Conduct Problems [CP]) were included as dependent variables of the models, whilst the three main indexes of the BRIEF (Behavioral, Emotional and Cognitive Regulation Indexes), the z-scores of the two subscales of the merged Empathy Questionnaire (Affective and Cognitive Empathy) and the SCQ total scores were used as independent variables of the models.

3. Results

3.1. Questionnaires

Scores obtained by the four clinical groups in the aforementioned questionnaires are reported in Figure 1A–C. No significant differences could be detected in the APSD (Figure 1A) and in the SCQ questionnaires (Figure 1B). Finally, no significant difference emerged neither in the Affective nor in the Cognitive Empathy subscales, neither of the two Empathy questionnaires considered individually (BES and IRI–data not shown) nor in the merged one (Figure 1C).

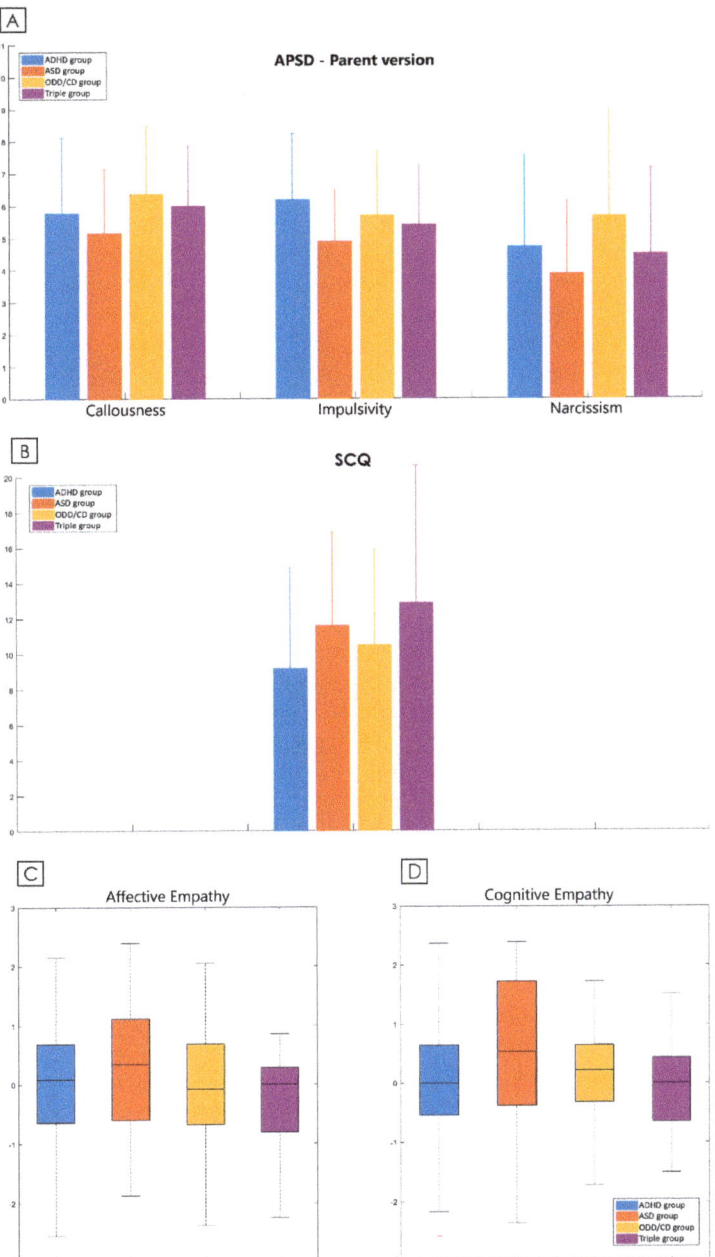

Figure 1. Questionnaires. Scores obtained by the four clinical groups in the Antisocial Process Screening Device (APSD, (**A**)), the Social Communication Questionnaire (SCQ, (**B**)) and the merged Empathy Questionnaire (**C**) are here illustrated. Scores are compared between ADHD group (blue bars), ASD group (red bars), ODD/CD group (yellow bars) and Triple group (purple bars). Graphs represent means with standard deviation bars, except for (**D**) where boxplots represent medians and first and third quartiles with minimum/maximum bars.

3.2. Correlations

Significant correlations between BRIEF-2-related subscales and APSD, SCQ and Empathy questionnaires are illustrated in Figure 2. Briefly, the Callousness subscale of the APSD was positively associated with the Inhibit and Self-Monitor scales of the BRIEF-2, while the Impulsivity subscale was positively correlated with all scales of the questionnaire. Similar findings were reported for the Narcissism subscale of the APSD, which was positively associated to most subscales of the BRIEF-2 across its three dimensions. The SCQ total score was positively associated to the Emotional and Behavioral Regulation related subscales of the BRIEF-2 and with the Initiate and Plan/Organize subscales. Finally, no significant correlations emerged for the Cognitive Empathy scale, while the Affective Empathy scale was negatively correlated with the Inhibit, the Self-Monitor and the Emotional Control subscales of the BRIEF-2.

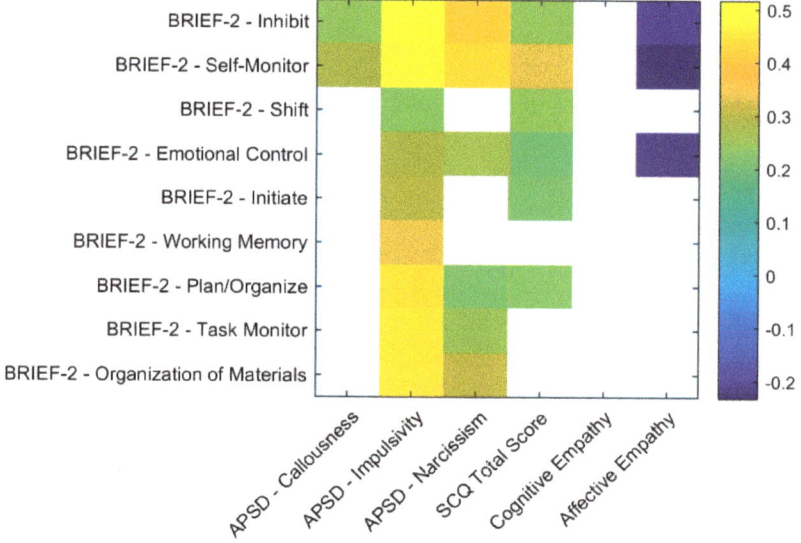

Figure 2. Correlations.

Pearson's linear correlation coefficients were here represented as colored boxes to show only significant relationships between continuous variables of selected questionnaires. The traditional significance level of 5% was corrected by means of Bonferroni's correction method for multiple comparisons. A color legend bar is displayed on the right.

3.3. Regression Models

Finally, a linear regression model was applied to identify statistical relationships between four aggressive/disruptive behavior-related CBCL subscales (AB, RBB, ODP, CP), as dependent variables, and several subscales from the other questionnaires, as independent variables, namely: the three main indexes of the BRIEF-2 (Behavioral, Emotional and Cognitive Regulation Indexes), the two Empathy subscales (Affective and Cognitive Empathy scales) and the SCQ total score.

As displayed in Table 1A–D, a significant positive association was found between both AB (Table 1A) and ODP (Table 1B) subscales of the CBCL, and the Behavioral and Emotional Regulation Indexes of the BRIEF-2. A significant positive relationship emerged, instead, between the RBB (Table 1C) and the CP (Table 1D) subscales of the CBCL, and the Behavioral—but not the Emotional—Regulation Index of the BRIEF-2, while a significant negative relationship was found for the Affective—but not the Cognitive—Empathy subscale.

Table 1. Linear Regression Models.

A. CBCL-AB	Estimates	β-Coefficients	Standard Errors	p-Values
Intercept	26.3134	0.0000	4.9028	4.21×10^{-7} ***
BRIEF-2-BRI	0.7645	0.3891	0.1843	6.49×10^{-5} ***
BRIEF-2-CRI	0.0667	0.2932	0.0715	0.3525
BRIEF-2-ERI	0.4610	0.0753	0.1481	0.0023 **
Affective Empathy	−1.2782	−0.1137	0.9909	0.1996
Cognitive Empathy	0.6295	0.0580	0.9616	0.5139
SCQ Score	−0.0541	−0.0306	0.1317	0.6816
B. CBCL-ODP	**Estimates**	**β-Coefficients**	**Standard Errors**	**p-Values**
Intercept	35.6661	0.0000	3.8429	1.23×10^{-15} ***
BRIEF-2-BRI	0.5471	0.3891	0.1445	0.0002 ***
BRIEF-2-CRI	0.0535	0.2932	0.0560	0.3420
BRIEF-2-ERI	0.3042	0.0753	0.1161	0.0099 **
Affective Empathy	−0.9299	−0.1137	0.7767	0.2336
Cognitive Empathy	0.1635	0.0580	0.7537	0.8285
SCQ Score	0.0105	−0.0306	0.1032	0.9186
C. CBCL-RBB	**Estimates**	**β-Coefficients**	**Standard Errors**	**p-Values**
Intercept	38.4738	0.0000	3.6169	$<2 \times 10^{-16}$ ***
BRIEF-2-BRI	0.6978	0.3891	0.1355	1.11×10^{-6} ***
BRIEF-2-CRI	0.0355	0.2932	0.0526	0.5008
BRIEF-2-ERI	0.0637	0.0753	0.1091	0.5606
Affective Empathy	−1.5698	−0.1137	0.7326	0.0343 *
Cognitive Empathy	−0.0574	0.0580	0.7121	0.9359
SCQ Score	−0.0296	−0.0306	0.0968	0.7599
D. CBCL-CP	**Estimates**	**β-Coefficients**	**Standard Errors**	**p-Values**
Intercept	37.5833	0.0000	3.7916	$<2 \times 10^{-16}$ ***
BRIEF-2-BRI	0.7870	0.3891	0.1424	2.12×10^{-7} ***
BRIEF-2-CRI	−0.0062	0.2932	0.0547	0.9096
BRIEF-2-ERI	0.1749	0.0753	0.1165	0.1359
Affective Empathy	−1.7449	−0.1137	0.7665	0.0247 *
Cognitive Empathy	−0.3663	0.0580	0.7409	0.6220
SCQ Score	−0.1235	−0.0306	0.1008	0.2229

Estimates, standard errors and p-values are here presented for four linear regression models between selected subscales of the administered questionnaires. Four subscales of the Child Behavior Checklist questionnaire, namely Aggressive Behaviors (**A**), Oppositional-Defiant Problems (**B**), Rule-Breaking Behaviors (**C**), and Conduct Problems (**D**), were included as dependent variables of the models. The three main indexes of the Behavior Rating Inventory of Executive Functions-Second version (Behavioral, Emotional and Cognitive Regulation Indexes), the two subscales of the Empathy questionnaire (Affective and Cognitive Empathy), and the Social Communication Questionnaire total scores were used as independent variables of the model. * p-values < 0.05, ** p-values < 0.01, *** p-values < 0.001.

4. Discussion

The first aim of the present study was to explore possible relationships between the different aspects of empathy and specific subcomponents of EF in children and adolescents with ADHD alone, ADHD and ODD/CD and/or ASD. To this aim, our effort was to achieve at least three major objectives: (1) to assess empathic attitudes, CU traits, antisocial behaviors and socio-relational skills in our four groups of patients; (2) to identify potential relationships between these variables and the EF profiles; (3) to explore the interrelated role of the cognitive and affective dimensions of empathy and the EF in regulating antisocial behaviors and aggressiveness. To the best of our knowledge, this is the first study of the kind performed in such a multi-structured sample of children and adolescents.

First, none of the questionnaires used in our study was individually able to discriminate between the four clinical groups. The SCQ is a clinical checklist, based on parents or caregivers report, aimed at identifying the presence of abnormal social and communicative behaviors. Although the SCQ is used as a screening tool for ASD symptoms, the lack of significant differences in our sample between ADHD patients with or without ASD suggests that the social functioning deficits reported in ADHD patients [21], at least in their parents' judgement, were severe enough to mitigate the difference among groups. It is also likely, however, that, since parents of ADHD children, with or without ASD, are usually more aware of, and worried about, the behavioral consequences of the disorder, socio-communication difficulties could go unnoticed even in patients with a confirmed diagnosis of ASD. A complementary but not alternative explanation may be that our high-functioning ASD patients did not exhibit such a great severity of social and communicative symptoms [66,67], so that caregivers could not be fully aware of their functional consequences.

Similarly, no significant differences emerged between groups in the two questionnaires assessing CU traits. Our finding may suggest that these traits may be trans-nosographic and thus be present not exclusively in ODD/CD, but also in ADHD [68] and in ASD patients [69]. As for the Empathy questionnaires, neither the BES and IRI nor the merged version of the two, did show any significant differences between the four clinical groups. Unfortunately, few data are available in the literature on the empathic attitudes of ADHD children with comorbid psychiatric conditions [70]. One would expect, based on previous findings on non-comorbid conditions, a greater impairment of the affective component for subjects with ADHD in comorbidity with behavioral disorders [17], while a greater impairment of the cognitive component in subjects with ADHD+ASD [10,18]. Our results could be interpreted in light of the subtle complexity of empathy deficits in these neurodevelopmental disorders, which limited the likelihood to find significant differences among comorbid conditions. It should be also taken into account that all our subjects were diagnosed with ADHD and this shared clinical condition may have obscured possible differences among groups. However, this finding further supports the notion that comorbid conditions are not the simple summation of two different disorders. In light of this, ADHD + ASD patients are not simply ASD patients with an additional ADHD, but a specific phenotype, possibly with a lesser cognitive empathic deficit or greater affective empathic impairment. Similarly, ADHD + ODD/CD patients may present a lesser affective empathic deficit or greater cognitive empathic impairment. This hypothesis should be tested by comparing "pure" ASD and ODD/CD with patients with ADHD and comorbidity conditions. Interestingly, recent studies shed some light on future research about specific empathy impairments in ASD and ODD/CD individuals, suggesting that different mechanisms and factors may be involved in empathic problems in such conditions [71,72].

The principal goal of the present study was to assess the reciprocal relationship between empathic attitudes and EF in ADHD patients. A recent meta-analysis [29], mainly including studies performed on healthy subjects, found positive correlations between empathic competences and EF. Gökçen et al. [43,44] reported similar findings in individuals with ASD traits, suggesting the role of EF in regulating empathic competences in neurodevelopmental disorders. Similarly, a more recent study by Abdel-Hamid et al., 2019 [47], identified in ADHD patients, but not in healthy controls, overlapping significant correlations between theory of mind and empathy measures and EF performances at the Trail Making Test, which specifically assesses Cognitive Flexibility and Working Memory skills. As for the so-called "hot" EF, that is the process underlying the affective modulation of behavioral responses [73,74], Miranda et al., 2017 [75], observed significant correlations between social cognition deficits, assessed by means of a specific subscale of the NEPSY–II test [76], and the BRIEF inhibition and emotional control scales in an ADHD sample, while the former are linked to metacognitive deficits in high functioning ASD patients.

In our sample, affective empathic competences, assessed through the BES and the IRI questionnaires, are negatively correlated with Emotional and Behavioral Regulation impairments, identified through the BRIEF-2 questionnaire. The greater the difficulties in "hot" EF, the lower the empathic attitudes, or, in other words, individuals with severe deficits in the EF profile exhibited lower scores on Empathy questionnaires. Nonetheless, no significant correlations were found neither for EF metacognitive domains nor with the cognitive empathy subscale.

Our results suggest that inhibitory and emotional control play an important role in regulating externalizing behavior, even controlling for empathic competences. As stated above, empathic attitudes are activated through an emotional processing which is regulated both by bottom-up and top-down circuitry within the prefrontal and limbic cortex [29,77]. This effective control is achieved through EF modulation, allowing for a fine adjustment of the sharing experience [33]. It should be noted that bottom-up and top-down processes are hardly separable when examined on a behavioral level. Nonetheless, the Russian Doll Model by Preston and de Waal [31] recently posited that top-down executive regulation of empathic processing develops later than bottom-up routes, which are responsible for uncontrolled empathic responses that operates automatically. This model is in line with the Hoffman's developmental theory of empathy [37], according to which Emotional Contagion would develop earlier than more regulated forms of empathic attitude towards the others.

Our results indicate that EF are more strongly related to the affective empathy than to the cognitive one, which is in disagreement with the results of the aforementioned meta-analysis [29]. Nonetheless, it should be emphasized that the studies of this meta-analysis did not include ADHD patients, who could exhibit such a severe impairment in their EF and a deficit in their cognitive empathic competences, that reciprocal associations would not result in statistical significance. In other words, we posit that ADHD patients are somewhat constrained by their executive dysfunction in an underdevelopment of their empathic attitude, which would be limited to the expression of an emotional contagion from the other.

Furthermore, significant positive relationships were found between several variables of the APSD questionnaire and the BRIEF-2 subscales related to the Emotional and Behavioral Regulation domains. Namely, the higher the scores in CU traits-related questionnaires, the higher the impairment in the Emotional-Behavioral Regulation competences. This finding is in line with a recent study assessing the relationship between CU traits and parent ratings of EF [78]. In particular, this study [78] highlights how CU traits are related to emotional self-regulation, but not to the EF performance scales. Since parental ratings are believed to capture EF behavioral representations, these clinical ratings may be more closely associated with behavioral representations of CU traits, which are also identified by the parents' report [78].

Finally, in our research, we tried to investigate, in a clinical sample of ADHD patients with psychiatric comorbidities, the relationships between two of the fundamental psychological grounds in the neuropsychologic developmental milestones of children and adolescents, namely EF and empathic attitudes, and how they reciprocally interact to regulate behavioral self-regulation and aggressiveness. Our results confirm a strong and finely structured relationship between these variables, being aggressive behaviors and related disturbances significantly influenced by these underlying processes. Our work highlights two different interactions between EF and empathy to regulate social behaviors in ADHD, where a dysfunction of these elements is essential for aggressive and antisocial behaviors to be carried out towards the others.

A first model identifies aggressiveness and oppositional problems, as indexed through the CBCL questionnaire, mainly associated with difficulties in executive emotional-behavioral regulation processes (such as impulse control and the ability to appropriately regulate one's behavior according to the context), but not with dimensions of empathy. Interestingly, reactive aggressiveness usually emerges as an impulsive response to hostile-perceived environmental events, often precipitated by irritability and tantrums [79]. This type of aggressiveness has been related to an orbito-frontal cortical dysfunction, for its primary role in adapting system reactivity to stress events [9,17,80].

On the other hand, rule-breaking behaviors and conduct disorders, as indexed through the CBCL questionnaire, likely relate to a proactive type of aggressiveness, which is associated to the activation of self-oriented behaviors to take advantage for personal purposes to the achievement of benefits at the emotional expense of the others' perspective [79]. Our study confirms that these aspects possibly relate to low levels of affective, but not cognitive, empathy and to impaired behavioral, but not emotional, regulation functioning. It has been hypothesized that proactive aggressiveness might be caused by dysfunctional mechanisms of violence inhibition, which are usually activated by others' discomfort signs, such as fear and sadness [15]. A deficient activation of this self-control mechanism is usually attributed to abnormal responses of the limbic system, particularly of the amygdala, which have been linked to antisocial behaviors in psychopathy [14,15].

Our results are thus in line with previous studies and further elucidate the complex and intriguing relationships between empathic attitudes and EF. In other words, it seems that both impaired behavioral self-regulation and difficulties in the emotional sharing of others' internal state may lead to a down-regulation of proactive aggressiveness inhibition systems, while emotional and behavioral regulation functioning systems are essential in preventing more reactive forms of aggressiveness towards the others. Thus, the multifaceted interactions of both "hot" EF and empathic attitudes have a central role in regulating prosocial behaviors.

Our study displays, however, a number of limitations that might undermine the robustness of our conclusions; notably, a marked discrepancy in group size, particularly between the "pure" ADHD and ADHD+ODD/CD+ASD groups, and the absence of a control group of healthy children. The purpose of this preliminary study was, indeed, to explore the issues addressed above; therefore, further studies on larger samples, possibly including heathy controls, a greater number of girls and ASD patients, and children with limited prosocial emotions, will be performed to confirm the results.

5. Conclusions

In conclusion, our study provides a further contribution for a better understanding of the complex and intriguing relationship between empathic competence and executive skills. These evidences could be beneficial for the definition of treatment strategies aimed at attenuating externalizing behaviors. Aggressive behaviors would, indeed, be modified by an empathic attitude-oriented approach, which should focus on the underlying executive dysfunction. To sum up, we showed that executive functioning and empathic attitudes interact with each other to regulate aggressive behaviors, being the former more related to reactive aggressiveness and the latter to proactive aggressiveness.

Author Contributions: Conceptualization: C.C., G.S., P.C., P.F., E.I., P.M., A.N., S.P., G.M. and A.M.; methodology: C.C., G.S., P.F., E.I., A.N., C.P., L.P., L.R., E.V., G.M. and A.M.; writing draft: C.C., G.S., P.C., P.F., P.M., A.N., S.P., G.M. and A.M. All authors have read and agreed to the published version of the manuscript.

Funding: This research was funded by the Italian Ministry of the Health RC2019 and 5 × 1000 founds

Acknowledgments: We wish to acknowledge all the patients, family members and research staff from all the units that participated in the study.

Conflicts of Interest: Masi has received research grants from Lundbeck and Humana, was in an advisory board for Angelini, and has been speaker for Angelini, FB Health, Janssen, Lundbeck, and Otsuka. All the other authors do not have conflicts of interest to declare.

References

1. Decety, J.; Moriguchi, Y. The empathic brain and its dysfunction in psychiatric populations: Implications for intervention across different clinical conditions. *Biopsychosoc. Med.* **2007**, *1*, 22. [CrossRef] [PubMed]
2. Zahn-Waxler, C.; Robinson, J.L.; Emde, R.N. The development of empathy in twins. *Dev. Psychol.* **1992**, *28*, 1038–1047. [CrossRef]
3. Knafo, A.; Zahn-Waxler, C.; Van Hulle, C.; Robinson, J.A.L.; Rhee, S.H. The developmental origins of a disposition toward empathy: Genetic and environmental contributions. *Emotion* **2008**, *8*, 737–752. [CrossRef] [PubMed]
4. Singer, T.; Seymour, B.; O'Doherty, J.P.; Stephan, K.E.; Dolan, R.J.; Frith, C.D. Empathic neural responses are modulated by the perceived fairness of others. *Nature* **2006**, *439*, 466–469. [CrossRef]
5. Muratori, P.; Lochman, J.E.; Lai, E.; Milone, A.; Nocentini, A.; Pisano, S.; Righini, E.; Masi, G. Which dimension of parenting predicts the change of callous unemotional traits in children with disruptive behavior disorder? *Compr. Psychiatry* **2016**, *69*, 202–210. [CrossRef]
6. Gonzalez-Liencres, C.; Shamay-Tsoory, S.G.; Brüne, M. Towards a neuroscience of empathy: Ontogeny, phylogeny, brain mechanisms, context and psychopathology. *Neurosci. Biobehav. Rev.* **2013**, *37*, 1537–1548. [CrossRef]

7. Vellante, M.; Baron-Cohen, S.; Melis, M.; Marrone, M.; Petretto, D.R.; Masala, C.; Preti, A. The "Reading the Mind in the Eyes" test: Systematic review of psychometric properties and a validation study in Italy. *Cogn. Neuropsychiatry* **2013**, *18*, 326–354. [CrossRef]
8. Preti, A.; Vellante, M.; Baron-Cohen, S.; Zucca, G.; Petretto, D.R.; Masala, C. The Empathy Quotient: A cross-cultural comparison of the Italian version. *Cogn. Neuropsychiatry* **2011**, *16*, 50–70. [CrossRef]
9. Blair, R.J.R. Responding to the emotions of others: Dissociating forms of empathy through the study of typical and psychiatric populations. *Conscious. Cogn.* **2005**, *14*, 698–718. [CrossRef]
10. Bons, D.; van den Broek, E.; Scheepers, F.; Herpers, P.; Rommelse, N.; Buitelaaar, J.K. Motor, emotional, and cognitive empathy in children and adolescents with autism spectrum disorder and conduct disorder. *J. Abnorm. Child Psychol.* **2013**, *41*, 425–443. [CrossRef]
11. Mazza, M.; Pino, M.C.; Mariano, M.; Tempesta, D.; Ferrara, M.; De Berardis, D.; Masedu, F.; Valenti, M. Affective and cognitive empathy in adolescents with autism spectrum disorder. *Front. Hum. Neurosci.* **2014**, *8*, 791. [CrossRef] [PubMed]
12. Jolliffe, D.; Farrington, D.P. Development and validation of the Basic Empathy Scale. *J. Adolesc.* **2006**, *29*, 589–611. [CrossRef] [PubMed]
13. Loney, B.R.; Frick, P.J.; Clements, C.B.; Ellis, M.L.; Kerlin, K. Callous-Unemotional Traits, Impulsivity, and Emotional Processing in Adolescents With Antisocial Behavior Problems. *J. Clin. Child Adolesc. Psychol.* **2003**, *32*, 66–80. [CrossRef] [PubMed]
14. Dadds, M.R.; Perry, Y.; Hawes, D.J.; Merz, S.; Riddell, A.C.; Haines, D.J.; Solak, E. Attention to the eyes and fear-recognition deficits in child psychopathy. *Br. J. Psychiatry* **2006**, *189*, 280–281. [CrossRef]
15. Blair, R.J.R. Neurocognitive models of aggression, the antisocial personality disorders, and psychopathy. *J. Neurol. Neurosurg. Psychiatry* **2001**, *71*, 727–731. [CrossRef] [PubMed]
16. Blair, R.J.R. The amygdala and ventromedial prefrontal cortex in morality and psychopathy n.d. *Trends Cogn. Sci.* **2007**, *11*, 387–392. [CrossRef]
17. Milone, A.; Cerniglia, L.; Cristofani, C.; Inguaggiato, E.; Levantini, V.; Masi, G. Empathy in youths with conduct disorder and callous-unemotional traits. *Neural Plast.* **2019**, *2019*. [CrossRef]
18. Jones, A.P.; Happé, F.G.E.; Gilbert, F.; Burnett, S.; Viding, E. Feeling, caring, knowing: Different types of empathy deficit in boys with psychopathic tendencies and autism spectrum disorder. *J. Child Psychol. Psychiatry* **2010**, *51*, 1188–1197. [CrossRef]
19. Ashwin, C.; Chapman, E.; Colle, L.; Baron-Cohen, S. Impaired recognition of negative basic emotions in autism: A test of the amygdala theory. *Soc. Neurosci.* **2006**, *1*, 349–363. [CrossRef]
20. Braaten, E.; Rosen, L.A. Self-regulation of affect in attention deficit-hyperactivity disorder (ADHD) and non-ADHD boys: Differences in empathic responding. *J. Consult. Clin. Psychol.* **2000**, *68*, 313–321. [CrossRef]
21. Nijmeijer, J.S.; Minderaa, R.B.; Buitelaar, J.K.; Mulligan, A.; Hartman, C.A.; Hoekstra, P.J. Attention-deficit/hyperactivity disorder and social dysfunctioning. *Clin. Psychol. Rev.* **2008**, *28*, 692–708. [CrossRef] [PubMed]
22. Abikoff, H.; Hechtman, L.; Klein, R.G.; Gallagher, R.; Fleiss, K.; Etcovitch, J.; Cousins, L.; Greenfield, B.; Martin, D.; Pollack, S. Social functioning in children with ADHD treated with long-term methylphenidate and multimodal psychosocial treatment. *J. Am. Acad. Child Adolesc. Psychiatry* **2004**, *43*, 820–829. [CrossRef] [PubMed]
23. Cordier, R.; Bundy, A.; Hocking, C.; Einfeld, S. Empathy in the play of children with attention deficit hyperactivity disorder. *OTJR Occup. Particip. Health* **2010**, *30*, 122–132. [CrossRef]
24. Maoz, H.; Gvirts, H.Z.; Sheffer, M.; Bloch, Y. Theory of Mind and Empathy in Children With ADHD. *J. Atten. Disord.* **2019**, *23*, 1331–1338. [CrossRef] [PubMed]
25. Davis, A. multidimensional approach to individual difference in empathy. *JSAS Cat. Sel. Doc. Psychol.* **1980**, *10*, 85.
26. Maoz, H.; Tsviban, L.; Gvirts, H.Z.; Shamay-Tsoory, S.G.; Levkovitz, Y.; Watemberg, N.; Bloch, Y. Stimulants improve theory of mind in children with attention deficit/hyperactivity disorder. *J. Psychopharmacol.* **2014**, *28*, 212–219. [CrossRef]
27. Uekermann, J.; Kraemer, M.; Krankenhaus, A.K.; Abdel-Hamid, M.; Hebebrand, J.; Daum, I.; Wiltfang, J.; Kis, B. Social cognition in attention-deficit hyperactivity disorder (ADHD). *Neurosci. Biobehav. Rev.* **2009**, *34*, 734–743. [CrossRef]

28. Barkley, R.A. The relevance of the Still lectures to attention-deficit/hyperactivity disorder: A commentary. *J. Atten. Disord.* **2006**, *10*, 137–140. [CrossRef]
29. Yan, Z.; Hong, S.; Liu, F.; Su, Y. A meta-analysis of the relationship between empathy and executive function. *PsyCh J.* **2020**, *9*, 34–43. [CrossRef]
30. Preston, S.D.; de Waal, F.B.M. Empathy: Its ultimate and proximate bases. *Behav. Brain Sci.* **2002**, *25*, 1–20. [CrossRef]
31. de Waal, F.B.M.; Preston, S.D. Mammalian empathy: Behavioural manifestations and neural basis. *Nat. Rev. Neurosci.* **2017**, *18*, 498–509. [CrossRef] [PubMed]
32. Decety, J.; Meyer, M. From emotion resonance to empathic understanding: A social developmental neuroscience account. *Dev. Psychopathol.* **2008**, *20*, 1053–1080. [CrossRef] [PubMed]
33. Heyes, C. Empathy is not in our genes. *Neurosci. Biobehav. Rev.* **2018**, *95*, 499–507. [CrossRef] [PubMed]
34. de Waal, F.B.M. Putting the altruism back into altruism: The evolution of empathy. *Annu. Rev. Psychol.* **2008**, *59*, 279–300. [CrossRef]
35. Hoffman, M.L. Prosocial behavior and empathy: Developmental processes. *Int. Encycl. Soc. Behav. Sci.* **2001**, 12230–12233. [CrossRef]
36. Shamay-Tsoory, S.G. The neural bases for empathy. *Neuroscientist* **2011**, *17*, 18–24. [CrossRef]
37. Hoffman, M.L. The contribution of empathy to justice and moral judgment. In *Empathy and Its Development*; Eisenberg, N., Strayer, J., Eds.; University of Cambridge Press: Cambridge, UK, 1987; pp. 47–80.
38. Ze, O.; Thoma, P.; Suchan, B. Cognitive and affective empathy in younger and older individuals. *Aging Ment. Health* **2014**, *18*, 929–935. [CrossRef]
39. Valiente, C.; Eisenberg, N.; Fabes, R.A.; Shepard, S.A.; Cumberland, A.; Losoya, S.H. Prediction of children's empathy-related responding from their effortful control and parents' expressivity. *Dev. Psychol.* **2004**, *40*, 911–926. [CrossRef]
40. Spinella, M. Self-rated executive function: Development of the executive function index. *Int. J. Neurosci.* **2005**, *115*, 649–667. [CrossRef]
41. Eisenberg, N.; Okun, M.A. The relations of dispositional regulation and emotionality to elders' empathy-related responding and affect while volunteering. *J. Pers.* **1996**, *64*, 157–183. [CrossRef]
42. Gao, Z.; Ye, T.; Shen, M.; Perry, A. Working memory capacity of biological movements predicts empathy traits. *Psychon. Bull. Rev.* **2016**, *23*, 468–475. [CrossRef] [PubMed]
43. Gökçen, E.; Petrides, K.V.; Hudry, K.; Frederickson, N.; Smillie, L.D. Sub-threshold autism traits: The role of trait emotional intelligence and cognitive flexibility. *Br. J. Psychol.* **2014**, *105*, 187–199. [CrossRef] [PubMed]
44. Gökçen, E.; Frederickson, N.; Petrides, K.V. Theory of mind and executive control deficits in typically developing adults and adolescents with high levels of autism traits. *J. Autism Dev. Disord.* **2016**, *46*, 2072–2087. [CrossRef] [PubMed]
45. Huang, H.; Su, Y.; Jin, J. Empathy-related responding in chinese toddlers: Factorial structure and cognitive contributors. *Infant Child Dev.* **2017**, *26*, e1983. [CrossRef] [PubMed]
46. Jenkins, L.N.; Demaray, M.K.; Tennant, J. Social, emotional, and cognitive factors associated with bullying. *School Psych. Rev.* **2017**, *46*, 42–64. [CrossRef]
47. Abdel-Hamid, M.; Niklewski, F.; Heßmann, P.; Guberina, N.; Kownatka, M.; Kraemer, M.; Scherbaum, N.; Dziobek, I.; Bartels, C.; Wiltfang, J.; et al. Impaired empathy but no theory of mind deficits in adult attention deficit hyperactivity disorder. *Brain Behav.* **2019**, *9*, e01401. [CrossRef]
48. Pineda-Alhucema, W.; Aristizabal, E.; Escudero-Cabarcas, J.; Acosta-López, J.E.; Vélez, J.I. Executive function and theory of mind in children with ADHD: A systematic review. *Neuropsychol. Rev.* **2018**, *28*, 341–358. [CrossRef]
49. Andreou, M.; Skrimpa, V. Theory of mind deficits and neurophysiological operations in autism spectrum disorders: A review. *Brain Sci.* **2020**, *10*, 393. [CrossRef]
50. Goldberg, E.; Podell, K. Adaptive decision making, ecological validity, and the frontal lobes. *J. Clin. Exp. Neuropsychol.* **2000**, *22*, 56–68. [CrossRef]
51. Gioia, G.; Isquith, P.; Guy, S.; Kenworthy, L. *BRIEF-2: Behavior Rating Inventory of Executive Function: Professional Manual*; Psychological Assessment Resources: Lutz, FL, USA, 2015.
52. Van der Meere, J.; Marzocchi, G.M.; De Meo, T. Response inhibition and attention deficit hyperactivity disorder with and without oppositional defiant disorder screened from a community sample. *Dev. Neuropsychol.* **2005**, *28*, 459–472. [CrossRef] [PubMed]

53. Willcutt, E.G.; Doyle, A.E.; Nigg, J.T.; Faraone, S.V.; Pennington, B.F. Validity of the executive function theory of attention-deficit/hyperactivity disorder: A meta-analytic review. *Biol. Psychiatry* **2005**, *57*, 1336–1346. [CrossRef] [PubMed]
54. Marton, I.; Wiener, J.; Rogers, M.; Moore, C.; Tannock, R. Empathy and social perspective taking in children with attention-deficit/ hyperactivity disorder. *J. Abnorm. Child Psychol.* **2009**, *37*, 107–118. [CrossRef] [PubMed]
55. American Psychological Association. *Diagnostic and Statistical Manual of Mental Disorders*, 5th ed.; American Psychological Association: Washington, DC, USA, 2013.
56. Kaufman, J.; Birmaher, B.; Brent, D.; Rao, U.; Flynn, C.; Moreci, P.; Williamson, D.; Ryan, N. Schedule for affective disorders and schizophrenia for school-age children-present and lifetime version (K-SADS-PL): Initial reliability and validity data. *J. Am. Acad. Child Adolesc. Psychiatry* **1997**, *36*, 980–988. [CrossRef]
57. Pandolfi, V.; Magyar, C.I. Child behavior checklist for ages 6–18. In *Encyclopedia of Autism Spectrum Disorders*; Volkmar, F.R., Ed.; Springer: New York, NY, USA, 2013; pp. 581–587. [CrossRef]
58. Achenbach, T.; Rescorla, L. *Manual for the ASEBA School-Age Forms and Profiles: An Integrated System of Multi-Informant Assessment*; Research Center for Children, Youth, & Families, University of Vermont: Burlington, VT, USA, 2001.
59. Rutter, M.; Bailey, A.; Lord, C. *The Social Communication Questionnaire Manual*; Western Psychological Services: Los Angeles, CA, USA, 2003.
60. Rutter, M.; LeCouteur, A.; Lord, C. *Autism Diagnostic Interview-Revised*; Western Psychological Services: Los Angeles, CA, USA, 2003.
61. Lord, C.; Rutter, M.; DiLavore, P.; Risi, S.; Gotham, K.; Bishop, S. *Autism Diagnostic Observation Schedule (ADOS-2)*, 2nd ed.; Western Psychological Services: Los Angeles, CA, USA, 2012; Available online: https://www.wpspublish.com/ados-2-autism-diagnostic-observation-schedule-second-edition (accessed on 22 February 2020).
62. Frick, P.; Hare, R. *Antisocial Process. Screening Device: APSD*; Multi-Health Systems: Toronto, ON, Canada, 2001.
63. Masi, G.; Milone, A.; Brovedani, P.; Pisano, S.; Muratori, P. Psychiatric evaluation of youths with disruptive behavior disorders and psychopathic traits: A critical review of assessment measures. *Neurosci. Biobehav. Rev.* **2018**, *91*, 21–33. [CrossRef] [PubMed]
64. Litvack-Miller, W.; McDougall, D.; Romney, D.M. The structure of empathy during middle childhood and its relationship to prosocial behavior. *Genet. Soc. Gen. Psychol. Monogr.* **1997**, *123*, 303–324.
65. Benjamini, Y.; Hochberg, Y. Controlling the false discovery rate: A practical and powerful approach to multiple testing. *J. R. Stat. Soc.* **1995**, *57*, 289–300. [CrossRef]
66. Mouti, A.; Dryer, R.; Kohn, M. Differentiating autism spectrum disorder from ADHD using the social communication questionnaire. *J. Atten. Disord.* **2019**, *23*, 828–837. [CrossRef]
67. Narzisi, A.; Posada, M.; Barbieri, F.; Chericoni, N.; Ciuffolini, D.; Pinzino, M.; Romano, R.; Scattoni, M.L.; Tancredi, R.; Calderoni, S.; et al. Prevalence of autism spectrum disorder in a large Italian catchment area: A school-based population study within the ASDEU project. *Epidemiol. Psychiatr. Sci.* **2018**, *29*, e5. [CrossRef]
68. Tye, C.; Bedford, R.; Asherson, P.; Ashwood, K.L.; Azadi, B.; Bolton, P.; McLoughlin, G. Callous-unemotional traits moderate executive function in children with ASD and ADHD: A pilot event-related potential study. *Dev. Cogn. Neurosci.* **2017**, *26*, 84–90. [CrossRef]
69. Herpers, P.C.M.; Rommelse, N.N.J.; Bons, D.M.A.; Buitelaar, J.K.; Scheepers, F.E. Callous-unemotional traits as a cross-disorders construct. *Soc. Psychiatry Psychiatr. Epidemiol.* **2012**, *47*, 2045–2064. [CrossRef]
70. Ay, M.G.; Kiliç, B.G. Factors associated with empathy among adolescents with attention deficit hyperactivity disorder. *Turk Psikiyatr. Derg.* **2019**, *30*, 260–267. [CrossRef]
71. Song, Y.; Nie, T.; Shi, W.; Zhao, X.; Yang, Y. Empathy impairment in individuals with autism spectrum conditions from a multidimensional perspective: A meta-analysis. *Front. Psychol.* **2019**, *10*, 1902. [CrossRef] [PubMed]
72. Pijper, J.; de Wied, M.; van Rijn, S.; van Goozen, S.; Swaab, H.; Meeus, W. Executive attention and empathy-related responses in boys with oppositional defiant disorder or conduct disorder, with and without comorbid anxiety disorder. *Child Psychiatry Hum. Dev.* **2018**, *49*, 956–965. [CrossRef] [PubMed]
73. Zelazo, P.D.; Carlson, S.M. Hot and cool executive function in childhood and adolescence: Development and plasticity. *Child Dev. Perspect.* **2012**, *6*, 354–360. [CrossRef]

74. Zelazo, P.D. Executive function and psychopathology: A neurodevelopmental perspective. *Annu. Rev. Clin. Psychol.* **2020**, *16*, 431–454. [CrossRef]
75. Miranda, A.; Berenguer, C.; Roselló, B.; Baixauli, I.; Colomer, C. Social cognition in children with high-functioning autism spectrum disorder and attention-deficit/hyperactivity disorder. associations with executive functions. *Front. Psychol.* **2017**, *8*, 1035. [CrossRef]
76. Brooks, B.L.; Sherman, E.M.S.; Strauss, E. NEPSY-II: A Developmental neuropsychological assessment, second edition. *Child Neuropsychol.* **2010**, *16*, 80–101. [CrossRef]
77. Fassino, S. Empatia e strategie dell'incoraggiamento nel processo di cambiamento. *Riv. Psicol. Indiv.* **2009**, *63*, 49–63.
78. Rizeq, J.; Toplak, M.E.; Ledochowski, J.; Basile, A.; Andrade, B.F. Developmental neuropsychology callous-unemotional traits and executive functions are unique correlates of disruptive behavior in children. *Dev. Neuropsychol.* **2020**, *45*, 154–166. [CrossRef]
79. Lambruschi, F.; Muratori, P. *Psicopatologia e Psicoterapia dei Disturbi della Condotta*; Carocci: Rome, Italy, 2013.
80. Blair, R.J.R.; Peschardt, K.S.; Budhani, S.; Mitchell, D.G.V.; Pine, D.S. The development of psychopathy. *J. Child Psychol. Psychiatry* **2006**, *47*, 262–276. [CrossRef]

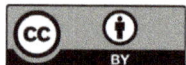

© 2020 by the authors. Licensee MDPI, Basel, Switzerland. This article is an open access article distributed under the terms and conditions of the Creative Commons Attribution (CC BY) license (http://creativecommons.org/licenses/by/4.0/).

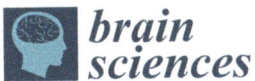 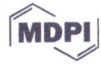

Communication

Association of Autism Onset, Epilepsy, and Behavior in a Community of Adults with Autism and Severe Intellectual Disability

Stefano Damiani [1,*], Pietro Leali [2], Guido Nosari [3], Monica Caviglia [4], Mariangela V. Puci [5], Maria Cristina Monti [5], Natascia Brondino [1] and Pierluigi Politi [1]

1. Department of Brain and Behavioral Sciences, University of Pavia, 27100 Pavia, Italy; natascia.brondino@unipv.it (N.B.); pierluigi.politi@unipv.it (P.P.)
2. Faculty of Medicine, University of Pavia, 27100 Pavia, Italy; leali.pietro@gmail.com
3. Department of Neurosciences and Mental Health, IRCCS Ca' Granda Ospedale Maggiore Policlinico, 20122 Milan, Italy; guido.nosari@gmail.com
4. RSD Cascina Rossago, 27050 Ponte Nizza, Italy; mo.caviglia@gmail.com
5. Department of Public Health, Experimental and Forensic Medicine, University of Pavia, 27100 Pavia, Italy; mariangela.puci@unipv.it (M.V.P.); cristina.monti@unipv.it (M.C.M.)
* Correspondence: stefano.damiani01@ateneopv.it; Tel.: +39-3400760002

Received: 22 May 2020; Accepted: 22 July 2020; Published: 27 July 2020

Abstract: Autism spectrum disorders (ASDs) are hard to characterize due to their clinical heterogeneity. Whether epilepsy and other highly prevalent comorbidities may be related to specific subphenotypes such as regressive ASD (i.e., the onset of symptoms after a period of apparently typical development) is controversial and yet to be determined. Such discrepancies may be related to the fact that age, level of cognitive functioning, and environmental variables are often not taken into account. We considered a sample of 20 subjects (i) between 20 and 55 years of age, (ii) with severe/profound intellectual disability, (iii) living in the same rural context of a farm community. As a primary aim, we tested for the association between epilepsy and regressive ASD. Secondly, we explored differences in behavioral and pharmacological profiles related to the presence of each of these conditions, as worse behavioral profiles have been separately associated with both epilepsy and regressive ASD in previous studies. An initial trend was observed for associations between the presence of epilepsy and regressive ASD (odds ratio: 5.33; 95% CI: 0.62–45.41, *p*-value: 0.086). Secondly, subjects with either regressive ASD or epilepsy showed worse behavioral profiles (despite the higher pharmacotherapy they received). These preliminary results, which need to be further confirmed, suggest the presence of specific associations of different clinical conditions in subjects with rarely investigated phenotypes.

Keywords: autism in adulthood; intellectual disability; regressive autism; epilepsy; challenging behaviors

1. Introduction

Autism spectrum disorder (ASD) is a neurodevelopmental condition whose phenotype encompasses various degrees of disability. Its growing prevalence has recently reached an estimate of 1 over 40 children [1]. ASD is associated with a wide range of comorbidities, among which intellectual disability (ID) or "low-functioning" ASD, epilepsy, and psychiatric disorders are the most frequent [2,3]. Compared to their "high-functioning" counterparts, low-functioning ASD individuals tend to exhibit more severe symptomatology and represent approximately 50% of the ASD population [4]. Few studies have been conducted on this 50% of the ASD population with comorbid ID, with its poor clinical outcomes and, thus, higher need for effective therapeutical strategies [5]. Similar to ID, epilepsy is also associated with challenging behaviors in individuals with ASD and ID [6]. Moreover, congenital autism spectrum disorders (CASD, when the core symptoms are evident from the very early life stages) may show different clinical presentations from regressive autism disorders (RASD, when the child loses abilities and milestones that were already achieved) [7]. In spite of the well-established presence of shared mechanisms between epilepsy and the autism spectrum being taken as a whole [8], the degree of association between epilepsy and RASD is not fully understood, with the few studies on this topic mostly focused on children [9,10].

A categorization of ASD subphenotypes is highly needed. This explorative study describes the clinical profile of 20 adults with ASD and severe/profound ID by assessing the presence of epilepsy and their history of RASD. The primary aim is to assess (i) the chance of these two conditions occurring together and (ii) the impact of each condition over the clinical picture in order to test whether epilepsy or RASD may be associated with the individuals' behavior. Both these features are hence compared to individual behaviors and pharmacotherapy, expecting worse profiles in subjects with epilepsy or RASD.

2. Materials and Methods

2.1. Study Design

This work is an observational retrospective study. We conducted a thorough data collection for each subject in two ways: (i) The number of seizures and sleep-disturbed nights were collected from the clinical records of each subject from January 2012 to December 2017 and sorted in 72 monthly timepoints for a total of 6 years; (ii) at the end of this time-window, behavioral profiles were assessed with the aberrant behavior checklist (ABC) [11] and data concerning antipsychotic, antidepressant, benzodiazepine, and anticonvulsant therapy were recorded.

2.2. Participants

Participants were recruited from Cascina Rossago, a farm community located in a rural area in the province of Pavia, Italy. For each subject, the legal representative gave his informed consent for inclusion before participation in the study. The study was conducted in accordance with the Declaration of Helsinki, and the protocol was approved by the Ethics Committee of IRCSS San Matteo, Pavia, Italy. This facility setting is meant to promote the active involvement of the user in farming activities such as fruit harvesting, breeding, and gardening. Moreover, sports and artistic workshops such as painting and drawing, music courses, pottery, basketball, and pool swimming are provided. The location is surrounded by nature: a rural environment was chosen both to avoid external disturbing factors such as city-life distress and to favor natural circadian and seasonal rhythms. This community was considered ideal for the purpose of our research for multiple reasons. Firstly, it is committed to offering lifelong care and working plans to adult ASD patients with severe to profound ID. The same living environment, activities, and diet are hence available for all the subjects. Secondly, each patient was constantly monitored by healthcare professionals, with accurate and detailed medical records. The main sample characteristics are shown in Table 1. RASD and epilepsy were considered as primary factors to present more specific information regarding the subsamples.

Table 1. Sample characteristics.

	All Subjects	Groups Stratified by Absence/Presence of Epilepsy			Groups Stratified by Autism Onset		
	(n = 20)	Absence (n = 9)	Presence (n = 11)	Absence vs. Presence p-Value	CASD (n = 9)	RASD (n = 11)	CASD vs. RASD p-Value
Age—mean ± SD	37.5 ± 9.5	36.33 ± 3.9	38.5 ± 2.4	0.632 †	36.6 ± 8.1	38.3 ± 10.8	0.698 †
Sex—n (%)							
Male	15 (75.0)	6 (66.7)	9 (81.8)	0.617 #	5 (55.6)	10 (90.9)	0.127 #
BMI (kg/m^2)—mean ± SD	25.3 ± 4.2	24.8 ± 3.8	25.7 ± 4.7	0.649 †	26.1 ± 3.3	25.4 ± 4.6	0.553 †
Drug therapy—n (%)							
anticonvulsant	12 (60.0)	4 (44.4)	8 (72.7)	0.362 #	4 (44.4)	8 (72.7)	0.362 #
benzodiazepine	11 (55.0)	3 (33.3)	8 (72.7)	0.175 #	3 (33.3)	8 (72.7)	0.175 #
Antidepressant	6 (30.0)	2 (22.2)	4 (36.4)	0.642 #	2 (22.2)	4 (36.4)	0.642 #
antipsychotic	10 (50.0)	4 (44.4)	6 (54.6)	0.999 #	4 (44.4)	6 (54.6)	0.999 #

† Student's t-test # Fisher's exact test; CASD = congenital autism spectrum disorder; RASD = regressive autism spectrum disorder.

2.3. Materials

Epilepsy—A subject was considered epileptic if the diagnosis from a specialized neurological center was present. The patient's legal representatives were contacted to further confirm the anamnestic data and to provide the official documentation confirming the clinical history. The retrospective analysis of the data allowed us to reconstruct the number of seizures suffered by each subject monthly. Taking into account the numerical limits of the sample in contrast with the detailed temporal data, a graphic illustration of the epilepsy trends was produced as a useful tool to promptly understand and visualize the differences between the two cohorts.

CASD/RASD—In relation to the diagnosis of RASD, early life medical records were available for all the subjects. According to the commonly agreed definition [12], we classified patients who initially reached cognitive and behavioral milestones but experienced a setback before the age of 3 as RASD.

2.4. Pharmacological Treatments

In our sample, 18 of the 20 participants were on psychopharmacological therapy. Antipsychotics were necessary for 10 subjects to support educational interventions for challenging behaviors. Anticonvulsants and benzodiazepines were used to control seizures in the majority of cases. In subjects without epilepsy (4 cases), these drugs were administered with the aim of controlling impulsive and self-harming behaviors [13].

2.5. Data Analyses

To describe the sample, we calculated summary statistics that are expressed as means, standard deviations (SD), median and 25th–75th percentiles or percentages, as appropriate. A Shapiro–Wilk test was used to test the normality of the data. We used Fisher's exact test for categorical variables and Student's t-test or the Mann–Whitney test, as appropriate, for the quantitative ones. Odds ratio (OR) with 95% confidence interval (CI) was calculated to evaluate the associations between epilepsy and RASD/CASD. Statistical analysis was conducted using STATA/SE for Windows, version 15 (StataCorp, College Station, TX, USA). A *p*-value <0.05 was considered significant.

3. Results

The mean age of the whole sample was 37.5 ± 9.48 years (range 23–55 years), 15 (75%) were males. For all patients, the mean BMI was 25.30 ± 4.21 kg/m^2. Information about drug therapy revealed that 60% of patients consumed antiepileptic drugs, 55% benzodiazepines, 30% antidepressants, and 50%

psychiatric drugs (Table 1). Table 1 shows patient characteristics for all subjects, stratified by the presence of epilepsy and CASD/RASD conditions. The history of registered epileptic seizures is graphically reported in Figure 1.

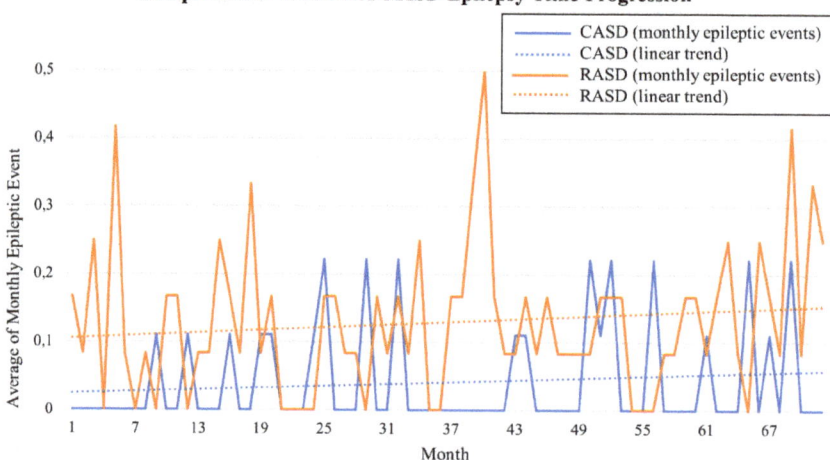

Figure 1. The graph represents oscillations in the presentation of epileptic events in CASD and RASD groups during the 6-year interval. The more frequent and higher spikes suggest a greater occurrence of seizures in the RASD group. Conversely, the seizure-free period reaches the zero level more often and for longer timespans in the CASD group. This trend tends to remain stable across the period of observation.

Six subjects had no history of epilepsy or RASD, three had only epilepsy, three had only RASD, and eight had both epilepsy and RASD (Figure 2A). The odds ratio was computed to check for associations between the presence of epilepsy and RASD (OR: 5.33; 95% CI: 0.62–45.41, p-value: 0.086).

The ABC median subscores were higher in epileptic patients versus nonepileptic patients and in the RASD group versus the CASD group (Table 2). No statistically significant difference was appreciated, but a trend was observed, for which each condition tends to increase the severity of challenging behaviors (all the ABC median subscores are higher in both epilepsy and RASD groups; see Figure 2).

Table 2. Aberrant behavior checklist (ABC) subscales scores.

	All Subjects	Groups Stratified by Absence/Presence of Epilepsy			Groups Stratified by Autism Onset		
	(n = 20)	Absence (n = 9)	Presence (n = 11)	Absence vs. Presence p-Value	CASD (n = 9)	RASD (n = 11)	CASD vs. RASD p-Value
Hyperactivity							
Mean ± SD	21.05 ± 7.56	19.0 ± 9.0	22.73 ± 6.08	0.270	17.56 ± 8.29	23.9 ± 5.80	0.056
Median (IQR)	21.0 (16.0–25.5)	17.0 (15.0–25.0)	22.0 (18.0–26.0)		17.0 (14.0–23.0)	24.0 (19.0–30.0)	
Irritability							
Mean ± SD	22.25 ± 8.65	19.67 ± 10.37	24.36 ± 6.73	0.209	19.56 ± 10.19	24.45 ± 6.87	0.261
Median (IQR)	21.5 (18.0–29.0)	18.0 (15.0–29.0)	23.0 (19.0–29.0)		18.0 (13.0–26.5)	23.0 (19.0–32.0)	
Lethargy							
Mean ± SD	20.65 ± 9.45	19.22 ± 11.34	21.82 ± 7.96	0.469	18.56 ± 11.86	22.36 ± 7.06	0.370
Median (IQR)	19.5 (16.5–26.0)	17.0 (11.0–25.0)	20.0 (18.0–26.0)		17.0 (9.0–29.5)	22.0 (18.0–26.0)	

Table 2. Cont.

	All Subjects	Groups Stratified by Absence/Presence of Epilepsy			Groups Stratified by Autism Onset		
	(n = 20)	Absence (n = 9)	Presence (n = 11)	Absence vs. Presence p-Value	CASD (n = 9)	RASD (n = 11)	CASD vs. RASD p-Value
Stereotypy							
Mean ± SD	11.15 ± 3.99	10.22 ± 4.71	11.91 ± 3.33	0.377	9.89 ± 4.51	12.18 ± 3.37	0.230
Median (IQR)	11.0 (7.0–14.0)	10.0 (7.0–14.0)	12.0 (9.0–14.0)		10.0 (7.0–13.0)	13.0 (9.0–14.0)	
Inappropriate speech							
Mean ± SD	5.85 ± 3.10	5.0 ± 2.92	6.55 ± 3.21	0.267	4.67 ± 2.50	6.82 ± 3.31	0.175
Median (IQR)	5.0 (4.0–7.5)	5.0 (4.0–6.0)	6.0 (4.0–9.0)		5 (2.5–6.5)	6.0 (4.0–11.0)	

p-values obtained from Mann–Whitney U-tests. CASD = congenital autism spectrum disorder; RASD = regressive autism spectrum disorder.

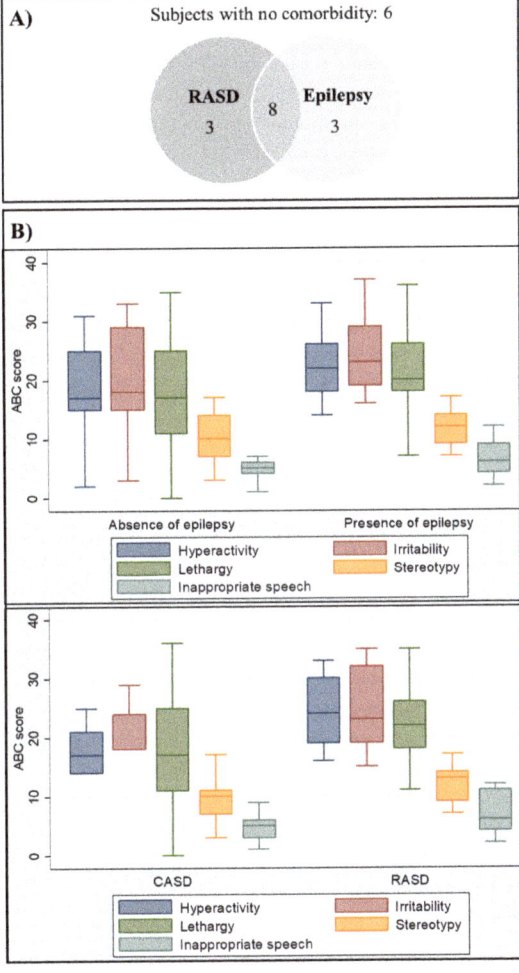

Figure 2. (**A**) Number of subjects with RASD, epilepsy, and both conditions are displayed. (**B**) Boxplots representing the difference of ABC median scores and the 25th–75th percentile of ABC scores in subjects stratified by epilepsy absent/present and CADS/RASD.

4. Discussion

We analyzed a sample of adult patients with ASD and ID who are stably living within the setting of a farm community. The main purpose of our study is to assess the association between autism onset and epilepsy and the impact of these conditions on behavioral profiles. Even though limitations such as the sample size did not allow the emergence of statistically significant results, the RASD subjects were 5 times more likely to also have a diagnosis of epilepsy.

We retrospectively measured the average of monthly epileptic events, i.e., any type of seizure, to better describe the presence of epileptic events and their frequency. RASD patients experienced a greater number of events, with fewer and shorter epilepsy-free periods. The three CASD subjects with epilepsy seemed to respond better to pharmacotherapy, with better control of the seizures.

Concerning behavioral profiles, even if differences in the ABC domains did not reach statistical significance, both RASD and epilepsy groups scored higher in each of these subscores. This trend is important, especially considering that the behavioral impairments are observed despite the higher pharmacotherapy that the RASD and epilepsy groups are undergoing. In fact, these subjects are more likely to consume not only anticonvulsants/mood stabilizers and benzodiazepines (which would be intuitive due to the epileptic risk), but also antipsychotics and antidepressants, which were initiated to better control problem behaviors and dysregulated moods, respectively. Autism and epilepsy share several neurobiological pathways [14]. An increased association between RASD and epilepsy may be determined by severe brain damage (for instance, after encephalitis, which is a risk factor for both autism [15] and epilepsy [16]) occurring in the first years of life. For instance, in our sample, two subjects suffered acute infection-related, early age neuroinflammation, after which seizures and regression arose.

The main limitation of this study is the low sample size, which does not allow us to hypothesize more complex assumptions based on the statistical significance of the findings due to excessively wide confidence intervals. The restrictive inclusion criteria and the same living and care conditions allowed to exclude several confounding factors, such as the variability given by differences in cognitive profiles, environments, diets, and therapeutical/educational approaches. However, high intersubject variability in behavioral and pharmacological profiles was measured despite these highly specific criteria.

5. Conclusions

Our findings show that (i) RASD and epilepsy tend to present together in a subsample of subjects with ASD and ID, (ii) RASD is associated with poorer control of epileptic symptoms, and (iii) RASD and epilepsy tend to worsen the behavioral prognosis, requiring more psychopharmacological therapies to compensate the clinical problems. Even though previous studies concerning the association between RASD and epilepsy yielded controversial results, the apparently contrasting findings may be attributed to the often-neglected differences between different life-phases (children versus adults) and levels of cognitive functioning. Carefully considering age and the presence of ID as influencing factors may hence help to shed light on this relatively uncharted but promising field of investigation in order to refine clinical classifications and tailor individualized treatments. These results invite us to further explore the subject, with the aim of determining whether the occurrence of different symptoms in autistic subpopulations may eventually lead to the individuation of ASD phenotypes.

Author Contributions: Conceptualization, S.D.; methodology, M.V.P. and M.C.M.; formal analysis, M.V.P. and M.C.M.; investigation, P.L. and N.B.; resources, M.C.; data curation, G.N.; writing—original draft preparation, P.L.; writing—review and editing, S.D. and G.N.; visualization, S.D. and P.L.; supervision, M.C. and P.P.; project administration, P.P. All authors have read and agreed to the published version of the manuscript.

Funding: This research received no external funding.

Conflicts of Interest: The authors declare no conflict of interest.

References

1. Xu, G.; Strathearn, L.; Liu, B.; O'brien, M.; Kopelman, T.G.; Zhu, J.; Snetselaar, L.G.; Bao, W. Prevalence and treatment patterns of autism spectrum disorder in the United States, 2016. *JAMA Pediatrics* **2019**, *173*, 153–159. [CrossRef] [PubMed]
2. Cervantes, P.E.; Matson, J.L. Comorbid symptomology in adults with autism spectrum disorder and intellectual disability. *J. Autism Dev. Disord.* **2015**, *45*, 3961–3970. [CrossRef] [PubMed]
3. Mannion, A.; Leader, G. Comorbidity in autism spectrum disorder: A literature review. *Res. Autism Spectr. Disord.* **2013**, *7*, 1595–1616. [CrossRef]
4. Matson, J.L.; Shoemaker, M. Intellectual disability and its relationship to autism spectrum disorders. *Res. Dev. Disabil.* **2009**, *30*, 1107–1114. [CrossRef] [PubMed]
5. Feldman, M.; Bosett, J.; Collet, C.; Burnham-Riosa, P. Where are persons with intellectual disabilities in medical research? A survey of published clinical trials. *J. Intellect. Disabil. Res.* **2014**, *58*, 800–809. [CrossRef] [PubMed]
6. Smith, K.R.; Matson, J.L. Behavior problems: Differences among intellectually disabled adults with co-morbid autism spectrum disorders and epilepsy. *Res. Dev. Disabil.* **2010**, *31*, 1062–1069. [CrossRef] [PubMed]
7. Rogers, S.J. Developmental regression in autism spectrum disorders. *Ment. Retard. Dev. Disabil. Res. Rev.* **2004**, *10*, 139–143. [CrossRef] [PubMed]
8. Richard, A.E.; Scheffer, I.E.; Wilson, S.J. Features of the broader autism phenotype in people with epilepsy support shared mechanisms between epilepsy and autism spectrum disorder. *Neurosci. Biobehav. Rev.* **2017**, *75*, 203–233. [CrossRef] [PubMed]
9. Hrdlicka, M. EEG abnormalities, epilepsy and regression in autism: A review. *Neuroendocrinol. Lett.* **2008**, *29*, 405. [PubMed]
10. Trauner, D.A. Behavioral correlates of epileptiform abnormalities in autism. *Epilepsy Behav.* **2015**, *47*, 163–166. [CrossRef] [PubMed]
11. Kaat, A.J.; Lecavalier, L.; Aman, M.G. Validity of the aberrant behavior checklist in children with autism spectrum disorder. *J. Autism Dev. Disord.* **2014**, *44*, 1103–1116. [CrossRef] [PubMed]
12. Stefanatos, G.A. Regression in autistic spectrum disorders. *Neuropsychol. Rev.* **2008**, *18*, 305–319. [CrossRef] [PubMed]
13. Ji, N.Y.; Findling, R.L. Pharmacotherapy for mental health problems in people with intellectual disability. *Curr. Opin. Psychiatry* **2016**, *29*, 103–125. [CrossRef] [PubMed]
14. Lee, B.H.; Smith, T.; Paciorkowski, A.R. Autism spectrum disorder and epilepsy: Disorders with a shared biology. *Epilepsy Behav.* **2015**, *47*, 191–201. [CrossRef] [PubMed]
15. Kern, J.K.; Geier, D.A.; Sykes, L.K.; Geier, M.R. Relevance of neuroinflammation and encephalitis in autism. *Front. Cell. Neurosci.* **2015**, *9*, 519. [CrossRef]
16. Klein, P.; Dingledine, R.; Aronica, E.; Bernard, C.; Blumcke, I.; Boison, D.; Brodie, M.J.; Brooks-Kayal, A.R.; Engel, J., Jr.; Forcelli, P.A.; et al. Commonalities in epileptogenic processes from different acute brain insults: Do they translate? *Epilepsia* **2018**, *59*, 37–66. [CrossRef]

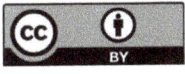

© 2020 by the authors. Licensee MDPI, Basel, Switzerland. This article is an open access article distributed under the terms and conditions of the Creative Commons Attribution (CC BY) license (http://creativecommons.org/licenses/by/4.0/).

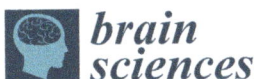 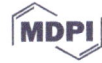

Article

Explaining Age at Autism Spectrum Diagnosis in Children with Migrant and Non-Migrant Background in Austria

Patricia Garcia Primo [1], Christoph Weber [1,2], Manuel Posada de la Paz [3,*], Johannes Fellinger [1,4,5], Anna Dirmhirn [4] and Daniel Holzinger [1,4,6]

1. Research Institute of Developmental Medicine, Johannes Kepler University, 4020 Linz, Austria; patricia.garcia_primo@jku.at (P.G.P.); christoph.weber@ph-ooe.at (C.W.); Johannes.Fellinger@bblinz.at (J.F.); Daniel.Holzinger@bblinz.at (D.H.)
2. Department for Inclusive Education, University of Education Upper Austria, 4020 Linz, Austria
3. Institute of Rare Diseases Research (IIER) & CIBERER, Instituto de Salud Carlos III, 28029 Madrid, Spain
4. Institut für Sinnes- und Sprachneurologie, Konventhospital Barmherzige Brüder, 4020 Linz, Austria; Anna.Dirmhirn@bblinz.at
5. Division of Social Psychiatry, Medical University of Vienna, 1010 Vienna, Austria
6. Institute of Linguistics, Karl-Franzens University of Graz, 8010 Graz, Austria
* Correspondence: mposada@isciii.es

Received: 26 May 2020; Accepted: 9 July 2020; Published: 14 July 2020

Abstract: This study explored (i) differences in age at Autism Spectrum Disorder (ASD) diagnosis between children with and without a migrant background in the main diagnostic centre for ASD in Upper Austria (ii) factors related to the age at diagnosis and (iii) whether specific factors differed between the two groups. A retrospective chart analysis included all children who received their first diagnosis before the age of 10 years ($n = 211$) between 2013 and 2018. Children with a migrant background were diagnosed 13 months earlier than those without ($r = 0.278$, $p < 0.001$), and had more severe delays in language, more severe autism, no Asperger's syndrome, lower parental educational level and more frequent referrals by paediatricians. For the total sample, expressive language delay, severity of restricted and repetitive behaviours, higher nonverbal development, and paediatric referrals explained earlier diagnoses. There was a stronger effect of parental education and weaker effect of language impairment on age at ASD diagnosis in children with a migrant background. In conclusion, no delay in diagnosing ASD in children with a migrant background in a country with universal health care and an established system of paediatric developmental surveillance was found. Awareness of ASD, including Asperger's syndrome, should be raised among families and healthcare professionals.

Keywords: migration; autism; diagnosis; Europe; health system

1. Introduction

(1) Prevalence of Autism Spectrum Disorder (ASD): The prevalence of ASD has risen in the last decade, with current rates of 1/59 in North America [1] and similar rates reported in Europe [2–5]. In the absence of ASD prevalence studies in Austria, epidemiological studies must be consulted [6], which would indicate a number of approximately 80,000 individuals with ASD diagnosis in this country—clearly a number that has a considerable impact on the national health and social systems. *ASD and migration.* A growing number of European studies, particularly from Nordic countries, suggests an increased frequency of autism in children of immigrant parents [7–10]. However, a recent systematic review of ASD prevalence and migration status in Europe has shown no simple, linear relationship between prevalence or risk of ASD and immigrant status [11,12]. Earlier data from North

American studies tend not to support this finding [13,14], whereas a recent ADDM (Autism and Developmental Disabilities Monitoring Network) study has shown a higher ASD prevalence in black children as compared to their white peers [15]. In Europe, the number of immigrants is substantial and also on the rise. In 2018, 22.3 million people with citizenship of a non-member country (4.4% of the EU-28 population) resided in an EU member state. Additionally, 17.6 million people in the EU were citizens of another EU member state [16]. Within the EU, Austria has one of the highest proportions of migrants (23.3%) [17]. The proportion of children who do not use German as their primary family language is 26% across all school types and 31% in primary schools [18].

(2) Age at ASD diagnosis and predictors: The increase in ASD prevalence has been accompanied by a decrease in the age at diagnosis in many countries [11,19], although there are exceptions [9]. Early ASD diagnosis is the gateway to support services [20] and interventions. Growing evidence points to the beneficial effects of enrolment at younger age in autism intervention on (a) the child's long-term outcomes [4,21,22], (b) the family's coping skills [23,24] and (c) costs to society [25,26]. Timely access to ASD diagnosis and support requires equitable access to health services, which is also one of the principles of the World Health Organisation (WHO) for universal health coverage [27]. Specific factors that affect the age at ASD diagnosis have been identified in several studies and are mainly related to clinical ASD presentation [28]. Severe language delay and more severe repetitive behaviours have been shown to be very common symptoms that prompt early medical consultation and diagnosis at a younger age. Hearing impairment and intellectual disability [28,29] have been found to delay identification of ASD in many cases. However, a low level of intellectual functioning can also stimulate earlier developmental investigation and earlier autism diagnosis [30–32]. Particular characteristics that are related to the child's family such as living in under-resourced or rural areas [28], low parental occupational level [33] and/or lower socioeconomic status [34,35] have more recently been identified as factors related to later ASD diagnosis. Furthermore, characteristics of the health system (mainly presence or absence of universal coverage), and whether it has a tradition of surveillance or screening programmes, must be considered.

(3) Migration and age at diagnosis: Lastly, migration status may also be a cause of delayed diagnosis [28,36–41]. Several studies in the USA have shown that children from immigrant families are more likely to be diagnosed later (mostly after the age of 4) than their non-migrant peers [28,33,37,39,41]. Although these data show an association between parental immigration and delay of autism diagnosis in North America, a limited number of studies has investigated this outside the United States [42]. To our knowledge, in Europe only one study in the Netherlands has explored this research question; the authors concluded that the immigrant sample did not differ in age at ASD diagnosis from the non-immigrant sample [43]. The following specific factors related to the age at ASD diagnosis in children from immigrant families have been reported [44]: firstly, a lack of knowledge of the host country language can restrict access to ASD awareness campaigns and education about ASD [44–47]. In addition, culture-related differences, such as parental feelings of shame and guilt related to child disability, have been described between families of children with developmental disabilities and the values and expectations of service providers [48–50]. A lack of understanding of the host country's health care system and community stigma can also prevent parents from seeking care [49,51]. Negative perceptions of services and a poor understanding of rehabilitation concepts can also delay access to specialised health services, and parents with a migration background have reported perceived discrimination by service providers [52]. Furthermore, culturally shaped interpretations of child behaviours (e.g., social communication) can influence the parents' seeking of medical advice [53]. As a consequence, professional organisations such as the American Psychological Association increasingly emphasise the importance of accounting for cultural differences in both professional practices and research [54].

(4) Health Care Services for Children with ASD in Upper Austria: The Austrian federal state of Upper Austria (1.48 million inhabitants) has a high proportion of immigration. In Upper Austria, 31% of all primary school children have a family language other than German [18]. The Austrian federal state

of Upper Austria provides an extensive network of healthcare institutions and a universal-coverage health insurance system. The social system in Austria offers free public early intervention for all children with developmental delays. In Upper Austria, a paediatric well-baby check-up program is provided free of charge from birth to school entry (at the age of 6 years) and is well accepted by families. An important element of this programme is a specific language screening programme (SPES) that was developed in 2007 by the Institute of Neurology of Language and Senses (ISSN) to identify children with increased risk for persisting language difficulties at the 2- and 3-year paediatric check-ups. The SPES language screening is used on a voluntary basis by the majority of paediatricians. Children who fail the short assessment of receptive vocabulary are referred for further neurodevelopmental assessment. By use of this screening the age of autism diagnosis could be significantly decreased within the last decade. About 50% of all children live in rural areas (i.e., thinly populated areas; 12% of these children do not use German as their primary family language), 13% live in the city of Linz, where the proportion of children with a family language other than German is 56% [55].

The out-patient clinic of the ISSN, situated within a public general hospital in the city of Linz, has been the major clinical focus for developmental disorders for the local community in Upper Austria in the last decade. It is the main centre where the complex multidisciplinary diagnostic evaluation needed for ASD diagnosis is regularly conducted [56]. In the associated Autism Centre, ASD-specific early intervention—following primarily the Early Start Denver Model—is provided [57]. In the last decade, the percentage of patients with a migrant background using the diagnostic clinic has risen from about 40% to 50%. Thus, data from this clinic's medical charts lend themselves to investigating factors that may determine a possible relationship between immigrant status and access to diagnosis.

Aim and Hypotheses

This study aimed to explore (i) whether there are differences in terms of age at ASD diagnosis between children with or without a migrant background at the principal diagnostic centre for ASD in Upper Austria, (ii) what factors might be correlated with the age at diagnosis of these children and (iii) whether predictors of age at diagnosis differ between children with and without a migrant background.

2. Methods

2.1. Study Design

A cross sectional study was used. All children of parents with and without a migrant background (see definition below) who attended the diagnostic centre of the ISSN in the study period (01-01-2013 to 31-12-2018) and received an ICD-10- diagnosis (International Classification of Diseases, 10th Revision [58]) of ASD (F84) for the first time before the age of 10 years were considered in the study.

Migration background cannot be sufficiently defined by citizenship, since there are many families with parents born outside Austria (and even more second-generation families) who have Austrian citizenship. The ISSN medical records did not contain systematic information on the parents' and children's places of birth, but detailed information about the language(s) spoken in the family. Therefore, a family was considered to have a migrant background if both parents (or one parent in a single-parent family) used a language other than German as their primary language in the family. There were no members of Austria's autochthonous ethnic minorities in the study sample.

Age of diagnosis was limited to a maximum of 10 years for both samples, since there were only few individual children in our clinical population who received an ASD diagnosis after that age. All ASD cases were evaluated at the ISSN by a developmental paediatrician, a clinical psychologist and a clinical linguist using various standardised tests depending on each child's developmental level and a clinical (non-standardised) interview. The ICD-10 [58] was used as a basis for clinical diagnosis of ASD and for the classification codes in the reports. All clinicians had been trained in the implementation and scoring of the ADOS-2 [59], which was applied in the majority of cases. Main outcomes were summarised in a comprehensive medical report.

2.2. Study Variables

Dependent variable: chronological age of the child at first ASD diagnosis. Independent variables: grouped by (a) sociodemographic, (b) clinical characteristic and (c) referral to diagnosis.

(a) Sociodemographic characteristics: Migration background status was based on language(s) predominantly spoken by the parents in the family as reported by the parents themselves. A family was considered to have a migrant background if both mother and father (or a single parent) used a language other than German as their primary language at home. The languages reported as being used at home by the study population were then categorised into five geographical regions: South-Eastern and Eastern Europe, Western and Northern Europe, Middle and East Asia, West Asia, and others (see Supplement S3). No parent was excluded due to insufficient language skills since translators were always available within the health system. Parental educational level was derived from the information provided by the parents in the registration form prior to clinical evaluation. Parents reported their current occupational level and/or educational background, and this information was then categorised into two levels of education: with or without high school diploma. For the analysis the highest parental educational level (i.e., of either father or mother) was used. Location of family residence was also elicited from the information provided by the parents in the registration form. This data was used to determine the degree of urbanisation of the place of residence (densely populated urban areas vs. thinly populated areas) and to estimate the distance between family residence and diagnostic clinic (in kilometres).

(b) Clinical characteristics: Gender was extracted from the medical record of the child. The non-verbal IQ score is the standardised non-verbal quotient of the child at the time of ASD diagnosis, either extracted directly from the evaluation report or calculated using the well-known quotient formula with the non-verbal developmental age of the child divided by the chronological age indicated in the report. The most common standardised cognitive tests reported were Mullen Scales of Early Learning (MSEL) [60], the Bayley Scales of Infant Development III [61] and the Hamburg-Wechsler Intelligenz test IV [62], depending on the child's age and level of functioning. Language Scores (Receptive and Expressive): receptive (RL) and expressive (EL) language developmental quotient scores, usually assessed by use of the MSEL, were either obtained directly from the diagnostic report or calculated from age-equivalent scores (age-equivalent scores/chronological age $\times$ 100) when the clinician indicated the language level of the child in months (usually based on a standardised language test, but also according to clinical picture when administration of a test was not possible due to the characteristics of the child) (PGP and DH). Language skills where assessed by linguists experienced in multilingualism in the child's primary language. If necessary, interpreters were used and parental observations were taken into consideration. Children with a developmental quotient below 50 were considered to have a moderate or severe delay. Variables of ASD Subtype: ICD-10 Code diagnosis of ASD (F84) ADOS Calibrated Severity Scores (CSS) for Social Affect (SA) and Restricted and Repetitive Behaviours (RRB) were transformed as appropriate from the original SA and RRB raw scores of the clinical report, following the indications of Gotham et al. [63], based on the child age, module and/or version of ADOS administered and reported in the clinical record (PGP and DH). A change in the clinical diagnostic procedure within the study period (from ADOS-G to ADOS-2) [64] was taken into account by the calibrated severity scores.

(c) Referral to diagnosis was either directly stated by the parents in the registration form or reported to the clinician at the evaluation (and therefore included in the diagnostic report).

2.3. Procedures

The clinical charts of all cases were revised and abstracted by researchers with considerable knowledge and experience in the field of neurodevelopmental disorders. To ensure accuracy, reliability and consistency in data abstraction, we developed, tested and revised a Record Review Protocol (RCR) following best practice [65,66]. An initial list of variables to be captured was tested in a small pilot study, discussed by the research team, and adjusted where necessary. In the case of conflicting or uncertain information in the medical charts, consensus decisions (PGM, DH) were made. The information that was reviewed referred to demographic and clinical characteristics of the children and their families and to the system of referral for ASD diagnosis.

Ethics: This study was approved by the ethics committee (Ethikkommission der Medizinischen Fakultät der Johannes Kepler Universität), Nr. 1140/2020 Version 3, following the rules of the Declaration of Helsinki of 1975 revised in 2013 [67].

2.4. Statistical Analysis

First, we separately calculated descriptive statistics (means, standard deviations for continuous variables and percentages for categorical variables) of all study variables for children with and without a migration background. Second, bivariate correlations were calculated between the age at diagnosis and the sociodemographic and clinical variables. This was done for the total sample and also separately according to migration status. In order to test for differences in correlations between the migrant and non-migrant groups, a Wald χ^2-test was carried out. Correlations were also calculated for different age groups in order to identify possible age-dependent predictors of the age at diagnosis. For all bivariate analyses we calculated effect size measures in a correlation metric, more specifically, Pearson's r for the association between continuous variables, point biserial correlation for the association between binary variable and continuous variables and phi or Cramer's V for the association between categorical variables. Finally, we used linear regression models to evaluate the effects of all predictors simultaneously. We also tested whether the association between predictors and age at diagnosis differed by migrant status. This was achieved by including interaction terms (e.g., migrant × sex) in the regression models [68]. We report unstandardised regression coefficients (b) and their standard errors (SE) and standardised coefficients (β) that have the same metric as correlation coefficients and could likewise be interpreted as effect size measures [69,70]. Several study variables had a high number of missing values (e.g., 42% missing values for parental education; see also Table 1). Preliminary analysis indicated that missingness depended on other variables (i.e., missing at random [71]). For example, children with missing values for parental education were diagnosed later (M = 52 months vs. M = 44 months). Thus, in order to avoid bias and a loss of statistical power, we used multiple imputation (MI)—a state-of-the-art technique for dealing with missing data—to replace missing values [71]. Firstly, the missing data was imputed by available data, and several imputed data sets were generated. Secondly, analyses were carried out for all data sets, and lastly the results of all data sets were pooled and final coefficients and standard errors were computed according to Rubin's combination rules [72]. Specifically, we used the blimp software [71,73], which implements a multiple imputation by chained equations (MICE) algorithm. All study variables were used for the imputation models, and imputations were carried out separately for the migrant and non-migrant groups. In order to obtain accurate standard errors, 200 imputed data sets were generated [74]. M*plus* 8.2. [75] was used for all analyses based on imputed data. Due to the non-normal distribution of the dependent variable of age at diagnosis (skewness = 1.411, kurtosis = 1.424), a maximum-likelihood estimation with robust standard errors (MLR) was used. Only descriptive results are reported for non-imputed data. These analyses were carried out using SPSS 26 and Jamovi [76].

Table 1. Sample characteristics by migration status.

	Values	%M	Total (n = 211) M (SD) or n (%)	Non-Migrants (n = 91) M (SD) or n (%)	Migrants (n = 120) M (SD) or n (%)	Difference ES r^a	p
Age at Diagnosis	12–119 m.o.	0%	46.7 (22.80)	53.96 (26.86)	41.19 (17.33)	0.278	<0.001
Sociodemographic Characteristics							
Family Residence in Urban Area	No/Yes	0%	148 (70.1%)	51 (56.0%)	97 (80.8%)	0.268	<0.001
Distance to Hospital	0–187 km	0%	38.27 (37.50)	49.27 (41.67)	29.93 (31.73)	0.256	<0.001
Parental Level of Education above High School	No/Yes	41%	37 (30.1%)	23 (42.6%)	14 (20.3%)	0.241	0.007
Clinical Characteristics							
Male Gender	No/Yes	0%	174 (82.5%)	77 (84.6%)	97 (80.8%)	0.049	0.474
Non-Verbal Developmental Quotient, (D/IQ)	16–122	13%	62.26 (18.89)	65.5 (21.15)	59.67 (16.56)	0.155	0.036
D/IQ 50 or Below	No/Yes	13%	37 (20.1%)	16 (19.8%)	21 (20.4%)	0.008	0.915
Expressive Language Quotient (ELQ)	13–128	15%	46.38 (24.44)	57.42 (28.93)	39.34 (18.46)	0.340	<0.001
ELQ 50 or Below	No/Yes	15%	118 (65.9%)	37 (49.3%)	81 (77.90%)	0.297	<0.001
Receptive Language Quotient (RLQ)	15–133	15%	48.25 (24.65)	59.6 (29.04)	40.75 (18.23)	0.355	<0.001
RLQ Score 50 or Below	No/Yes	15%	116 (64.8%)	36 (47.4%)	80 (77.70%)	0.314	<0.001
ADOS-Calibrated Severity Scores—Total CSS	1–10	18%	6.35 (2.19)	5.83 (2.16)	6.71 (2.15)	0.591	0.041
Social Affect—CSS	1–10	18%	5.85 (1.8)	5.76 (1.86)	5.91 (1.86)	0.009	0.198
Repetitive Behaviour—CSS							
ICD-10 ASD Code		0%				0.385	<0.001
Autism Disorder			122 (57.80%)	38 (41.8%)	84 (70.00%)		
Asperger's Disorder			21 (10%)	20 (22%)	1 (0.80%)		
PDD-nos			68 (32.20%)	33 (36.2%)	35 (29.20%)		
Referral to Diagnosis							
Referred by Paediatrician	No/Yes	27%	76 (36%)	23 (25.3%)	53 (44.2%)	0.289	<0.001

Note. %M = percentage missing values, M = mean, SD = standard deviation. [a] Effect size estimates for differences between migrants and non-migrants in a correlation metric.

3. Results

3.1. Descriptive Results

In Table 1 the descriptive results (based on non-imputed data) both for the total sample and for the non-migrant and migrant subsamples separately are shown. Results based on imputed data are provided in the Supplement (S1).

Of the 211 children in the sample, 58% received a diagnosis of autistic disorder, 10% of Asperger's disorder, and 32% of Pervasive Developmental Disorder–Not Otherwise Specified (PDD-NOS). Children with autistic disorder were diagnosed at an average age of 39.4 months, followed by children with PDD-NOS (50.8 months) and children with Asperger's disorder (75.9 months). Notably, children with Asperger's disorder were almost exclusively from the non-migrant group; only one case in the children with migrant background subsample had received an Asperger's disorder diagnosis. The difference in the ICD-10 ASD type between the non-migrant and migrant groups is highly significant (Cramer's V = 0.385, $p < 0.001$).

The mean age at diagnosis was 46.7 months (SD = 22.8) for the total sample. Values ranged from 12 to 119 months. The non-migrant group was diagnosed at a mean age of 54 months as compared to 41.2 months for the migrant group. Thus, children with a migration background received their autism diagnosis significantly earlier (difference of about 13 months) than those without ($r = 0.278$, $p < 0.001$). The distributions of the age at diagnosis for the total sample and the migration-status subsamples are shown in Figure 1. The sample with a migrant background is characterised by a reduced distribution with a stronger concentration around ages 2–4 and a smaller proportion of children diagnosed with ASD at a later age.

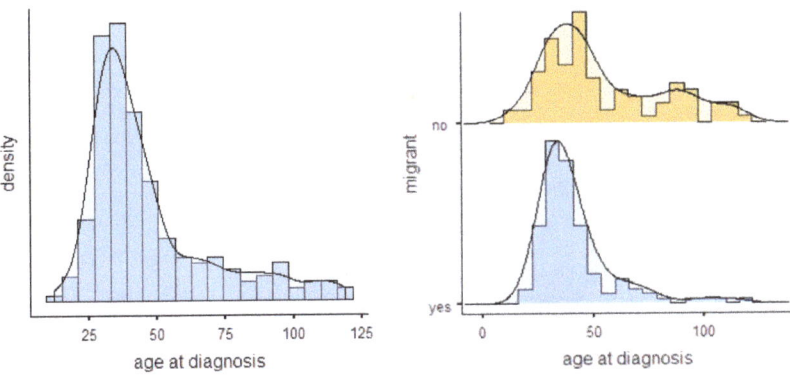

Figure 1. Age at diagnosis distribution histogram and density plot for total sample and split by migrant status.

3.2. Bivariate Analysis

In the total sample, there are moderate correlations between age at diagnosis and language scores. Children with lower expressive ($r = 0.423$, $p < 0.001$) and receptive ($r = 0.355$, $p < 0.001$) language scores were diagnosed significantly earlier. There is also a moderate correlation between RB-CSS and age at diagnosis ($r = -0.370$, $p < 0.001$). Children with higher RB-CSS received their diagnosis significantly earlier than those with lower RB-CSS. Similarly, analysis revealed a weak correlation between SA-CSS and age at diagnosis ($r = -0.158$, $p < 0.05$); more specifically, diagnosis occurred earlier in the case of higher severity scores for social affect. Finally, children who were referred by a paediatrician received their diagnoses earlier ($r = -0.255$, $p < 0.001$, M 40.78 months) than the rest of the sample (M 51.16 months). Table 2 shows the correlations between age at diagnosis and predictor variables for the total sample and the migration-status subsamples.

Table 2. Correlations between sample characteristics and age at diagnosis separated by migration status.

	Total	Non-Migrants	Migrants	Correlation Difference between Groups [a]
Sociodemographic Characteristics	r	r	r	p
Family Residence in Urban Area	−0.132	−0.073	−0.047	0.684
Distance Between Home And Hospital in Km	0.031	−0.050	−0.034	0.740
Parental Level of Education above High School	0.100	0.198	−0.169 *	0.035
Clinical Characteristics				
Male Gender	0.011	0.095	−0.048	0.252
Non-Verbal Developmental Quotient (IQ)	0.065	0.123	−0.131	0.136
Expressive Language Quotient (ELQ)	0.423 ***	0.443 ***	0.216	0.014
Receptive Language Quotient (RLQ)	0.355 ***	0.341 ***	0.177	0.059
ADOS-Calibrated Severity Scores—Total CSS				
Social Affect—CSS	−0.158 *	0.011	−0.263 **	0.206
Repetitive Behaviour—CSS	−0.370 ***	−0.446 ***	−0.326 ***	0.186
Referred by Paediatrician	−0.255 ***	−0.195	−0.220 *	0.707

Note. Correlations are based on multiple imputed data. [a] p-values for correlation differences between migrants and non-migrants are based on a Wald χ^2-Test. *** $p < 0.001$, ** $p < 0.01$, * $p < 0.05$.

There are some notable differences between the strengths of the correlations with age of diagnosis between children with and without a migrant background. First, for migrant-background children there is a negative association between age at diagnosis and parental education (r = −0.169, p < 0.05). Thus, children of parents with migrant status who had at least graduated high school were diagnosed at an earlier age than children of parents with migration background who had no high school diploma. In contrast, this association is of comparable strength but of opposite direction and not statistically significant in the non-migrant subsample (r = 0.198, p > 0.05). Second, the correlations between both ELQ and RLQ and age at diagnosis are of moderate strength and statistically significant for the non-migrant group (ELQ, r = 0.443, p < 0.001; RLQ, r = 0.341, p < 0.001), but weaker and non-significant for the migrant group (ELQ, r = 0.216, p < 0.10; RLQ, r = 0.177, p > 0.05). Finally, it is interesting to note that the correlation between SA-CSS and age at diagnosis is significant for the migrant subsample (r = −0.263, p < 0.01), but not for non-migrant subsample (r = 0.011, p > 0.05). However, these two correlations do not differ significantly.

Table 3 presents the results of exploring age effects on the correlations between the predictors and age at diagnosis for two subsamples defined by age at diagnosis (<48 months vs. ≥48 months) and migration status. Note that these analyses suffer somewhat from small sample sizes (e.g., n = 23 for the migrant group in the "age at diagnosis ≥ 48 months" subsample). Nonetheless, there are several interesting results. First, there is no significant correlation between age at diagnosis and ELQ and RLQ, respectively, in the younger subsample, neither for children with nor for those without a migrant background. These correlations are only significant for non-migrant-background children in the older group (ELQ, r = 0.462, p < 0.001; RLQ, r = 0.346, p < 0.05). Thus, non-migrant-background children aged ≥ 48 months at diagnosis received their diagnoses earlier, the lower their language scores were. A somewhat similar pattern—although individual correlations are not significant—was found for the correlations between RLQ and age at diagnosis in the migrant group. RLQ and age at diagnosis correlate moderately (r = 0.332; p < 0.10) for migrant-background children aged ≥ 48 months at diagnosis, but not for those who received their diagnosis before 48 months (r = −0.122; p > 0.05). Second, the RB-CSS is only correlated with age at diagnosis for children who received their diagnosis at the age of 48 months or later. In detail, there are moderate to strong correlations between RB-CSS and age at diagnosis for children both with (r = −0.530, p < 0.01) and without (r = −0.477, p < 0.001) a migrant background. In the subsample of children who were younger at diagnosis, these correlations are much smaller and not significant (correlation differences between age subsamples are significant). Finally, there is a negative and significant small correlation between age at diagnosis and distance between home and hospital in the older non-migrant subsample (r = −0.282, p < 0.05). Thus, children from this subsample received their diagnoses later, the closer they lived to the hospital. For children with a migrant background in this age group, the correlation is not significant and positive (r = 0.179, p > 0.05). The correlations differ marginally (p < 0.10).

Table 3. Correlations between sample characteristics and age at diagnosis according to migration status and age-at-diagnosis subsample.

	Age at Diagnosis < 48 Months		Age at Diagnosis ≥ 48 Months		Correlation Differences between Groups (p-Values) [a]			
	(1) Non-Migrants (n = 50)	(2) Migrants (n = 97)	(3) Non-Migrants (n = 41)	(4) Migrants (n = 23)				
	r	r	r	r	1, 2	3, 4	1, 3	2, 4
Sociodemographic Characteristics								
Family Residence in Urban Area	−0.079	0.167	0.033	−0.114	0.244	0.597	0.700	0.461
Home Distance to Hospital in km	−0.009	−0.122	−0.282 *	0.179	0.711	0.059	0.118	0.265
Parental Level of Education above High School	0.037	−0.094	0.167	−0.197	0.574	0.204	0.418	0.559
Clinical Characteristics								
Male Gender	0.090	0.034	−0.124	−0.200	0.680	0.848	0.355	0.204
Non-Verbal Developmental Quotient (IQ)	0.066	−0.150	0.168	0.235	0.305	0.989	0.371	0.213
Expressive Language Quotient (ELQ)	0.097	−0.172	0.462 ***	0.186	0.249	0.158	0.006	0.284
Receptive Language Quotient (RLQ)	0.007	−0.122	0.346 *	0.332	0.662	0.659	0.037	0.097
ADOS-Calibrated Severity Scores—Total CSS								
Social Affect—CSS	−0.111	−0.128	0.144	0.023	0.916	0.623	0.294	0.779
Repetitive Behaviour—CSS	0.125	0.002	−0.477 ***	−0.530 **	0.531	0.989	0.003	0.045
Referred by Paediatrician	−0.085	−0.026	−0.087	−0.148	0.702	0.836	0.785	0.550

Note. Correlations are based on multiple imputed data. [a] p-values for correlation differences between groups are based on a Wald χ^2-Test. *** $p < 0.001$, ** $p < 0.01$, * $p < 0.05$.

3.3. Regression Analysis

The results of the regression models are shown in Table 4. Due to the high correlation between ELQ and RLQ (r = 0.84), a unique composite language score (Language Quotient, LQ = (RLQ + ELQ)/2) was used in the regression models. All 10 predictors explain 34.6% of the variance in age at diagnosis. In accordance with the bivariate results, the LQ turned out to be the best predictor ($\beta = 0.389$, $p < 0.001$), followed by RB-CSS ($\beta = -0.301$, $p < 0.001$) and referral by paediatrician ($\beta = -0.206$, $p < 0.01$). Interestingly, the association between IQ and age at diagnosis, which was not significant in the bivariate analysis, is negative and statistically significant ($\beta = -0.175$, $p < 0.05$), when we control for other predictors. In fact, the association becomes significant as soon as we control for LQ; thus, given a constant LQ, the higher the IQ, the younger the child at diagnosis.

Table 4. Regression model for age at diagnosis.

	b (SE)	β	95%-CI
Sociodemographic Characteristics			
Family Residence in Urban Area	1.139 (3.457)	0.023	(−0.113, 0.159)
Distance between Home and Hospital in km	−0.020 (0.038)	−0.033	(−0.156, 0.089)
Parental Level of Education above High School	−3.719 (4.103)	−0.073	(−0.231, 0.085)
Migration Status	−6.228 (3.305)	−0.136	(−0.275, 0.004)
Clinical Characteristics			
Male Gender	1.539 (3.433)	0.026	(−0.087, 0.138)
Non-Verbal Developmental Quotient	−0.219 * (0.098)	−0.175	(−0.336, −0.014)
Language Composite (Expressive and Receptive)	0.363 *** (0.090)	0.389	(0.204, 0.574)
ADOS-Calibrated Severity Scores—Total CSS			
Social Affect—CSS	−0.133 (0.739)	−0.013	(−0.157, 0.131)
Repetitive Behaviour—CSS	−3.575 *** (0.941)	−0.301	(−0.452, −0.150)
Referred by Paediatrician	−9.370 ** (3.375)	−0.206	(−0.349, −0.063)
R^2		0.346	

Note. Results are based on multiple imputed data. 95%-CI = 95% confidence interval for β. *** $p < 0.001$, ** $p < 0.01$, * $p < 0.05$.

The regression model shows that migrant status is only marginally significantly associated with age at diagnosis ($\beta = -0.136$, $p < 0.10$) once other predictors have been controlled for. In detail, the difference in age at diagnosis, which amounted to about 13 months in the bivariate case (see Table 1), decreases to 6 months (b = −6.228) when other predictors are being controlled for. Again, the LQ is primarily responsible for differences between the bivariate and the multivariate analyses. Once we control for LQ, the difference between migration status and age at diagnosis decreases to roughly 7 months (b = −6.686, $p < 0.05$). Thus, about half of the difference in the age at diagnosis between the migrant and non-migrant groups is due to lower language scores of the migrant subsample.

In order to analyse possible differences in the associations between age at diagnosis and the independent variables between the migrant and non-migrant groups, we applied a series of regression models including interaction terms (for detailed results see Supplement S2). None of the interaction effects were significant. Thus, in contrast to the bivariate results (Table 2), no differences between the migrant and non-migrant subsamples in the associations between age at diagnosis and independent variables were found in the multivariate models.

Finally, some further analyses were performed to better understand the negative IQ effect in the multivariate regression model. In detail, we included an interaction term between IQ and LQ, which turned out to be statistically significant (b = 0.007, $p < 0.01$). In order to interpret this interaction, we plotted the simple slopes, that is, the associations of IQ and age at diagnosis for both high (=M + SD) and low (=M − SD) levels of LQ. Figure 2 shows that there is no association between IQ and age at diagnosis for children with high LQ. This association is negative and significant at low LQ levels. Thus, children with high IQ and low LQ were diagnosed the earliest.

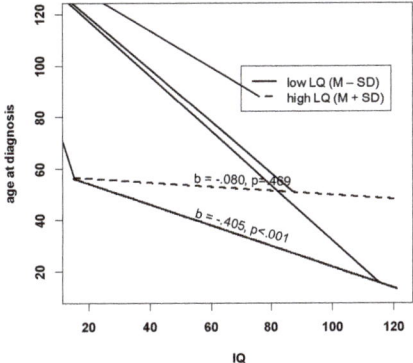

Figure 2. Interaction between LQ and IQ. Note. M = mean, SD = standard deviation. IQ = Non-Verbal Developmental Quotient. LQ = composite language score. b = unstandardised regression coefficient for IQ at high levels of LQ (M + SD) and low levels of LQ (M − SD).

4. Discussion

The aim of this study was to investigate and compare age at diagnosis of autism spectrum disorders in children with or without a migrant background from an intake population of an outpatient clinic for developmental disorders in Austria and to examine the impact of sociodemographic variables, child characteristics and referral factors on age at diagnosis. We carried out a retrospective chart analysis including all children who received an ASD diagnosis before the age of 10 years for the first time.

Notably, our results demonstrate a higher percentage of children with (57%) than without (43%) a migrant background being diagnosed with ASD in our clinic. This contrasts with a reverse ratio of about 30:70 of primary non-German to German family language in Austria. On the one hand, this might be explained by the high percentage of immigrant families (56%) in the city of Linz and a closer distance to the diagnostic centre facilitating service use. On the other hand, the high percentage of children with migrant background might also be due to a higher prevalence of ASD in migrant populations, as described by some of the European studies [8,10]. Additionally, clinical experience shows a high uptake of medical referrals among families with a migrant background. In our sample, a significantly higher number of migrant- than non-migrant-background families reported that their child had been referred to the clinic by a paediatrician. There also seems to be a general tendency for families with a migrant background to use primary paediatric care more often and longer [77] than non-migrant-background families; the latter are more likely to consult general practitioners, who are often less well trained in identifying developmental disorders. Finally, the large proportion of ASD diagnoses in children with a migrant background is probably also related to free access to health care in Austria. Studies in countries without universal health care have shown that children with ethnic and racial differences are less often diagnosed with ASD [78].

Our main finding is that for the total study sample, children with a migrant background received the ASD diagnosis significantly earlier than the rest of the sample. However, in the younger subsample, diagnosed before 48 months of age, the mean age at diagnosis was almost identical for the migrant and non-migrant groups (34.4 and 34.6 months, respectively). For the total sample, the significantly younger mean age at diagnosis in the subsample with a migrant background is due to a lack of children with less severe autism symptomatology (Asperger disorder), who are usually presented to the clinic at an age older than 4 years. In any case, contrary to findings in other health systems [78], there are no disparities in early access to diagnosis of ASD in Austria, where free health care and a medical surveillance system (preventive medical check-ups) are provided for all.

In accordance with the literature [8,79,80], we found significant differences in clinical symptomatology between migrant- and non-migrant-background children diagnosed with ASD. The sample with a migrant background demonstrated significantly longer delays in language as well as more severe autism and tended to be more delayed in their nonverbal cognitive development. The differences in language development persisted after reducing the sample to those diagnosed before the age of 4 years. A comparison of the distribution of autism subtypes (according to ICD_10) showed an almost complete absence of diagnoses of Asperger's disorder in children with a migrant background ($n = 1$) in contrast to the non-migrant subsample ($n = 21$). This accords with the results of Lehti et al. in 2015 [10], who found in a national birth cohort study of children diagnosed with Asperger's disorder in Finland a significantly decreased likelihood of diagnosis in children whose parents were immigrants (adjusted odds ratio 0.2, 95% CI 0.1–0.4). The higher likelihood of childhood autism versus Asperger's disorder syndrome in children with a migrant background might be related to specific risk factors associated with childhood autism (but not with Asperger's disorder) that occur more frequently in the migrant population, such as perinatal complications, low birth weight and lower gestational age [9,81]. However, we strongly suspect that our results also reflect service utilisation. Underdiagnoses might be due to less awareness of milder forms of ASD in the migrant-background subsample with a significantly lower level of parental education. In addition, the culturally shaped appearance of Asperger's disorder and communication problems between health professionals and parents and children might be other reasons for a lower number of this type of diagnosis.

Bivariate and multivariate analyses that identified factors correlated with delayed age at diagnosis for the total sample demonstrated a strong impact of the severity of language problems (expressive and/or receptive) on earlier ASD diagnosis. Severe delays in expressive language are easily noticed both by parents and by professionals in health and education systems and have been described as the most frequently observed symptoms of ASD that prompt medical consultation [82]. They have also been shown to be an important marker of non-apparent (invisible) developmental disorders [83]. In concordance with the findings of other studies, the severity of restricted and repetitive behaviours is another factor significantly related to earlier diagnosis of ASD, which is most likely a consequence of their obvious character compared to the often more subtle peculiarities in social communication. In addition, RBBs are often perceived as a cause of stress by the families and might therefore lead to external help being sought. The third-strongest factor related to earlier diagnosis was referral by a primary care paediatrician. Despite possible challenges in providing language- and culturally appropriate screening [78], well-trained paediatricians play an important role in reducing barriers to (early) ASD diagnosis. Finally, higher levels of intellectual functioning were found to be correlated with younger age at diagnosis, especially in children with seriously delayed language development, but it is also seen with average language scores. A severe language delay combined with significantly higher cognitive development may be even more obvious to parents and referring primary care professionals than a generalised developmental delay associated with a stronger need for explanation. With an expected majority of male gender in the sample, gender was not found to correlate significantly with age at diagnosis. Interestingly, parental education and the distance between the family's place of residence and the diagnostic centre did not add significantly to explaining the variance in age at ASD diagnosis.

A comparison of factors related to age at identification of ASD in the migrant and non-migrant samples mostly showed significantly stronger effects of parental education in the group with a migration background. However, the correlation was small. In migrant-background families, educational disparities are often linked to pronounced deficits in (spoken and written) language that might have a particularly strong effect on access to health information.

The severity of (primarily expressive) language delay had significantly stronger effects on delayed ASD diagnosis in the non-migrant sample. This effect is almost exclusively observed in the older subsample (>4 years), where—due to the much higher number of children with Asperger's disorder—variance in language development was significantly higher in the non-migrant sample. In school children with a migrant background, parents and professionals in health and education might ascribe language difficulties to bilingual language acquisition rather than to a developmental disorder. However, given the small size of the sample of older children with a migrant background ($n = 23$), results must be interpreted with caution. The minimal differences in factors explaining age at autism diagnosis between children with and without a migrant background are most likely a consequence of equitable access to medical care and a model of early identification with strong involvement of primary paediatric care that is well accepted.

The almost complete lack of significant effects of variables associated with age at diagnosis in the younger subsample is surprising at first glance. However, the variance in age at diagnosis was very small in the group aged younger than 4 years and probably related to the fact that paediatric screenings (mainly for expressive and receptive language) are usually offered at the ages of 2 and 3 years. Earlier referrals are highly unlikely. Furthermore, kindergarten, where autistic symptoms might be noticed, typically starts at the age of three. Long waiting periods for diagnostic services due to insufficient resources can cause inequalities and might be another reason that complicates the finding of significant predictors. The retrospective medical chart analysis presented has some limitations. Firstly, due to sample recruitment from a single clinic, effects of specific clinic-related factors on the age at diagnosis cannot be excluded. Secondly, another limitation of this study is its reliance on self-reported data about the parental level of occupation, since other information about Socioeconomic Status (SES), such as income or highest parental education, was not included in the medical charts. Even for information on parental occupation, data extracted from medical reports were very incomplete. Missing data, including those for other variables, were reported, and multiple imputations was used for missing values to avoid bias. Analyses of correlates of age at diagnosis by splitting the sample into two age subsamples and by migration status were interpreted with caution due to the small sizes of some of the subsamples.

5. Conclusions

This is one of the rare studies investigating age at diagnosis in children with a migrant background in Europe. Our findings highlight that for them the diagnosis of ASD is not delayed in Upper Austria, where universal health care includes a system of preventive medical check-ups provided mainly by paediatricians during the first years of life. Specific effects of lower parental education on age at diagnosis in families with a migrant background point to the importance of utilising existing preventive systems for systematic ASD screening and to the need to improve parent education on child development and health care services. The almost complete absence of diagnoses of milder forms of ASD (Asperger's disorder) in children with a migrant background demonstrates the need for improving awareness of the whole autism spectrum by training professionals in health care and education and extending education to parents. Restricted and repetitive behaviours, language delay, and the combination of severe language delay with a relatively higher nonverbal development are possible symptoms of autism that can be used to identify ASD by observation by parents or professionals and by their inclusion in systematic screening tools.

For children both with and without a migrant background, referrals by primary care paediatricians significantly decreased age at diagnosis. A universal implementation of a streamlined model from systematic screening to timely diagnosis is expected to further reduce age at ASD diagnosis and to facilitate earlier access to specialised intervention.

Supplementary Materials: The following are available online at http://www.mdpi.com/2076-3425/10/7/448/s1, Table S1: Sample characteristics by migration status based on multiple imputed data, Table S2: Regression models including interactions for age at diagnosis, Table S3: Languages reported as the primary language in the families with migrant background grouped by geographical areas ($n = 120$).

Author Contributions: P.G.P. and D.H. designed the study; P.G.P. and D.H. did the retrospective data analysis; C.W. did the statistical analysis; P.G.P., D.H. and C.W. wrote the paper; M.P.d.l.P. and J.F. were advising, all authors contributed with the revisions. All authors have read and agreed to the published version of the manuscript.

Acknowledgments: We thank the Federal Institute for Education Research, Innovation and Development of the Austrian School System for providing some statidistical information included in the introduction.

Conflicts of Interest: The authors declare no conflict of interest.

References

1. Christensen, D.L.; Maenner, M.J.; Bilder, D.; Constantino, J.N.; Daniels, J.; Durkin, M.S.; Fitzgerald, R.T.; Kurzius-Spencer, M.; Pettygrove, S.D.; Robinson, C.; et al. Prevalence and Characteristics of Autism Spectrum Disorder Among Children Aged 4 Years-Early Autism and Developmental Disabilities Monitoring Network, Seven Sites, United States, 2010, 2012, and 2014. MMWR. *Surveill. Summ.* **2019**, *68*, 1–19. [CrossRef] [PubMed]
2. Atladottir, H.O.; Schendel, D.E.; Henriksen, T.B.; Hjort, L.; Parner, E.T. Gestational Age and Autism Spectrum Disorder: Trends in Risk Over Time. *Autism Res.* **2016**, *9*, 224–231. [CrossRef] [PubMed]
3. Boilson, A.M.; Staines, A.; Ramirez, A.; Posada, M.; Sweeney, M.R. Operationalisation of the European Protocol for Autism Prevalence (EPAP) for Autism Spectrum Disorder Prevalence Measurement in Ireland. *J. Autism Dev. Disord.* **2016**, *46*, 3054–3067. [CrossRef]
4. Reichow, B. Overview of meta-analyses on early intensive behavioral intervention for young children with autism spectrum disorders. *J. Autism Dev. Disord.* **2012**, *42*, 512–520. [CrossRef] [PubMed]
5. Rydzewska, E.; Hughes-McCormack, L.A.; Gillberg, C.; Henderson, A.; MacIntyre, C.; Rintoul, J.; Cooper, S.-A. Age at identification, prevalence and general health of children with autism: Observational study of a whole country population. *BMJ Open* **2019**, *9*, e025904. [CrossRef]
6. Bejarano-Martin, A.; Canal-Bedia, R.; Magan-Maganto, M.; Fernandez-Alvarez, C.; Cilleros-Martin, M.V.; Sanchez-Gomez, M.C.; Garcia-Primo, P.; Rose-Sweeney, M.; Boilson, A.; Linertova, R.; et al. Early Detection, Diagnosis and Intervention Services for Young Children with Autism Spectrum Disorder in the European Union (ASDEU): Family and Professional Perspectives. *J. Autism Dev. Disord.* **2019**. [CrossRef]
7. Allison, C.; Williams, J.; Scott, F.; Stott, C.; Bolton, P.; Baron-Cohen, S.; Brayne, C. The Childhood Asperger Syndrome Test (CAST): Test-Retest Reliability in a High Scoring Sample. *Autism Int. J. Res. Pract.* **2007**, *11*, 173–185. [CrossRef]
8. Bolton, S.; McDonald, D.; Curtis, E.; Kelly, S.; Gallagher, L. Autism in a recently arrived immigrant population. *Eur. J. Pediatr.* **2014**, *173*, 337–343. [CrossRef]
9. Haglund, N.G.S.; Kallen, K.B.M. Risk factors for autism and Asperger syndrome. Perinatal factors and migration. *Autism Int. J. Res. Pract.* **2011**, *15*, 163–183. [CrossRef]
10. Lehti, V.; Hinkka-Yli-Salomaki, S.; Cheslack-Postava, K.; Gissler, M.; Brown, A.S.; Sourander, A. The risk of childhood autism among second-generation migrants in Finland: A case-control study. *BMC Pediatr.* **2013**, *13*, 171. [CrossRef]
11. Fuentes, J.; Basurko, A.; Isasa, I.; Galende, I.; Muguerza, M.D.; García-Primo, P.; García, J.; Fernández-Álvarez, C.J.; Canal-Bedia, R.; La Posada de Paz, M. The ASDEU autism prevalence study in northern Spain. *Eur. Child Adolesc. Psychiatry* **2020**. [CrossRef]
12. Kawa, R.; Saemundsen, E.; Loa Jonsdottir, S.; Hellendoorn, A.; Lemcke, S.; Canal-Bedia, R.; Garcia-Primo, P.; Moilanen, I. European studies on prevalence and risk of autism spectrum disorders according to immigrant status-a review. *Eur. J. Public Health* **2017**, *27*, 101–110. [CrossRef]
13. Croen, L.A.; Grether, J.K.; Hoogstrate, J.; Selvin, S. The changing prevalence of autism in California. *J. Autism Dev. Disord.* **2002**, *32*, 207–215. [CrossRef] [PubMed]
14. Yeargin-Allsopp, M.; Rice, C.; Karapurkar, T.; Doernberg, N.; Boyle, C.; Murphy, C. Prevalence of autism in a US metropolitan area. *JAMA* **2003**, *289*, 49–55. [CrossRef] [PubMed]
15. Nevison, C.; Zahorodny, W. Race/Ethnicity-Resolved Time Trends in United States ASD Prevalence Estimates from IDEA and ADDM. *J. Autism Dev. Disord.* **2019**, *49*, 4721–4730. [CrossRef]
16. EUROSTAT. Migration and Migrant Population Statistics. Available online: https://ec.europa.eu/eurostat/statistics-explained/index.php/Migration_and_migrant_population_statistics#Migrant_population:_22.3_million_non-EU_citizens_living_in_the_EU_on_1_January_2018 (accessed on 4 April 2020).
17. Bundesministerium Europäische und Internationale Angelegenheiten. Statistisches Jahrbuch "migration & Integration 2019": Integrationsbericht 2019. Available online: https://www.bmeia.gv.at/integration/integrationsbericht/ (accessed on 4 April 2020).

18. Bundesministerium Europäische und Internationale Angelegenheiten. Österreich Integrationsbericht 2019: Integrationsbericht 2019: Integration in Österreich-Zahlen, Entwicklungen, Schwerpunkte. Available online: https://www.bmeia.gv.at/fileadmin/user_upload/Zentrale/Integration/Integrationsbericht_2019/Migration-Integration-2019.pdf (accessed on 4 April 2020).
19. Hertz-Picciotto, I.; Delwiche, L. The rise in autism and the role of age at diagnosis. *Epidemiology* **2009**, *20*, 84–90. [CrossRef]
20. Russell, G.; Norwich, B. Dilemmas, diagnosis and de-stigmatization: Parental perspectives on the diagnosis of autism spectrum disorders. *Clin. Child Psychol. Psychiatry* **2012**, *17*, 229–245. [CrossRef]
21. Dawson, G. Recent advances in research on early detection, causes, biology, and treatment of autism spectrum disorders. *Curr. Opin. Neurol.* **2010**, *23*, 95–96. [CrossRef]
22. Warren, Z.; McPheeters, M.L.; Sathe, N.; Foss-Feig, J.H.; Glasser, A.; Veenstra-Vanderweele, J. A systematic review of early intensive intervention for autism spectrum disorders. *Pediatrics* **2011**, *127*, e1303–e1311. [CrossRef]
23. Hayes, S.A.; Watson, S.L. The impact of parenting stress: A meta-analysis of studies comparing the experience of parenting stress in parents of children with and without autism spectrum disorder. *J. Autism Dev. Disord.* **2013**, *43*, 629–642. [CrossRef]
24. Koegel, L.K.; Koegel, R.L.; Ashbaugh, K.; Bradshaw, J. The importance of early identification and intervention for children with or at risk for autism spectrum disorders. *Int. J. Speech-Lang. Pathol.* **2014**, *16*, 50–56. [CrossRef] [PubMed]
25. Horlin, C.; Falkmer, M.; Parsons, R.; Albrecht, M.A.; Falkmer, T. The cost of autism spectrum disorders. *PLoS ONE* **2014**, *9*, e106552. [CrossRef] [PubMed]
26. Jacobson, J.W.; Mulick, J.A. System and cost research issues in treatments for people with autistic disorders. *J. Autism Dev. Disord.* **2000**, *30*, 585–593. [CrossRef] [PubMed]
27. Evans, D.B.; Hsu, J.; Boerma, T. Universal health coverage and universal access. *Bull. World Health Organ.* **2013**, *91*, 546–546A. [CrossRef]
28. Mandell, D.S.; Novak, M.M.; Zubritsky, C.D. Factors associated with age of diagnosis among children with autism spectrum disorders. *Pediatrics* **2005**, *116*, 1480–1486. [CrossRef]
29. Szymanski, C.A.; Brice, P.J.; Lam, K.H.; Hotto, S.A. Deaf children with autism spectrum disorders. *J. Autism Dev. Disord.* **2012**, *42*, 2027–2037. [CrossRef]
30. Bickel, J.; Bridgemohan, C.; Sideridis, G.; Huntington, N. Child and family characteristics associated with age of diagnosis of an autism spectrum disorder in a tertiary care setting. *J. Dev. Behav. Pediatr.* **2015**, *36*, 1–7. [CrossRef]
31. Eriksson, M.A.; Westerlund, J.; Hedvall, Å.; Åmark, P.; Gillberg, C.; Fernell, E. Medical conditions affect the outcome of early intervention in preschool children with autism spectrum disorders. *Eur. Child Adolesc. Psychiatry* **2013**, *22*, 23–33. [CrossRef]
32. Simonoff, E.; Pickles, A.; Charman, T.; Chandler, S.; Loucas, T.; Baird, G. Psychiatric disorders in children with autism spectrum disorders: Prevalence, comorbidity, and associated factors in a population-derived sample. *J. Am. Acad. Child Adolesc. Psychiatry* **2008**, *47*, 921–929. [CrossRef]
33. Harstad, E.; Huntington, N.; Bacic, J.; Barbaresi, W. Disparity of care for children with parent-reported autism spectrum disorders. *Acad. Pediatr.* **2013**, *13*, 334–339. [CrossRef]
34. Delobel-Ayoub, M.; Ehlinger, V.; Klapouszczak, D.; Maffre, T.; Raynaud, J.-P.; Delpierre, C.; Arnaud, C. Socioeconomic Disparities and Prevalence of Autism Spectrum Disorders and Intellectual Disability. *PLoS ONE* **2015**, *10*, e0141964. [CrossRef] [PubMed]
35. Durkin, M.S.; Maenner, M.J.; Meaney, F.J.; Levy, S.E.; DiGuiseppi, C.; Nicholas, J.S.; Kirby, R.S.; Pinto-Martin, J.A.; Schieve, L.A. Socioeconomic inequality in the prevalence of autism spectrum disorder: Evidence from a U.S. cross-sectional study. *PLoS ONE* **2010**, *5*, e11551. [CrossRef] [PubMed]
36. Chaidez, V.; Hansen, R.L.; Hertz-Picciotto, I. Autism spectrum disorders in Hispanics and non-Hispanics. *Autism Int. J. Res. Pract.* **2012**, *16*, 381–397. [CrossRef] [PubMed]
37. Daniels, A.M.; Mandell, D.S. Explaining differences in age at autism spectrum disorder diagnosis: A critical review. *Autism Int. J. Res. Pract.* **2014**, *18*, 583–597. [CrossRef]

38. Mandell, D.S.; Listerud, J.; Levy, S.E.; Pinto-Martin, J.A. Race differences in the age at diagnosis among medicaid-eligible children with autism. *J. Am. Acad. Child Adolesc. Psychiatry* **2002**, *41*, 1447–1453. [CrossRef]
39. Mandell, D.S.; Morales, K.H.; Xie, M.; Lawer, L.J.; Stahmer, A.C.; Marcus, S.C. Age of diagnosis among Medicaid-enrolled children with autism, 2001–2004. *Psychiatr. Serv.* **2010**, *61*, 822–829. [CrossRef]
40. Rivard, M.; Millau, M.; Magnan, C.; Mello, C.; Boulé, M. Snakes and Ladders: Barriers and Facilitators Experienced by Immigrant Families when Accessing an Autism Spectrum Disorder Diagnosis. *J. Dev. Phys. Disabil.* **2019**, *31*, 519–539. [CrossRef]
41. Valicenti-McDermott, M.; Hottinger, K.; Seijo, R.; Shulman, L. Age at diagnosis of autism spectrum disorders. *J. Pediatr.* **2012**, *161*, 554–556. [CrossRef]
42. Samadi, S.A.; McConkey, R. Autism in developing countries: Lessons from iran. *Autism Res. Treat.* **2011**, *2011*, 145359. [CrossRef]
43. VanDenHeuvel, A.; Fitzgerald, M.; Greiner, B.; Perry, I.J. Screening for autistic spectrum disorder at the 18-month developmental assessment: A population-based study. *Ir. Med. J* **2007**, *100*, 565–567.
44. Liptak, G.S.; Benzoni, L.B.; Mruzek, D.W.; Nolan, K.W.; Thingvoll, M.A.; Wade, C.M.; Fryer, G.E. Disparities in diagnosis and access to health services for children with autism: Data from the National Survey of Children's Health. *J. Dev. Behav. Pediatr.* **2008**, *29*, 152–160. [CrossRef] [PubMed]
45. Hussein, A.M.; Pellicano, E.; Crane, L. Understanding and awareness of autism among Somali parents living in the United Kingdom. *Autism Int. J. Res. Pract.* **2019**, *23*, 1408–1418. [CrossRef] [PubMed]
46. Sritharan, B.; Koola, M.M. Barriers faced by immigrant families of children with autism: A program to address the challenges. *Asian J. Psychiatry* **2019**, *39*, 53–57. [CrossRef]
47. Zuckerman, K.E.; Sinche, B.; Mejia, A.; Cobian, M.; Becker, T.; Nicolaidis, C. Latino parents' perspectives on barriers to autism diagnosis. *Acad. Pediatr.* **2014**, *14*, 301–308. [CrossRef] [PubMed]
48. Bailey, D.B.; Skinner, D.; Correa, V.; Arcia, E.; Reyes-Blanes, M.E.; Rodriguez, P.; Vázquez-Montilla, E.; Skinner, M. Needs and supports reported by Latino families of young children with developmental disabilities. *Am. J. Ment. Retard.* **1999**, *104*, 437–451. [CrossRef]
49. Dyches, T.T.; Wilder, L.K.; Sudweeks, R.R.; Obiakor, F.E.; Algozzine, B. Multicultural issues in autism. *J. Autism Dev. Disord.* **2004**, *34*, 211–222. [CrossRef]
50. Rogers-Dulan, J.; Blacher, J. African American families, religion, and disability: A conceptual framework. *Ment. Retard.* **1995**, *33*, 226–238.
51. Matson, J.L.; Matheis, M.; Burns, C.O.; Esposito, G.; Venuti, P.; Pisula, E.; Misiak, A.; Kalyva, E.; Tsakiris, V.; Kamio, Y.; et al. Examining cross-cultural differences in autism spectrum disorder: A multinational comparison from Greece, Italy, Japan, Poland, and the United States. *Eur. Psychiatry J. Assoc. Eur. Psychiatr.* **2017**, *42*, 70–76. [CrossRef]
52. Pondé, M.P.; Rousseau, C.; Carlos, M.A.C. Pervasive developmental disorder in the children of immigrant parents: Comparison of different assessment instruments. *Arq. Neuropsiquiatr.* **2013**, *71*, 877–882. [CrossRef]
53. Carruthers, S.; Kinnaird, E.; Rudra, A.; Smith, P.; Allison, C.; Auyeung, B.; Chakrabarti, B.; Wakabayashi, A.; Baron-Cohen, S.; Bakolis, I.; et al. A cross-cultural study of autistic traits across India, Japan and the UK. *Mol. Autism* **2018**, *9*, 52. [CrossRef]
54. American Psychological Association. Ethical Principles of Psychologists and Code of Conduct (2002, Amended Effective 1 June 2010, and 1 January 2017). 2017. Available online: https://www.apa.org/ethics/code/ethics-code-2017.pdf (accessed on 14 July 2020).
55. STATcube- Statistical Database of STATISCS AUSTRIA. Available online: http://www.statistik.at/web_en/publications_services/statcube/index.html (accessed on 14 July 2020).
56. Fellinger, J.; Holzinger, D. Creating innovative clinical and service models for communication: Institut fuer Sinnes- und Sprachneurologie. *J. Dev. Behav. Pediatr.* **2014**, *35*, 148–153. [CrossRef] [PubMed]
57. Holzinger, D.; Laister, D.; Vivanti, G.; Barbaresi, W.J.; Fellinger, J. Feasibility and Outcomes of the Early Start Denver Model Implemented with Low Intensity in a Community Setting in Austria. *J. Dev. Behav. Pediatr.* **2019**, *40*, 354–363. [CrossRef] [PubMed]
58. World Health Organization; Ebrary, Inc. *The ICD-10 Classification of Mental and Behavioural Disorders: Diagnostic Criteria for Research*; World Health Organization: Geneva, Switzerland, 1993; ISBN 9789241544559.
59. Poustka, L. *ADOS-2: Diagnostische Beobachtungsskala für Autistische Störungen 2*; Hogrefe: Göttingen, Germany, 2015.

60. Mullen, E.M. *Mullen Scales of Early Learning (AGS ed.)*; American Guidance Service Inc.: Circle Pines, MN, USA, 1995.
61. Bayley scales of infant and toddler development. In *Harcourt Assessment*; Springer: Boston, MA, USA, 2006.
62. Petermann, F.; Petermann, U.J. *Hamburg Wechsler Intelligenztest für Kinder IV (HAWIK-IV)*; Huber: Bern, Switzerland, 2008.
63. Gotham, K.; Pickles, A.; Lord, C. Standardizing ADOS scores for a measure of severity in autism spectrum disorders. *J. Autism Dev. Disord.* **2009**, *39*, 693–705. [CrossRef] [PubMed]
64. Lord, C.; Rutter, M.; Le, C.A. Autism Diagnostic Interview-Revised: A revised version of a diagnostic interview for caregivers of individuals with possible pervasive developmental disorders. *J. Autism Dev. Disord.* **1994**, *24*, 659–685. [CrossRef] [PubMed]
65. Gearing, R.E.; Mian, I.A.; Barber, J.; Ickowicz, A. A methodology for conducting retrospective chart review research in child and adolescent psychiatry. *J. Can. Acad. Child Adolesc. Psychiatry = J. de l'Academie canadienne de psychiatrie de l'enfant et de l'adolescent* **2006**, *15*, 126–134.
66. Vassar, M.; Holzmann, M. The retrospective chart review: Important methodological considerations. *J. Educ. Eval. Health Prof.* **2013**, *10*, 12. [CrossRef]
67. The World Medical Association, Inc. (WMA). WMA DoH Übersetzung DE_Rev 190905: Declaration of Helsinki of 1975, 2013 Reviewed 2013. Available online: https://www.wma.net/policy/hb-e-version-2019/ (accessed on 14 July 2020).
68. Cohen, J.; Cohen, P.; West, S.G.; Aiken, L.S. *Applied Multiple Regression/Correlation Analysis for the Behavioral Sciences*, 3rd ed.; Routledge, Taylor & Francis Group: New York, NY, USA; London, UK, 2003; ISBN 9780805822236.
69. Kelley, K.; Preacher, K.J. On effect size. *Psychol. Methods* **2012**, *17*, 137–152. [CrossRef]
70. Peterson, R.A.; Brown, S.P. On the use of beta coefficients in meta-analysis. *J. Appl. Psychol.* **2005**, *90*, 175–181. [CrossRef]
71. Enders, C.K. Multiple imputation as a flexible tool for missing data handling in clinical research. *Behav. Res. Ther.* **2017**, *98*, 4–18. [CrossRef]
72. Rubin, D.B. *Multiple Imputation for Nonresponse in Surveys, [Book on Demand]*; John Wiley: Hoboken, NJ, USA, 2011; ISBN 978-0-471-65574-9.
73. Keller, B.T.; Enders, C.K. Blimp User's Manual (Version 1.0), Los Angeles, CA, USA. 2017. Available online: http://www.appliedmissingdata.com/blimpuserguide-4.pdf (accessed on 14 July 2020).
74. von Hippel, P.T. How Many Imputations Do You Need? A Two-stage Calculation Using a Quadratic Rule. *Sociol. Methods Res.* **2018**. [CrossRef]
75. Muthén, L.K.; Muthén, B.O. *Mplus User's Guide*, 8th ed.; Muthén & Muthén: Los Angeles, CA, USA, 1998–2017.
76. The Jamovi Project. Jamovi. (Version 1.1), 2019, Sydney, Australia. Available online: https://www.jamovi.org/about.html (accessed on 14 July 2020).
77. Schenk, L.; Kamtsiuris, P.; Ellert, U. Ambulante Versorgung von Kindern mit Migrationshintergrund–Inanspruchnahme und Zufriedenheit. *Gesundheitswesen* **2009**, *71*. [CrossRef]
78. Zuckerman, K.E.; Mattox, K.; Donelan, K.; Batbayar, O.; Baghaee, A.; Bethell, C. Pediatrician identification of Latino children at risk for autism spectrum disorder. *Pediatrics* **2013**, *132*, 445–453. [CrossRef] [PubMed]
79. Magnusson, C.; Rai, D.; Goodman, A.; Lundberg, M.; Idring, S.; Svensson, A.; Koupil, I.; Serlachius, E.; Dalman, C. Migration and autism spectrum disorder: Population-based study. *Br. J. Psychiatry* **2012**, *201*, 109–115. [CrossRef] [PubMed]
80. Magnusson, M.; Rasmussen, F.; Sundelin, C. Early identification of children with communication disabilities–evaluation of a screening programme in a Swedish county. *Acta Paediatr.* **1996**, *85*, 1319–1326. [CrossRef] [PubMed]
81. Lampi, K.M.; Lehtonen, L.; Tran, P.L.; Suominen, A.; Lehti, V.; Banerjee, P.N.; Gissler, M.; Brown, A.S.; Sourander, A. Risk of autism spectrum disorders in low birth weight and small for gestational age infants. *J. Pediatr.* **2012**, *161*, 830–836. [CrossRef]

82. Kiing, J.S.H.; Neihart, M.; Chan, Y.-H. Teachers' role in identifying young children at risk for developmental delay and disabilities: Usefulness of the Parents Evaluation of Developmental Status tool. *Child Care Health Dev.* **2019**, *45*, 637–643. [CrossRef]
83. Henrichs, J.; Rescorla, L.; Donkersloot, C.; Schenk, J.J.; Raat, H.; Jaddoe, V.W.V.; Hofman, A.; Verhulst, F.C.; Tiemeier, H. Early Vocabulary Delay and Behavioral/Emotional Problems in Early Childhood: The Generation R Study. *J. Speech Lang. Hear. Res.* **2013**, *56*, 553–566. [CrossRef]

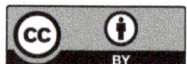

© 2020 by the authors. Licensee MDPI, Basel, Switzerland. This article is an open access article distributed under the terms and conditions of the Creative Commons Attribution (CC BY) license (http://creativecommons.org/licenses/by/4.0/).

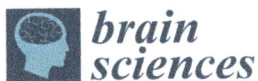 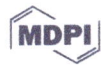

Article

"Mom Let's Go to the Dentist!" Preliminary Feasibility of a Tailored Dental Intervention for Children with Autism Spectrum Disorder in the Italian Public Health Service

Antonio Narzisi [1,†], Mariasole Bondioli [2,†], Francesca Pardossi [3,†], Lucia Billeci [4], Maria Claudia Buzzi [5], Marina Buzzi [5], Martina Pinzino [6], Caterina Senette [5], Valentina Semucci [7], Alessandro Tonacci [4], Fabio Uscidda [2], Benedetta Vagelli [8], Maria Rita Giuca [3,9] and Susanna Pelagatti [2,10,*]

1. IRCCS Stella Maris Foundation, 56018 Pisa (Calambrone), Italy; antonio.narzisi@fsm.unipi.it
2. Department of Informatics, University of Pisa, 56127 Pisa, Italy; mariasole.bondioli@gmail.com (M.B.); fabio.usc@gmail.com (F.U.)
3. Unit of Odontostomatology and Oral Surgery, University Hospital of Pisa, 56126 Pisa Italy; f.pardossi@yahoo.it (F.P.); mariarita.giuca@med.unipi.it (M.R.G.)
4. Institute of Clinical Physiology, National Research Council of Italy, (IFC-CNR), 56124 Pisa, Italy; lucia.billeci@ifc.cnr.it (L.B.); atonacci@ifc.cnr.it (A.T.)
5. Institute of Informatics and Telematics, National Research Council of Italy, (IIT-CNR), 56125 Pisa, Italy; claudia.buzzi@iit.cnr.it (M.C.B.); marina.buzzi@iit.cnr.it (M.B.); caterina.senette@iit.cnr.it (C.S.)
6. Institute of Neuroscience, National Research Council of Italy of Italy, (IN-CNR), 56125 Pisa, Italy; martinapinzino@outlook.it
7. UFSMIA, Zona Livorno, Azienda USL Toscana Nord Ovest, 57124 Livorno, Italy; valentina.semucci@uslnordovest.toscana.it
8. UFSMIA, Zona Pisana, Azienda USL Toscana Nord Ovest, 56121 Pisa, Italy; benedetta.vagelli@uslnordovest.toscana.it
9. Department of Surgical, Medical and Molecular Pathology and Critical Care Medicine, University of Pisa, 56126 Pisa, Italy
10. Autismo Pisa APS, Autism Parents Association, 56100 Pisa, Italy
* Correspondence: susanna.pelagatti@unipi.it; Tel.: +39-050-2212772
† These authors contributed equally to this work.

Received: 29 May 2020; Accepted: 10 July 2020; Published: 12 July 2020

Abstract: Children with autism spectrum disorder (ASD) show worse oral health than their peers. Their access to health services is, at present, inadequate: few high-quality interventions have been designed and implemented to improve their care procedures so far. The purpose of this study is to describe an experience of dental care supported by Information and Communication Technologies (ICT), for children with ASD in a public health service. In our study, 59 children (mean age 9.9 years; SD = 5.43) participated in the MyDentist project. It integrates classic dental care techniques with new practices for desensitization and fear control, delivered through an enhanced customized ICT-based intervention aiming at familiarizing the child with ASD with the medical setting and procedures. Two questionnaires were filled out by parents to describe the acceptability of the MyDentist experience for their children. Significant results were shown from T0 (before initiating MyDentist) to T1 (after 6 months of the MyDentist experience) regarding improved oral hygiene and cooperation during dental treatments. Families positively assessed the use of ICT support. In conclusion, the project demonstrated acceptability by parents, suggesting that public health dental care and prevention can be successfully implemented without resorting to costly pharmacological interventions (with potential side effects), taking better care of children's health.

Keywords: autism; dental care; oral health; medical procedures; ICT; wearable sensors

1. Introduction

Autism spectrum disorder (ASD) is a severe multifactorial disorder characterized by an umbrella of specific symptoms in the areas of social communication, restricted interests, and repetitive behaviors [1]. The incidence of ASD is worldwide and recent epidemiological data estimated it to be 1/54 in United States and 1/87 in Italy [2,3]. ASD varies greatly in the severity of associated socio-communicative impairments and in the degree of cognitive and language development [4]. Although there is no specific relationship between ASD and oral disease, it is well-recognized that many individuals with ASD have much worse oral health than non-autistic people [5–10]. This may be related to barriers to dental services, sensory sensitivities and heightened levels of stress and anxiety during care; these factors may affect the level of cooperation of individuals with ASD in regard to daily hygiene routines, oral exams, and dental care [11–17]. The presence of comorbid self-injurious behaviors, poor oral care at home and specific dietary habits that can favor tooth decay should also be considered [17,18].

Sensory sensitivity is extremely heterogeneous in subjects with ASD [19,20]. It can include hyper-sensitivity to specific sensory input. Subjects with ASD can also experience sensory overload, becoming overwhelmed by incoming stimuli. In these situations, sights, sounds, smells, tastes, touch, balance and body awareness can feel like real physical pain [19,20].

These children can also present intellectual disabilities and significant behavioral issues [21].

These features make it difficult for dentists to assess and treat children with ASD; due to sensory sensitivity and/or intellectual disability, it may be necessary to resort to general anesthesia or sedation (conscious or deep) for dental care or invasive treatment [22–24].

Unfortunately, the professional training offered by most university programs does not deal specifically with people with ASD, so it is necessary to teach dental professionals how to treat them correctly [22]. Children with ASD need to be supported and guided during the visit by an interdisciplinary plan of action that takes into account their specific needs in order to promote better dental health [22,25,26]. Therefore, to increase the probability of successful dental treatment for patients with ASD, dentists should have an in-depth interdisciplinary understanding of ASD in terms of symptomatology and functional profiles [27,28]. However, as highlighted by the World Health Organization (WHO) and American Academy of Pediatric Dentistry, access to services and support for people with ASD is presently inadequate [29,30].

In order improve cooperation of patients with ASD in a dental setting, a link between the behavioral approach and the personalized use of information and communication technologies (ICT) could be efficacious. According to previous studies conducted on children with ASD, it is possible to achieve improved oral hygiene also with both Augmentative Alternative Communication (AAC) and online video modeling sessions [31,32]. The AAC encompasses the communication methods used to supplement speech for those with specific impairments in the production or comprehension of spoken language. Specifically, AAC technologies support children with ASD to (a) enhance language learning, (b) facilitate social interaction and (c) teach interaction strategies to communication partners [31]. Video modeling is a mode for teaching behaviors that uses video recording to provide a visual model of the targeted behavior or skill. Video modeling could include basic video modeling, video self-modeling, point-of-view video modeling, and video prompting [32].

This type of studies [31,32] provides preliminary support for the use of ICT-enhanced interventions to improve oral hygiene for children with autism [33,34]. Providing dental care to patients with ASD may require modifying the traditional treatment plans and settings [33,34], which include many sensory stimuli that may affect the way children behave. Therefore, it is extremely important to think about functional ways to reduce these users' anxiety and sensory hypersensitivity in order to increase their compliance with procedures and to carry out dental care as planned. Despite the high prevalence of issues in treating people with ASD, only few randomized controlled pilot studies have been designed and implemented to improve their dental care procedures so far [17,35–37]. The extreme importance of oral health in children with ASD is due to the potential beneficial effects on chewing/eating, language disorder and dental traumas [30].

The aim of this paper is to describe the first results of the project MyDentist, an in-the-field experience of dental care for children with ASD in an Italian public health service, with the support of a web application that includes various digital materials (video models, social stories, photos, and games), which can be personalized for each patient.

From a clinical point of view, the two specific aims of the MyDentist project were to provide adequate dental care for subjects with ASD and to support and motivate their maintaining acceptable oral health at home. The first aim focused on increasing the patient's collaboration when sitting in the dentist chair, considering the time needed by each specific patient when performing from the simplest to the most complex therapeutic treatment. In this way, it would be possible to reduce the use of general anesthesia, at least for those treatments that generally do not need it, thus lowering economic and psychological costs.

The second aim was choosing the most appropriate method to guide the patient during their oral hygiene routine at home. The selected strategies included teaching patients and parents and/or caregivers how to brush one's teeth, identifying the most suitable tool to reinforce motivation in taking care of oral health.

Confidence is achieved both during dental sessions at the clinic and at home, using games, videos and other digital activities personalized for each patient. Exploiting the combination of these techniques, we managed to first approach the simplest medical procedures (sitting in the dental chair, opening the mouth, having the oral cavity checked first only visually and then using tools such as mirror and explorer), and then to integrate increasingly complex instruments and methods.

At the same time, the project explored the use of wearable sensors to assess subjects' physiological response before and after the dental procedure by applying commercial devices and analyzing, ex-post, the modification of the Autonomic Nervous System activity via signal processing related to electrocardiogram (ECG) and Galvanic Skin Response (GSR), two significant, well-known physiological indicators of psychological stress, which will be better defined in Section 4.

2. Method

2.1. Sample

The total sample included 59 subjects (45 males; 14 females) aged between 4 and 16 years (mean age = 9.9 years; SD = 5.43) who were sequentially recruited at the Department of Pediatric Odontoiatry of Santa Chiara Hospital in Pisa during the period January 2019–October 2020. Inclusion criteria were a diagnosis of autism spectrum disorder (ASD) according to DSM-5 criteria [1] and pediatric age. The diagnosis was certified by the Italian Mental Health System. All subjects with ASD were native Italian speakers (Table 1).

The study was approved by the local Ethics Committee (Prot. N. 10–06/05/2019 AOUP, Pisa, Italy,) and was in accordance both with the ethical standards of the 1964 Declaration of Helsinki and the Italian Association of Psychology (AIP). The protocol for data acquisition with wearable sensors was approved by the Institutional Ethical Clearance board of CNR.

Table 1. Socio-demographic characteristics and functional profile of the sample.

Age	(in Years)
Mean	9.9
SD	5.43
Gender	*n*
Males	45
Females	14
DSM-5–ASD Severity Levels	
Level 1	5
Level 2	37
Level 3	17
Cognitive Functioning	
Normal range	5
Mild	4
Moderate	28
Severe	19
Language	
No words	29
2–3 words	14
Fluent	16

2.2. Intervention

2.2.1. MyDentist

MyDentist was developed as a multidisciplinary experimental approach to dental care and prevention for subjects with ASD, combining ICT, behavioral techniques and a specific clinical protocol designed for ASD. The protocol definition came from the combination of a special dentistry foundation, knowledge and previous experience on assistive technologies for people with ASD, and the crucial support from psychologists and speech therapists offering expert advice in the field of diagnosis of and intervention in ASD. The choice of a multidisciplinary approach derived from previous studies in the literature [24,29] and from a pilot study performed in 2017 [27].

The concepts on which MyDentist has been developed are the following: (i) the high frequency of use of general anesthesia; (ii) the difficulty to face a lack of collaboration when working with ASD patients; (iii) manifestations of anxiety in reaction to the context of the visit; (iv) the need to keep consistency between home oral hygiene and oral care at the clinic. Luckily, some recent experiences in this field have led to the development of new forms of intervention, constantly evolving and mainly focused on psychological approaches where dentists explore the use of different communication channels to enhance collaboration and interaction with children (reinforcement, costumes, play activities) [31,32].

For all these reasons, MyDentist builds on this preliminary literature to explore new forms of patient interaction with the clinical environment and with the medical staff. We propose digital activities to reduce anxiety during the visit, to teach medical procedures and familiarize the patient with the environment. Accessible training is delivered through multimodal activities and games based on AAC, exploiting the visual channel, usually the most effective sense in people with ASD [31]. ICT can facilitate the implementation of AAC, making it easy and comfortable to communicate anyplace, anytime through a mobile device (tablet, smartphone). Moreover, digital AAC (delivered via app) is highly scalable (vast amount of items vs. the paper/plastic version) and customizable, allowing one to add new (personalized) items.

A key feature of the MyDentist approach is the complete personalization of the medical protocol in order to adapt it to the particular needs of each ASD patient, to favor a relationship of trust between the patient and the health professional, and to positively exploit the digital activities.

2.2.2. The MyDentist Web Application

Several studies underline the positive effect of daily use of ICT tools with people with ASD, in both learning contexts and social situations [38–41]. As reported in these studies, people with ASD seem to like innovative educational approaches enhanced by ICT tools mainly because when using technology, they can avoid typical issues involved in human interaction, such as impatience, feelings of inadequacy, unpredictability of people's behavior, and poor recognition of emotions, irony, and figurative language.

The use of ICT to facilitate dental care delivered to patients with ASD is a relatively unexplored field. Isong et al. [35] and Barry et al. [42] both investigated the power of visual stimuli on achieving ASD patients 'cooperation during medical procedures. However, in both these studies ICT tools were not personalized and the children were passive users of digital content. Instead, during the MyDentist experience we tried to offer a personalization of the medical protocol in order to adapt it to the particular needs of each ASD patient, thus making it possible to favor a relationship of trust and to best take advantage of the digital activities proposed directly involving the patient, who become an active actor in the care protocol.

MyDentist delivers a large amount of digital material personalized for each patient: social stories and video models describing all the procedures, the behaviors at the dental clinic and the correct dental care at home, videos and photos taken during dental sessions, and serious games. Managing all this material is very complex and error prone, so MyDentist supports data management with a web application, accessible from any browser on both PCs and tablets. The application helps dentists to build personalized virtual paths following the intervention protocol of a single patient and to provide each patient with all the material needed to boost self-confidence, for instance the photos taken during previous sessions, homework to prepare for the next session and other relaxing and motivating material. The app can be used in many different ways:

- Digital Copybook mode (for all patients): during visits to collect photos and videos (selfies and not) that the child can review and show to family members once at home;
- Mirror mode: during the visits used in camera-selfie mode to allow the child to see himself during dental practices;
- Distractor mode: during the visit to distract or to relax with favorite videos/pictures;
- Reinforcement mode: at the end of the session to perform entertainment and play activities that work both as reinforcement and as consolidation of the activities carried out during the visit;
- Familiarization/learning mode: at home to recall previous visits, to prepare for the next one and to perform digital activities assigned by the dentist (playing games, watching videos, practicing social stories, etc.).

The Web Application (Figure 1) consists of two areas:

- Dentist Area: where the dentist creates the personalized profile of each patient, in order to schedule a visit, build a personalized clinical path, collect multimedia materials of visits, create personalized clinical programs by customizing games, share resources and assign home tasks.
- Patient Area: where each patient can access his/her personalized path. This includes games showing dental procedures in an amusing way (e.g., sequences, puzzles, memories); video models for dental procedures (for instance showing how to use a toothbrush), interactive PDF files to get used to dental clinic sounds, social stories that introduce the dental environment, procedures and/or objects and photos/videos collected during visits.

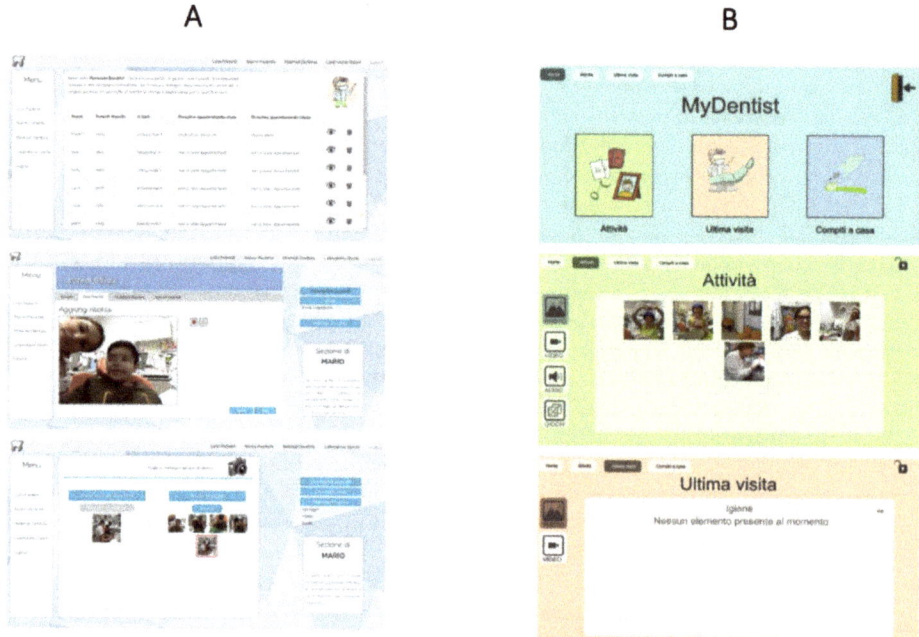

Figure 1. The MyDentist User Interfaces: the dentist's section (**A**) and the patient's section (**B**).

2.2.3. The MyDentist Intervention Protocol

In MyDentist each child follows a personalized path, which starts with one or more familiarization sessions, which goal is to make the child used to the people and the environment. After that, we applied one of three dental procedures. First, prophylaxis with either manual or ultrasonic instruments, which can be challenging for patients with ASD due to the sound of ultrasonic scalers, or noxious tasting prophylaxis paste with manual instruments. Second, fissure and pit sealing, which requires a degree of cooperation, are usually difficult for ASD people. This procedure, despite being a completely atraumatic and not painful, cannot be interrupted, and the patient must always keep their mouth open from beginning to end. In addition, the various materials used have a pronounced taste that may not be easily tolerated.

Third, dental treatment of deciduous and permanent elements is carried out using rotating instruments such as a dental drill and a micromotor. The use of instruments with diamond burrs is reserved for ASD patients with high collaboration skills, since these instruments could damage oral tissues in case of abrupt movements by the patient. In addition, these procedures are often preceded by injection of local anesthesia to cancel painful stimuli. Finally, restoration must be carried out using adhesive materials that require a dry oral setting and therefore a maximum control of salivation.

3. Procedure

3.1. MyDentist Intervention Path

All patients shared a basic path: a preliminary interview with parents, a first visit, some familiarization sessions via a psychological approach, and some operative sessions. A global vision of the MyDentist intervention, common to all the patients, is shown in Figure 2. However, for each step, a personalization of the path of prevention and treatment was defined, according to (1) the specific dental needs (urgent interventions/no urgency, need to improve and increase the norms of oral hygiene at home, need to familiarize the child with the dental clinic in order to be able to carry out preventive interventions); (2) the patient's needs (especially in relation to the educational/therapeutic paths that he/she was already following), also analyzing any manifestation of the spectrum in relation to the procedures carried out. The personalization path is created cooperating with parents and caregivers and based on observations during the sessions. Visits are basically setting adaptation sessions in which everyone arrives at a state of trust by progressively introducing him/her to the dental team, the clinical environment, the tools used, and the procedures to be implemented. It is fundamental not to force the subject to carry out certain actions but to perform them in their own time and way; it is also important to inform the parents/caregivers so that they also respect the chosen timing to proceed through the path.

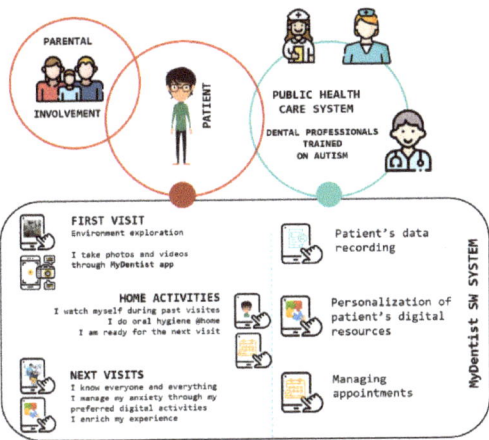

Figure 2. MyDentist global view.

3.1.1. Preliminary Interview with Parents

The interview with the parents takes place in the absence of the patient in order to collect as much information as possible about the child. During the interview, the patient's medical records are filled in with medical, family, and dental history data, which are essential in order to obtain the most complete patient profile. Eating habits (frequency and type of meals and snacks) including the use of sweetened drinks or soft drinks, are also noted. Moreover, oral hygiene habits at home are recorded: type of toothbrush and toothpaste, whether the patient is able to rinse, how many times a day the child brushes his/her teeth, whether alone or with the help of an adult, whether other aids are used (floss, mouthwash, etc.). We also record information about the neuropsychiatric assessment of the child: the diagnosis of ASD (when and by whom it was made, whether there are comorbidities) and the characteristics of the patient's communication (verbal or non-verbal subject, and if verbal whether structured or not), understanding, use of non-verbal language (e.g., pointing), presence of hyper-sensitivity. Next, we evaluate the potential use of images as communication support (what kind, in what way, with whom they are used), the use of ICT supports, the positive stimuli (e.g., music, cartoons) that can be used, and sports or hobbies if any. Finally, we collect information related to the child's present and past therapies (when, for how long).

The interview allows us to collect information about how to plan interventions and helps us to better identify the objectives to pursue, which must be tailored to fit the patient's needs. Finally, we explain to the parents what to do with their children (not to force children to do things they do not want to do during the initial meetings, prepare them with the material needed, communicate with the team periodically in order to record every change); we also instruct the parents on the correct habits to maintain for good oral health.

3.1.2. First Visit

The first visit helped the dentist to get to know each child and to test its reactions to simple requests such as to sit down on the dental chair or to open his/her mouth. During the visit, thanks to the parents' cooperation, we offered a kit of digital tools to the child to help him/her become familiar with the dentist and the clinical environment, before carrying out the medical intervention. The dentist (helped by the ICT mediator) personalized the kit's components in all the intervention phases depending on the child's needs. According to the indications of the parents and therapists, each visit (the first and the other ones) includes the possibility of familiarization at home with the dental activities to be performed in the following sessions through the use of ICT tools such as video modeling, social stories and cognitive learning games (puzzles, memories, sequences), also referring to photos and videos from previous sessions, with the aim of keeping anxiety under control.

3.1.3. Familiarization Session via a Psychological Approach

In order to facilitate the collaboration of the child during the visits we exploit the use of technological devices such as the tablet (as detailed below) as well the use of playful-communicative supports such as costumes and disguises (i.e., Snow White, Joy of Inside Out, Alice in Wonderland) and thematic songs (Figure 3).

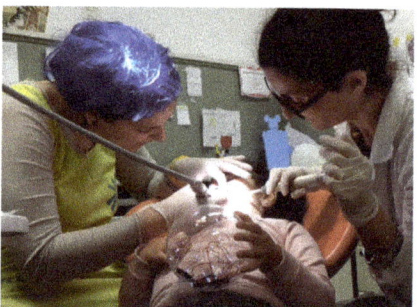

Figure 3. Dental room and the involved staff.

All the procedures, from the waiting room to the final greetings to the team, are carried out by having the child participate and making him/her aware of what the dentist is doing. This is done by communicating the steps of the operative phase. Usually, we adopted multiple strategies based on the child's skills: (a) supporting the verbal instructions with visual cues; (b) Augmentative and Alternative Communication (AAC) and video-modeling.

It is also particularly important to use positive reinforcement after reaching a specific objective and at the end of each session.

3.1.4. Operative Sessions

In the case of a familiarization visit (first visit or other visits if needed) the activities are more flexible but aim to keep to basic objectives such as sitting, collaborating, opening one's mouth, etc. Conversely, in the case of an operative session, such as the treatment of cavities or sealing molars, actions are more focused on small measures that increase attention and reduce distractors.

Whatever the type of visit, the MyDentist approach is based on reshaping the objectives of the session according to the collaboration shown by the patient, even during the visit itself, calibrating compliance with the needs expressed (directly or indirectly) by the child, with the aim of pushing the patient beyond his/her limits. The tablet is considered an integral part of the interaction with the patient but is also an advantage for the staff when collecting material for social stories, cognitive learning games, audio, and video archives.

Only when goals or sub-goals (at least one for each session) are considered achieved, the planned protocol moves to the reinforcement/play phase. Taking care to separate clearly these two stages, especially in the patient's perception, this final phase is devoted to reward the child with a prize such as listening to his/her favorite songs or watching his/her preferred video, playing or drawing with the tablet. Leveraging on the habits of the patient, this moment represents a particularly important ritual for the success of the visit, facilitating the maintenance of concentration even in the most operational sessions.

4. Instruments

4.1. Questionnaires

The research team developed the questionnaires to use in this study. Both questionnaires were pre/pilot tested on a subset of 10 parents. Two experts examined the questionnaires for face and content validation. One of the experts has 15 years of experience in the field of Autism Spectrum Disorder. Both experts have a master's degree in psychology and one of them has a PhD in Developmental Neurosciences. They have been involved in several national and European research projects. For face validity, the experts were asked if all questions were clearly worded and would not be misinterpreted. For content validity, the experts evaluated the relevance of the questions using a scale of 1 to 3, where 1 = not relevant, 2 = relevant but not necessary, and 3 = absolutely necessary. The experts were also asked if other questions should be added to the questions. The remarks of the two experts were collected and discussed and were used to revise the questionnaires. The experts examined the revised questionnaire and declared agreement with its content and clarity.

Parents anonymously completed two questionnaires in order to describe their personal experience with MyDentist. Questionnaire A was aimed at evaluating the approach of children to the dental experience. It was filled out two times, at T0 and after 6 months, T1. It is an 18-item parent-report measure designed to record the behaviors of subjects. Each item describes a specific behavior and the parent is asked to rate its frequency on a four-point Likert scale (0, never; 1, sometimes; 2, often; 3, regularly).

After 6 months of the MyDentist experience, a second questionnaire (Questionnaire B) was sent to the parents of children who participated in the MyDentist project. The questionnaire included 16 items with a positive or negative orientation toward the multi-media support. The questions regarded the evaluation of tablet use and the improvement (if present) in the child's skills. The parents had to answer through a Likert scale from 0 to 3 (0 = no, 1 = little, 2 = quite, 3 = very).

4.2. Psychophysiological Assessment

As mentioned in the previous sections, aside from observing a positive effect of the MyDentist approach as indicated by the results of the questionnaires, we would like to answer the following question: Is it possible to have an "objective" measure that provides an indicator of the effect of MyDentist on stress?

To answer such questions, our idea is to assess the response of the Autonomic Nervous System (ANS) using wearable devices. The ANS measurement is a useful instrument for evaluating the subject's stress and emotional state in ASD. Indeed, when perceiving a stressor, self-regulating processes start by automatically activating the ANS, its sympathetic component [43,44]. The ANS can be monitored non-invasively and reliably by means of wearable sensors, shown to be effective and useful even in young children and in children with disabilities [45–47].

Therefore, in order to be able to objectively evaluate the influence of the practice proposed with the MyDentist approach in modulating the anxiety state of subjects with ASD who undergo dental treatment, we intend to use non-invasive devices for recording ANS activity. Specifically, the idea is to assess the ANS activity before and after each dental session and to longitudinally monitor each child for an observation period of approximately 4–6 months. With this strategy, it would be possible to observe whether the dental session-associated stress is reduced as time passes thanks to the MyDentist application.

To assess the feasibility of applying such approach, we evaluated the ANS activity using wearable devices before and after the first dental session with MyDentist, with one child participating in the study (5-year-old child with ASD level 2 according to DSM-V criteria and an IQ in the "mild" range).

The child was equipped with two wearable sensors, the first of which for monitoring an electrocardiogram (ECG) and the other one devoted to galvanic skin response (GSR). The ECG signal was acquired through the Shimmer ECG sensor, v.2 (Shimmer Sensing, Dublin, Ireland) attached to a fitness-like chest strap manufactured by Polar Electro Oy (Kempele, Finland), in turn interfaced with the human body through two dry electrodes. The sampling frequency was set to 500 Hz. The GSR signal was captured by the Shimmer3 GSR+ sensor (Shimmer) by adhering to two neighboring fingers of the subject's non-dominant hand via comfortable rings embedding dry electrodes, with optimal comfort for the subject tested. As for the GSR, the sampling frequency was selected from among the ones available from the sensor firmware, set to 51.2 Hz. The signals were acquired while the subject was seated comfortably on a chair at a table in a quiet room for 5 min both before and after the session.

The acquired physiological signals were processed using Matlab (Mathworks, Natick, MA, USA). The ECG signal was analyzed for the calculation of the tachogram (RR series, i.e., the time elapsed between two successive R-waves), taking advantage of the Pan-Tompkins algorithm [48] and to extract both time- and frequency-domain features, including:

- Heart rate (HR): the number of contractions of the heart occurring per time unit, expressed in bpm;
- Root mean square of successive differences (RMSSD): measure of heart rate variability (HRV), specifically related to parasympathetic activity, expressed in ms;
- Normalized component of the power spectral density of the ECG signal at low frequency (0.04–0.15 Hz) (nLF); it is related both to the sympathetic and parasympathetic response;
- Normalized component of the power spectral density of the ECG spectrum at high frequency (0.15–0.4 Hz) (nHF); it is mainly related to the parasympathetic response;
- Low- vs. high-frequency components of the power spectral density of the ECG spectrum (LF/HF Ratio): under controlled conditions, it expresses the balance between the sympathetic and parasympathetic nervous system branches [49].

GSR signal was analyzed using Ledalab V3.4.9 (General Public License (GNU), Graz, Austria), a Matlab-based tool. The signal was first filtered by a moving average filter (n = 8) for artifact removal, followed by a continuous decomposition analysis (CDA) via the dedicated Ledalab function, leading to the extraction of tonic (and phasic, not used here) components. Indeed, just the tonic phase of the GSR signal was extracted and analyzed, since the main goal of the analysis was related to the assessment of slow changes in the autonomic activity rather than to the response of a single, time-defined stimulation that would have affected the phasic component of the GSR, as well [50].

5. Descriptive Analysis

Given the exploratory nature of the present study, there was no assumption of the sample size. Categorical data were summarized into frequency counts, percentages, and contingency tables, which were analyzed using chi-square analysis for both questionnaires. Analyses were carried out using SPSS version 21.0 for Windows (SPSS Inc. Chicago, IL, USA).

6. Results

6.1. Questionnaires

Significant results were shown from T0 (before initiating MyDentist) to T1 (after 6 months of MD experience) in 14 of the 18 questions to which the parent had replied (Table 2).

Table 2. Chi Square results between T0 and T1 at Questionnaire A.

	Never (0) t0 n	Never (0) t1 n	Sometimes (1) t0 n	Sometimes (1) t1 n	Often (2) t0 n	Often (2) t1 n	Regularly (3) t0 n	Regularly (3) t1 n	Chi Square $\chi^2; p$
Q.1 Does your child like to brush his teeth?	12	8	33	27	9	12	5	11	4.07; ns
Q.2 Is it possible to teach oral hygiene?	9	8	34	8	11	34	5	8	28.59; <0.001
Q.3 Is your child able to follow the rules for proper dental hygiene?	15	1	28	8	6	26	10	25	42.28; <0.001
Q.4 Is your child capable of using a toothbrush?	27	8	20	34	5	8	3	8	16.84; 0.001
Q.5 Is your child capable of putting toothpaste on the toothbrush?	32	17	16	8	6	17	5	17	19.06; <0.001
Q.6 Does the child use dental floss?	55	55	2	2	1	1	1	1	0; ns
Q.7 Does the child brush his teeth independently?	32	8	19	25	6	24	2	1	26.34; <0.001
Q.8 Is your child able to brush his teeth independently?	8	1	1	8	8	39	38	8	50.89; <0.001
Q.9 Is your child capable of brushing his teeth properly?	13	8	21	17	12	8	13	25	6.19; ns
Q.10 Is your child able to brush his teeth twice a day after meals?	13	25	26	8	11	24	9	1	24.54; <0.001
Q.11 Does the child brush his teeth after meals?	23	8	15	17	9	8	12	25	12; 0.007
Q.12 Does the child experience hypersensitivity (i.e., toothbrush)?	25	42	20	12	8	3	6	2	10.58; 0.014
Q.13 Has the child ever had dental treatment?	48	29	1	17	6	2	4	10	23.47; <0.001
Q.14 Has it ever been necessary to resort to general sedation?	29	1	9	1	5	1	15	56	58.87; <0.001
Q.15 Does the child have a dental visit at least once a year?	24	55	15	2	9	1	10	1	35.86; <0.001
Q.16 Does your child become upset when he has to go to the dentist?	30	1	20	7	7	25	2	25	63.10; <0.001
Q.17 Is your child collaborative during dental visits?	17	17	13	25	17	8	12	8	7.82; 0.049
Q.18 Does he have difficulty remaining seated for the duration of the visit?	12	9	33	29	9	11	5	9	2.02; ns

The result was significant at $p < 0.05$.

Families have positively assessed the use of multi-media support in MyDentist. Parents acknowledged that the multi-media supports were appropriately customized, facilitated a good compliance of the child with the dental setting and reduced the child's stress during the dental examination. According to parents' answers, the use of multi-media supports made children more familiar with dental hygiene, more adapted to and cooperative with the dental setting. Moreover, sensory issues and problematic behaviors appeared more manageable for the children. The multi-media supports helped children in translating acquired skills also out of the dental clinic and in learning the autonomous use of tools for dental hygiene. Parents evaluated the MyDentist project as useful, considered the advice received during the MyDentist experience to be applicable at home and recommended MyDentist to other parents of children with ASD. For only 1/3 of parents the multi-media support was considered hyper-stimulating (Table 3).

Table 3. Percentage of parents' answers to Questionnaire B.

	Questions	No	Little	Quite	Very
		%	%	%	%
Q.1	Was the multimedia support used in MyDentist (MD) useful?	0	0	40	60
Q.2	Was the multimedia support appropriately customized?	0	0	37.9	62.1
Q.3	Was the experience of MD appreciated by your child?	0	0	33.3	66.7
Q.4	Do you think that the tablet was hyper-stimulating for your child?	38.7	19.4	9.7	32.3
Q.5	Did the use of the tablet facilitate good compliance of the child with the dental setting?	0	0	35.5	64.6
Q.6	Did the use of the tablet reduce the child's stress during the dental examination?	14.2	0	42.9	42.9
Q.7	Did the child also use the tablet to become familiar with dental hygiene?	3.2	22.6	51.6	22.6
Q.8	Have you found the child to be better adapted to the dental setting?	0	0	71	29
Q.9	Is the child more cooperative during the dental examination?	0	6.2	25	68.8
Q.10	Is the child more able to control sensory issues during the dental examination?	0	0	48.9	51.6
Q.11	If present, have problematic behaviors during the dental examination decreased?	7.7	13.3	36.7	43.3
Q.12	Is the child more collaborative in performing home hygiene?	0	11.7	50	38.3
Q.13	Is the child more autonomous in the use of the suggested tools for dental hygiene?	9.4	15.6	46.9	28.1
Q.14	Was the MD project useful?	0	0	10.3	89.7
Q.15	Can you apply at home any advice received during the MD experience?	0	0	69	31
Q.16	Would you recommend MD to parents of children with autism?	0	0	0	100

6.2. Psychophysiological Assessment

Concerning the assessment through wearable sensors, in Figure 4 it can be observed that after the dental session, the parasympathetic contribution increased, as suggested by the rise in RMSSD, nHF and by the decrease of LF/HF. Accordingly, the tonic component of the GSR signal decreased with respect to the baseline pre-session after the dental session, as observed in Figure 5.

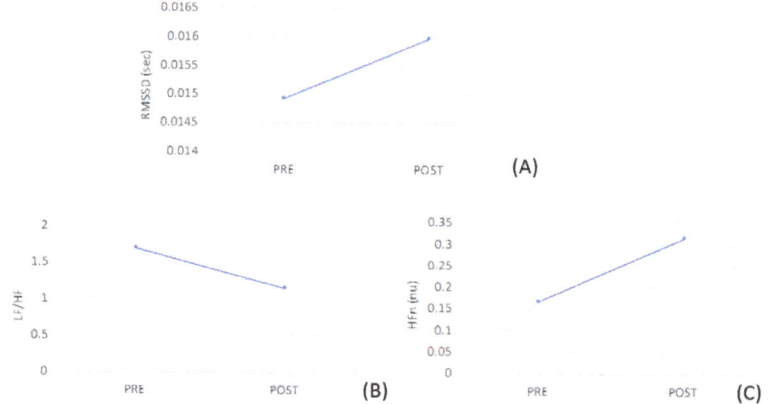

Figure 4. Trend of the features extracted from the R-R series: (**A**) Root Mean Square of the Successive Differences of the R-R signal (RMSSD), (**B**) LF/HF ratio, (**C**) normalized High Frequency component of the ECG signal.

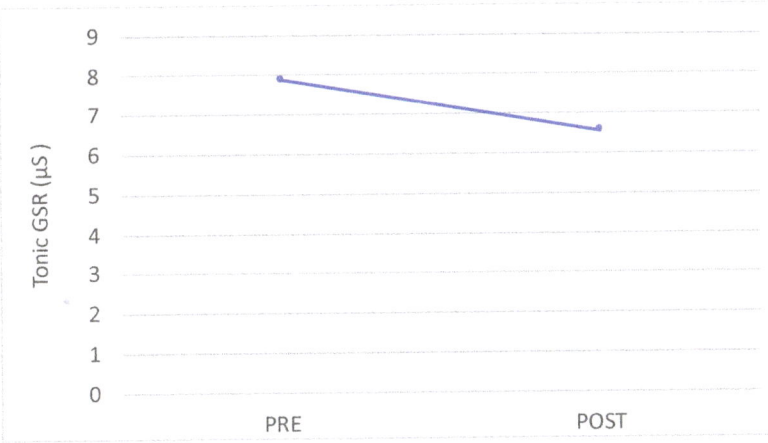

Figure 5. Trend of the tonic component of the Galvanic Skin Response (GSR) signal.

7. Discussion

Children with ASD have poor oral health and they present high care demands, which requires much time, effort, and patience [8,51]. Findings of this study suggest the feasibility of the MyDentist approach and the positive role of technology support [52]. Most of the families of the children involved in this study showed a positive level of involvement (there were no dropouts). Our descriptive data suggest that the children learned the basis of adequate oral care following the rules for proper dental hygiene, using a toothbrush and brushing teeth after meals. Moreover, they showed progressive compliance with the dental visits remaining in a seated position and managing their sensory issues better. Parents and caregivers alike manifested satisfaction for the MyDentist protocol and they strongly recommended it to parents of children with ASD. The ICT use in the MyDentist protocol was positively accepted by the families involved. They considered that the multimedia supports were appropriately customized to meet the child's needs; it facilitated good compliance of the child with the dental setting and reduced the child's stress during the dental examination. ICT has the potential to offer ASD users increased rehabilitation and support to empower their abilities, anytime, anyplace, and on any device (https://iite.unesco.org). Repetitive and predictable answers could help these patients control anxiety and accept new medical practices. Thus, to increase positive results, personalization becomes crucial for making the surrounding environment comfortable and user-friendly.

Our findings also underlined the importance of ICT as an important tool for teaching children with ASD better cooperative behaviors aiding them in the familiarization process with rules and techniques of appropriate oral hygiene. It is well-recognized that children with ASD experience challenges with communication which can negatively interfere with professional oral care [52]. However, most children with ASD tend to process visual information more efficiently than auditory information [53]. For these reasons, in our study AAC and video-modeling as teaching supports were used. Another key finding of the application of the MyDentist protocol is the improved collaborative behavior of the child in home oral hygiene practices. This suggests the potential translational effect of the MyDentist experience.

In addition, the preliminary investigation in a single subject regarding the use of wearable sensors to assess autonomic nervous system response suggested the feasibility of using this approach to evaluate the child's physiological response, thus confirming our previous studies [41–43]. This approach allows us to obtain useful information about the anxious response to a potentially stressful event [36]. In this specific child and for this specific session, it seemed that the child was more comfortable and relaxed after the session, expressing an increase in parasympathetic activity. It would be interesting to observe whether after using the MyDentist approach regularly, the child is more relaxed also before the session. In the near future, we intend to include a fairly large group of subjects compatibly with their profile in order provide more information about the response of the child than that merely obtained from behavioral observation. This would be extremely important for objectivizing the effect of the intervention and implementing more effective and individualized approaches.

In order to evaluate the cost for a generalization in other settings, we need to highlight that the MyDentist intervention differs from the regular dental care intervention for people with ASD in these aspects:

1. Professionals are trained in how to treat people with ASD. As mentioned in the Introduction, to increase the probability of successful dental treatment for patients with ASD, dentists should have an in-depth interdisciplinary understanding of ASD in terms of symptomatology and functional profiles, but unfortunately the professional training offered by most university programs does not deal specifically with people with ASD.
2. Professionals are also trained to use the MyDentist application, which helps to set up a personalized use of the ICT tools
3. In the first period of the intervention, an additional person acting as an ICT-mediator for both professionals and patients/caregivers joined the dental clinic staff.

Indeed, the cost of the MyDentist intervention can be estimated in:

- Cost for the design and development of the MyDentist application;
- Cost of the cloud-storage service;
- Cost of a tablet for the dental clinic;
- A 2-year employment contract for an ICT mediator.

Considering our experience, the professionals were already trained in how to interact with people with ASD and how to use the MyDentist application, since they participated in its design. Patients at home used their own mobile devices.

The estimated cost for replicating the MyDentist intervention in other settings should consider:

- For professionals:
  - Training regarding people with ASD and the most appropriate way to interact with them;
  - Training to use the MyDentist application: to this aim, we are finalizing all the documentation such as user manual, tutorials and demo, which will be freely available.
- For the clinic:
  - A 6- or 12-month employment contract for an ICT mediator.

The MyDentist application will be available for free, at no cost.

Regarding the training of dental staff, it depends on several factors such as the type of course, the duration and the organization that provides the course. However, in order to indicate in more detail what the cost may be, we believe it may be sufficient a brief training course with an ASD expert (e.g., psychologist, neuropsychologist or speech therapist). Furthermore, dental staff will also need an additional day for autonomously training on the MyDentist application reading the documentation and trying the app.

The ICT mediator is a person with skills on the use of digital tools in order to support the work of the dental staff showing how and when to use the application and the tablet. This does not require a very high technical ICT skills so a graduate person may be sufficient. However, the ICT mediator must also have ASD training, together with the dental staff, in order to know how to approach and interact with people with ASD.

In some cases, the treatment path may be longer than estimated, but there are benefits for both the patient, who could be treated while safely avoiding sedation for minor interventions, and presumably

8. Limits of the Study

In this preliminary study, some limitations must be acknowledged. The most relevant is undoubtedly the constrained dataset that strongly limits wide-ranging conclusions. In order to overcome the limits of our study, future investigations should consider: (1) a more systematic data about functional profiles of each experimental participant (ADOS/IQ scores; and robust characterization of the sample in terms of sensory sensitivity and co-morbid conditions; (2) the inclusion of a control group with ASD (e.g., assignment to routine/usual treatment) with a randomized assignment to conditions or, possibly, the adoption of a crossover strategy over the entire population of volunteers; (3) to collect pre- and post-intervention data on parents stress' degree; (4) the lack of a protocol or decision-making tree for the use of the MyDentist intervention.

Finally, a limit of our study was the evaluation of the autonomic nervous system response in only one child for a single session.

Thus, further research is needed to confirm our interesting preliminary (and descriptive) data to determine the effectiveness of the intervention. Moreover, in an upcoming study the enrollment of a larger number of subjects will be important in order to create subgroups of more homogeneous samples in terms of age range, IQ range and oral hygiene issues.

9. Future Direction

Given the overall encouraging results achieved by the exploratory study presented herein, we expect to extend the recording of physiological parameters to the visit phase, at least in a subgroup of individuals who might be more compliant with being equipped with wearables sensors, even during the visit, by the dentist. Such individuals, selected from among the subjects with high-functioning ASD, will compose the cohort for this further evaluation, and will be followed in the next study. This would enable comparing the compliance and the psychophysiological response, and therefore the overall benefit brought by the MyDentist App, with respect to the previous literature dealing with dental research, stress and ASD [54–57]. Finally, other parameters could be extracted from the physiological signals, including frequency of non-specific skin conductance responses (NS-SCRs) for the GSR.

10. Conclusions

Networking between families, caregivers and health providers should be activated with the aim of making everyone aware of the dental health problems that children with autism have to face [13,58,59].

It is essential to combine the efforts and professionalism of all the figures involved in helping a child with autism in order to draw up ad hoc guidelines for dental health in children with ASD.

In conclusion, these preliminary findings regarding the MyDentist project have shown the feasibility of dental care in children with ASD. Furthermore, the project showed the parents' acceptance of the MyDentist project and the feasibility of dental care in a public service without additional costs for families. In the first phase of the dental care program, an additional cost is required for dental clinics facilities to teach clinicians how to implement the intervention with persons with ASD, and to proficiently learn how to exploit the MyDentist program specificities. Moreover, an ICT mediator could be essential to provide the necessary technological support. However, also considering these constraints, we believe that the cost effectiveness is largely in favor of the intervention. Potential benefits for these special-needs patients are extremely important both in term of health (through prevention or treatment, if needed) and in terms of general wellbeing.

Author Contributions: Conceptualization, S.P., M.R.G.; Formal Analysis, A.N., L.B. A.T.; Data Curation, M.B., F.P., A.N., M.P.; Patient recruitment: M.B., F.P., B.V., V.S.; ICT developers: F.U., M.C.B., M.B., C.S.; Writing—Original Draft Preparation, A.N.; Writing—review and editing, A.N., L.B.; Supervision, S.P., M.R.G.; Project Writing, S.P., M.R.G. All authors have read and agreed to the published version of the manuscript.

Funding: This research received no external funding.

Acknowledgments: The authors wish to thank all the participants, the children and their parents.

Conflicts of Interest: The authors declare no conflict of interest.

References

1. American Psychiatric Association (APA). *Diagnostic and Statistical Manual of Mental Disorders*, 5th ed.; American Psychiatric Association: Washington, DC, USA, 2013.
2. Maenner, M.J.; Shaw, K.A.; Baio, J.; Washington, A.; Patrick, M.; DiRienzo, M.; Christensen, D.L.; Wiggins, L.D.; Pettygrove, S.; Andrews, J.G.; et al. Prevalence of Autism spectrum disorder Among Children Aged 8 Years—Autism and Developmental Disabilities Monitoring Network, 11 Sites, United States, 2016. *Mmwr Surveill. Summ.* **2020**, *69*, 1–12. [CrossRef] [PubMed]
3. Narzisi, A.; Posada, M.; Barbieri, F.; Chericoni, N.; Ciu_olini, D.; Pinzino, M.; Romano, R.; Scattoni, M.L.; Tancredi, R.; Calderoni, S.; et al. Prevalence of Autism spectrum disorder in a large Italian catchment area, a school-based population study within the ASDEU project. *Epidemiol. Psychiatr. Sci.* **2018**, *29*, e5. [CrossRef] [PubMed]
4. Levy, S.E.; Mandell, D.S.; Schultz, R.T. Autism. *Lancet* **2009**, *7*, 162738. [CrossRef]
5. Delli, K.; Reichart, P.A.; Bornstein, M.; Livas, C. Management of children with autism spectrum disorder in the dental setting: Concerns, behavioural approaches and Recommenda-tions. *Med. Oral Patol. Oral Y Cir. Bucal* **2013**, *18*, e862–e868. [CrossRef]
6. Gandhi, R.P.; Klein, U. Autism spectrum disorders: An update on oral health management. *J. Evid. Based Dent. Pract.* **2014**, *14*, 115–126. [CrossRef]
7. Lu, J.; Sun, C.A. Evaluation of the effect of concentrated growth factor in oral rehabilitation. *Shanghai Kou Qiang Yi Xue* **2018**, *27*, 93–95. [PubMed]
8. Robertson, M.D.; Schwendicke, F.; de Araujo, M.P.; Radford, J.R.; Harris, J.C.; McGregor, S.; Innes, N.P.T. Dental caries experience, care index and restorative index in children with learning disabilities and children without learning disabilities; a systematic review and meta-analysis. *BMC Oral Health* **2019**, *19*, 146. [CrossRef]
9. Chandrashekhar, S.; Bommangoudar, J.S. Management of Autistic Patients in Dental Office: A Clinical Update. *Int. J. Clin. Pediatr. Dent.* **2018**, *11*, 219–227. [CrossRef]
10. Du, R.Y.; Yiu, C.K.Y.; King, N.G. Oral Health Behaviours of Preschool Children with Autism Spectrum Disorders and Their Barriers to Dental Care. *J. Autism Dev. Disord.* **2019**, *49*, 453–459. [CrossRef]
11. Kuhaneck, H.M.; Chisholm, E.C. Improving Dental Visits for Individuals with Autism Spectrum Disorders Through an Understanding of Sensory Processing. *Spec. Care Dent.* **2012**, *32*, 229–233. [CrossRef]
12. Stein, L.I.; Polido, J.C.; Cermak, S.A. Oral care and sensory over-responsivity in children with autism spectrum disorders. *Pediatr Dent.* **2013**, *35*, 230–235. [PubMed]
13. Stein, L.I.; Lane, C.J.; Williams, M.E.; Dawson, M.E.; Polido, J.C.; Cermak, S.A. Physiological and behavioral stress and anxiety in children with autism spectrum disorders during routine oral care. *Biomed. Res. Int.* **2014**, *2014*, 694876. [CrossRef]
14. Khrautieo, T.; Srimaneekarn, N.; Rirattanapong, P.; Smutkeeree, A. Association of sensory sensitivities and toothbrushing cooperation in autism spectrum disorder. *Int. J. Paediatr Dent.* **2020**, *30*, 505–513. [CrossRef] [PubMed]
15. Bartolomé-Villar, B.; Mourelle-Martínez, M.R.; Diéguez-Pérez, M.; de Nova-García, M.J. Incidence of Oral Health in Paediatric Patients with Disabilities: Sensory Disorders and Autism Spectrum Disorder. Systematic Review II. *J. Clin. Exp. Dent.* **2016**, *8*, e344–e351. [CrossRef] [PubMed]
16. Neil, L.; Choque Olsson, N.; Pellicano, E. The Relationship between Intolerance of Uncertainty, Sensory Sensitivities, and Anxiety in Autistic and Typically Developing Children. *J. Autism Dev. Disord.* **2016**, *46*, 1962–1973. [CrossRef] [PubMed]

17. Cermak, S.A.; Stein Duker, L.I.; Williams, M.I.; Dawson, M.E.; Lane, C.J.; Polido, J.C. Sensory Adapted Dental Environments to Enhance Oral Care for Children with Autism Spectrum Disorders: A Randomized Controlled Pilot Study. *J. Autism Dev. Disord.* **2015**, *45*, 2876–2888. [CrossRef]
18. Duker, L.I.S.; Henwood, B.F.; Bluthenthal, R.N.; Juhlin, E.; Polido, J.C.; Cermak, S.A. Parents' perceptions of dental care challenges in male children with autism spectrum disorder: An initial qualitative exploration. *Res. Autism Spectr Disord.* **2017**, *39*, 63–67. [CrossRef]
19. Kilroy, E.; Aziz-Zadeh, L.; Cermak, S. Ayres Theories of Autism and Sensory Integration Revisited: What Contemporary Neuroscience Has to Say. *Brain Sci.* **2019**, *21*, 68. [CrossRef]
20. Robertson, C.E.; Baron-Cohen, S. Sensory perception in autism. *Nat. Rev. Neurosci.* **2017**, *18*, 671–684. [CrossRef]
21. Epitropakis, C.; DiPietro, E.A. Medication Compliance Protocol for Pediatric Patients with Severe Intellectual and Behavioral Disabilities. *J. Pediatr Nurs.* **2015**, *30*, 329–332. [CrossRef]
22. Rouches, A.; Lefer, G.; Dajean-Trutaud, S.; Lopez-Cazaux, S. Amélioration de la santé orale des enfants avec autisme: Les outils à notre disposition. *Arch. De Pédiatrie* **2018**, *25*, 145–149. [CrossRef] [PubMed]
23. Ferrazzano, G.F.; Salerno, C.; Bravaccio, C.; Ingenito, A.; Sangianantoni, G.; Cantile, T. Autism spectrum disorders and oral health status: Review of the literature. *Eur. J. Paediatr. Dent.* **2020**, *21*, 9–12. [PubMed]
24. Capp, P.L.; de Faria, M.E.; Siqueira, S.R.; Cillo, M.T.; Prado, E.G.; de Siqueira, J.T. Special care dentistry: Midazolam conscious sedation for patients with neurological diseases. *Eur J. Paediatr Dent.* **2010**, *11*, 162–164. [PubMed]
25. Summers, J.; Shahrami, A.; Cali, S.; D'Mello, C.; Kdako, M.; Palikucin-Reljin, A.; Lunsky, Y. Self-Injury in Autism spectrum disorder and intellectual disability: Exploring the role of reactivity to pain and sensory input. *Brain Sci.* **2017**, *7*, 140. [CrossRef]
26. Stiefel, D.J. Dental care considerations for disabled adults. Special care in dentistry. American Association of Hospital Dentists, the Academy of Dentistry for the Handicapped, and the American Society for Geriatric Dentistry. *Spec. Care Dent.* **2002**, *22* (Suppl. 3), 26S.
27. Bondioli, M.; Buzzi, M.C.; Buzzi, M.; Pelagatti, S.; Senette, C. ICT to aid dental care of children with autism. In Proceedings of the 19th International ACM SIGACCESS Conference on Computers and Accessibility, Baltimore, MD, USA, 30 October–1 November 2017.
28. da Silva, S.N.; Gimenez, T.; Souza, R.C.; Mello-Moura, A.C.V.; Raggio, D.P.; Morimoto, S.; Lara, J.S.; Soares, G.C.; Tedesco, T.K. Oral health status of children and young adults with autism spectrum disorders: Systematic review and meta-analysis. *Int. J. Paediatr. Dent.* **2017**, *27*, 388–398. [CrossRef]
29. WHO. *Sixty-Seventh World Health Assembly*; WHO: Geneva, Switzerland, 2014.
30. American Academy of Pediatric Dentistry. *Reference Manual 2010–2011*; American Academy of Pediatric Dentistry: Chicago, IL, USA, 2010.
31. Grewal, N.; Sethi, T.; Grewal, S. Widening horizons through alternative and augmentative communication systems for managing children with special health care needs in a pediatric dental setup. *Spec. Care Dent.* **2015**, *35*, 114–119. [CrossRef]
32. Popple, B.; Wall, C.; Flink, L.; Powell, K.; Discepolo, K.; Keck, D.; Mademtzi, M.; Volkmar, F.; Shic, F. Brief Report: Remotely Delivered Video Modeling for Improving Oral Hygiene in Children with ASD: A Pilot Study. *J. Autism Dev. Disord.* **2016**, *46*, 2791–2796. [CrossRef]
33. Bernard-Opitz, V.; Sriram, N.; Nakhoda-Sapuan, S. Enhancing social problem solving in children with autism and normal children through computer-assisted instruction. *J. Autism Dev. Disord.* **2001**, *31*, 377–384. [CrossRef]
34. Rank, R.C.I.C.; Vilela, J.E.R.; Rank, M.S.; Ogawa, W.N.; Imparato, J.C.P. Effect of awards after dental care in children's motivation. *Eur. Arch. Paediatr Dent.* **2019**, *20*, 85–93. [CrossRef]
35. Isong, I.A.; Rao, S.R.; Holifield, C.; Iannuzzi, D.; Hanson, E.; Ware, J.; Nelson, L.P. Addressing Dental Fear in Children With Autism Spectrum Disorders: A Randomized Controlled Pilot Study Using Electronic Screen Media. *Clin. Pediatr (Phila.)* **2014**, *53*, 230–237. [CrossRef]
36. Mah, J.W.; Tsang, P. Visual Schedule System in Dental Care for Patients with Autism: A Pilot Study. *J. Clin. Pediatr Dent.* **2016**, *40*, 393–399. [CrossRef] [PubMed]

37. Nilchian, F.; Shakibaei, F.; Jarah, Z.T. Evaluation of Visual Pedagogy in Dental Check-ups and Preventive Practices Among 6-12-Year-Old Children with Autism. *J. Autism Dev. Disord.* **2017**, *47*, 858–864. [CrossRef] [PubMed]
38. Prado, I.M.; Carcavalli, L.; Abreu, L.G.; Serra-Negra, J.M.; Paiva, S.M.; Martins, C.C. Use of distraction techniques for the management of anxiety and fear in paediatric dental practice: A systematic review of randomized controlled trials. *Int J. Paediatr Dent.* **2019**, *29*, 650–668. [CrossRef] [PubMed]
39. Charlop, M.H.; Milstein, J.P. Teaching autistic children conversational speech using video modeling. *J. Appl. Behav. Anal.* **1989**, *22*, 275–285. [CrossRef]
40. Da Silva, M.L.; Gonçalves, D.; Guerreiro, T.; Silva, H. A web-based application to address individual interests of children with autism spectrum disorders. *Procedia Comput. Sci.* **2012**, *14*, 20–27. [CrossRef]
41. Passerino, L.M.; Santarosa, L.M.C. Autism and digital learning environments: Processes of interaction and mediation. *Comput. Educ.* **2018**, *51*, 385–402. [CrossRef]
42. Barry, S.M. *Improving Access and Reducing Barriers to Dental Care for Children with Autism Spectrum Disorder*; University of Leeds: West Yorkshire, UK, 2012.
43. Porges, S.W. The polyvagal theory: Phylogenetic substrates of a social nervous system. *Int. J. Psychophysiol.* **2001**, *42*, 123–146. [CrossRef]
44. Porges, S.W. The Polyvagal Theory: Phylogenetic contributions to social behavior. *Physiol. Behav.* **2003**, *79*, 503–513. [CrossRef]
45. Billeci, L.; Tonacci, A.; Tartarisco, G.; Narzisi, A.; Di Palma, S.; Corda, D.; Baldus, G.; Cruciani, F.; Anzalone, S.M.; Calderoni, S.; et al. The MICHELANGELO Study Group. An Integrated Approach for the Monitoring of Brain and Autonomic Response of Children with Autism spectrum disorders during Treatment by Wearable Technologies. *Front. Neurosci.* **2016**, *10*, 276. [CrossRef]
46. Di Palma, S.; Tonacci, A.; Narzisi, A.; Domenici, C.; Pioggia, G.; Muratori, F.; Billeci, L. The MICHELANGELO Study Group. Monitoring of autonomic response to sociocognitive tasks during treatment in children with autism spectrum disorders by wearable technologies: A feasibility study. *Comp. Biol. Med.* **2017**, *85*, 143–152. [CrossRef] [PubMed]
47. Billeci, L.; Tonacci, A.; Narzisi, A.; Manigrasso, Z.; Varanini, M.; Fulceri, F.; Lattarulo, C.; Calderoni, S.; Muratori, F. Heart Rate Variability during a Joint Attention Task in Toddlers with Autism spectrum disorders. *Front. Physiol.* **2018**, *9*, 467. [CrossRef]
48. Pan, J.; Tompkins, W.J. A real-time QRS detection algorithm. *Ieee Trans. Biomed. Eng.* **1985**, *32*, 230–236. [CrossRef] [PubMed]
49. Shaffer, F.; Ginsberg, J.P. An Overview of Heart Rate Variability Metrics and Norms. *Front. Public Health* **2017**, *5*, 258. [CrossRef] [PubMed]
50. Boucsein, W. *Electrodermal Activity*; Springer Science & Business Media: Berlin, Germany, 2012.
51. Hoefman, R.; Payakachat, N.; van Exel, J.; Kuhlthau, K.; Kovacs, E.; Pyne, J.; Tilford, J.M. Caring for a Child with Autism spectrum disorder and Parents' Quality of Life: Application of the CarerQol. *J. Autism Dev. Disord.* **2014**, *44*, 1933–1945. [CrossRef]
52. Naidoo, M.; Singh, S. A Dental Communication Board as an Oral Care Tool for Children with Autism spectrum disorder. *J. Autism Dev. Disord.* **2020**, *5*, 1–13. [CrossRef]
53. Yamasaki, T.; Maekawa, T.; Takahashi, H.; Fujita, T.; Kamio, Y.; Tobimatsu, S. Electrophysiology of Visual and Auditory Perception in Autism Spectrum Disorders. *Compr. Guide Autism* **2014**, 791–808.
54. Fakhruddin, K.S.; El Batawi, H.Y. Effectiveness of audiovisual distraction in behavior modification during dental caries assessment and sealant placement in children with autism spectrum disorder. *Dent. Res. J.* **2017**, *14*, 177–182. [CrossRef]
55. Jaber, M.A. Dental caries experience, oral health status and treatment needs of dental pa-tients with autism. *J. Appl. Oral Sci.* **2011**, *19*, 212–217. [CrossRef]
56. Corridore, D.; Zumbo, G.; Corvino, I.; Guaragna, M.; Bossù, M.; Polimeni, A.; Vozza, I. Prevalence of oral disease and treatment types proposed to children affected by Autistic Spectrum Disorder in Pediatric Dentistry: A Systematic Review. *Clin. Ter.* **2020**, *171*, e275–e282.
57. Penmetsa, C.; Penmetcha, S.; Cheruku, S.R.; Mallineni, S.K.; Patil, A.K.; Namineni, S. Role of Dental Discomfort Questionnaire-Based Approach in Recognition of Symptomatic Expressions Due to Dental Pain in Children with Autism spectrum disorders. *Contemp Clin. Dent.* **2019**, *10*, 446–451. [PubMed]

58. Elmore, J.L.; Bruhn, A.M.; Bobzien, J.L. Interventions for the Reduction of Dental Anxiety and Corresponding Behavioral Deficits in Children with Autism Spectrum Disorder. *J. Dent. Hyg.* **2016**, *90*, 111–120. [PubMed]
59. Shah, A.; Singh, S.; Ajithkrishnan, C.G.; Bipinkumar Kariya, P.; Patel, H.; Ghosh, A. Caregiver's Sense of Coherence: A Predictor of Oral Health-Related Behaviors of Autistic Children in India. *Contemp. Clin. Dent.* **2019**, *10*, 197–202. [PubMed]

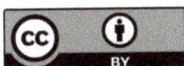

© 2020 by the authors. Licensee MDPI, Basel, Switzerland. This article is an open access article distributed under the terms and conditions of the Creative Commons Attribution (CC BY) license (http://creativecommons.org/licenses/by/4.0/).

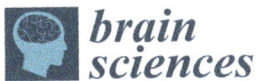 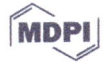

Communication

Effective Strategies for Managing COVID-19 Emergency Restrictions for Adults with Severe ASD in a Daycare Center in Italy

Natascia Brondino *, Stefano Damiani and Pierluigi Politi

Department of Brain and Behavioral Sciences, University of Pavia, via Bassi 21, 27100 Pavia, Italy; stefano.damiani01@ateneopv.it (S.D.); pierluigi.politi@unipv.it (P.P.)
* Correspondence: natascia.brondino@unipv.it; Tel.: +39-0382-987250

Received: 18 June 2020; Accepted: 7 July 2020; Published: 9 July 2020

Abstract: The COVID-19 pandemic has posed a serious challenge for the life and mental health of people with autism spectrum disorder (ASD). COVID-19 sanitary restrictions led to significant changes in the lives of people with ASD, including their routines; similarly, these modifications affected the daily activities of the daycare centers which they attended. The present retrospective study evaluated the impact of COVID-19 restrictions on challenging behaviors in a cohort of people with severe ASD attending a daycare center in Italy at the beginning of the pandemic. During the first two weeks of the pandemic, we did not observe variations in challenging behaviors. This suggests that adaptations used to support these individuals with ASD in adapting to the COVID-19 emergency restrictions were effective for managing their behavior.

Keywords: autism spectrum disorder; COVID-19; challenging behavior

1. Introduction

Autism spectrum disorders (ASDs) are complex neurodevelopmental conditions characterized not only by impairment in socio-emotional reciprocity and communication, but also by restrictive and repetitive patterns of behaviors (RRB) and interests [1]. Until recently, the RRB domain has received little attention compared to the social domain. Several mechanisms may underlie RRB, as they can act as a method of communicating needs or obtaining attention. In addition, RRB may often represent a self-regulatory system to modulate anxiety and the level of activation. While the exact mechanism underlying specific types of RRB may be relevant to guide treatment, the impact of RRB, irrespective of the etiopathogenesis, is particularly relevant in severe ASD with comorbid cognitive impairment: Individuals in this group often present an unpostponable adhesion to routines, rituals, and repetitive behaviors which could significantly impair the quality of life of both ASD subjects and caregivers [2]. Additionally, disruption of routines or, more generally, changes to expectations are usually correlated with a worsening in challenging behaviors [2,3] leading to bouts of self- and other-directed aggressiveness.

The emergence of the COVID-19 pandemic in Italy started in February and is still ongoing. At the beginning of the emergency, the Italian government promulgated several restrictions of increasing severity, starting on 23 February 2020, in order to flatten the curve of contagions. Firstly, the government closed schools, restaurants, malls (on the weekends), swimming pools, and gyms, forbade gatherings (no more than 8 people per room), and recommended social distancing of at least 1 m between each other. It was also recommended to frequently wash hands in order to contain the virus.

It is evident that the COVID-19 emergency restrictions resulted in many relevant changes in the lives of people with ASD and their families. Such a complex situation was extremely difficult to share with service users, especially when learning disabilities were present. Understanding why things were changing, why the sanitary limitations should be scrupulously followed, without losing hope that the emergency would end if everyone cooperates, has been a real challenge for people with developmental disabilities. Additionally, the recommended use of personal protective equipment (PPE) has been controversial among this population. In this paper we focus on a peculiar issue, the impact of COVID-19 restrictions on the routine of daycare centers for adults with ASD and cognitive impairment, which rely on maintaining predictability and an ecologically structured context. The application of governmental restrictions determined significant changes in the activities of the daycare center and a great effort from the healthcare workers to maintain the quality and specificity of services provided to people with ASD. In the end, the difficulties in applying COVID-19 emergency restrictions led to the closure of all daycare centers for people with developmental disabilities one week before total lockdown of the country, which happened on 10 March 2020. These changes may have had the potential to increase distress in our patients and, consequently, challenging behaviors and the need of psychotropic medications [4]. The countermeasures and modifications of daycare center activities were put in place in order to comply to COVID-19 restrictions. In spite of having been dictated by necessity, these restrictions were implemented and inspired by knowledge on management of RRB and problem behaviors. For instance, differential reinforcement of variability was put in place in order to reinforce changes in routine activities or in behavioral responding to ordinary situations. As the spontaneous rate of variability is extremely low in autism, therapists firstly reinforced non-repetitions, moving subsequently to reinforcing of behaviors that were not previously observed.

The aim of the present study is to evaluate the impact of restrictions on challenging behaviors in a sample of individuals with ASD and cognitive impairment attending a daycare center before complete lockdown.

2. Materials and Methods

We conducted a retrospective study evaluating medical charts in a daycare center for adolescents and adults with ASD.

The daycare center "Il Tiglio" is a day center specifically designed for individuals with severe ASD and comorbid cognitive impairment, located in the Lombardy Region, Italy, near a regional nature park. It accommodates 18 individuals with ASD, and the staff is composed of 7 therapists, 1 psychologist, 1 kinesiologist, 2 care assistants, 1 nurse, and 1 consultant psychiatrist. Weekly schedules for each individual are strictly monitored and kept consistent. Planned activities consist of physical activity (water-based activities in a nearby swimming pool once a week, trekking once a week, judo lessons once a week, adaptive physical activity twice a week—both at the daycare center and in a nearby gym), horticultural therapy (once a week), cognitive training for language production and augmentative and alternative communication (AAC) use (every day), occupational therapy (every day), and art therapy (twice a week). The center is open five days a week from 8:00 a.m. to 5:00 p.m.

To comply with COVID-19 emergency restrictions, several adjustments were adopted in order to maintain the best quality of life for individuals with ASD. Specifically, as swimming and physical contact sports were no longer possible to perform, we implemented trekking (which was done every day for at least 1–2 h). Laboratories were split so that no more than 4–5 people were in the same room at the same time. AAC and social stories were implemented in order to provide information about the virus and about specific restrictions (for instance, some of them usually went to malls on the weekends with their parents as part of their routine and, as shops were closed, this could have resulted in potential problem behaviors). All individuals with ASD had already learned how to wash their hands thanks to a behavioral treatment and positive reinforcement; therefore, this routine was increased in frequency and inserted in a visual agenda for each of them. To increase changes in routine behaviors, differential reinforcement of variability was implemented: During the time between the arrival at the day center and the beginning of activities, everyone had a specific routine which could include doing puzzles, drawing, or running in the field outside. Every time the individual with ASD changed his/her arrival routine, a reinforcement (consisting in the possibility to listen to music or watching preferred parts of movies or social reinforcement) was given.

2.1. Measures

As general clinical practice, each day care workers filled out the aberrant behavior checklist (ABC) [5] for each individual with ASD. The ABC is a scale empirically designed to measure psychiatric symptoms and problem behaviors in subjects with developmental disabilities. It is composed of 58 items, evaluating 5 domains: Irritability; lethargy/social withdrawal; stereotypic behavior; hyperactivity; and inappropriate speech. Higher scores indicate a higher level of problem behaviors. The ABC is generally completed by the primary caregiver and informants can complete the scale in 10–15 min the first time they fill it in; subsequently it is more rapid, and it is used in our daycare center on a daily basis. The ABC was specifically designed for subjects living in institutions and residential settings, and therefore appeared appropriate for our center.

2.2. Design

We retrospectively evaluated the effect of COVID-19 emergency restrictions and daycare center implementation on problem behaviors using our registry. We evaluated changes in ABC total scores between 19 February 2020 (the last day free from restrictions) and 4 March 2020 (two weeks after the full restrictions were applied).

2.3. Statistical Analysis

Differences between the two time points were evaluated by means of a paired-sample t-test after the normality of data was ascertained. To account for multiple comparison, Bonferroni's correction was applied. IBM SPSS Statistics for Windows, version 23 (IBM Corp., Armonk, NY, USA) was used for all statistical analyses. Two-tailed p-value < 0.06 was regarded as statistically significant.

3. Results

General characteristics of the sample are reported in Table 1. Our sample was composed of 18 young adults, of which 13 are males. All presented severe ASD; four individuals with ASD occasionally showed self-injurious behavior, while seven had severe bouts of aggression. All individuals were diagnosed during childhood. However, each of them was also re-evaluated by a senior psychiatrist with specific expertise in ASD in adulthood, according to the DSM 5 criteria. All individuals were rated as Level 3 of severity (requiring very substantial support). Diagnosis was supported by ADI-R [6] in all cases. ADOS 2 module 4 [7] was also performed in a verbal subject with mild cognitive impairment ($n = 1$). Cognitive impairment was evaluated by means of the Leiter 3 scale and by clinical judgment. Most of the sample subjects received stable psychiatric medications. Antipsychotics were administered to more than half of the sample (aripiprazole $n = 4$, risperidone $n = 1$, olanzapine $n = 1$, levomepromazine $n = 2$, clotiapine $n = 4$), while mood stabilizers were less frequently prescribed (valproate $n = 3$, gabapentin $n = 2$).

Overall, no significant differences in ABC scores were observed between the two time-points (24.83 ± 11.75 vs. 22.33 ± 12.18, $t = -1.07$, $p = 0.29$). In order to evaluate the generalizability of our findings, our baseline data (t0: 19 February 2020) were compared to the same period of the previous two years (19 February 2019 and 19 February 2018). No significant differences were found (2019 $t = -0.09$, $p = 0.43$; 2018 $t = 0.03$, $p = 0.46$). Additionally, we compared the 19 February 2020 ABC scores with ABC scores of the previous five days to determine if our baseline data were consistent with the previous week: No significant differences were found (p not significant for all the comparisons). We evaluated differences in ABC subscales: No statistically significant differences were found (see Table S1).

Table 1. General characteristics of the sample.

Variables	Mean ± SD or % (n)
Age	22.72 ± 4.75
Gender, male	72.2% (13)
DSM 5 level of severity	
Level 3	100% (18)
Verbal behavior	
Verbal	44.4% (8)
Minimally verbal	27.8% (5)
Non-verbal	27.8% (5)
Cognitive impairment	
Mild	5.6% (1)
Moderate	50% (9)
Severe	22.2% (4)
Profound	22.2% (4)
Medications	83.3% (15)
Antipsychotics	66.6% (12)
Mood stabilizers	27.8% (5)

4. Discussion

Our retrospective study did not show a significant change in problem behaviors in our individuals with ASD after COVID-19 restrictions were initiated. We could cautiously hypothesize that the preventive countermeasures we adopted were effective in reducing distress in individuals with ASD. This could be due to several reasons: First, maintaining the same amount of physical activity (increasing trekking over water-based activity or group contact sports) could have played a key role in controlling problem behaviors in individuals with ASD: It is well-known that physical activity can reduce aggressiveness, stereotyped and self-injurious behaviors, as well as self-stimulation [8]. Walking/trekking could be feasible for almost everyone, irrespective of physical fitness. It is cost-effective and it could be performed outdoors (both in winter and in summer), minimizing the risk of contagion connected with closed indoor environments, while enhancing health benefits connected with exposure to nature. Second, splitting the initial laboratory group into smaller groups (4 individuals or less) could have helped in maintaining the daily schedule without major deviations, allowing for social distancing at the same time. Third, smaller groups increased the ratio between therapists and individuals with ASD, leading to more personalized interventions. Fourth, reducing transfers to other facilities (like swimming pools, gyms) may have led to a lower sensory stimulation and therefore lower anxiety. Finally, AAC as well as social stories could have been a powerful instrument for changing the visual agenda of each individual and teaching new routines (i.e., wearing a facial mask) or enhancing already learned skills (i.e., hand washing).

Our retrospective study presents several limitations: The sample size is small, even if compatible with the average sample size of a daycare center. Another limitation is the lack of a control group. Unfortunately, the absence of a control group is inevitable, as sanitary restrictions were mandatory for all centers in the country. In the future we could design retrospective studies in order to evaluate time fluctuation in problem behaviors before and after the pandemic of COVID-19. In fact, the impact of COVID-19 after the lockdown and closure of daycare centers is yet to be determined. During lockdown, online interventions were implemented as suggested in [9] in order to help parents in caring for their loved ones, who did not have access to their daycare center. Additionally, the need for emergency home interventions, as well as dose-increases of psychiatric medications, were required in several cases. Another potential limitation regarded the care workers who filled the ABC and performed the intervention: Our implementation was designed by the coordinator of the daycare center who did not care directly for individuals with ASD and did not complete the ABC scores. All care workers were blind to the subsequent evaluation leading to the present study. Finally, the time interval chosen for the evaluation of the impact of COVID-19 restriction could have been longer in order to detect changes in behaviors; however, the ABC is designed to detect changes in a shorter period of time and the worsening of problem behaviors usually appear more rapidly than improvement.

At present, the COVID-19 emergency is still representing a massive psychological overload for all individuals, among whom we should not forget individuals with ASD, with their peculiar needs. Despite its limitations, our study may provide some important suggestions for the re-opening phase and the return to a "new normal": Daycare centers in Italy are still struggling to find a compromise between minimizing the risk of contagion and providing adequate care for individuals with severe ASD. In fact, the long-term lack of specific interventions in this group may have resulted in loss of skills, reduction of positive behaviors, and increases in maladaptive behaviors. Additionally, returning to the same level of activity as before the COVID-19 pandemic may not be easy. For instance, changes due to restrictions and the general disempowerment of the public care services may slow the return to normality for individuals with ASD. On the other hand, the slow progress may be supportive for individuals with ASD, allowing them to re-adapt to a full daycare schedule at a slower pace.

Supplementary Materials: The following are available online at http://www.mdpi.com/2076-3425/10/7/436/s1, Table S1: additional information about the sample.

Author Contributions: Conceptualization, formal analysis, and investigation, N.B.; writing—review and editing, N.B., S.D., P.P. All authors have read and agreed to the published version of the manuscript.

Funding: This research received no external funding.

Acknowledgments: We thank all health workers and therapists from our day center for their precious efforts. We thank all people with ASD and their families for their strength during this unprecedented crisis.

Conflicts of Interest: The authors declare no conflict of interest.

References

1. American Psychiatric Association. *Diagnostic and Statistical Manual of Mental Disorders*, 5th ed.; American Psychiatric Association: Washington, DC, USA, 2013.
2. Gomot, M.; Wicker, B. A challenging, unpredictable world for people with Autism Spectrum Disorder. *Int. J. Psychophysiol.* **2012**, *83*, 240–247. [CrossRef] [PubMed]
3. Bull, L.E.; Oliver, C.; Callaghan, E.; Woodcock, K.A.; Oliver, C. Increased Exposure to Rigid Routines can Lead to Increased Challenging Behavior Following Changes to Those Routines. *J. Autism Dev. Disord.* **2015**, *45*, 1569–1578. [CrossRef] [PubMed]
4. Courtenay, K.; Perera, B. COVID-19 and people with intellectual disability: Impacts of a pandemic. *Ir. J. Psychol. Med.* **2020**, 1–21. [CrossRef] [PubMed]
5. Aman, M. *Aberrant Behavior Checklist Manual*; Slosson Publications: East Aurora, NY, USA, 1986.
6. Lord, C.; Rutter, M.; Le Couteur, A. Autism Diagnostic Interview-Revised: A revised version of a diagnostic interview for caregivers of individuals with possible pervasive developmental disorders. *J. Autism Dev. Disord.* **1994**, *24*, 659–685. [CrossRef] [PubMed]
7. Lord, C.; Rutter, M.; DiLavore, P.C.; Risi, S.; Gotham, K.; Bishop, S.L. *Autism Diagnostic Observation Schedule*, 2nd ed.; Western Psychological Services: Torrance, CA, USA, 2012.
8. Srinivasan, S.M.; Pescatello, L.S.; Bhat, A.N. Current Perspectives on Physical Activity and Exercise Recommendations for Children and Adolescents with Autism Spectrum Disorders. *Phys. Ther.* **2014**, *94*, 875–889. [CrossRef] [PubMed]
9. Narzisi, A. Handle the Autism Spectrum Condition during Coronavirus (COVID-19) Stay at Home Period: Ten Tips for Helping Parents and Caregivers of Young Children. *Brain Sci.* **2020**, *10*, 207. [CrossRef] [PubMed]

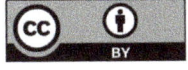

© 2020 by the authors. Licensee MDPI, Basel, Switzerland. This article is an open access article distributed under the terms and conditions of the Creative Commons Attribution (CC BY) license (http://creativecommons.org/licenses/by/4.0/).

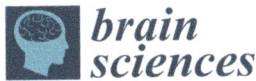 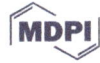

Article

Autistic Traits Differently Account for Context-Based Predictions of Physical and Social Events

Valentina Bianco [1,†], Alessandra Finisguerra [2,†], Sonia Betti [1,3], Giulia D'Argenio [1,4] and Cosimo Urgesi [1,2,*]

1. Laboratory of Cognitive Neuroscience, Department of Languages and Literatures, Communication, Education and Society, University of Udine, 33100 Udine, Italy; valentina.bianco@uniud.it (V.B.); sonia.betti@studenti.unipd.it (S.B.); GIULIA.D'ARGENIO@phd.units.it (G.D.)
2. Scientific Institute, IRCCS E. Medea, Pasian di Prato, 33037 Udine, Italy; alessandra.finisguerra@lanostrafamiglia.it
3. Department of General Psychology, University of Padova, 35131 Padova, Italy
4. PhD Program in Neural and Cognitive Sciences, Department of Life Sciences, University of Trieste, 34128 Trieste, Italy
* Correspondence: cosimo.urgesi@uniud.it
† These authors contributed equally to this work.

Received: 25 May 2020; Accepted: 18 June 2020; Published: 1 July 2020

Abstract: Autism is associated with difficulties in making predictions based on contextual cues. Here, we investigated whether the distribution of autistic traits in the general population, as measured through the Autistic Quotient (AQ), is associated with alterations of context-based predictions of social and non-social stimuli. Seventy-eight healthy participants performed a social task, requiring the prediction of the unfolding of an action as interpersonal (e.g., to give) or individual (e.g., to eat), and a non-social task, requiring the prediction of the appearance of a moving shape as a short (e.g., square) or a long (e.g., rectangle) figure. Both tasks consisted of (i) a familiarization phase, in which the association between each stimulus type and a contextual cue was manipulated with different probabilities of co-occurrence, and (ii) a testing phase, in which visual information was impoverished by early occlusion of video display, thus forcing participants to rely on previously learned context-based associations. Findings showed that the prediction of both social and non-social stimuli was facilitated when embedded in high-probability contexts. However, only the contextual modulation of non-social predictions was reduced in individuals with lower 'Attention switching' abilities. The results provide evidence for an association between weaker context-based expectations of non-social events and higher autistic traits.

Keywords: autistic traits; autism; action observation; action prediction; context; priors

1. Introduction

Autism spectrum disorder (ASD) consists of a range of neurodevelopment conditions characterized by deficits in reciprocal social behavior and communication, as well as by restrictive and repetitive behaviors and interests, which are present in the early developmental period [1]. Beside the other manifestations of this disorder, including social withdrawal and isolation [2], the presence of sensory abnormalities [3] and difficulties in mentalizing processes [4], it has been repeatedly shown that individuals with ASD struggle with making predictions or with deciding what to pay attention to on the basis of prior expectations about the sensory world [5]. The impairments in discerning the predictive relationships between events may not only compromise habituation processes [6], but they may also generate anxiety, resulting in the typical insistence of sameness usually observed in individuals with ASD [7].

This difficulty is further amplified when people are involved in social situations, where unpredictable interactions could take place. Indeed, dealing with social interactions in an effective way often requires the ability to anticipate others' behavior, predicting their intentions from observing their movements. Movement kinematic information, however, may be ambiguous in many (if not most) social situations [8,9]. Thus, a social observer needs to integrate this sensory evidence with knowledge of past experiences aiming at the same goal or with contextual cues facilitating action prediction [10–16].

According to predictive coding accounts [17], the brain works as a Bayesian inference machine, merging prior expectations with current evidence to assess the probability of future outcomes as a result of rule learning. For instance, in the visual domain, prior contextual information is responsible for the elementary regularities that bias our perception of shape and color [18] as well as for the effects of perceptual learning on the processing of visual objects [19]. Moving to the framework of social cognition, studies challenging the comprehension of social behavior showed that individuals with typical development strongly rely on prior knowledge regarding the context in which actions are usually observed in order to recognize action unfolding [13–16], especially when perceptual information is scarce [20]. The predictive coding account may explain the perceptual impairments of ASD individuals in both the social and non-social domains. Indeed, an impaired learning curve may generate deficits in picking up statistical constancies in the environment, favoring routine and attention to details at the price of the broad picture (see [21] for review). Accordingly, reduced reliance on prior expectations relative to sensory inputs has been shown to lead to a plethora of abnormalities consistently observed in ASD individuals [21,22]. In a similar vein, although the ability to read the goal of an action during action observation seems to be preserved in ASD ([23], but see also [24,25] for contrasting results), there is consistent evidence that, when the outcome of the action is ambiguous, individuals with ASD exhibit impairments in using contextual priors to predict action unfolding [20,26–28]. Collectively, these observations highlight the difficulties of ASD individuals in integrating the available sensory evidence with previous experience when dealing with the prediction of both physical and social stimuli.

ASD has been traditionally considered as a clinical condition distinct from typical-development functioning [29]; however, there is consistent consensus in considering the disorder as the upper extreme of a constellation of impairments that may be continuously distributed in nature [30–32]. Along this continuum, people can, indeed, be characterized to a different extent by the presence of subclinical autistic traits. These traits can be measured by a self-report questionnaire, the Autism-Spectrum Quotient (AQ, [30]), which is widely used in research and clinical practice to measure autistic traits in the general population (see [33] for a systematic review). The AQ describes the subclinical autistic impairments across different domains related to either social behavior (i.e., Social skills and Communication) or non-social aspects of cognition (i.e., Imagination, Attention to detail, and Attention Switching).

Previous studies measuring autistic traits in the general population showed that high autistic traits (i.e., AQ scores > 21, 1 standard deviation, s.d., above the group mean) are associated with altered perceptual adaptation for social objects [34]. Furthermore, either individuals with ASD or typical-development individuals high in autistic traits (i.e., AQ scores, Mean = 22.13, s.d. = 5.74) presented a reduced sensitivity to context-based integration of sensory feedback with prior expectation [35]. These observations supported the view of a greater reliance on new information relative to prior information in ASD and high-autistic–trait individuals. A recent study [15] extended these findings to action scenarios, by investigating the association between autistic traits and motor responses during the observation of others' actions embedded in contexts. Indeed, observing actions embedded in contexts that are congruent or incongruent with the unfolding kinematics, respectively, facilitated or inhibited discrimination performance and motor activation, as compared to observing actions embedded in an ambiguous context [14–16]. Notably, lower sensitivity to contextual information and higher reliance on the sensory evidence provided by kinematics were found in individuals with higher autistic traits [16], in particular in the domains of Social skills and Attention to details [16,36].

This points to an association between both social and non-social aspects of autistic traits and impairments in the integration of sensory evidence and contextual information.

Crucially, there is extensive evidence that the behavioral traits associated to social and non-social aspects of cognition may be independently distributed in the general population, pointing to different neurocognitive bases ([37] for review). However, it is still unclear how social and cognitive aspects of autistic traits might be related to the use of previous experience to predict social or non-social events. In the present study, we sought to investigate at what extent the presence of autistic traits might interfere with the ability to implicitly learn the associations between a contextual cue and a specific event (i.e., contextual priors), and to use this association in order to make predictions under perceptual uncertainty. The relation between the amount of social or cognitive autistic traits and context-based predictions were tested in a social domain pertaining the prediction of actions and in a non-social domain pertaining the anticipation of appearing objects. Specifically, concerning this latter domain, we used moving shapes as stimuli in order to manipulate arbitrary associations between a contextual cue and the moving shape, thus avoiding any previously-learned semantic associations that could affect context-based manipulations for everyday-life objects. It is noteworthy that moving shapes have been used as control stimulus for action observation in previous neuroimaging and brain stimulation studies. In particular, a study by Schubotz and co-workers [38] showed that sequential presentations of biological (i.e., action) and non-biological abstract stimuli (i.e., circles) share the recruitment of premotor regions, while triggering distinctive patterns of activations in other fronto-parietal areas. In a similar vein, a more recent study by Paracampo and co-workers [39] asked participants to predict the outcome of hand or shape movements and found that, in spite of comparable difficulty, only the first task was affected by interferential stimulation of the left primary motor cortex. In both of these studies, moving shapes were used as control stimuli for assessing the action-specific or the domain general brain involvement in predictive mechanisms. Capitalizing on these studies, here we adopted an action prediction and a shape prediction task to assess the use of prior information in driving prediction across the two domains.

In the present study, we hypothesized that, in both domains, participants should be biased towards the implicitly-learned contextual priors in order to compensate for perceptual uncertainty. Moreover, we hypothesized that the presence of autistic traits involving social aspects might relate to a reduced reliance on contextual priors to predict the unfolding of actions, while those involving non-social aspects of cognition, especially attention switching, might relate to a reduced reliance on contextual priors to predict the fate of physical events (i.e., object appearance).

2. Materials and Methods

2.1. Participants

Seventy-eight healthy young university students (49 Female, mean age = 24.12, s.d. = 6.06 years) participated in the study. We determined the sample size for testing the effects of a single predictor in the multiple regression design of our study (number of predictors = 5 AQ scales) through the G*POWER software [40]. Based on the results of a previous study on the predictive effects of the AQ subscales on action-context integration in adults with typical development [16], we estimated a medium effect size of $f^2 = 0.15$ [41] and set the significance level at $\alpha = 0.05$, and the desired power (1 − β) at 0.9. Participants were recruited at the University of Udine. All participants were right-handed [42] and had normal or corrected-to-normal vision. The study was approved by the local Ethics Committee (Prot. N. 47/2015/Sper, 26/05/2015 Comitato Etico Regionale Unico, Friuli Venezia Giulia, Italy) and was carried out in accordance with the ethical standards of the 1964 Declaration of Helsinki. All participants were naïve to the aims and hypothesis of the experiment and provided their written informed consent prior to the enrollment in the study. Only after the end of the whole experiment, participants were debriefed about the experimental hypothesis.

2.2. General Design

We used two separate prediction tasks, requiring participants to observe videos of social actions, in an action prediction task, or videos showing moving geometrical shapes, in a shape prediction task. In particular, we presented these videos in two different alternative force choice (2AFC) tasks in a paradigm including a probabilistic learning (familiarization) phase followed by a prediction (testing) phase and allowing the assessment of contextual prior in making predictions [20] when sensory evidence is scarce. Notably, the strength of priors in driving prediction is thought to be especially brought into play in 2AFC, given that top-down signals encoding conditional expectations might influence obliged decisions regarding the physical nature of sensory input [43].

A within-subject design was used. For each participant, the experiment consisted of two separate experimental sessions during which the action prediction task and the shape prediction task were administered, respectively. Each task session lasted around 20 min. The familiarization phase comprised a total of 160 trials equally divided into 4 identical familiarization blocks, while the testing phase was made of a total of 80 trials, presented in 2 identical testing blocks of 40 trials. Each testing block was administered after two familiarization blocks, allowing a few minutes' rest between blocks. The order of the two tasks was counterbalanced across participants. At the end of the two task sessions, participants' autistic traits were assessed by administering the AQ questionnaire (AQ, [30]).

2.3. Stimuli and Tasks

Action Prediction Task. For the action prediction task, the same videos and paradigm proposed by Amoruso et al. [20] were used. During this task, participants watched videos showing a male child (10 years old) who was sitting in front of a peer and was grasping with his right hand an object, an apple or a glass, to perform either an individual action (to eat, to drink) or an interpersonal one (to offer). Based on the kinematics of the hand approaching the object, two possible hints could be suggested: reaching for grasping the object from its side signaled the action of moving the object toward the mouth with the individual intention of eating or drinking, while reaching for grasping the object from its top prompted the interpersonal action of offering the object. Notably, each action was performed in the presence of specific contextual cues: for actions performed upon the apple, the two possible contextual cues were a violet or an orange dish; for the actions performed with the glass, the two possible cues were a white or a blue tablecloth. In this way, stimuli consisted of a total of 8 different videos (Figure 1a).

For both phases (familiarization and testing phase) of this task, participants were asked to watch the videos and to predict the action unfolding (eat/drink versus offer). However, videos of the familiarization and testing phase dramatically differed in their length and thus in the amount of visual information provided. Indeed, videos of the familiarization phase were interrupted after the hand pre-shaping and the reaching phase, two frames before the hand contact with the object, when the amount of visual information was sufficient to distinguish the individual from the interpersonal action (Figure 1b). Differently, videos of the testing phase were interrupted during the hand pre-shaping phase, thus when the movement kinematic was still ambiguous (Figure 1c). It is important to note that, even though participants watched only the initial part of the videos, when these were originally recorded, the child was asked to perform the complete action in order to provide reliable kinematics information. For further details on video recording, please refer to [19].

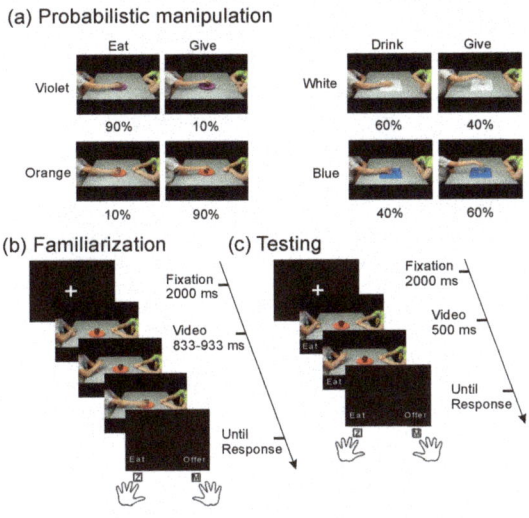

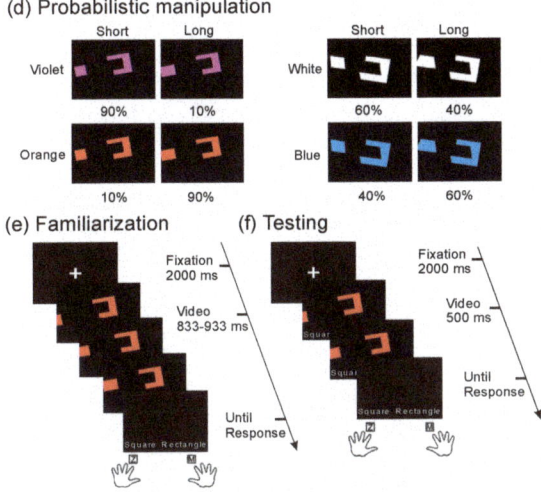

Figure 1. Stimuli and Experimental tasks. Action prediction task: (**a**) sketch of probabilities manipulation for the familiarization phase. Action-context associations were manipulated in terms of their probability of co-occurrence to 90%, 10%, 60%, and 40%; (**b**) familiarization phase showing videos of a child performing individual or interpersonal actions. Participants had to predict action unfolding; (**c**) testing phase showing the same videos during familiarization but of shortened duration. Participants had to predict action unfolding, as during the familiarization phase. Shape prediction task; (**d**) sketch of probabilities manipulation for the familiarization phase. Shapes-context associations were manipulated in terms of their probability of co-occurrence to 90%, 10%, 60% and 40%; (**e**) familiarization phase showing videos of moving shapes approaching the receptor shape. Participants had to predict shape identity; (**f**) testing phase showing the same videos during familiarization but of shortened duration. Participants had to predict shape identity, as during the familiarization phase.

Crucially, during the familiarization phase, we manipulated the probability of co-occurrence between each action and the contextual cues. More specifically, the probability of co-occurrence was set in order to have the 90%, 60%, 40% or 10% of trials representing an action-contextual cue association (namely, for 36, 24, 16, and 4 trials, respectively). For instance, an apple presented on a violet plate could be grasped 90% of the time to eat and 10% of the time to offer. In the same block, an apple presented on an orange plate could be grasped 90% of the time to offer and 10% of the time to eat. For the actions performed on the glass presented in the same block, a glass presented on a white tablecloth could be grasped 60% of the time to drink and 40% of the time to offer. Conversely, in the same block, a glass presented on a blue tablecloth was grasped 60% of the time to offer and 40% of the time to drink (Figure 1a). In this way, we sought to implicitly manipulate prior expectations regarding the action unfolding, based on the presence of these contextual cues. Importantly, the probabilistic manipulation was kept identical across the two repetitions of the familiarization phase within each participant, but we counterbalanced across participants the probability of associations between each action and a given contextual cue.

The same instructions were given during the familiarization and the testing phases. However, according to Amoruso et al. [20], in this last phase during which video duration was drastically reduced, given the perceptual uncertainty generated by the ambiguity of action kinematics, a response bias towards previously acquired contextual priors should occur. Notably, during this phase, all possible action-contextual cues associations were equally presented, thus 10 trials for each of the 8 action-contextual cue video associations were included in the whole testing phase. Before the beginning of the task, participants received information regarding the identity of the objects and demonstrations of the different possible ways of manipulating them. More specifically, we provided participants with specific examples with the original objects used in the videos (e.g., 'this is how we grasp an apple when we want to offer it'). However, explicit information about the associations between contextual cues and actions were not provided.

Shape Prediction Tasks

We developed this task to compare context-based predictions in social and non-social domains. To this aim, the same logic of the action prediction task was followed in designing the task.

Video frames were created in Power Point (Microsoft Corporation, Redmond, WA, USA). They depicted colored geometric shapes appearing from the left side of the screen and moving toward the right, where a still complementary receptor figure was presented. The moving geometric shapes could be a right-angle polygon (a square or a rectangle) or an acute-angle polygon (a parallelogram or a trapezoid). The shapes of each pair of polygons looked similar on their right side, which was immediately visible at the beginning of the movement. However, with the increased visibility of the horizontal segments during the movement, the identity of the specific polygon could be detected according to the ratio between the major and minor axis of the figure, thus according to whether the horizontal segment was longer than (i.e., rectangle or trapezoid) or equal to (i.e., square or parallelogram) the visible right vertical segment. The still receptor hosted, on its left side, a concavity that was suited for binding the moving shape (Figure 1d). As in the action prediction task, we manipulated specific contextual cues based on the color of the moving shape and receptor. In particular, the square and the rectangle could be colored either in orange or in violet, while the parallelogram and the trapezoid could be colored either in white or in blue. This way, 8 different videos were created (Figure 1d). The receptor always had the same color of the moving shape, thus facilitating the salience of the color cue since the very beginning of the video.

For both the familiarization and the testing phases of this task, participants were asked to observe the videos and to predict the moving shape. Importantly, during the familiarization phase, the shapes fully appeared on the screen and thus could be easily identified (Figure 1e). Conversely, during the testing phase, videos were interrupted just one frame after the halfway appearance of the horizontal segment, thus providing minimal information about the ratio of the major-minor axis of the shape and its identity (Figure 1f). In both phases, we varied, across participants, two different response modality versions of the same task. For a first response modality (position response), which was administered to 38 participants, the left side of each complementary receptor contained two concavities, respectively, in its lower and upper parts; each concavity could host only a specific moving shape. Participants were required to report the upper or lower position of the receptor that could host the moving shape. For the second response modality (naming response), which was administered to 40 participants, the receptor presented only one concavity that could bind both possible shapes in each pair (i.e., the square or the rectangle, for one receptor, and the parallelogram or the trapezoid for the other). Participants were required to report the polygon name of the moving shape (please refer to the *Procedure and trial structure* section for further details). This way, we manipulated the contribution of the spatial and verbal ability demands that could affect the difficulty of the shape prediction task and that could be differently loaded in the two tasks.

Crucially, during the familiarization phase, we manipulated the probability of co-occurrence between each polygon and its color, using the same probability settings of the action prediction task. For instance, a violet shape could end up appearing as a square 90% of the time and as a rectangle 10% of the time. Conversely, an orange shape could end up appearing as a rectangle 90% of the time and as a square the remaining 10% of the time. In the same block, a blue shape could be a trapezoid 60% of the time and a 40% of the time, while a white shape could be a parallelogram 60% of the time a trapezoid 40% of the time (Figure 1d).

The same instructions were given in both phases. However, as in the testing phase, video duration was drastically reduced and therefore the shape identity was more ambiguous; we expected participants' responses to be biased towards the contextual priors (i.e., shape–color associations) acquired during the familiarization phase. Notably, during this phase, all possible shape–color associations were equally presented, namely 10 trials for each of the 8 shape–color associations.

As in the action prediction task, the probabilistic manipulation was kept identical across the two repetitions of the familiarization phase within each participant, but we counterbalanced the probability of associations between each polygon and a given color across participants. Before performing the tasks, participants received information regarding the identity of all the possible geometric figures by using two-dimensional paper figures. More specifically, we provided participants with specific hints regarding the similarity of the right side but different major-minor axis ratio of the two shapes in each pair. The possible associations between color and shapes, however, were never explicitly acknowledged.

2.4. Procedure and Trial Structure

The same procedure and trial structure were used in the two tasks. Participants were seated in front of a computer screen at a distance of about 60 cm, with their arms positioned palm down on the keyboard. Stimuli were presented using the E-Prime software (version 2.0, Psychology Software Tools, Inc., Pittsburgh, PA, USA). Video resolution was set at 1280 × 768 pixels, with a refresh rate of 60 Hz. Trials started with the presentation of a central fixation cross (remaining on the screen for 2000 ms), which was followed by video presentation (Figure 1). Videos were presented frame-by frame at a rate of 30 Hz. In the familiarization phase, videos lasted 833–933 ms (25–28 frames), while in the testing phase videos were interrupted after 500 ms (i.e., after the initial 15 frames). For the familiarization phase, at the end of each video, a response prompt was presented at the bottom of the screen until participant's response. It showed, respectively, at the left and right of the screen, the verbal descriptors of the two possible actions (the Italian verbs "mangiare/bere" or "offrire"; in English "to eat/drink" or "to offer") or the position/name of the two possible concavities/polygons (the Italian adverbs "sopra" and "sotto", in English "up" and "down"; the Italian names "quadrato" and "rettangolo", or "trapezio" and "parallelogramma", in English "square" and "rectangle", or "trapezoid" and "parallelogram"). For the testing phase, the response prompt appeared at video onset and remained on the screen until the participant's response; this way, participants could provide their response as soon as they were able to guess the correct response. Participants were asked to respond with their index fingers using the left

(Z) or the right (M) keys corresponding to the left or right location of the descriptors. The position of the descriptors was counterbalanced between participants. An empty black screen was presented for 1000 ms between each consecutive trial.

2.5. Autistic Traits Measure

At the end of the two experimental sessions, participants completed the Italian version of the Autism-Spectrum Quotient (AQ, [30,44]), a self-report questionnaire measuring autistic traits in the general population that is widely used in research and clinical practice. The AQ consists of 50 items divided into five subscales. The Attention switching subscale measures deficits in control processes of cognition and measures the ability to switch rapidly between multiple tasks. This ability is crucial in real life scenarios, where we are challenged by a constantly changing environment and we have to adapt accordingly, frequently switching attention among multiple sources of salient events. This subscale includes items such as: "I prefer to do things the same way over and over again"; "If there is an interruption, I can switch back to what I was doing very quickly". The Attention to Detail subscale measures the tendency to focus more on individual pieces of information at the expense of perceiving the global picture. Typical items are: "I notice patterns in things all the time"; "I usually concentrate more on the whole picture, rather than on the small details". The Communication subscale measures deficits in the skill to properly provide and receive different kinds of information and includes items like: "I frequently find that I don't know how to keep a conversation going"; "I find it easy to read between the lines when someone is talking to me". The Imagination subscale covers deficits in the ability to form sensory images and experiences in the mind. Example items are: "If I try to imagine something, I find it very easy to create a picture in my mind"; "I find it difficult to imagine what it would be like to be someone else". Finally, the Social Skills subscale concerns deficits in knowing how to act in different types of social situations and is measured with items such as: "I prefer to do things with others rather than on my own"; "I find it difficult to work out people's intentions". For each item, participants are required to provide one of four responses: 'definitely agree', 'slightly agree', 'slightly disagree', and 'definitely disagree'. Answers are scored 1 or 0 indicating the presence or absence of autistic traits. Higher scores reflect higher autistic traits, thus greater impairment in attention switching, imagination, communication and social skills abilities, as well as a perceptual bias toward details in spite of a deficit in global processing for the Attention to Detail subscale. Individual AQ total scores range between 0 and 50, while subscale scores range between 0 and 10.

2.6. Data Handling

Individual AQ total and subscale scores were calculated according to standard procedures [30,44]. Independent sample *t*-test (two-tailed) was used to compare the score of male and female participants within our sample and with those reported in age-, education-, and gender-matched Italian samples reported a previous study [45].

Individual performance in the familiarization and prediction phase was expressed as d prime (d'), a bias corrected measure of sensitivity in discriminating between two categories, and as response criterion (c), which checks for the existence of a bias in providing a specific response (see [46]). For the action prediction task, individual actions identified as individual were considered 'hits', while interpersonal actions identified as individual were considered 'false alarms'. For both versions of the shape prediction task, short shapes identified as short were considered 'hits', while long shapes identified as short were considered 'false alarms'.

Individual d' and c values for the familiarization phase were entered into separate 2 × 2 mixed repeated measure analysis of variance (RM-ANOVA), with Task (Action vs. Shape prediction) as within-subject variable and shape-prediction Response Modality (Position vs. Naming) as between-subject factor. For the familiarization phase, the d' and c values were averaged across the four probability conditions due to their unequal number of trials generated by the probabilistic manipulation. For the testing phase, the d' and c values were subjected to mixed 2X2X4 RM-ANOVAs with Task and Probability (10%, 40%, 60%, 90%) as within-subject variables and shape-prediction Response Modality as between-subject factor. Estimates of the effect size were obtained using the partial η squared (η_p^2, [41]). *Post-hoc* pairwise comparisons were carried out using the Newman–Keuls test.

Based on the results of the RM-ANOVA, we calculated, for the testing phase of each task, a facilitation index by subtracting, for each participant, the d' value obtained in the condition of lowest probability (10%) from the average d' values obtained in the other probabilities of association (40%, 60%, 90%). In this way, we obtained individual measures of the reliance in using contextual priors to predict the unfolding action or shape.

Then, standard multiple linear regression models were tested to assess whether the individual level of contextual modulation in the two tasks was predicted by autistic traits. Scores at the five AQ subscales (Attention switching, Attention to detail, Communication, Imagination, Social skills) were entered as independent variables, while the Action or Shape d' Facilitation indexes were entered as dependent variables. The assumptions for multiple regression analysis were met, given the presence of linear relationships between the dependent and the independent variables, and all variables were also checked for homoscedasticity and collinearity.

All analyses were implemented in Statistica software (Version number 12, Statsoft, Tulsa, OK, USA). The alpha value for all statistical tests was set at 0.05.

3. Results

3.1. AQ Scores

Analysis of the distribution of the AQ total score revealed that it was normally distributed, with skewness of 0.41 (s.e. = 0.27) and kurtosis of −0.44 (s.e. = 0.53). The individual AQ total scores ranged between 3 and 36 (Mean = 16.4, s.d. = 7.5), spanning from low (i.e., < 13) to high (i.e., > 18) levels of autistic traits [30]. As expected [30], men (N = 30; Mean = 18.3, s.d. = 8.56) tended to have higher AQ scores than women (N = 48, Mean = 15.21, s.d. = 6.58), but the difference between the two gender groups did not reach significance (t_{76} = 1.8, p = 0.076). Importantly, a recent study [45] describing a sample of Italian University students of fact-based humanities, which best matched our sample for age, study-field, and gender, revealed comparable distributions of AQ scores for both men (N = 29; Mean = 17.9, s.d. = 6; t_{57} = -0.21, p = 0.837) and women (N = 30; Mean = 17.5, s.d. = 6.9; t_{68} = 1.41, p = 0.163). Table 1 describes the statistics for each AQ subscale.

Table 1. Distribution and collinearity indexes of the AQ subscale scores.

AQ Subscale	Mean	St. Dev.	Range	Skewness	Kurtosis	Tolerance
Attention Switching	4.3	2.2	0–9	−0.08	−0.75	0.507
Attention to detail	4.8	2.2	0–10	0.05	−0.45	0.847
Communication	2.0	2.0	0–8	0.87	−0.17	0.463
Imagination	2.7	1.8	0–7	0.35	−0.65	0.750
Social skills	2.3	2.2	0–9	1.03	0.30	0.413

3.2. Behavioral Results: ANOVA

For the familiarization phase, the RM-ANOVA on d' values did not report any significant effects for Task ($F_{1,76}$ = 0.86, p = 0.355), Response Modality ($F_{1,76}$ = 3.60, p = 0.061) and their interaction ($F_{1,76}$ = 0.68, p = 0.411). Similarly, the RM-ANOVA on c values did not report any significant effects for Task ($F_{1,76}$ = 2.12, p = 0.149), Response Modality ($F_{1,76}$ = 0.89, p = 0.348) and Interaction ($F_{1,76}$ = 1.87, p = 0.175).

For the testing phase, the RM-ANOVA on d' values yielded a main effect of Probability ($F_{3,228}$ = 12.28, p < 0.001, η_p^2 = 0.13). Post-hoc comparisons revealed that d' values were lower for the 10% (mean = 1.653; s.e. = 0.12) than the 40% (mean = 2.020; s.e. = 0.081), 60% (mean = 2.133; s.e. = 0.086) and 90% (mean = 2.242; s.e. = 0.076) conditions, thus suggesting a decreased sensitivity in target discrimination under low predictability based on the contextual cues. No significant differences were observed among the 40%, 60%, and 90% conditions (all $ps > 0.07$). Importantly, the main effect of Task ($F_{1,76} = 0.49$, $p = 0.484$) and the Task × Probability Interaction ($F_{3,228} = 1.03$, $p = 0.376$) were not significant, suggesting that the two tasks were matched for prediction difficulty and that no differences in prior modulation were present between the Action Prediction and the Shape Prediction tasks (see Figure 2). Regarding the Response Modality of the Shape Prediction Task, a main effect emerged ($F_{1,76} = 16.14$, $p < 0.001$, $\eta_p^2 = 0.17$), since we found that performing the prediction tasks was easier in Position Response (mean = 2.285; s.e. = 0.097) than in Naming Response (mean = 1.738; s.e. = 0.095). Importantly, no interaction between Response Modality and the other factors was found (Task × Response Modality: $F_{1,76} = 3.77$, $p = 0.056$, Probability × Response Modality: $F_{3,228} = 1.11$, $p = 0.342$, Task × Probability × Response Modality, $F_{3,228} = 0.07$ $p = 0.974$), thus ruling out a possible influence of relative difficulty of task performance due to response modality on context probability modulation.

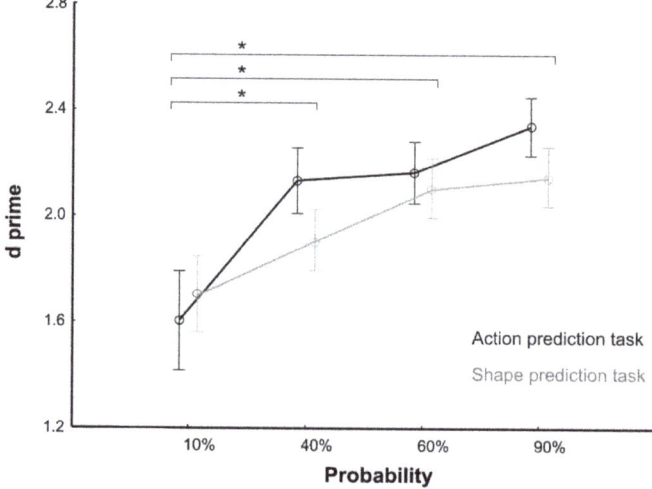

Figure 2. Behavioral results. Participants' performance in predicting the action (black line) and the shape identity (grey line) for the four probability conditions (10%, 40%, 60%, 90%) expressed as d'. Data points represent group averages. Asterisks indicate significant comparisons ($p < 0.05$). Error bars represent SEM.

With respect to the response criterion, the RM-ANOVA on c values yielded a main effect of Task ($F_{1,76} = 5.40$, $p = 0.023$, $\eta_p^2 = 0.06$), showing a negative criterion in the Shape Prediction Task (mean = −0.046; s.e. = 0.034) and a positive criterion in the Action Prediction Task (mean = 0.045; s.e. = 0.021, $p = 0.03$). This suggests that participants were differently biased in reporting one of the two outcomes in the two tasks. This, however, did not interact with Probability ($F_{3,228} = 0.29$, $p = 0.833$), nor was the main effect of Probability significant ($F_{3,228} = 0.34$, $p = 0.799$), ruling out a change in responses bias depending on the strength of the contextual prior (see Figure 3). We also found a main effect of Response Modality ($F_{1,76} = 12.83$, $p = 0.008$, $\eta_p^2 = 0.14$), further modulated by a significant Response Modality X Task Interaction ($F_{1,76} = 20.51$, $p < 0.001$ $\eta_p^2 = 0.21$). Post-hoc comparisons showed lower c values in Position Response (mean = −0.21; s.e. = 0.049) than Naming Response (mean = 0.117; s.e. = 0.047) for the Shape ($p < 0.001$), but not for the Action Prediction Task (Position response: mean = 0.062; s.e. = 0.031; Naming response: mean = 0.029; s.e. = 0.03, $p = 0.567$). This shows that the different response modalities of the two shape prediction versions led to a different bias in reporting the appearance of a long or a short shape. Importantly, no interaction with Probability was found ($F_{3,228} = 0.85$, $p = 0.470$), ruling out that the contextual modulation was affected by changes in responses bias across the two task versions.

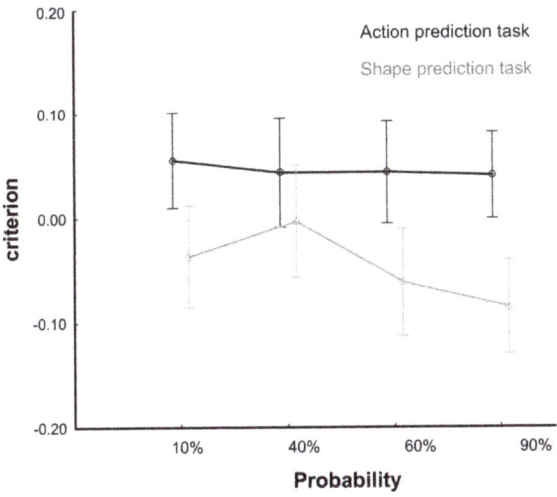

Figure 3. Behavioural results. Participants' response biases in predicting the action (black line) and the shape identity (grey line) for the four probability conditions (10%, 40%, 60%, 90%) expressed as criterion (c). Data points represent group averages. Error bars represent SEM.

3.3. Behavioral Results: Regression Analysis

Table 2 shows the summary statistics of standard multiple regression analyses conducted separately for Action d' Facilitation and Shape d' Facilitation indices. Multicollinearity statistics confirmed that the assumption was not violated (Tolerance > 0.4). For the Action d' Facilitation index, none of the subscale scores was a significant predictor (whole model: adjusted $R^2 = -0.0461$; $F_{5,72} = 0.70$; $p = 0.628$). Interestingly, for the Shape d' Facilitation index, the Attention switching subscale score was a significant predictor ($p = 0.019$; whole model: adjusted $R^2 = 0.035$; $F_{5,72} = 1.561$; $p = 0.181$). All the other subscale scores were not reliable predictors (all $ps > 0.407$). Thus, a higher level of cognitive autistic trait reflecting Attention Switching deficits were associated with a lower contextual prior modulation for the non-social, but not for the social task. This result was corroborated by the one-tailed Fisher transformation test, which showed that the negative correlation between Attention Switching and the Shape facilitation index (r = −0.270, Figure 4b) was significantly ($p = 0.046$) lower than the non-significant correlation between Attention Switching and the Action facilitation index (r = −0.007, Figure 4a).

Table 2. *p*-Values are marked as bold, for $p < 0.05$.

Action Facilitation Index			
Coefficients	β	t	*p*-Level
Attention Switching	0.051	0.316	0.752
Attention to detail	−0.073	−0.589	0.557
Communication	−0.146	−0.864	0.390
Imagination	0.219	1.648	0.103
Social skills	−0.045	−0.251	0.802
Shape Facilitation Index			
Coefficients	β	t	*p*-Level
Attention Switching	**−0.375**	**−2.392**	**0.019**
Attention to detail	0.022	0.185	0.853
Communication	0.143	0.875	0.384
Imagination	−0.077	−0.597	0.552
Social skills	0.081	0.469	0.639

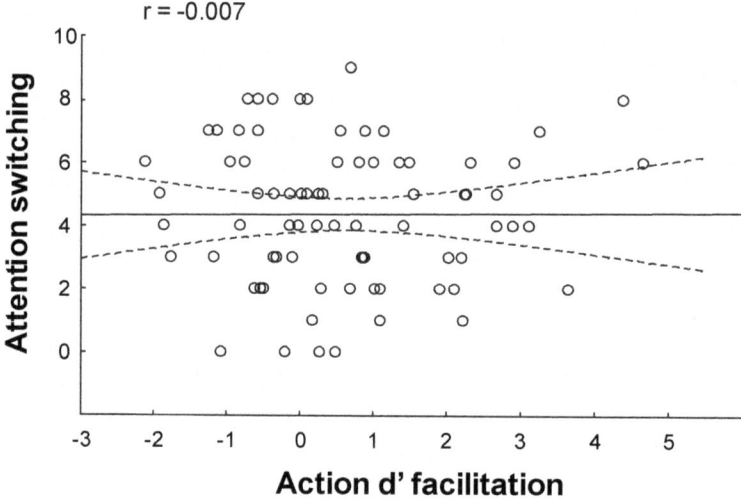

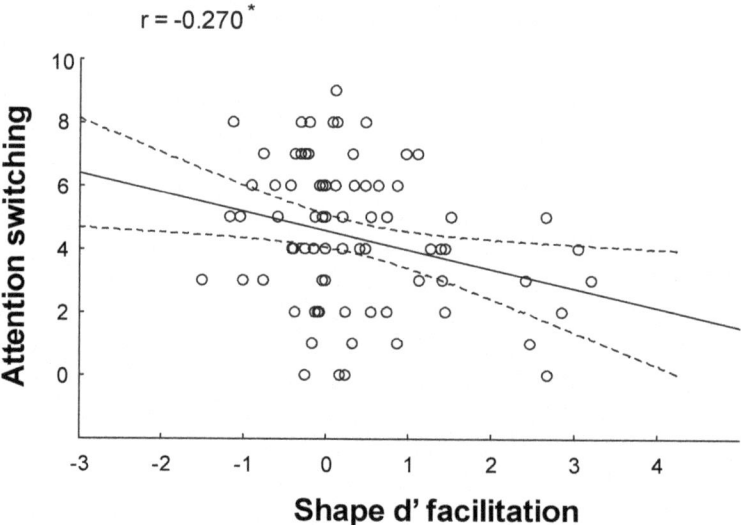

Figure 4. Correlational results. (**a**) lack of significant correlation between facilitation index for the action prediction task and attention switching scores; (**b**) significant negative correlation between facilitation index for the shape prediction task and attention switching scores.

4. Discussion

The present study tested to which extent the level of autistic traits in a general (i.e., non ASD) population could be associated with the ability to learn and use contextual priors to make predictions of social and non-social events. In line with the predictive coding account [17], we expected that contextual priors should modulate the precision of both action and shape predictions. Furthermore, in line with studies showing poor use of contextual priors for actions in ASD individuals [20] and poorer integration of action-context cues in individuals with higher autistic traits [16], we expected that social and cognitive aspects of the autistic traits should differently account for the use of contextual priors to predict the outcomes of social and physical events, respectively. In keeping with the first hypothesis, we showed that behavioral performance in predicting action and shape unfolding was significantly influenced by the strength of the contextual priors: the more the probabilities of co-occurrence of a contextual cue and a given event, the more participants were accurate in performing the tasks. This modulation was independent from the social nature of the task, since it was detected for both the action and shape prediction tasks. Moreover, it was independent from task difficulty, since we found comparable modulation for the two versions of the shape prediction task where the response modality was manipulated to load more spatial or verbal abilities. Crucially, the second hypothesis was only partially supported, since we found that cognitive (i.e., Attention Switching), but not social (i.e., Social Skills or Communication) aspects of the autistic traits accounted for the strength of contextual prior in the shape prediction task. However, we failed to find an association between either social or non-social autistic traits and use of contextual prior in the action prediction task.

4.1. Contextual Modulation of Social and Physical Event Prediction

The ideomotor theory [47] and forward models of action [48]) claim that the ability to predict action intention represents a crucial aspect of motor control and relies on previously learnt bidirectional associations between the motor act and its consequent sensory effects [49]). Action prediction mechanisms have been studies using different techniques. For instance, paradigms investigating the processing of anticipated action effects showed that self-generated stimuli are perceived as less intense than externally-triggered stimuli, resulting in sensory attenuation [50]. Other neurophysiological studies focused on the brain correlates of the anticipated action effects [51]. Here, we addressed action prediction from a Bayesian perspective related to the associations between action observation and contextual priors.

Using the same action prediction task of this study, a recent study [20] showed that children with typical development were able to use previously learned contextual information to successfully predict an ongoing action. In contrast, despite similar performance of children with typical development and children with ASD in discriminating fully observed actions, children with ASD did not leverage priors to predict action unfolding when visual information was ambiguous. The present study replicated the same pattern of findings in a large sample of young adult observers with typical development, thus providing evidence for consisting reliance on contextual priors in action perception across the lifespan. A recent study [52] also found that, in conditions of impoverished kinematic information available to an observer, explicit verbal information concerning the ongoing action strongly biased action prediction. In contrast, when kinematics was fully visible, the explicit verbal information had little, if no effect, with informative kinematics overriding the verbal information. The condition of fully visible kinematics was comparable to our familiarization condition, in which the unfolding action was clearly showed until one frame before the hand–object contact. Indeed, our participants could easily recognize the action outcome and used this experience in the testing phase, when kinematic information was reduced. Still, differently than in Koul et al. [52]'s study, some action-specific kinematic cues were still available during the testing phase and participants integrated this information with that provided by contextual priors, rather than overwriting kinematic evidence with the contextual prior. Thus, prediction performance was not completely biased to the contextual prior and even in the lowest probability condition participant's sensitivity was well above 0. Of note, given that sensitivity was defined based on kinematics and not on the context, this means that kinematics was correctly identified, but performance was modulated by contextual priors. In keeping with the predictive coding view of action processing [53,54], when observing someone performing an action, our brain generates top-down expectations to explain away the perceptual kinematics. In this recursive processing, incoming kinematic evidence is continuously matched with experiential or contextual priors in order to reduce the prediction error and reach a more precise model of the perceived action. Evidence for the integration of contextual prior and kinematic information has come from neuroimaging [13] and neurophysiological [12,14–16,54] investigations of modulation of motor activity according to the compatibility between the observed action and the embedding context.

The present study extended the same implicit learning of stimulus-context associations to a non-social domain, namely the prediction of an appearing object based on its color. Results provided evidence of prior-related perceptual advantages in the prediction of this physical event. In line with the predicting coding theory [17], it appeared that, when observing ambiguous moving geometric shapes, our brain generates predictions to guess in a proactive way the identity of the observed stimulus, leading to a modulation of perceptual areas according to the compatibility between the object identity and the embedding context (see [55]). In this sense, future studies are needed to clarify whether the context-based modulation of motor activity during action observation is specific for actions or rather reflects a general mapping of predictability [38].

4.2. Attention Switching Accounts for Context-Based Prediction of Physical Events

Several studies have provided evidence of altered perception of the world in individuals with autism [56–60] and in typically-developing individuals with high autistic traits [61–63].

Three main theories have been proposed to explain the abnormalities associated with atypical visual processing in autism. The Weak Central Coherence model [64] highlights the superior focus on the local aspects of a scene at the expense of the global "bigger picture". The Enhanced Perceptual Functioning model [65] emphasizes the enhancement in the detection of visual features. Interestingly, in a predictive coding account [65], these abnormalities may stem from an unbalance in the integration of top-down and bottom-up signals for the perception of the external world. Indeed, individuals with autism or high autistic traits may rely less on priors and more on sensorial evidence, showing a 'hypo-priors' mode of processing [66]. Empirical studies, however, have provided contrasting findings on whether the perceptual abnormalities of autism-like perception are due to weaker prior (e.g., [67,68]) or more precise sensorial information (e.g., [63,69]). Nevertheless, all these theories share the notion that individuals with autism-like perception do not integrate visual information in an optimal manner, thus perceiving an overwhelming sense of 'sensory overload' when dealing with the environment [70].

Using a task tapping the implicit learning of arbitrary shape–color associations, here we showed that high autistic traits accounted for a reduced ability to use the expectations arising from previous experience in order to discriminate among geometric shapes in situations of reduced visual information. In particular, individuals with less attention switching abilities tended not to take advantage of previously learned shape–color associations to disambiguate the appearing shape, pointing to a role of weak contextual priors in an autism-like perception of the world.

The role of a specific autistic trait linked to executive function deficits is consistent with a seminal work by Courchesne et al. [71] where authors showed an impaired ability of individuals with ASD to execute rapid attention switches during an attention shifting paradigm. Furthermore, as also demonstrated by a functional neuroimaging study using an adaptive version of the embedded figure test (EFT, [72]), participants with ASD are more dependent on perception, thus adopting a more local approach when faced with a task, compared to typically developing individuals. Notably, given the involvement of distinct cortical activations in individuals with ASD and individuals with typical development, the differences in behavioral performance seemed to be associated with different underlying neural systems, suggesting that individuals with and without autism use different cognitive strategies and engage different neural networks in performing the same task.

4.3. Autistic Traits Accounts for Context-Based Prediction of Actions

Several studies showed that, in individuals with ASD, although action understanding is preserved ([23] but see also [24,25] for contrasting results), impairments arise when the goal of the action has to be inferred on the basis of contextual cues [27,73], pointing to a reduced reliance on prior knowledge as the core of social interaction deficits in ASD. Therefore, we expected an association between the AQ measures of social behavior (i.e., communication, social skills) and the context-based predictions of social events. Contrary to these expectations, however, we did not find any correlation between any AQ subscales and the advantage provided by contextual cues during the performance of the action prediction task. The lack of significant results might also seem partially in contrast to previous study [16], where the authors found a negative correlation between the AQ subscales social skills and communication and neurophysiological correlates of the integration between top-down contextual expectations and movement kinematics. However, similar to the present study, the authors failed to find significant correlations between behavioral performance and AQ scores. In a similar vein, while a deficit in using contextual priors to predict action unfolding was observed in children with ASD as compared to those with typical development, the relative distribution of the deficit was not accounted for by their deficits in social perception abilities, but by their behavioral problems [20]. This might reflect that, while autistic traits may be associated with a different neural processing of social actions, this does not necessarily lead to an action prediction failure.

Otherwise, the lack of association between autistic traits and context-based predictions in individuals with either typical development or in ASD, despite the deficits shown by the last group as a whole, might reflect the dissociation between ASD and autistic traits. Consolidated views support the proposal of considering ASD as a dimensional rather than categorical disorder, with blurry and quantitative distinctions between subclinical autistic traits observed in the general population and individuals diagnosed as ASD [31,74]). Following this view, previous investigations have demonstrated the existence of a significant correlation between autistic traits and the sensory and perceptual alterations found in clinical autism [75]. Crucially, individuals with high autistic-trait scores showed similar perceptual difficulties in global processing often associated with clinical ASD than individuals with low-autistic trait scores [76]. Conversely, contrary evidence has been provided by Silverman et al. [77], who showed that autistic traits related to communication and social skills in ASD are not strongly correlated with the symptoms of stereotyped and repetitive behaviors. This is in line with the alternative view proposed by genetic studies (e.g., [78]) suggesting that ASD is best characterized as a category distinct from autistic traits [79]. Notably, to reconcile these two positions and explain contrasting findings, a categorical-dimensional hybrid model of ASD has been proposed [80,81]). This model, which has been also considered for defining the ASD diagnostic criteria in the fifth edition of the Diagnostic and Statistical Manual for Mental Disorder, has conceived the presence of either a categorical distinction between individuals with and without ASD or a dimensional representation of ASD symptoms. However, by assessing the associations between naturally varying levels of autistic traits on the ability to make experience-dependent predictions on upcoming events, without testing individuals with an ASD diagnosis, the present study does not allow establishing the extent at which clinical forms of ASD and autistic-like behaviors overlap.

5. Conclusions and Limitations

In conclusion, we showed that, while ASD has been associated to deficits linked to the context-based prediction of actions, the distribution of autistic traits in the general population is related to the strength of contextual priors only in the prediction of physical events. This conclusion, however, needs to be commensurate with the limitations of this study. First of all, while we powered our study to detect significant AQ prediction effects based on previous studies, it is possible that the relative uniformity of the sample, all young university students mainly enrolled in fact-based-humanities courses, might have shrunk the range of AQ variations, thus limiting predictive power. Furthermore, the unbalanced representations of male and female participants in our sample, partly related to the distribution of male and female students in the sampled university courses, might have also biased the distribution of AQ scores to lower levels of autistic traits, thus masking a possible association between action prediction and high autistic traits. Indeed, a recent study has documented an interactive effect of gender and study field on the AQ distribution in a large sample of university students [44]. In addition, using action videos depicting child models might have altered the type of action processing in our adult sample. Furthermore, we did not test here individuals with ASD and could not verify whether and how ASD and autistic traits are differently associated with context-based prediction of physical and social events. Finally, while the non-social task was designed to match the social one for difficulty and general procedure, it mapped less on everyday-life situations, thus lacking ecological validity as compared to the social task. Future studies are needed to couple the present behavioral data with neurophysiological measures and to include both behavioral and neural measures of individuals with ASD, in order to advance our understanding of the relation between object and action prediction, autistic traits, and ASD.

Author Contributions: Conceptualization, A.F. and C.U.; Methodology, A.F. and C.U.; Formal Analysis, V.B., A.F., and C.U.; Investigation, V.B., A.F., S.B., G.D., and C.U.; Data Curation, V.B.; Writing—Original Draft Preparation, V.B. and A.F.; Writing—Review and Editing, S.B., G.D., and C.U.; Supervision, C.U.; Funding Acquisition, C.U. and A.F. All authors have read and agree to the published version of the manuscript.

Funding: This work was supported by grants from the Italian Ministry of University and Research (PRIN 2017, Prot. 2017N7WCLP; to C.U.), the Italian Ministry of Health (Bando Ricerca Finalizzata, Prot. GR-2016-02363640; to C.U.; Ricerca Corrente 2020, Scientific Institute, IRCCS E. Medea; to A.F.), and by the Department of Languages and Literatures, Communication, Education and Society, University of Udine (PRID 2018; to C.U.).

Acknowledgments: We thank Eva Francesca Sponton and Valentina Azzano Cantarutti for their contribution in data collection.

Conflicts of Interest: The authors declare no conflict of interest.

References

1. American Psychiatric Association. *Diagnostic and Statistical Manual of Mental Disorders*, 5th ed.; DSM-5; Psychiatric Association: Washington, DC, USA; Burbank, CA, USA, 2013.
2. Orsmond, G.I.; Shattuck, P.T.; Cooper, B.P.; Sterzing, P.R.; Anderson, K.A. Social participation among young adults with an autism spectrum disorder. *J. Autism Dev. Disord.* **2013**, *43*, 2710–2719. [CrossRef] [PubMed]
3. Leekam, S.R.; Nieto, C.; Libby, S.J.; Wing, L.; Gould, J. Describing the sensory abnormalities of children and adults with autism. *J. Autism Dev. Disord.* **2007**, *37*, 894–910. [CrossRef] [PubMed]
4. White, S.; Hill, E.; Happé, F.; Frith, U. Revisiting the strange stories: Revealing mentalizing impairments in autism. *Child Dev.* **2009**, *80*, 1097–1117. [CrossRef] [PubMed]
5. Sinha, P.; Kjelgaard, M.M.; Gandhi, T.K.; Tsourides, K.; Cardinaux, A.L.; Pantazis, D.; Diamond, S.P. Held RM. Autism as a disorder of prediction. *Proc. Natl. Acad. Sci. USA* **2014**, *111*, 15220–15225. [CrossRef] [PubMed]
6. Kleinhans, N.M.; Johnson, L.C.; Richards, T.; Mahurin, R.; Greenson, J.; Dawson, G.; Aylward, E. Reduced neural habituation in the amygdala and social impairments in autism spectrum disorders. *Am. J. Psychiatry* **2009**, *166*, 467–475. [CrossRef]
7. Gillott, A.; Furniss, F.; Walter, A. Anxiety in high-functioning children with autism. *Autism* **2001**, *5*, 277–286. [CrossRef]
8. Amoruso, L.; Finisguerra, A. Low or high-level motor coding? The role of stimulus complexity. *Front. Hum. Neurosci.* **2019**, *13*, 332. [CrossRef]
9. Finisguerra, A.; Amoruso, L.; Makris, S.; Urgesi, C. Dissociated representations of deceptive intentions and kinematic adaptations in the observer's motor system. *Cerebral Cortex* **2018**, *28*, 33–47. [CrossRef]
10. Iacoboni, M.; Molnar-Szakacs, I.; Gallese, V.; Buccino, G.; Mazziotta, J.C.; Rizzolatti, G. Grasping the intentions of others with one's own mirror neuron system. *PLoS Biol.* **2005**, *3*, e79. [CrossRef]
11. Ansuini, C.; Giosa, L.; Turella, L.; Altoè, G.; Castiello, U. An object for an action, the same object for other actions: Effects on hand shaping. *Exp. Brain Res.* **2008**, *185*, 111–119. [CrossRef]
12. Amoruso, L.; Finisguerra, A.; Urgesi, C. Contextualizing action observation in the predictive brain: Causal contributions of prefrontal and middle temporal areas. *NeuroImage* **2018**, *177*, 68–78. [CrossRef] [PubMed]

13. Wurm, M.F.; Schubotz, R.I. 2016 What's she doing in the kitchen? Context helps when actions are hard to recognize. *Psychon. Bull Rev.* **2016**, *24*, 503–509. [CrossRef] [PubMed]
14. Amoruso, L.; Urgesi, C. Contextual modulation of motor resonance during the observation of everyday actions. *NeuroImage* **2016**, *134*, 74–84. [CrossRef] [PubMed]
15. Amoruso, L.; Finisguerra, A.; Urgesi, C. Tracking the time course of top-down contextual effects on motor responses during action comprehension. *J. Neurosci.* **2016**, *36*, 11590–11600. [CrossRef] [PubMed]
16. Amoruso, L.; Finisguerra, A.; Urgesi, C. Autistic traits predict poor integration between top-down contextual expectations and movement kinematics during action observation. *Sci. Rep.* **2018**, *8*, 16208. [CrossRef] [PubMed]
17. Friston, K. The free-energy principle: A unified brain theory? *Nat. Rev. Neurosci.* **2010**, *11*, 127–138. [CrossRef] [PubMed]
18. Land, E.H. The retinex theory of color vision. *Sci. Am.* **1977**, *237*, 108–129. [CrossRef]
19. Gilbert, C.D.; Sigman, M.; Crist, R.E. The neural basis of perceptual learning. *Neuron* **2001**, *31*, 681–697. [CrossRef]
20. Amoruso, L.; Narzisi, A.; Pinzino, M.; Finisguerra, A.; Billeci, L.; Calderoni, S.; Urgesi, C. Contextual priors do not modulate action prediction in children with autism. *Proc. R. Soc. Lond.* **2019**, *286*, 20191319. [CrossRef]
21. Van de Cruys, S.; Evers, K.; Van der Hallen, R.; Van Eylen, L.; Boets, B.; de-Wit, L.; Wagemans, J. Precise minds in uncertain worlds: Predictive coding in autism. *Psychol. Rev.* **2014**, *121*, 649. [CrossRef]
22. Lawson, R.P.; Rees, G.; Friston, K.J. An aberrant precision account of autism. *Front. Hum. Neuroscience* **2014**, *8*, 302.
23. Hamilton, A.F.D.C. Research review: Goals, intentions and mental states: Challenges for theories of autism. *J. Child Psychol. Psychiatry* **2009**, *50*, 881–892. [CrossRef] [PubMed]
24. Iacoboni, M.; Dapretto, M. The mirror neuron system and the consequences of its dysfunction. *Nat. Rev. Neurosci.* **2006**, *7*, 942–951. [CrossRef] [PubMed]
25. Zalla, T.; Labruyere, N.; Georgieff, N. Goal-directed action representation in autism. *J. Autism Dev. Disord.* **2006**, *36*, 527–540. [CrossRef] [PubMed]
26. Cattaneo, L.; Fabbri-Destro, M.; Boria, S.; Pieraccini, C.; Monti, A.; Cossu, G.; Rizzolatti, G. Impairment of actions chains in autism and its possible role in intention understanding. *Proc. Natl. Acad. Sci. USA* **2007**, *104*, 17825–17830. [CrossRef]
27. Chambon, V.; Farrer, C.; Pacherie, E.; Jacquet, P.O.; Leboyer, M.; Zalla, T. Reduced sensitivity to social priors during action prediction in adults with autism spectrum disorders. *Cognition* **2017**, *160*, 17–26. [CrossRef]
28. Gomot, M.; Wicker, B. A challenging, unpredictable world for people with autism spectrum disorder. *Int. J. Psychophysiol.* **2012**, *83*, 240–247. [CrossRef]
29. Volkmar, F.R.; Cohen, D.J.; Paul, R. An evaluation of DSM-III criteria for infantile autism. *J. Am. Acad. Child Psy.* **1986**, *25*, 190–197. [CrossRef]
30. Baron-Cohen, S.; Wheelwright, S.; Skinner, R.; Martin, J.; Clubley, E. The autism-spectrum quotient (AQ): Evidence from Asperger syndrome/high-functioning autism, males and females, scientists and mathematicians. *J. Autism Dev. Disord.* **2001**, *31*, 5–17. [CrossRef]
31. Constantino, J.; Todd, R. Autistic traits in the general population—A twin study. *Arch. Gen. Psychiatry* **2003**, *60*, 524–530. [CrossRef]
32. Posserud, M.B.; Lundervold, A.J.; Gillberg, C. Autistic features in a total population of 7–9-year-old children assessed by the ASSQ (Autism Spectrum Screening Questionnaire). *J. Child Psychol. Psychiatry* **2006**, *47*, 167–175. [CrossRef] [PubMed]
33. Ruzich, E.; Allison, C.; Smith, P.; Watson, P.; Auyeung, B.; Ring, H.; Baron-Cohen, S. Measuring autistic traits in the general population: A systematic review of the Autism-Spectrum Quotient (AQ) in a nonclinical population sample of 6900 typical adult males and females. *Mol. Autism* **2015**, *6*, 2. [CrossRef] [PubMed]
34. Miu, A.C.; Pană, S.E.; Avram, J. Emotional face processing in neurotypicals with autistic traits: Implications for the broad autism phenotype. *Psychiatry Res.* **2012**, *198*, 489–494. [CrossRef] [PubMed]
35. Palmer, C.J.; Paton, B.; Kirkovski, M.; Enticott, P.G.; Hohwy, J. Context sensitivity in action decreases along the autism spectrum: A predictive processing perspective. *Proc. R. Soc. B-Biol. Sci.* **2015**, *282*, 20141557. [CrossRef]

36. Amoruso, L.; Finisguerra, A.; Urgesi, C. Spatial frequency tuning of motor responses reveals differential contribution of dorsal and ventral systems to action comprehension. *Proc. Natl. Acad. Sci. USA* **2020**, *117*, 13151–13161. [CrossRef]
37. Happé, F.; Ronald, A.; Plomin, R. Time to give up on a single explanation for autism. *Nat. Neurosci.* **2006**, *9*, 1218–1220. [CrossRef]
38. Schubotz, R.I.; Von Cramon, D.Y. Sequences of abstract nonbiological stimuli share ventral premotor cortex with action observation and imagery. *J. Neurosci.* **2004**, *24*, 5467–5474. [CrossRef]
39. Paracampo, R.; Montemurro, M.; de Vega, M.; Avenanti, A. Primary motor cortex crucial for action prediction: A. tDCS study. *Cortex* **2018**, *109*, 287–302. [CrossRef]
40. Faul, F.; Erdfelder, E.; Lang, A.G.; Buchner, A. G* Power 3: A flexible statistical power analysis program for the social, behavioral, and biomedical sciences. *Behav. Res. Methods* **2007**, *39*, 175–191. [CrossRef]
41. Cohen, J. The effect size. *Stat. Power Anal. Behav. Sci.* **1988**, *2*, 77–83.
42. Oldfield, R.C. The assessment and analysis of handedness: The Edinburgh inventory. *Neuropsychologia* **1971**, *9*, 97–113. [CrossRef]
43. Summerfield, C.; Koechlin, E. A neural representation of prior information during perceptual inference. *Neuron* **2008**, *59*, 336–347. [CrossRef] [PubMed]
44. Ruta, L.; Mazzone, D.; Mazzone, L.; Wheelwright, S.; Baron-Cohen, S. The Autism-Spectrum Quotient—Italian version: A cross-cultural confirmation of the broader autism phenotype. *J. Autism Dev. Disord.* **2012**, *42*, 625–633. [CrossRef] [PubMed]
45. Conson, M.; Senese, V.P.; Baiano, C.; Zappullo, I.; Warrier, V.; Salzano, S.; Baron-Cohen, S. The effects of autistic traits and academic degree on visuospatial abilities. *Cogn. Process.* **2020**, *21*, 127–140. [CrossRef] [PubMed]
46. Stanislaw, H.; Todorov, N. Calculation of signal detection theory measures. *Behav. Res. Methods* **1999**, *31*, 137–149. [CrossRef]
47. Shin, Y.K.; Proctor, R.W.; Capaldi, E.J. A review of contemporary ideomotor theory. *Psychol. Bull.* **2010**, *136*, 943. [CrossRef] [PubMed]
48. Pickering, M.J.; Clark, A. Getting ahead: Forward models and their place in cognitive architecture. *Trends Cogn. Sci.* **2014**, *18*, 451–456. [CrossRef]
49. Waszak, F.; Cardoso-Leite, P.; Hughes, G. Action effect anticipation: Neurophysiological basis and functional consequences. *Neurosc. Biobehav. Rev.* **2012**, *36*, 943–959. [CrossRef]
50. Cardoso-Leite, P.; Mamassian, P.; Schütz-Bosbach, S.; Waszak, F. A new look at sensory attenuation: Action-effect anticipation affects sensitivity, not response bias. *Psychol. Sci.* **2010**, *21*, 1740–1745. [CrossRef]
51. Blakemore, S.J.; Wolpert, D.M.; Frith, C.D. Central cancellation of self-produced tickle sensation. *Nat. Neurosci.* **1998**, *1*, 635–640. [CrossRef]
52. Koul, A.; Soriano, M.; Tversky, B.; Becchio, C.; Cavallo, A. The kinematics that you do not expect: Integrating prior information and kinematics to understand intentions. *Cognition* **2019**, *182*, 213–219. [CrossRef] [PubMed]
53. Kilner, J.M.; Friston, K.J.; Frith, C.D. Predictive coding: An account of the mirror neuron system. *Cogn. Process* **2007**, *8*, 159–166. [CrossRef] [PubMed]
54. Kilner, J.M. More than one pathway to action understanding. *Trends Cogn. Sci.* **2011**, *15*, 352–357. [CrossRef] [PubMed]
55. Bar, M. Visual objects in context. *Nat. Rev. Neurosci.* **2004**, *5*, 617–629. [CrossRef]
56. Ego, C.; Bonhomme, L.; de Xivry, J.J.O.; Da Fonseca, D.; Lefèvre, P.; Masson, G.S.; Deruelle, C. Behavioral characterization of prediction and internal models in adolescents with autistic spectrum disorders. *Neuropsychologia* **2016**, *91*, 335–345. [CrossRef]
57. Tewolde, F.G.; Bishop, D.V.; Manning, C. Visual motion prediction and verbal false memory performance in autistic children. *Autism Res.* **2018**, *11*, 509–518. [CrossRef]
58. Balsters, J.H.; Apps, M.A.; Bolis, D.; Lehner, R.; Gallagher, L.; Wenderoth, N. Disrupted prediction errors index social deficits in autism spectrum disorder. *Brain* **2017**, *140*, 235–246. [CrossRef]

59. Goris, J.; Braem, S.; Nijhof, A.D.; Rigoni, D.; Deschrijver, E.; Van de Cruys, S.; Wiersema, J.R.; Brass, M. Sensory prediction errors are less modulated by global context in autism spectrum disorder. *Biol. Psychiatry Cogn. Neurosci. Neuroimaging* **2018**, *3*, 667–674. [CrossRef]
60. Turi, M.; Burr, D.C.; Igliozzi, R.; Aagten-Murphy, D.; Muratori, F.; Pellicano, E. Children with autism spectrum disorder show reduced adaptation to number. *Proc. Natl. Acad. Sci. USA* **2015**, *112*, 7868–7872. [CrossRef]
61. Braukmann, R.; Ward, E.; Hessels, R.S.; Bekkering, H.; Buitelaar, J.K.; Hunnius, S. Action prediction in 10-month-old infants at high and low familial risk for Autism Spectrum Disorder. *Res. Autism Spectrum Disord.* **2018**, *49*, 34–46. [CrossRef]
62. Karvelis, P.; Seitz, A.R.; Lawrie, S.M.; Seriès, P. Autistic traits, but not schizotypy, predict increased weighting of sensory information in Bayesian visual integration. *ELife* **2018**, *7*, e34115. [CrossRef] [PubMed]
63. Skewes, J.C.; Jegindø, E.-M.; Gebauer, L. Perceptual inference and autistic traits. *Autism* **2015**, *19*, 301–307. [CrossRef] [PubMed]
64. Frith, U.; Happé, F. Autism: Beyond "theory of mind". *Cogn. Cogn.* **1995**, 13–30. [CrossRef]
65. Mottron, L.; Burack, J.A. Enhanced perceptual functioning in the development of autism. In *The Development of Autism: Perspectives from Theory and Research*; Lawrence Erlbaum Associates Publishers: Mahwah, NJ, USA, 2001; pp. 131–148.
66. Pellicano, E.; Burr, D.C. When the world becomes 'too real': A Bayesian explanation of autistic perception. *Trends Cogn. Sci.* **2012**, *16*, 504–510. [CrossRef] [PubMed]
67. Lawson, R.P.; Aylward, J.; White, S.; Rees, G. A striking reduction of simple loudness adaptation in autism. *Sci. Rep.* **2015**, *5*, 16157. [CrossRef] [PubMed]
68. Lawson, R.P.; Mathys, C.; Rees, G. Adults with autism overestimate the volatility of the sensory environment. *Nat. Neurosci.* **2017**, *20*, 1293–1299. [CrossRef]
69. Manning, C.; Kilner, J.M.; Neil, L.; Karaminis, T.; Pellicano, E. Children on the autism spectrum update their behaviour in response to a volatile environment. *Dev. Sci.* **2017**, *20*, e12435. [CrossRef]
70. Simmons, D.R.; Robertson, A.; McKay, L.S.; Toal, E.; McAleer, P.; Pollick, F.E. Vision in autism spectrum disorders. *Vis. Res.* **2009**, *49*, 2705–2739. [CrossRef]
71. Courchesne, E.; Townsend, J.; Akshoomoff, N.; Saitoh, O.; Yeung-Courchesne, R.; Lincoln, A.J.; James, H.E.; Haas, R.H.; Schreibman, L.; Lau, L. Impairment in shifting attention in Autistic and Cerebellar Patients'. *Behav. Neurosci.* **1994**, *108*, 848–865.
72. Ring, H.; Baron-Cohen, S.; Wheelwright, S.; Williams, S.C.; Brammer, M.; Andrew, C.; Bullmore, E.T. Cerebral correlates of preserved cognitive skills in autism: A functional MRI study of embedded figures task performance. *Brain* **1999**, *122*, 1305–1315. [CrossRef]
73. Schuwerk, T.; Sodian, B.; Paulus, M. Cognitive Mechanisms Underlying Action Prediction in Children and Adults with Autism Spectrum Condition. *J. Autism Dev. Disord.* **2016**, *46*, 3623–3639. [CrossRef]
74. Spiker, D.; Lotspeich, L.J.; DiMiceli, S.; Myers, R.M.; Risch, N. Behavioral phenotypic variation in autism multiplex families: Evidence for a continuous severity gradient. *Am. J. Med. Genet.* **2002**, *114*, 129–136. [CrossRef] [PubMed]
75. Robertson, A.; Simmons, D. The Relationship between Sensory Sensitivity and Autistic Traits in the General Population. *J. Autism Dev. Disord.* **2013**, *43*, 775–784. [CrossRef] [PubMed]
76. Grinter, E.J.; Maybery, M.; Van Beek, P.L.; Pellicano, E.; Badcock, J.C.; Badcock, D.R. Global Visual Processing and Self-Rated Autistic-like Traits. *J. Autism Dev. Disord.* **2009**, *39*, 1278–1290. [CrossRef] [PubMed]
77. Silverman, J.M.; Smith, C.J.; Schmeidler, J.; Hollander, E.; Lawlor, B.A.; Fitzgerald, M.; Buxbaum, J.D.; Delaney, K.; Galvin, P. the Autism Genetic Research Exchange Consortium Symptom domains in autism and related conditions: Evidence for familiality. *Am. J. Med. Genet.* **2002**, *114*, 64–73. [CrossRef] [PubMed]
78. Abrahams, B.S.; Geschwind, D.H. Advances in autism genetics: On the threshold of a new neurobiology. *Nat. Rev. Genet.* **2008**, *9*, 341–355. [CrossRef] [PubMed]
79. Frazier, T.W.; Youngstrom, E.A.; Sinclair, L.; Kubu, C.S.; Law, P.; Rezai, A.; Constantino, J.N.; Eng, C. Autism Spectrum Disorders as a Qualitatively Distinct Category From Typical Behavior in a Large, Clinically Ascertained Sample. *Assessment* **2010**, *17*, 308–320. [CrossRef]

80. Elton, A.; Di Martino, A.; Hazlett, H.C.; Gao, W. Neural Connectivity Evidence for a Categorical-Dimensional Hybrid Model of Autism Spectrum Disorder. *Boil. Psychiatry* **2016**, *80*, 120–128. [CrossRef]
81. Frazier, T.W.; Youngstrom, E.A.; Speer, L.; Embacher, R.; Law, P.; Constantino, J.; Findling, R.L.; Hardan, A.Y.; Eng, C. Validation of Proposed DSM-5 Criteria for Autism Spectrum Disorder. *J. Am. Acad. Child Adolesc. Psychiatry* **2012**, *51*, 28–40. [CrossRef]

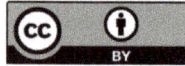

© 2020 by the authors. Licensee MDPI, Basel, Switzerland. This article is an open access article distributed under the terms and conditions of the Creative Commons Attribution (CC BY) license (http://creativecommons.org/licenses/by/4.0/).

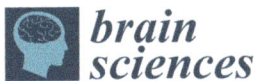 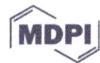

Article

Autism in Adulthood: Clinical and Demographic Characteristics of a Cohort of Five Hundred Persons with Autism Analyzed by a Novel Multistep Network Model

Roberto Keller [1], Silvia Chieregato [1], Stefania Bari [1], Romina Castaldo [1], Filippo Rutto [2], Annalisa Chiocchetti [3] and Umberto Dianzani [3,*]

[1] Adult Autism Center, Mental Health Department, Health Unit ASL Città di Torino, 10138 Turin, Italy; rokel2003@libero.it (R.K.); chieregato.s@gmail.com (S.C.); stefania.bari@aslcittaditorino.it (S.B.); romina.castaldo@aslcittaditorino.it (R.C.)
[2] Department of Psychology, University of Turin, 10100 Turin, Italy; filipporutto@gmail.com
[3] Department of Health Sciences, Universita' del Piemonte Orientale, 28100 Novara, Italy; annalisa.chiocchetti@med.uniupo.it
* Correspondence: umberto.dianzani@med.uniupo.it

Received: 20 May 2020; Accepted: 27 June 2020; Published: 1 July 2020

Abstract: Autism spectrum disorder (ASD) is a neurodevelopmental disorder characterized by deficits in communication and relational skills, associated with repetitive verbal and motor behaviors, restricted patterns of interest, need for a predictable and stable environment, and hypo- or hypersensitivity to sensory inputs. Due to the challenging diagnosis and the paucity of specific interventions, persons with autism (PWA) reaching the adult age often display a severe functional regression. In this scenario, the Regional Center for Autism in Adulthood in Turin seeks to develop a personalized rehabilitation and enablement program for PWA who received a diagnosis of autism in childhood/adolescence or for individuals with suspected adulthood ASD. This program is based on a Multistep Network Model involving PWA, family members, social workers, teachers, and clinicians. Our initial analysis of 500 PWA shows that delayed autism diagnosis and a lack of specific interventions at a young age are largely responsible for the creation of a "lost generation" of adults with ASD, now in dire need of effective psychosocial interventions. As PWA often present with psychopathological co-occurrences or challenging behaviors associated with lack of adequate communication and relational skills, interventions for such individuals should be mainly aimed to improve their self-reliance and social attitude. In particular, preparing PWA for employment, whenever possible, should be regarded as an essential part of the intervention program given the social value of work. Overall, our findings indicate that the development of public centers specialized in assisting and treating PWA can improve the accuracy of ASD diagnosis in adulthood and foster specific habilitative interventions aimed to improve the quality of life of both PWA and their families.

Keywords: autism spectrum disorder; adulthood; diagnosis; intervention

1. Introduction

Autism spectrum disorder (ASD) is a neurodevelopmental disorder with a prevalence ranging from 1% in the general population to ~1.9% in specific population groups [1,2]. ASD is typically characterized by deficits in socio-emotional reciprocity, impaired verbal and non-verbal communication skills, and an inability to develop and maintain adequate social relationships with peers, often associated with repetitive verbal and motor behaviors, restricted patterns of interest, need for a predictable and stable environment, and hypo- or hypersensitivity to sensory inputs. The onset of clinical symptoms occurs during the early years of life [1].

A large number of persons with autism (PWA) also meet criteria for co-occurring psychiatric conditions at a significantly higher rate compared to non-autistic populations [3,4]. Consequently, the socio-economic impact of ASD has become an increasing concern for public healthcare systems, which are now oriented toward an early diagnosis and intervention to improve ASD patient management while reducing the costs related to ASD care. However, there is paucity of guidelines for the diagnosis and management of PWA in adulthood. This aspect is of particular relevance in light of the detrimental effect that functional regression in these patients can exert on their psychosocial and work wellbeing. Indeed, PWA and their families are exposed to a "lifetime of difficult transitions" due to a limited number of service providers and resources alongside stringent and restrictive program funding criteria. As a result, there is widespread concern about the ability of some individuals with ASD to establish meaningful lives in adulthood [5].

Adolescents and adults with ASD are largely an underserved population. In a survey in Poland, the vast majority of parents of young PWA complained about the lack of assistance and support for PWA (93.5%) and the many difficulties in accessing the available services (82.7%) [6]. Indeed, low-income families and those living outside large cities have to deal more frequently with barriers to service access. This is particularly important in light of the fact that adult ASD patients need targeted psychosocial support to meet increasing social demands related to independent living, personal relationships, and successful employment. It is estimated that no more than 20% of adults with ASD have good or very good outcomes in these areas [7–9].

Studies from the US and Canada have reported that the number of outpatient services used by PWA decreases from childhood to adulthood and continues to decrease until late adulthood, while the use of medications and in-patient services increases [7–9], with very limited social integration, poor job prospects and high rates of mental health problems [10]. Indeed, the ensuing social isolation and unemployment further contribute to high rates of depression, anxiety, and other psychiatric disorders [11,12].

Qualitative studies have shown that transition outcomes among ASD patients are negatively affected by several factors such as poor person-environment fit, uncertainty about the roles of parents and the lack of comprehensive or integrated services. These findings have also revealed the aspects of familial, organizational and policy contexts that may be targeted for interventions. In this regard, stakeholders emphasize that supports should be individualized and focused on the changing aspects of the young adult's social and physical environment rather than on behavioral changes [12–14]. Thus, there is widespread consensus that policymakers should address economic, regional, and age-related inequities in access to services among PWA [6,15]. Furthermore, adult-oriented healthcare services should work directly with PWA and their support networks to facilitate successful engagement with services and enable adults to manage their mental health needs [16].

To address these challenges, in 2009, a specialized Regional Center for Autism in Adulthood has been established at the department of Mental Health in Turin. The aim of the Center is to follow up PWA who received a diagnosis of autism in childhood/adolescence or individuals with suspected adulthood ASD, with the aim of improving the accuracy of ASD diagnosis and identifying a personalized rehabilitation and enablement program and this study describes the clinical and demographic characteristics of the participants in the survey outcomes of the diagnostic path.

2. Materials and Methods

Participants were adults referred to the Regional Center for Autism in Adulthood in Turin by general psychiatrists across the Piedmont region—the region has an adult population of 3,600,000 inhabitants—due to ASD or suspected autism, with the aim of designing a personalized intervention plan. Each participant was evaluated using a model developed by the center, namely the Multistep Network Model. This tool consists of a multistep diagnostic and evaluation assessment that combines diagnostic evaluation with a personalized life project devised by a team of psychiatrists and psychologists of the center, the PWA and their family members, social workers, members of the educational and vocational services (i.e., teachers and job trainers) and employment agencies (i.e., job-brokers). The main goal of the approach is to set up a network of integrated services to serve the needs of PWA in the Piedmont region.

All clinical evaluations, testing and treatments were conducted in the center upon written informed consent signed directly by the participants or their guardians, authorizing data collection and processing as well. Not requiring a specific authorization from the Ethics Committee during the course of daily clinical activity, all clinical and research activities described in this study were authorized by the Medical Director of the Local Health Unit DSM To2 in 2009. Such authorization was subsequently confirmed by the Director of the Local Health Unit Città di Torino in 2019. The research was also authorized by the Institutional Board of the Piedmont Public Health Agency by means of two Regional Council Resolutions (DGR) No. 22-7178, 3 March 2014 and No. 88-8997, 16 May 2019.

Multistep Network Model:

Step required for diagnosis and individualized project:

(a) First meeting with the parents: (i) careful collection of life history, (ii) all interventions carried out, (iii) needs and expectations—the direct meeting with the subject to be evaluated takes place only in the case of suspected high functioning PWA;

(b) Meeting with the PWA or individual with suspected autism: (i) welcoming and creating a human supporting relationship, (ii) clinical evaluation of the symptoms presented, (iii) clinical evaluation of any psychopathological symptom in co-occurrence, (iv) objective neurological evaluation, and (v) clinical evaluation of cognitive functioning;

(c) Assessment of the intellectual profile by using appropriate tests for the level of clinical functioning (Wechsler Adult Intelligence Scale IV edition; Raven; Leiter) and, if necessary, neuropsychological testing [17–19];

(d) Evaluation tests for suspected autism. The choice of tests to be performed is based on the clinical functioning and cognitive profile—Autism Diagnostic Interview-revised (ADIr) for all; Ritvo Autism and Asperger's Diagnostic Scale-revised (RAADS) or Autism Diagnostic Observation Shedule-2nd Edition (ADOS 2) or Childhood Autism Rating Scale, Second Edition (CARS2-ST)depending on the level of functioning defined according to the clinical level and cognitive profile) [20–23];

(e) Evaluation of the adaptive functioning profile (e.g., Vineland/Adaptive Behavior Assessment System – Second Edition) [24,25]; Test evaluation of psychopathological functioning—if there is a clinical suspicion—with scales for intellectual functioning evaluation (Structured Clinical Interview, Minnesota Multiphasic Personality Inventory-2, Systematic Psychopathological Assessment for persons with Intellectual and Developmental Disabilities - General screening, Rorschach) [26];

(f) Medical evaluation focused on general health and specific conditions of neurodevelopment, including neuroimaging, genetic, metabolic evaluation, Electroencephalogram (EEG), depending on the individual's situation;

(g) Network meetings between operators of the Center for Autism in Adulthood and the patient's family members. When possible, there should also be meetings between the PWA and the operators involved in the clinical management of the patient, i.e., the child neuropsychiatrist, and if in transition age, social workers, school teachers, job trainers, and educators. In addition, all personal information and that related to the life context should be collected. These meetings should ultimately lead to the creation of a life project through the integration of clinical information and that derived from the care network, above all taking into account the preferences and wishes of the PWA and their families;

(h) The activation of a habilitative path provided directly by the center and/or presentation of the project to a Medico-Legal/Social Health Assessment Committee for evaluation of its appropriateness and allocation of the budget for the projects that will be delivered by accredited private healthcare centers.

3. Results

We performed a descriptive analysis of our cohort consisting of 500 participants. The sample of participants is described in Table 1.

Table 1. Description of the participants.

Sample	n	%	
Male	388	77.5	
Female	112	22.5	
Age	M = 31.7	SD = 10.7	Range: 18–82 years
Place of Residence	n	%	
Turin	262	52.9	
(Rural) Canavese Area	34	6.9	
Nichelino/Moncalieri and Carmagnola (Periurban areas)	55	11.1	
Medico-Legal Assessment of Professional Competences	n	%	
	302	65.4	
In Details			
46% civil disability level (CD)		2.1	
67% civil disability level (CD)		0.9	
75% civil disability level (CD)		7.1	

According to DSM5 criteria, ASD levels diagnosed in adult patients were as follows: level 1 in 39% (n = 193), level 2 in 27.1% (n = 135), level 3 in 18% (n = 90), neurodevelopmental disorder NOS not otherwise specified in 3% (n = 15), personality disorder (no autism) in 2.8% (n = 14) and psychosis (no autism) in 2.2% (n = 11). Additionally, 67.2% (n = 336) of participants displayed psychiatric and neurological co-occurrences, as shown in Tables 2 and 3 [1].

Intellectual disability was found in 53% (n = 265), which was mild in 35.8% of cases (n = 95), moderate in 34% (n = 90), and severe in 30.2% (n = 80), while 11% of the sample (n = 55) had a speech disorder.

Concerning therapies, 42% (n = 207) received psychotropic drugs and 14% anti-epileptic drugs (n = 69). Relevant medical comorbidities were epilepsy (16.6%; n = 82), allergies (8.4%; n = 39), and gastrointestinal complaints (21.3%; n = 99).

Table 2. Psychopathological and neurological co-occurrence in the study participants with autism.

Co-Occurrence	n	%
personality disorders	79	24%
challenging/problem behaviour	66	19.6%
Attention Deficit Hyperactivity Disorder (ADHD)	32	9.5%
epilepsy	23	6.8%
obsessive compulsive disorder	23	6.8%
major depressive disorder	21	6.3%
psychosis	19	5.7%
bipolar disorder	8	2.4%
anxiety disorder	6	1.8%

Table 2. Cont.

Co-Occurrence	n	%
specific learning disorder.	6	1.8%
tic disorder	6	1.8%
oppositional defiant disorder	5	1.5%
deafness	5	1.5%
Down syndrome	5	1.5%
social phobia	5	1.5%
Tourette syndrome	5	1.5%
eating disorder	4	1.2%
blindness	3	0.9%
movement disorder	3	0.9%
substance abuse disorder	3	0.9%
dyspraxia	2	0.6%
language disorder	2	0.6%
X fragile syndrome	2	0.6%
tuberous sclerosis	1	0.3%
Turner syndrome	1	0.3%
XXY syndrome	1	0.3%

Table 3. Personality disorders in the study participants with autism.

Personality Disorders Co-Occurrence in ASD (PD)	n	%
paranoid PD	19	5.7%
borderline PD	18	5.4%
personality disorder not otherwise specified	7	2.1%
schizotypical PD	7	2.1%
avoidant PD	6	1.8%
obsessive PD	6	1.8%
narcissistic PD	5	1.5%
schizoid PD	5	1.5%
aggressive passive PD	3	0.9%
histrionic PD	2	0.6%
dependant PD	1	0.3%
Total	**79**	**24%**

The parent's age at the time of birth ranged 17–48 years (mean ± SD: 30.72 ± 5.4) for the mothers, and 18–60 (mean ± SD: 34.21 ± 6.3) for the fathers; 15.5% of mothers experienced complications during pregnancy ($n = 72$) (Table 4). Moreover, 27.8% of the mothers had complications during delivery ($n = 130$).

Table 4. Prenatal and perinatal complications.

Complications	n	%	Note
During pregnancy	72	15.5	including 5.8% risk of abortion ($n = 27$)
Gestosis	12	2.5	
Twin pregnancy	7	1.5	
Depressive disorder	3	0.6	
Diabetes	1	0.2	
Thyroid disorder	1	0.2	
Toxoplasmosis	2	0.4	

With regard to neurodevelopmental stages, language skills on average appeared at 25.1 months (SD 19.94, range 6–180 months), and walking skills were achieved at 15.7 months (SD 6.3, range 8–60 months).

Table 5 reports the ages of PWA when the first symptoms became worrisome for the PWA's family. The average age of symptom recognition was 41.6 months (SD 54.3), with the most delayed recognition occurring at the age of 50 years.

Table 5. Age of PWA when the first ASD symptoms worried the family.

The Age When Symptoms Worried the Family	% PWA
6 Months	3.8
12 Months	11.3
18 Months	19.5
24 Months	42.6
30 Months	47.2
42 Months	80.3
48 Months	84.3
60 Months	97.8
72 Months	93.8

Symptoms at onset ranged from social-relational isolation in 38.1% of cases ($n = 166$), delay in the appearance of language in 25.7% ($n = 112$), inadequate relationship with peers in 15.1% ($n = 66$), stereotypies in 8.7% ($n = 38$), loss of language in 5.5% ($n = 24$), subjective experience of diversity (in individuals with high functioning autism in 3.2% ($n = 14$), and motor-coordination difficulties in 3.2% ($n = 14$).

First diagnosis of autism was made at the average age of 10.8 years (SD 12.3), but the diagnosis was revised in 49.4% of cases ($n = 246$), with an average of 26.5 years (SD 10.5). In 24.8% of cases ($n = 123$) the diagnosis was changed. Of note, during childhood only a small proportion of participants received medical assessment: 26.1% ($n = 126$) were evaluated with MRI (Magnetic resonance imaging) brain scan, 13.5% ($n = 65$) with cranial computed axial tomography, 16.8 ($n = 81$) with genetic analysis, and 16.2 ($n = 78$) with metabolic screening.

The types of intervention administered during childhood and adolescence are described in Table 6. No specific interventions were prescribed in 23.4% of cases ($n = 117$).

Table 6. Intervention administered during childhood and adolescence.

Intervention Type	n	%
Psychotherapy	143	29.9
Speech Therapy	200	42.1
Educational Interventions	117	24.6
Psychomotor skills Treatment	183	38.6
Delacato method	4	0.8
Portage method	13	2.7

The analysis of schooling revealed that 6 out of 500 participants had an elementary education degree without completing middle school (1.2%), whereas 137 subjects (27.4%) finished middle school but did not pursue secondary education. Fifty-seven participants (11.4%) started a secondary education program but dropped out. Thus, 38.8% of participants earned a middle school diploma, while 52.2% of them completed successfully a secondary school program. Only 4.4% of subjects enrolled in a post-secondary program. Notably, 70.1% of participants ($n = 337$) needed additional teaching support at school, and 31.7% of subjects were bullied ($n = 146$). Unfortunately, bullying occurred in almost all situations related to Level 1 Autism (DSM5 criteria, ASD Requiring support) [1].

Neuropsychiatric disorders were reported in 53% of family members—familiarity up to III degree—$n = 265$. The most frequent disorders were depression (21%; $n = 56$), autism (16.2%; $n = 43$), psychosis (14%; $n = 37$), intellectual disability (13.2%; $n = 35$), dementia (5.3%; $n = 14$), Parkinson's disease (4.2%; $n = 11$), specific learning disability (3.8%; $n = 10$), drug abuse 3.8% ($n = 10$) and Down syndrome (3.4%; $n = 9$).

After the evaluation, 189 out of 500 people (37.8%) received interventions directly delivered by the Center for Autism in Adulthood. Specifically, study participants were administered social skills interventions (37%; $n = 69$), cognitive-behavioral psychotherapy (26%; $n = 50$), expressiveness through visual art (9%; $n = 17$), parenting support group programs (9%; $n = 17$), body-vocal expressiveness (7%; $n = 13$), cognitive enhancement (Feuerstein method) (6%; $n = 12$), neuropsychological rehabilitation (3%; $n = 6$), habilitative intervention with animals (2%; $n = 3$) and musical expressiveness (1%; $n = 2$).

Indirect interventions were provided by accredited private centers as follows: 50.4% of patients ($n = 143$) attended a daily center, 31% ($n = 88$) underwent psychoeducational intervention and 7.4% ($n = 21$) followed a work-oriented training path. From the psychiatric standpoint, 6% ($n = 17$) were assisted by a mental health center due to the presence of severe psychopathological co-occurrences.

Finally, analyzing the housing situation, most PWA still lived with their families, with only 8.1% ($n = 40$) living in a residential structure offering around-the-clock assistance. Only 1% ($n = 5$) shared an apartment with few other disabled people, whereas 11% ($n = 54$) lived independently.

4. Discussion

Autism in adulthood is a complex condition that should be distinguished from ASD in childhood and adolescence, especially for high level of co-occurrence and specific needs [9,27,28]. In this regard, there are several reasons that prompted us to develop a new integrated assessment models, termed the Multistep Network Model, able to improve the accuracy of autism diagnosis in adults, a growing concern for public healthcare systems, with the ultimate goal of developing personalized rehabilitation and enablement programs. Firstly, there are a number of undiagnosed PWA, especially among women with ASD, that need to be detected [29–31]. Secondly, the transition to adulthood needs to be built by means of a habilitative program specific for adult (personalized life-project). Thirdly, we can clinically observe high rates of psychiatric comorbidities, requiring specific treatment. Finally, as caregivers become older, there is a marked decrease in family resources, which translates into a higher level of concern for the future of PWA [9,27].

Currently, PWA can follow a wide range of pathways during their transition to adulthood, such as attending college, entering the labor force, and achieving a degree of independent living. Less cognitively able individuals, on the other hand, may be eligible for state benefits or may access supported employment programs. Thus, clinicians need to familiarize with the unique needs of adults with ASD to be able to administer specific supports and interventions to these patients to ensure their best possible social integration in the community [28].

Among high functioning PWA, our study shows that these patients, especially women, are more likely to experience feeling different. This awareness begins at an early age—"I have always felt different from others" is a frequently used expression among adults with autism—, suggesting a more internalized autism syndrome [31]. Considering the possibility to decrease the risk of ASD, we can observe that prenatal, perinatal, and postnatal factors have been associated with autism [32]. The average age of parents at the time of birth, which could have increased the genetic risk in our sample, is in line with that of the general population—i.e., 30 years for the mother and 34 years for the father in PWA vs. 30.6 years for the mother and 34.2 years for the father in the general population. The role of pregnancy and delivery with respect to the pathogenesis appears to be relevant as 15.5% of PWA had complicated pregnancies and 27.8% had complications at delivery. These elements may therefore have been decisive for the development of hypoxic brain injuries with neuronal damages. According to a meta-analysis by Wang et al., during the prenatal period, the factors associated with autism risk were maternal and paternal age ≥ 35 years, mother's and father's ethnicity (i.e., Caucasian and Asian), gestational hypertension, gestational diabetes, maternal and paternal education level (i.e., college graduation), threatened abortion and antepartum hemorrhage. During the perinatal period, the factors associated with autism risk were caesarian delivery, gestational age ≤ 36 weeks, parity ≥ 4, spontaneous labor, induced labor, no labor, breech presentation, preeclampsia, and fetal distress. During the postnatal period, the factors associated with autism risk were low birth weight, postpartum hemorrhage, male gender, and brain anomaly [32]. Thus, health policy programs aimed at improving pre-natal and peri-natal conditions, including environmental factors that may preclude a safe pregnancy, may play an important role in decreasing ASD incidence.

Therefore, the implementation of training programs for teachers of nursery and primary schools together with routine screening by pediatricians is highly recommended to improve ASD diagnosis at an early age.

It is also important to point out that language problems in ASD patients are not only related to onset delay but also to semantic deficits: children with ASD produced more global, rather than local, semantic features in their definitions than children with normal language. An over-reliance on global, rather than local, features in children with ASD may reflect in-depth deficits of word knowledge [33].

The need for a diagnostic revaluation over time during the transition to adulthood is clearly documented by the fact that almost half of the PWA (49.4%) required revision of diagnosis—mostly due to changes of the clinical picture, nosographic reference parameters, cognitive functioning, psychopathological co-occurrences, etc.—, which was modified in 24.8% of PWA. The revaluation is particularly useful in detecting not only modifications of cognitive level of functioning but also the co-occurrence of a psychiatric disorder. Consistently, ASD diagnoses were confirmed in all PWA if made previously. Co-occurring mental health conditions are more prevalent in ASD than in the general population and a careful assessment of mental health is an essential component of care for all PWA and should be integrated into clinical practice with specific assessment [34–38]. Given that the co-occurrence of personality disorders is typically related to young adulthood but not childhood, the assessment should also explore personality in ASD. Psychopathological co-occurrences were present in 67.2% of the sample. They included the high prevalence of challenging behavior/problem behavior, which constitutes one of the main issues in family management. For this purpose, adequate diagnostic methods should be implemented, aimed primarily at excluding organic causes, with a subsequent activation of response programs, possibly behavioral, limiting psychopharmacological intervention as much as possible. The co-occurrence of Attention Deficit Hyperactivity Disorder (ADHD, 9.5%) is likely underestimated because of difficulty in making ADHD diagnosis in severe cases of autism and the presence of overlapping symptoms in both disorders. However, these should be regarded as continuous neurodevelopmental disorders instead of categorical comorbidities [39]. Generally, obsessive-compulsive disorders (OCD, 6.8%) are difficult to diagnose in PWA due to the presence of autistic rituals that, even though they may seem obsessive, represent an epiphenomenon of the primary disorder [40]. Major depressive disorder (6.3%) has a lower prevalence in our sample than what reported in the literature. This may be due to an increase in diagnostic performance that allowed us to rule out major depression forms belonging to other nosographic pictures. However, we did find a co-occurrence of psychosis and paranoid personality disorder in 5.7% of cases: psychotic forms were represented by both reactive forms with paranoid characteristics, often activated by triggers, such as bullyism and mobbing, and an interpretative deficit of reality, alongside rare forms of the schizophrenic type [41]. The latter is probably ascribable to a common genetic load with respect to the neurodevelopmental disorder, which expresses a first autistic phase and a second phase of schizophrenic deterioration [42–44]. Concerning the structuring of a paranoid personality disorder, we identified several situations fueling a chronic persecutory reading of the external human environment, such as the inability to read the surrounding environment, experience of exclusion, distress originated from bullying and mobbing episodes, and problems with social and work insertion. Use of psychotropic drugs is reported in 42% of the sample, and antiepileptics in 14%, with the presence of comorbidity for epilepsy in 16.6% of subjects. In a large cohort in the UK, approximately one-third of the identified cohort was prescribed at least one psychotropic medication and the prevalence increased 3.3-fold from 0.109 per 100 persons in 2009 to 0.355 per 100 persons [45]. More recently, a survey carried out in the Emilia Romagna region in Italy showed that 74.5% of adults with ASD were being treated with a psychotropic drug, with 41.6% of the participants using an antipsychotic drug, 15.19% two or more antipsychotic drugs and 5.17% a long-acting antipsychotic drug [46]. This large increase in psychotropic drug use among PWA calls for strict monitoring of drug prescriptions by healthcare services. Regarding psychopathology, in particular neurodevelopmental disorders, we found that a high proportion (53%) of family members of PWA (up to the third degree) report neuropsychiatric disorders, with one family member out of five expressing a depressive disorder, partly reactive to chronic stress and partly independent. With respect to neurodevelopmental disorders, 16% of family members display forms of autism—therefore, at least 16 folds more frequently than the general population—, while others show intellectual disability, specific learning disorders, Down syndrome, ADHD, stereotypes, with a cumulative percentage for neurodevelopment disorders reaching 39.6%. These data underscore the importance of providing genetic-metabolic evaluation also in adulthood PWA, since a transgenerational transmission of the vulnerability to neurodevelopmental disorders is highly likely [47,48]. Psychotic disorders were reported in 14% of family members, raising a question with respect to common biological/genetic factors shared between autism spectrum disorders and psychotic disorders [49]. Another interesting observation regards the high incidence of neurodegenerative disorders, such as dementia—Parkinson's disease is present in 4.2% of the participants—which warrants further in-depth studies aimed to elucidate its potential pathogenetic ramifications.

At the somatic level, the most evident finding is the lower prevalence of allergies in PWA compared to that of the general population (8.4% vs. ~30%, respectively), indicating substantial differences in the immune system response to allergens between the two groups. Furthermore, we recorded gastrointestinal disorders in 21.3% of cases, which are often the basis of behavioral disturbances, especially in seriously affected PWA experiencing difficulties in communicating. Medical evaluation plays a key role in ASD, especially during the developmental age, since it can rule out secondary forms of autism that could be specifically treated. Metabolic and genetic evaluations were observed in 6.2% and 16.8% of PWA, respectively. This may be the result of both the scarce attention paid to the organic aspects of autism and the attribution of autism pathogenesis to poor parental relationships in that historical period [50]. Consequently, even the interventions that PWA received during their developmental age often lacked specificity. In our sample, we recorded the following types of intervention: psychotherapy—rarely cognitive behavioral and more frequently psychoanalytic—in 29.9% of cases, speech therapy in 41.1%, psychomotor skill training in 38.6%, and non-specific psychoeducational interventions in 24.6%. In this context, speech and psychomotor therapies represented for years the standardized response offered by public services to autistic or disabled children.

A relevant finding in this study is represented by the high levels of co-occurrence of intellectual disability in more than a half of PWA. This percentage is seemingly higher than that recently reported by a study on childhood autism. If confirmed, this co-occurrence may be ascribable to the inadequate treatments received by PWA during their childhood, which presumably contributed to worsen their cognitive and functional abilities. This percentage may also indicate a general improvement in the diagnosis of high functioning forms of autism, which probably went undiagnosed in the past, especially in females [3].

Bullying is a trigger for psychopathology in adolescence and adulthood. One-third (31.7%) of PWA reported to have been bullied. This occurred to almost all PWA with the best functioning level (ASD level 1, DSM 5), which appear to be at high risk of psycho-traumatic events especially if undiagnosed. In keeping with other studies, autism severity did not significantly predict bullying-related behaviors. Consequently, secondary psychopathological comorbidity (e.g., anxiety, depression, etc.) may arise. Furthermore, this represents the level of autism in which the diagnostic evaluation is often lacking, as shown by those children mistaken for "little geniuses", whose socio-relational deficit is seen as a side effect of academic excellence [51,52]. With regard to the severity of the ASD, since we are a public health assessment center, our PWA sample included all forms of autism, with 39% of minor forms, i.e., ASD level 1 DSM 5, including previously defined forms of high-functioning autism and Asperger's syndrome—27.1% of level 2 autism (DSM 5), and 18% of severe forms of autism (ASD level 3 DSM 5) [1]. A small proportion included participants with neurodevelopmental disorders but with no sufficient information to categorize them in a specific subtype. The lack of information was due, for example, to the old age of PWA, which made it extremely difficult to gain information about his/her childhood from the parents. The few participants that did not meet the diagnostic criteria for autism were found to match those related to personality disorders (2.8%) and psychosis (2.2%), thus providing a bona fide of the assessment carried out by the Regional Center for Autism in Adulthood and the screening made by the general psychiatrists. Our organization is in fact based on a screening performed by a general psychiatrist to detect relevant psychiatric disorders before sending the patients to the Center. This triage policy has allowed us to save a considerable amount of clinical resources that would have otherwise been used to assess non-ASD patients. Our results also point out that the transition from childhood to adulthood in PWA represents a critical step for their families, whose management requires an overall re-evaluation, both at the clinical and project level. Consistently, the clinical evaluation model applied in this study is based not just on a process of progressive and deeper evaluation of the PWA or people with suspected autism and their families, but also on the available network of services that may be involved to formulate a personalized life-project (multistep network model). This personalized project is based on the information collected during the evaluation and may be delivered by the Regional Center for Autism in Adulthood or accredited private social centers. In the latter case, the project would need to be evaluated by a commission composed by members of the Health Public Agency and Public Social Services of the municipality of residence, which verifies the validity of the project and allocates a budget to support the external project. The interventions delivered directly by the Regional Center for Autism in Adulthood included paths for the improvement of social skills (social skill training) and cognitive-behavioral therapy. Group or individual support paths were activated for parents upon request. Another area of intervention concerned the improvement of expression and relationship skills, with activities aimed at improving communication through figurative arts—particularly for people with verbal communication impairment—and vocal-bodily expressive activities, using theater-based techniques. A subgroup of PWA, with medium-level autistic functioning and cognitive difficulties, followed a path specifically dedicated to improving cognitive functioning through structured learning techniques, such as Feuerstein or neuropsychological rehabilitation. Only in specific and selected exceptional situations, in the presence of severe communication deficits, interventions included the support of animals (three participants included) or communication through music (two participants). By analyzing the interventions provided indirectly by the accredited private partner, most PWA attended an educational activity covering most of the day and organized in groups (daily center; 50.4%), offering educational qualification courses and laboratories. In 31% of the participants, the activated path was instead based on individual educational activities or performed in small groups, delivering projects targeting specific skills of individual autonomy. For 7.4% of PWA, pre-work paths were activated: these consisted of training courses dedicated to PWA, lasting one to two years, made up of a theoretical part delivered in a classroom and a practical part via company internships. This type of path was dedicated to PWA with real job placement opportunities, thus needing less support, and managed by a professional school with teachers trained on autism and specifically dedicated to this type of course. In addition, the courses were prescribed provided that the PWA had followed a clinical path to improve and test his/her social skills and abilities to avoid stress deriving from real-life failures. Indeed, a person with autism needs to be adequately trained before being exposed to potentially harmful situations [53,54]. A small percentage of PWA (6%) was also followed by a Mental Health Center because these patients displayed a level of severity of the psychopathological comorbidity requiring a second parallel intervention dedicated to its management. This usually took place in outpatient clinics or day hospitals, but it may sometime require admission to the psychiatric ward. With regard to the housing situation, most PWA lived with their family of origin, whereas a small fraction (8%) lived in a community for disabled people with round-the-clock assistance. Only 1% of PWA resided in an apartment with other disabled people, while 11% achieved enough skills to live an independent life. Based on our findings, we propose a model for ASD in adulthood where public health and private services are integrated, and where the Regional Center for Autism in Adulthood plays a key role in managing PWA patients thanks to a joint effort between the private and public health sectors.

5. Conclusions

Among the several important aspects highlighted by our PWA analysis, the late age of autism diagnosis and the non-specific interventions provided during the developmental age are of particular relevance. As the current adult generation of PWA is apparently "lost", it urgently needs a very complex intervention program [34]. Indeed, these are PWA who have often developed other psychopathological co-occurrences or manifest a challenging behavior/problem behavior usually associated with lack of adequate communication and relational skills, never taught to them during their educational path.

Altogether, our findings call for a radical improvement of the accuracy and timeliness of the diagnosis of ASD in adulthood and the implementation of specific interventions in favor of this often-neglected population. Such interventions should address as much as possible the autonomy and communication dimensions, especially in those individuals that did not received any specific interventions during their developmental age. Also, preparing PWA for employment is of the utmost importance, if possible, given the social value of work. In conclusion, the implementation of public centers dedicated to PWA represents a viable solution for improving the diagnosis of ASD in adulthood and ameliorating the quality of life of PWA and their families through specific habilitative interventions. These interventions, in accordance with the Autism Guidelines, should merge multidisciplinary professional teams, formed by psychiatrists, clinical psychologists, educators and rehabilitation therapists, with other entities, such as social services, schools and job agencies, all forming a network capable of assisting autistic children and adults along their social integration path. In light of hypotheses regarding developmental and environmental influences on the course of ASD, future studies should compare the changes in symptoms and presentation across adulthood to those occurring in childhood.

Author Contributions: Conceptualization R.K.; methodology R.K.; software F.R., S.C.; validation, U.D., A.C.; formal analysis F.R.; investigation, S.B., R.C., R.K.; resources, A.C., U.D.; data curation, F.R., R.K., S.C.; writing—original draft preparation, R.K.; writing—review and editing, R.K., U.D., A.C., S.B.; visualization, R.K., F.R.; supervision, U.D., A.C.; project administration R.K., U.D., A.C.; funding acquisition, U.D., A.C. All authors have read and agreed to the published version of the manuscript.

Funding: This research received no external funding.

Conflicts of Interest: The authors declare no conflict of interest.

References

1. American Psychiatric Association. *Author Diagnostic and Statistical Manual of Mental Disorders*, 5th ed.; American Psychiatric Association: Arlington, VA, USA, 2013.
2. Maenner, M.J.; Shaw, K.A.; Baio, J. Prevalence of Autism Spectrum Disorder Among Children Aged 8 Years—Autism and Developmental Disabilities Monitoring Network, 11 Sites, United States, 2016. *MMWR Surveill. Summ.* **2020**, *69*, 1–12. [CrossRef]
3. Bertelli, M.O. Autism spectrum disorder and intellectual disability. In *Psychopathology in Adolescents and Adults with Autism Spectrum Disorders*; Keller, R., Ed.; Springer Nature Switzerland: Basel, Switzerland, 2019; pp. 111–130.
4. Simonoff, E.; Jones, C.R.G.; Baird, G.; Pickles, A.; Happé, F.; Charman, T. The persistence and stability of psychiatric problems in adolescents with autism spectrum disorders: Stability of psychiatric symptoms in autism spectrum disorders. *J. Child Psychol. Psychiatry* **2013**, *54*, 186–194. [CrossRef]
5. Milen, M.T.; Nicholas, D.B. Examining transitions from youth to adult services for young persons with autism. *Soc. Work Health Care* **2017**, *56*, 636–648. [CrossRef]
6. Płatos, M.; Pisula, E. Service use, unmet needs, and barriers to services among adolescents and young adults with autism spectrum disorder in Poland. *BMC Health Serv. Res.* **2019**, *19*, 587. [CrossRef]
7. Eaves, L.C.; Ho, H.H. Young adult outcome of autism spectrum disorders. *J. Autism Dev. Disord.* **2008**, *38*, 739–747. [CrossRef]
8. Howlin, P.; Moss, P.; Savage, S.; Rutter, M. Social outcomes in mid- to later adulthood among individuals diagnosed with autism and average nonverbal IQ as children. *J. Am. Acad. Child Adolesc. Psychiatry* **2013**, *52*, 572–581. [CrossRef]

9. Howlin, P.; Magiati, I. Autism spectrum disorder: Outcomes in adulthood. *Curr. Opin. Psychiatry* **2017**, *30*, 69–76. [CrossRef]
10. Lugnegård, T.; Hallerbäck, M.U.; Gillberg, C. Psychiatric comorbidity in young adults with a clinical diagnosis of Asperger syndrome. *Res. Dev. Disabil.* **2011**, *32*, 1910–1917. [CrossRef]
11. Hofvander, B.; Delorme, R.; Chaste, P.; Nydén, A.; Wentz, E.; Ståhlberg, O.; Herbrecht, E.; Stopin, A.; Anckarsäter, H.; Gillberg, C.; et al. Psychiatric and psychosocial problems in adults with normal-intelligence autism spectrum disorders. *BMC Psychiatry* **2009**, *9*, 1–9. [CrossRef]
12. Anderson, K.A.; Sosnowy, C.; Kuo, A.A.; Shattuck, P.T. Transition of Individuals With Autism to Adulthood: A Review of Qualitative Studies. *Pediatrics* **2018**, *141*, S318–S327. [CrossRef]
13. Cidav, Z.; Lawer, L.; Marcus, S.C.; Mandell, D.S. Age-Related Variation in Health Service Use and Associated Expenditures Among Children with Autism. *J. Autism Dev. Disord.* **2013**, *43*, 924–931. [CrossRef] [PubMed]
14. Turcotte, P.; Mathew, M.; Shea, L.L.; Brusilovskiy, E.; Nonnemacher, S.L. Service needs across the lifespan for individuals with autism. *J. Autism Dev. Disord.* **2016**, *46*, 2480–2489. [CrossRef] [PubMed]
15. Lord, C.; Elsabbagh, M.; Baird, G.; Veenstra-Vanderweele, J. Autism spectrum disorder. *Lancet* **2018**, *392*, 508–520. [CrossRef]
16. King, C.; Merrick, H.; Le Couteur, A. How should we support young people with ASD and mental health problems as they navigate the transition to adult life including access to adult healthcare services. *Epidemiol. Psychiatr. Sci.* **2020**, *29*, e90. [CrossRef]
17. Wechsler, D. *Wechsler Adult Intelligence Scale-Fourth Edition (WAIS-IV)*; NCS Pearson: San Antonio, TX, USA, 2008.
18. Raven, J.C. Standardization of progressive matrices, 1938. *Br. J. Med. Psychol.* **1941**, *19*, 137–150. [CrossRef]
19. Roid, G.H.; Miller, L.J. *Leiter International Performance Scale-Revised (Leiter-R)*; Stoelting: Wood Dale, IL, USA, 1997.
20. Rutter, M.; Le Couteur, A.; Lord, C. *ADI-R. Autism Diagnostic Interview Revised. Manual*; Western Psychological Services: Los Angeles, CA, USA, 2003.
21. Ritvo, R.A.; Ritvo, E.R.; Guthrie, N.; Ritvo, M.J.; Hufnagel, D.H.; McMahon, W.; Tonge, B.J.; Mataix-Cols, D.; Jassi, A.; Attwood, T.; et al. The Ritvo Autism Asperger Diagnostic Scale-Revised (RAADS-R): A Scale to Assist the Diagnosis of Autism Spectrum Disorder in Adults: An International Validation Study. *J. Autism Dev. Disord.* **2011**, *41*, 1076–1089. [CrossRef]
22. Lord, C.; Rutter, M.; DiLavore, P.C.; Risi, S.; Gotham, K.; Bishop, S. *Autism Diagnostic Observation Schedule: ADOS*; Western Psychological Services: Los Angeles, CA, USA, 2002.
23. Schopler, E.; Reichler, R.J.; DeVellis, R.F.; Daly, K. Toward objective classification of childhood autism: Childhood Autism Rating Scale (CARS). *J. Autism Dev. Disord.* **1980**, *10*, 91–103. [CrossRef]
24. Sparrow, S.S.; Cicchetti, D.V.; Balla, D.A. The Vineland Adaptive Behavior Scales. *Major Psychol. Assess. Instrum.* **1989**, *2*, 199–231.
25. Harrison, P.; Oakland, T. *ABAS-3: Adaptive Behavior Assessment System*; Western Psychological Services: Los Angeles, CA, USA, 2015.
26. Keller, R.; Bari, S.; Fratianni, B.; Piedimonte, A.; Freilone, F. Response to Rorschach test in autism spectrum disorders in adulthood: A pilot study. *J. Psychopathol.* **2018**, *24*, 224–229.
27. Bennett, A.E.; Miller, J.S.; Stollon, N.; Prasad, R.; Blum, N.J. Autism Spectrum Disorder and Transition-Aged Youth. *Curr. Psychiatry Rep.* **2018**, *20*, 103. [CrossRef]
28. Van Schalkwyk, G.I.; Volkmar, F.R. Autism Spectrum Disorders: Challenges and Opportunities for Transition to Adulthood. *Child Adolesc. Psychiatr. Clin. N. Am.* **2017**, *26*, 329–339. [CrossRef]
29. Baron-Cohen, S. Empathizing, systemizing, and the extreme male brain theory of autism. *Prog. Brain Res.* **2010**, *186*, 167–175.
30. Rynkiewicz, A.; Janas-Kozik, M.; Słopień, A. Girls and women with autism. *Psychiatr. Pol.* **2019**, *53*, 737–752. [CrossRef]
31. Lai, M.-C.; Lombardo, M.V.; Auyeung, B.; Chakrabarti, B.; Baron-Cohen, S. Sex/gender differences and autism: Setting the scene for future research. *J. Am. Acad. Child Adolesc. Psychiatry* **2015**, *54*, 11–24. [CrossRef]
32. Wang, C.; Geng, H.; Liu, W.; Zhang, G. Prenatal, perinatal, and postnatal factors associated with autism. *Medicine* **2017**, *96*, e6696. [CrossRef]

33. Gladfelter, A.; Barron, K.L. How Children with Autism Spectrum Disorder, Developmental Language Disorder, and Typical Language Learn to Produce Global and Local Semantic Features. *Brain Sci.* **2020**, *10*, 231. [CrossRef]
34. Lai, M.-C.; Baron-Cohen, S. Identifying the lost generation of adults with autism spectrum conditions. *Lancet Psychiatry* **2015**, *2*, 1013–1027. [CrossRef]
35. Valkanova, V.; Rhodes, F.; Allan, C.L. Diagnosis and management of autism in adults. *Practitioner* **2013**, *257*, 13–16.
36. Luciano, C.; Keller, R. Misdiagnosis of High Function Autism Spectrum Disorders in Adults: An Italian Case Series. *Autism Open Access* **2014**, *4*, 2. [CrossRef]
37. Sistema Italiano Linee Guida. *Linea Guida n. 21, Il Trattamento dei Disturbi Dello Spettro Autistico nei Bambini e Negli Adolescent*; Sistema Italiano Linee Guida: Roma, Italy, 2011.
38. Lai, M.C.; Kassee, C.; Besney, R.; Bonato, S.; Hull, L.; Mandy, W.; Szatmari, P.; Ameis, S.H. Prevalence of co-occurring mental health diagnoses in the autism population: A systematic review and meta-analysis. *Lancet Psychiatry* **2019**, *6*, 819–829. [CrossRef]
39. Craig, F.; Lamanna, A.L.; Margari, F.; Matera, E.; Simone, M.; Margari, L. Overlap Between Autism Spectrum Disorders and Attention Deficit Hyperactivity Disorder: Searching for Distinctive/Common Clinical Features. *Autism Res.* **2015**, *8*, 328–337. [CrossRef] [PubMed]
40. Postorino, V.; Kerns, C.M.; Vivanti, G.; Bradshaw, J.; Siracusano, M.; Mazzone, L. Anxiety Disorders and Obsessive-Compulsive Disorder in Individuals with Autism Spectrum Disorder. *Curr. Psychiatry Rep.* **2017**, *19*, 92. [CrossRef] [PubMed]
41. Keller, R.; Bari, S. Psychosis and Autism Spectrum Disorder. In *Psychopathology in Adolescents and Adults with Autism Spectrum Disorders*; Keller, R., Ed.; Springer Nature Switzerland: Basel, Switzerland, 2019; pp. 51–65.
42. Cauda, F.; Nani, A.; Costa, T.; Palermo, S.; Tatu, K.; Manuello, J.; Duca, S.; Fox, P.T.; Keller, R. The morphometric co-atrophy networking of schizophrenia, autistic and obsessive spectrum disorders. *Hum. Brain Mapp.* **2018**, *39*, 1898–1928. [CrossRef] [PubMed]
43. Cauda, F.; Costa, T.; Nani, A.; Fava, L.; Palermo, S.; Bianco, F.; Duca, S.; Tatu, K.; Keller, R. Are schizophrenia, autistic, and obsessive spectrum disorders dissociable on the basis of neuroimaging morphological findings?: A voxel-based meta-analysis. *Autism Res.* **2017**, *10*, 1079–1095. [CrossRef]
44. Keller, R.; Piedimonte, A.; Bianco, F.; Bari, S.; Cauda, F. Diagnostic Characteristics of Psychosis and Autism Spectrum Disorder in Adolescence and Adulthood. A Case Series. *Autism Open Access* **2015**, *6*, 159. [CrossRef]
45. Alfageh, B.H.; Man, K.K.C.; Besag, F.M.C.; Alhawassi, T.M.; Wong, I.C.K.; Brauer, R. Psychotropic Medication Prescribing for Neuropsychiatric Comorbidities in Individuals Diagnosed with Autism Spectrum Disorder (ASD) in the UK. *J. Autism Dev. Disord.* **2020**, *50*, 625–633. [CrossRef]
46. Di Sarro, R.; Varrucciu, N.; Di Santantonio, A.; Fioritti, A. Indagine sulle terapie farmacologiche e sulle diagnosi psichiatriche nei pazienti con diagnosi di disturbo dello spettro autistico registrati nei sistemi informativi territoriali. *G. Ital. Disturbi Neurosviluppo* **2020**, *5*, 100–107.
47. Keller, R.; Basta, R.; Salerno, L.; Elia, M. Autism, epilepsy, and synaptopathies: A not rare association. *Neurol. Sci.* **2017**, *38*, 1353–1361. [CrossRef]
48. Biamino, E.; Di Gregorio, E.; Belligni, E.F.; Keller, R.; Riberi, E.; Gandione, M.; Calcia, A.; Mancini, C.; Giorgio, E.; Cavalieri, S.; et al. A novel 3q29 deletion associated with autism, intellectual disability, psychiatric disorders, and obesity. *Am. J. Med Genet. Part B Neuropsychiatr. Genet.* **2016**, *171*, 290–299. [CrossRef]
49. Bertelli, M.; Merli, M.P.; Bradley, E.; Keller, R.; Varrucciu, N.; Del Furia, C.; Panocchia, N. The diagnostic boundary between autism spectrum disorder, intellectual developmental disorder and schizophrenia spectrum disorders. *Adv. Ment. Heal. Intellect. Disabil.* **2015**, *9*, 243–264. [CrossRef]
50. Deslauriers, N. The Empty Fortress: Infantile Autism and the Birth of the Self. *Arch. Gen. Psychiatry* **1967**, *17*, 510–512. [CrossRef]
51. Fink, E.; Olthof, T.; Goossens, F.; Van Der Meijden, S.; Begeer, S. Bullying-related behaviour in adolescents with autism: Links with autism severity and emotional and behavioural problems. *Autism* **2018**, *22*, 684–692. [CrossRef]
52. Smith, I.C.; White, S.W. Socio-emotional determinants of depressive symptoms in adolescents and adults with autism spectrum disorder: A systematic review. *Autism* **2020**, *24*, 995–1010. [CrossRef] [PubMed]
53. Bari, S.; Tisci, R.; Burlando, R.; Keller, R. Caring for Autistic Adults. A Qualitative Analysis Under the Lens of Capability Approach. *Ital. Sociol. Rev.* **2018**, *8*, 243–264.

54. Gorenstein, M.; Giserman-Kiss, I.; Feldman, E.; Isenstein, E.L.; Donnelly, L.; Wang, A.T.; Foss-Feig, J. Brief Report: A Job-Based Social Skills Program (JOBSS) for Adults with Autism Spectrum Disorder: A Pilot Randomized Controlled Trial. *J. Autism Dev. Disord.* **2020**, 1–8. [CrossRef] [PubMed]

© 2020 by the authors. Licensee MDPI, Basel, Switzerland. This article is an open access article distributed under the terms and conditions of the Creative Commons Attribution (CC BY) license (http://creativecommons.org/licenses/by/4.0/).

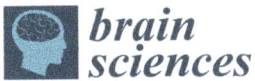 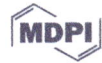

Article

Human Figure Drawings in Children with Autism Spectrum Disorders: A Possible Window on the Inner or the Outer World

Pamela Papangelo [1], Martina Pinzino [1], Susanna Pelagatti [2], Maddalena Fabbri-Destro [1,†,*] and Antonio Narzisi [3,†]

1. Institute of Neuroscience, National Research Council (CNR), Via Volturno 39/E, 43125 Parma, Italy; pamela.papangelo@gmail.com (P.P.); martinapinzino@outlook.it (M.P.)
2. Department of Informatics, University of Pisa, 56126 Pisa, Italy; susanna.pelagatti@gmail.com
3. IRCCS Stella Maris Foundation, 56126 Pisa, Italy; antonio.narzisi@fsm.unipi.it
* Correspondence: maddalena.fabbridestro@gmail.com; Tel.: +39-0521-903881
† Both authors contributed equally to this work.

Received: 25 May 2020; Accepted: 17 June 2020; Published: 23 June 2020

Abstract: Background: Tests based on human figure drawings (HFD) have captured the attention of clinicians and psychologists for a long time. The aim of the present study was to evaluate the performance of HFD of children with autism spectrum disorders (ASDs) relative to typically developing (TD) controls. Methods: All children were asked to draw three human figures (man, woman, self-portrait) and were evaluated with a neuropsychological battery. HFD were scored according to the Maturity Scale, and correlative approaches testing maturity against neuropsychological scores were applied. Results: ASDs presented marked deficits in maturity. No significant correlation emerged for both groups between maturity and the theory of mind test. On the contrary, positive and significant correlations between maturity and the affect recognition test (AR) were found, with group-specific patterns. In TD, this result regarded drawings of others, but not self-portraits, while an opposite pattern emerged for ASD, whose sole maturity in self-portraits significantly correlated with the AR scores. Conclusion: These findings suggest that the use of HFD tests with individuals with autism may not be used in clinical practices. However, in basic research, HFDs could be used to highlight dependencies between drawing performance and neuropsychological features, thus possibly providing hints on the functioning of autism.

Keywords: human figure drawings; Draw-a-Man; drawings maturity; autism spectrum disorders; social perception

1. Introduction

Children have been using drawings to express themselves since ancient times and this topic has captured the interest of scientists since the late 19th century. Indeed, by analyzing the presence/absence of graphical aspects like details, colors, proportions, and shapes, it is possible to trace a developmental maturation trajectory based on children's drawings [1]. Historically, the Draw-a-Man test (DAMT) developed by Goodenough [2] represents the first systematic scoring system for children's drawings, devised with the intent to provide a surrogate measure of children's intelligence. Scores were initially based on the number of details and the accuracy of placement of each body part. DAMT was later revised by Harris [3], who proposed that children should be asked to draw not just one but three human figures: a generic man, a generic woman, and a self-portrait. The scoring system for the maturity estimation was updated, accounting also for the precision of details, and proportions.

Since these initial pioneering studies, several revisions and applications have been conducted to enhance the utility of DAMT, and more generally of human figure drawing (HFD) tests, in virtue of their versatility and usability also with children with limited attention span and language difficulties. There is no exception for the use of the HFD in the field of autism.

As far as autism spectrum disorders (ASDs) drawings are concerned, children with autism were reported to have an unusual drawing ability, far beyond their general intelligence level [4–6], and drawing skills not impaired relative to age-matched typical peers [7,8]. However, Lee and Hobson [9] reported slightly lower global scores in HFD for children with ASD relative to children with learning difficulties, whereas the same pattern did not emerge across groups in drawings of houses. Similarly, Lim and Slaughter [10] indicated that in HFD, children with autism are generally less sophisticated and detailed than children without autism. Given this controversial pattern of results, whether children with autism differ from age-matched TD peers is still a matter of debate, leaving open the question whether human figure drawings could be useful in the clinical practice of autism. Indeed, while international guidelines [11] excluded tests based on drawings from the batteries used for the diagnosis of ASDs, it is possible that the maturity score covaries in association with other neuropsychological indices not easily obtainable in children with ASDs.

Autism spectrum disorders (ASDs) are a severe multifactorial disorder characterized by an umbrella of peculiarities in the areas of social communication, restricted interests, and repetitive behaviors [12]. The incidence of ASDs is worldwide and recent epidemiological data estimated it to be higher than 1/100 [13]. ASDs vary greatly in the severity of their socio-communicative impairments [14] as well as in cognitive and language development.

Many of the social interpersonal difficulties in ASD derive to some extent from weaknesses in the children's social perception, which in turn relies on both cognitive [15] and motor processes [16]. Social perception refers to children's ability to represent and understand others, their mental states, emotions, and beliefs. Concerning theory of mind (ToM), several studies demonstrated that individuals with ASDs have performance lower than individuals with typical development [17]. These deficits are reported using different versions of ToM tasks, including those examining false beliefs [18], cartoon animations [19], or inferences of mental states from photographs [20].

A key aspect of social perception in ASDs pertains to emotion and affect recognition, yet inconsistent findings have been reported so far. Indeed, while Kuusikko et al. [21] and Krebs et al. [22] pointed to an impairment of children with ASDs in emotion recognition, other studies [23–25] failed to report such a deficit. To date, no evidence has been provided about the possible relationship between social perception scores and performance in human figure drawing tests.

Starting from these premises, in the present study we evaluated the performance of the Draw-a-Man test in a group of children with ASDs, and compared them against a group of age-matched typically developing controls. In particular, we tested two hypotheses: (1) ASDs have lower maturity scores in DAMT, and (2) performance at DAMT differs according to the subjects to-be-depicted (self vs. representation of others). The value of such an investigation is that if a difference is highlighted (i.e., ASDs present lower scores relative to TD), tests based on human figure drawings should not be considered in ASDs as indexing maturity, unless a proper normative ASD population is acquired. In addition to factorial contrasts, the clinical value of the HFD test could be further characterized by correlative approaches testing maturity against neuropsychological scores most common in the clinical practice of autism.

2. Materials and Methods

2.1. Participants

Twenty-one typically developing boys (TD, age M = 8.7, SD = 1.8) and 22 boys with autism spectrum disorders (ASDs, age M = 9.2, SD = 1.7) were included in the study. Groups resulted matched for chronological age ($p = 0.30$) and nonverbal IQ assessed by Raven's Colored Progressive Matrices [26] ($p = 0.72$).

Concerning the ASD group, inclusion criteria were: (a) diagnosis of autism spectrum disorder according to DSM-V/ICD-10 criteria and certified by the Italian Mental Health System (acknowledgement of handicap through Italian law n. 104/1992); (b) age 6–12 years; (c) non-verbal intelligence quotient within the 90–130 range; (d) capacity to adhere to experimental procedures; and (e) lack of comorbidities according to their medical records. Exclusion criteria consisted of (a) presence or history of any other axis I mental disorder; or (b) history of traumatic brain injury or any other neurological disorder as by their medical record. Participants with ASDs were all children with high functioning autism and were recruited via the parents' association "Autismo Pisa APS" sited in Pisa. TD were recruited in primary schools in Parma as children matching the same age criterion used for the ASDs group. Children with a history of neurological or psychiatric disorders were not enrolled, as well as those whose parents or teachers expressed concerns about their development.

Informed written consent was obtained from the parents of all participants, and oral consent from each child. This study was approved by the Local Ethical Committee (Comitato Etico Area Vasta Emilia Nord, prot.n.13051) and was conducted according to the Helsinki Declaration.

2.2. Procedures

2.2.1. Neuropsychological Evaluation

All children were evaluated with a neuropsychological battery including social perception and visuo-spatial domains. Both of them were indexed by subscales of the NEPSY-II test [27].

2.2.2. Social Perception

Social perception domain is evaluated by two different subtests of NEPSY-II [27]: theory of mind and affect recognition. Each subtest is designed to measure a different set of skills necessary for understanding the feelings, perceptions, and intentions of others.

Theory of mind (ToM) includes two tasks. In the verbal task, scenarios or pictures are shown to the child, who has later to answer questions that require knowledge of another individual's perspective. In the contextual task, the child is shown a picture depicting a social situation in which the face of the target individual is not shown. The child is then asked to select one out of four photographs, as the one depicting the most appropriate affect for the target individual in the picture. Overall, theory of mind evaluates the ability to comprehend others' perspectives, intentions, and beliefs.

The affect recognition (AR) test assesses the ability to recognize affects (happiness, sadness, anger, fear, disgust, and neutral) from photographs of children's faces in different tasks like same–different, on-line, and delayed similarity recognition.

2.2.3. Visuo-Spatial Processing

The evaluation of the visuo-spatial domain was limited to the design copying (DC) test from NEPSY-II [27], aimed at assessing motor and visual-perceptual skills associated with the ability to copy two-dimensional geometric figures. It returns a global score (general score), as well as sub-scores measuring the degree of motor abilities, global attributes of the design, and local elements or details of the design. Taken together, these latter three sub-scores form the so-called design copying process score.

2.2.4. Human Figure Drawing (HFD) Test

At the end of the neuropsychological evaluation, each participant was tested with the human figure drawing test, according to the procedures proposed by Royer [28]. HFD allows to explore the child's level of intellectual maturity.

Each participant was given seven colored crayons (blue, green, red, yellow, purple, brown, and black), one pencil, one eraser, and 3 sheets of paper (21 × 29.5 cm) placed vertically. He was requested to draw, on the first sheet, a person. Upon completion of the first drawing, the participant was asked to indicate its gender, and the drawing was removed. Of note, most participants (36 out of

43) started from a male drawing. On the second sheet, the participant was then asked to draw a person of the opposite gender. Upon completion of the second human figure, the drawing was removed and a third sheet provided on which the child was invited to "draw a self-portrait". Children were left free to choose the size and position in the sheet of their drawings. No time limit was imposed.

2.2.5. Non-Human Figure Drawings

Subsequently, children were asked to accomplish a similar task, but depicting three houses (one house, another house, and their own one) rather than human figures. In this way, we obtained a second set of drawings allowing to test two interconnected hypotheses: first, whether children with ASD have peculiar features relative to TD, in particular in terms of similarity among drawings; second, whether such features are specific for human figures, or generalizable also to other subjects.

2.3. Coding of Drawings

The human figure drawings were scored according to the Maturity Scale [28]. This scale accounts for the presence of evolutionary details of the drawing, further grouped in the evaluation of head (23 items), body (32 items) and clothing (14 items), and color use. No Maturity Scale has been validated to date for houses, thus we limited its use to HFD.

To evaluate the differences among the human figure drawings, a similarity score was calculated [29]. The judgement of similarity was evaluated in parallel for three aspects, i.e., dimensions (height and width), body (shapes and colors), and attributes (shapes and colors of clothes and accessories). For each aspect, a score from zero (marked difference) to two (maximum similarity) was assigned. Such a score was evaluated among the three drawings, coupled two-by-two, thus obtaining 3 different scores. The similarity score was also calculated for the house drawings by adapting the scale of similarity used for the human figure drawings, and still comparing the houses to each other, two-by-two. Three different subscales (dimensions, attributes, and accessories) were considered.

We also calculated for the human figure drawings the value score [29]. This evaluates the presence of biases in the representational appearance between two drawings; for example, in the case of a colorful and richly decorated suit versus a monochromatic suit, the value score is greater for the former. The value score was evaluated in parallel for four aspects, i.e., the space occupied by each figure, the articulation of the body, the number of attributes, and the number of colors. These subscales were used to establish whether two figures were equally valued. For each subscale, scores from zero (equality) to two (marked or very marked difference) were assigned.

Two experimenters evaluated the drawings following strictly the guidelines indicated in Royer [28] for the maturity score, and in Bombi and Pinto [29] for the similarity and value scores. In the case of agreement between the two judgments, the agreed score was noted. Conversely, in the case of disagreement between the two experimenters, the final score was obtained after a joint evaluation among the two scorers and the senior author.

2.4. Statistical Analysis

All collected variables (see Table 1) underwent the Shapiro–Wilk's W-test for verifying the assumption of normality. Parametric (one-way ANOVA, Bonferroni post-hoc) or non-parametric tests (Kruskal–Wallis, Mann–Whitney post-hoc) were applied accordingly. Eta-squared (η^2) was calculated as a measure of effect size.

The factorial analysis was intended at verifying the homogeneity among groups in terms of age and non-verbal IQ. The same analysis on the neuropsychological scores and Maturity Scale aimed at evaluating the differences between groups.

Table 1. Main scores for each test and group. Each cell contains the average score (M) and its standard deviation (SD).

	Non-Verbal IQ	Theory of Mind (ToM)	Affect Recognition (AR)	Design Coping (General- DCG)	Design Copying Process (DCP)		
					Motor Ability (DCP-M)	Global Attributes (DCP-Glob)	Local Elements (DCP-Loc)
TD	M = 113.3 SD = 13.2	M = 12.7 SD = 2.9	M = 9.4 SD = 3.3	M = 9.4 SD = 2.4	M = 33.4 SD = 4.4	M = 29.4 SD = 5.1	M = 20.3 SD = 4.5
ASD	M = 112.3 SD = 11.1	M = 6.5 SD = 3.9	M = 7.8 SD = 4.3	M = 5.8 SD = 3.3	M = 28.5 SD = 7.1	M = 25.1 SD = 8.2	M = 16.2 SD = 6.6

Similarity and value scores spanned over a discrete and very narrow range (0, 1, 2), so a factorial analysis was not applicable. To evaluate comparatively these scores between groups, we then carried out a chi-squared tests inserting the count of each score for both ASD and TD, and evaluating whether their distribution varied across groups. In the case of a significant chi test, individual chi values were calculated to highlight which elements carried most of this disproportion.

Finally, we carried out correlation analyses testing the link between the Maturity Scale on one side, and indices of the social perception domain on the other. As we had no assumption on the linearity of such a relationship, we opted for using a Spearman rank correlation. In addition, the analysis was conducted separately for each group so to test the within-group dependency and not just a macroscopic between-group co-difference.

3. Results

Figure 1 reports the drawings from the HFDs of four participants, spanning over age (two 8 years old, two 11 years old) and groups (two TD and two ASDs).

We evaluated on the Maturity Scale and non-verbal IQ the presence of outliers as those subjects exceeding ±2 standard deviations of the sample's mean. Two ASDs and one TD children were outliers for the human figure drawings Maturity Scale, while two children with ASDs were outliers for the non-verbal IQ scores. Then, the final sample consisted of 21 TD and 22 ASD children. Table 1 recaps the average scores for each test and group.

The matching between populations was witnessed by the lack of significant difference between groups, as returned by the Mann–Whitney test, in terms of age (U(22, 21) = 188, Z = 1.04, $p = 0.30$) and non-verbal IQ (U(22, 21) = 216.5, Z = −0.36, $p = 0.72$).

The Maturity Scale resulted as highly significant between groups, as by the one-way ANOVA, for each HDF (HDF-1, $F(1, 41) = 12.67$, $p < 0.001$, $\eta^2 = 0.23$; HFD-2, $F(1, 41) = 15.86$, $p < 0.001$, $\eta^2 = 0.38$; HFD-self, $F(1, 41) = 11.73$, $p = 0.001$, $\eta^2 = 0.22$) (see Figure 2).

The same analysis returned a significant difference for ToM ($F(1, 41) = 34.68$, $p < 0.001$) indicating a marked difference between groups in the ability to comprehend others perspectives, intentions, and beliefs, with TD scores double relative to the ASD ones (TD M = 12.7, ASD M = 6.5). Similar results were obtained for the design copying general (DCG) score ($F(1, 41) = 16.53$, $p < 0.001$). When focusing on the subscale composing the design copy process (DCP), no difference between groups was found neither for DCP-global (TD M = 29.4, ASD M = 25.0) nor for DCP-local (TD M = 20.3, ASD M = 16.2). However, the motor subscale of copy design resulted to be significantly different between the two groups (DCP-motor: U(22, 21) = 127, Z = −2.51, $p = 0.01$) indicating that most of the difference in the DC performance between TD and ASDs relies on a poorer set of motor abilities of the latter group (TD M = 33.4, ASD M = 28.5). No difference emerges for scores at the AR test (U(22, 21) = 177, Z = −1.3, $p = 0.19$).

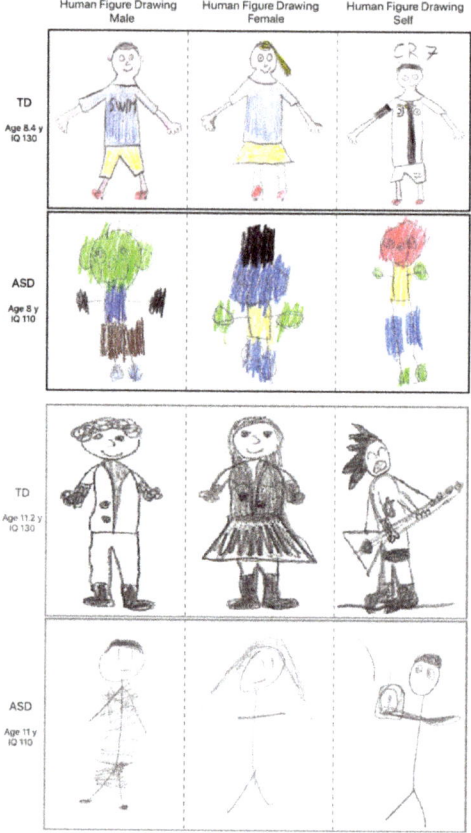

Figure 1. Examples of HFDs by ASD and TD children matched for age. Upper strips (black frame) relate to young children (8 years old), lower strips (grey frame) relate to older children in our range (11 years old). The triplets of maturity scores for the four subjects are (136.9, 125.0, 136.9), (72.4, 71.2, 76.2), (102.3, 112.1, 102.3), and (52.9, 50.1, 49.2), respectively.

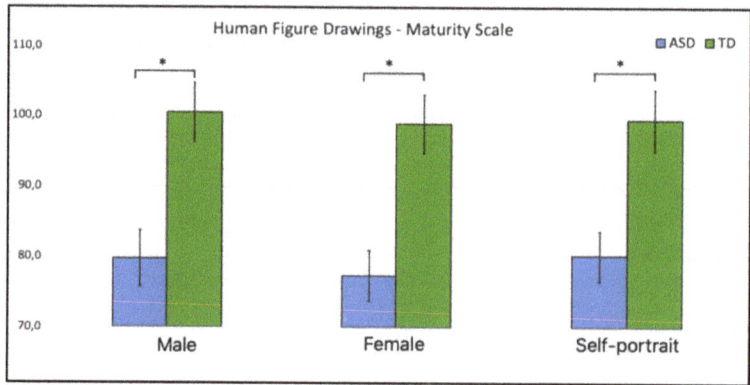

Figure 2. Maturity scale in the three drawings across ASDs and TD children. Bars indicate standard errors; asterisks a p-value < 0.01.

Concerning similarity, a chi-square test was applied to the three possible couples of human figure drawings (HFD-male vs. HFD-self, HFD-female vs. HFD-self, HFD-male vs. HFD-female). A significant difference emerged only in similarity between HFD-male and HFD-female (χ^2 (2, N = 43) = 7.39, p = 0.02). Examining individual chi values, this significance appears mostly due to an over-presence of score 2 (maximum similarity) in ASDs (26 vs. 19.4 expected, χ^2 = 2.2), while TD presented a lower rate of such a score (12 vs. 18.6 expected, χ^2 = 2.3). No other HFD comparison turned out significant. The same procedure was applied to the similarity scores obtained for the houses, so to evaluate whether the tendency to hyper-similarity was specific for human figures, or generalizable also to other subjects. Of note, none of the three house comparisons returned significant results (all p > 0.4).

Despite the correlation analysis between the maturity at HFD and ToM scores resulted as not significant for both groups in all the three drawings, a different pattern emerged between TD and ASDs. Indeed, while TD showed a tendency towards significance in all drawings (all p around 0.08) and r coefficients around 0.4, ASDs fell apart from significance, with r values around 0.

Concerning the correlation between maturity and affect recognition, TD exhibited significant and positive findings for HFD-male and HFD-female, while no link was found for HDF-self. Of note, this pattern was fully reversed examining children with ASDs, who exhibited a significant correlation in HFD-self vs. AR, while non-significant results for HFD-male and HFD-female were found. The results of the correlation analysis are reported in Table 2.

Table 2. Spearman correlation analysis between maturity and affect recognition scores, reporting (r) and p-values in the TD and ASD groups. Significant correlations (p < 0.05) are highlighted in grey.

Group	HFD	r (Spearman)	p-Value
TD	Male	0.53	0.015
	Female	0.53	0.012
	Self	0.33	0.14
ASD	Male	0.20	0.36
	Female	0.32	0.13
	Self	0.45	0.03

4. Discussion

Tests based on human figure drawings have captured the attention of clinicians and psychologists for a long time, likely due to the easiness and ecologicy of their administration, with the aim to achieve a surrogate measurement of children intelligence [30]. However, a non-negligible body of literature has repeatedly challenged the validity of HFD tests [31,32], in particular when non-neurotypical individuals are investigated. The lack of firm guidelines about this matter, moreover, leads to inconsistencies in clinical neurodevelopmental practice, where HFD tests are treated with a relevance spanning over a spectrum from negligible to over-rated.

Pertaining to children with ASDs, although several researchers have suggested the utility of HFD tests in assessing this population [9,33], there are several well-known case studies in which children with autism accompanied by severe cognitive deficits have exhibited a superior drawing ability [34,35]. The findings of the present study align with the view that ASDs have lower maturity in drawings than TD. In line with the revision of the DAMT by Harris (1963) [3], we requested participants to draw three different human figures, yet no substantial differences appeared across these, suggesting a globally lower functioning in drawing rather than a hallmark specific for a given subject (see for example [36]).

These findings suggest that the use of HFD tests with individuals with autism may be not warranted, failing to provide elements suited to drive clinical routines. Indeed, maturity scores are obtained via a normalization against a TD normative population which has—on average—higher scores. To be usable and informative at the individual level, data from a normative population including only children with ASDs should be collected, or at least reference values should be provided to clinicians about the range of maturity scores specific for autistic individuals.

Once ascertained that to date maturity cannot inform about an individual child with ASDs, it is still possible that scores at HFD correlate with the functioning of specific domains. This is why we tested in the same participants the construct of social perception that reflects a variety of psychological processes, mostly involved in ASD symptomatology, i.e., ToM and AR. ToM is defined as the cognitive ability leading to the awareness that others have minds with mental states, information, and motivations that may differ from one's own, allowing an individual to cognitively explain others behaviors [37]. In our study, coherently with previous literature [see 17], ToM scores resulted as highly segregated between ASDs and TD, yet no correlation emerged within both groups with HFD performance. This suggests a certain independency between performance in HFD and ToM tests, in turn reflecting a segregation between the underlying functions.

Concerning affective recognition, a completely different pattern was highlighted. Indeed, no difference appeared at the factorial analysis, suggesting a globally preserved (or restored via a rehabilitation intervention) ability of children with ASDs to explicitly recognize emotional expressions relative to control peers. Our results are in line with Narzisi et al., [38] who found that children with ASDs performed equally well as TD children in the affect recognition test (see also [39]), and with Tracy et al., [40], in which participants with ASDs succeeded in deciding whether an emotional photograph matched a target emotion. However, there is some evidence of atypical face perception processes in individuals with ASDs [41,42]. Indeed, while a deficit in face processing is not pathognomonic (meaning that it is not a definitive diagnostic sign), many children show a significant impairment in encoding facial features. In addition, Kuusikko et al. [21] indicated that despite that emotion recognition may improve with age in children with ASDs, it never completely achieves the level of typically developing individuals. Difficulties with social cognition do not always emerge in structured test situations, especially in high-functioning individuals with ASDs, and this may explain these inconsistent results. According to Harms et al., [43], some individuals with ASDs may utilize compensatory mechanisms (such as explicit cognitive processes) making the performance on facial emotion recognition tasks adequate in test situations, while atypical processing of stimuli is shown in neuroimaging studies [44] and difficulties in emotion recognition in real-life situations [45] are well-known.

Beyond the factorial analysis, we conducted a correlation analysis between scores obtained in HFD in the Maturity Scale and those obtained in the affective recognition test for both groups in order to get insights on the possible link between emotion recognition and drawing performance across multiple to-be-drawn subjects. Our results indicated not only the presence of positive and significant correlations, but also that they largely differed between groups. TD children showed a maturity score significantly associated with affect recognition in drawing other individuals, but not in self-portraits. An opposite pattern emerged for children with ASDs, whose sole maturity in self-portraits significantly correlated with the affective recognition scores.

Such a result could be interpreted in a very fascinating manner: in TD children, the capability to recognize others' emotions could underlie the competence to graphically represent others. In turns, in children with ASDs, emotion recognition is not associated with maturity in the representation of others, but rather it correlates only with maturity in the self-representation. In other words, affective recognition skills might be used by TD to decode the outer social world, but by ASD only to express/represent themselves.

One could speculate that this selective link reflects a lack of experience of the social world in ASD [10], due to their socio-communicative atypicalities and relational poverty further impacting on their cognitive style [46]. The link between maturity and social communicative skills is very interdependent in children with ASDs and it has been the subject of extensive theoretical and empirical investigations [47]. In children with TD, the goodness of early social experiences has been linked to later maturity outcomes [48,49]. As reported by Vivanti (2016) [47], on the contrary, it is plausible that an altered sociability during early development may uniquely impact social dimensions of learning, including de facto the ingredients underlying affective recognition.

Despite only partially covering the abilities underlying the human figure drawing test, we evaluated the design copying test from NEPSY-II [27] to collect an index of an overall drawing performance, comparative between the two groups. The factorial analysis showed a significant difference between children with ASDs and TD children with a difficulty in the global ability to copy two-dimensional geometric figures for the first group, suggesting a weakness in visuomotor integration. The global ability to copy is generally associated with preserved visual-perceptual skills, and our findings are consistent with the validation study of the NEPSY-II by Korkman et al. [27] and with the more recent study by Narzisi et al. [38]. A similar difference was found for the design copy process, and this effect resulted mainly due to one of its subscales, namely the motor subtest. Further, in this case, the group with ASD presented difficulties in fine motor control, in line with a large body of literature pointing at motor disorganization as one of the determinant features in autism [50].

5. Conclusions

In conclusion, our study indicates that children with ASDs have a marked deficit in the human figure drawing test. The lack of a global consensus in the interpretation of HFD results, as well as of normative data peculiar for autism, advocate for an effort, joint by developmental psychology and neuropsychiatry, to achieve a reliable framework for the assessment of individuals with ASDs.

However, out of the clinical practice, tests based on HFD could be considered in basic research for revealing dependencies between drawing performance and neuropsychological features, thus possibly providing hints on the functioning of autism. We hereby showed the existence of a link between maturity in HFD and affect recognition, but the specificity of this result for autism across neurodevelopmental disorders as well as the neural mechanisms at the basis of this alteration have yet to be ascertained. To answer these points, future studies might consider to test additional groups of patients, possibly involving affective disturbances, and accompanying HFD with neurophysiological recordings.

Author Contributions: P.P., M.F.-D. designed the experiment. P.P., M.P., S.P. and A.N. collected data, P.P., M.P. and M.F.-D. analyzed data. M.F.-D. and A.N. wrote the paper. All authors have contributed to, seen and approved the manuscript. All authors have read and agreed to the published version of the manuscript.

Funding: This research received no external funding.

Acknowledgments: P.P. was financially supported by "Soremartec Italia Srl" (Alba, Cuneo, Italy). We wish to thank Pietro Avanzini for his statistical help and comments to the manuscript. Last but not least we wish to thank the families of the children participating to the study for their passionate and active participation.

Conflicts of Interest: No author has any competing interests.

References

1. Wittmann, B. A Neolitich childwood: Children's drawings as prehistoric sources. *Res. Anthropol. Aesthet.* **2013**, *63/64*, 125–142. [CrossRef]
2. Goodenough, F.L. *Measurement of Intelligence by Drawings*; World Book: New York, NY, USA, 1926.
3. Harris, E.B. *Children's Drawings as Measures of Intellectual Maturity: A Revision of the Goodenough Draw-a-Man Test*; Harcourt, Brace & World: New York, NY, USA, 1963.
4. O'Connor, N.; Hermelin, B. Low intelligence and special abilities. *Child Psychol. Psychiatry Allied Discip.* **1988**, *29*, 391–396. [CrossRef] [PubMed]
5. Sacks, O. *An Anthropoligist on Mars*; Knopf: New York, NY, USA, 1995.
6. Selfe, L. *Nadia: A Case of Extraordinary Drawing Ability in an Autistic Child*; Academic Press: New York, NY, USA, 1977.
7. Charman, T.; Baron-Cohen, S. Drawing development in autism: The intellectual to visual realism shift. *Br. J. Dev. Psychol.* **1993**, *11*, 171–185. [CrossRef]
8. Eames, K.; Cox, M.V. Visual realism in the drawings of autistic, Down's syndrome and normal children. *Br. J. Dev. Psychol.* **1994**, *12*, 235–239. [CrossRef]

9. Lee, A.; Hobson, P.R. Drawing self and others: How do children with autism differ from those with learning difficulties? *Br. J. Dev. Psychol.* **2006**, *24*, 547–565. [CrossRef]
10. Lim, H.K.; Slaughter, V. Brief report: Human figure drawings by children with Asperger's syndrome. *J. Autism Dev. Disord.* **2008**, *38*, 988–994. [CrossRef] [PubMed]
11. Volkmar, F.; Siegel, M.; Woodbury-Smith, M.; King, B.; McCracken, J. State M, American Academy of Child and Adolescent Psychiatry (AACAP). Practice parameter for the assessment and treatment of children and adolescents with autism spectrum disorder. *J. Am. Acad. Child Adolesc. Psychiatry* **2014**, *53*, 237–257. [CrossRef] [PubMed]
12. American Psychiatric Association. *Diagnostic and Statistical Manual of Mental Disorders*, 5th ed.; American Psychiatric Pub: Washington, DC, USA, 2013.
13. Maenner, M.J.; Shaw, K.A.; Baio, J. Prevalence of Autism Spectrum Disorder Among Children Aged 8 Years—Autism and Developmental Disabilities Monitoring Network, 11 Sites, United States, 2016. *MMWR Surveill. Summ.* **2020**, *69*, 1. [CrossRef]
14. Lord, C.; Petkova, E.; Hus, V.; Gan, W.; Lu, F.; Martin, D.M.; Ousley, O.; Guy, L.; Bernier, R.; Gerdts, J.; et al. A multisite study of the clinical diagnosis of different autism spectrum disorders. *Arch. Gen. Psychiatry* **2012**, *69*, 306–313. [CrossRef]
15. Baron-Cohen, S.; Leslie, A.M.; Frith, U. Does the autistic child have a "theory of mind". *Cognition* **1985**, *21*, 37–46. [CrossRef]
16. Rizzolatti, G.; Fabbri-Destro, M.; Cattaneo, L. Mirror neurons and their clinical relevance. *Nat. Clin. Pr. Neurol.* **2009**, *5*, 24–34. [CrossRef] [PubMed]
17. Kimhi, Y. Theory of mind abilities and deficits in autism spectrum disorders. *Top. Lang. Disord.* **2014**, *34*, 329–343. [CrossRef]
18. Kimhi, Y.; Shoam-Kugelmas, D.; Ben-Artzi, G.A.; Ben-Moshe, I.; Bauminger-Zviely, N. Theory of mind and executive function in preschoolers with typical development versus intellectually able preschoolers with autism spectrum disorder. *J. Autism Dev. Disord.* **2014**, *44*, 2341–2354. [CrossRef]
19. Salter, G.; Seigal, A.; Claxton, M.; Lawrence, K.; Skuse, D. Can autistic children read the mind of an animated triangle? *Autism* **2008**, *12*, 349–371. [CrossRef] [PubMed]
20. Rosset, D.B.; Rondan, C.; Da Fonseca, D.; Santos, A.; Assouline, B.; Deruelle, C. Typical emotion processing for cartoon but not for real faces in children with autistic spectrum disorders. *J. Autism Dev. Disord.* **2008**, *38*, 919–925. [CrossRef]
21. Kuusikko, S.; Haapsamo, H.; Jansson-Verkasalo, E.; Hurtig, T.; Mattila, M.-L.; Ebeling, H.; Jussila, K.; Bölte, S.; Moilanen, I.; Miettunen, H. Emotion recognition in children and adolescents with autism spectrum disorders. *J. Autism Dev. Disord.* **2009**, *39*, 938–945. [CrossRef]
22. Krebs, J.F.; Biswas, A.; Pascalis, O.; Kamp-Becker, I.; Remschmidt, H.; Schwarzer, G. Face processing in children with autism spectrum disorder: Independent or interactive processing of facial identity and facial expression? *J. Autism Dev. Disord.* **2011**, *41*, 796–804. [CrossRef]
23. Grossman, J.B.; Klin, A.; Carter, A.S.; Volkmar, F.R. Verbal bias in recognition of facial emotions in children with Asperger syndrome. *J. Child Psychol. Psychiatry Allied Discip.* **2000**, *41*, 369–379. [CrossRef]
24. Braverman, M.; Fein, D.; Lucci, D.; Waterhouse, L. Affect comprehension in children with pervasive developmental disorders. *J. Autism Dev. Disord.* **1989**, *19*, 301–315. [CrossRef]
25. Boucher, J.; Lewis, V. Unfamiliar face recognition in relatively able autistic children. *J. Child Psychol. Psychiatry* **1992**, *33*, 843–859. [CrossRef]
26. Raven, J.C. *CPM (Coloured Progressive Matrices)*; Giunti O.S.: Firenze, Italy, 1984.
27. Korkman, M.; Kirk, U.; Kemp, S. *NEPSY-II*; Giunti O.S. Psycometrics: Firenze, Italy, 2011.
28. Royer, J. *La Personnalité de L'enfant à Travers le Dessin du Bonhomme*; Editest: Bruxelles, Belgium, 1977.
29. Bombi, A.S.; Pinto, G. *I Colori Dell'amicizia. Studi Sulle Rappresentazioni Pittoriche Dell'amicizia tra Bambini*; Il Mulino: Bologna, Italy, 1993.
30. Abell, S.C.; Wood, W.; Liebman, S.J. Children's Human Figure Drawings as Measures of Intelligence: The Comparative Validity of Three Scoring Systems. *J. Psychoeduc. Assess.* **2001**, *19*, 204–215. [CrossRef]
31. Camara, W.J.; Nathan, J.S.; Puente, A.E. Psychological test usage: Implications in professional psychology. *Prof. Psychol. Res. Pract.* **2000**, *31*, 141–154. [CrossRef]
32. Cashel, M.L. Child and adolescent psychological assessment: Current clinical practices and the impact of managed care. *Prof. Psychol. Res. Pract.* **2002**, *33*, 446–453. [CrossRef]

33. Reynolds, C.R.; Hickman, J.A. *Draw-A-Person Intellectual Ability Test for Children, Adolescents, and Adults Examiner's Manual*; Pro-ed: Austin, TX, USA, 2004.
34. Mottron, L.; Belleville, S. Perspective production in a savant autistic draughtsman. *Psychol. Med.* **1995**, *25*, 639–648. [CrossRef] [PubMed]
35. O'Connor, N.; Hermelin, B. Visual and graphic abilities of the idiot savant artist. *Psychol. Med.* **1987**, *17*, 79–90. [CrossRef]
36. Nuara, A.; Papangelo, P.; Avanzini, P.; Fabbri-Destro, M. Body representation in children with unilateral cerebral palsy. *Front. Psychol.* **2019**, *10*, 354. [CrossRef]
37. Korkmaz, B. Theory of mind and neurodevelopmental disorders of childhood. *Pediatric Res.* **2011**, *69*, 101–108. [CrossRef]
38. Narzisi, A.; Muratori, F.; Calderoni, S.; Fabbro, F.; Urgesi, C. Neuropsychological profile in high functioning autism spectrum disorders. *J. Autism Dev. Disord.* **2013**, *43*, 1895–1909. [CrossRef]
39. Barron-Linnankoski, S.; Reinvall, O.; Lahervuori, A.; Voutilainen, A.; Lahti-Nuuttila, P.; Korkman, M. Neurocognitive performance of children with higher functioning autism spectrum disorders on the NEPSY-II. *Child Neuropsychol.* **2015**, *21*, 55–77. [CrossRef]
40. Tracy, J.L.; Robins, R.W.; Schriber, R.A.; Solomon, M. Is emotion recognition impaired in individuals with autism spectrum disorders? *J. Autism Dev. Disord.* **2011**, *41*, 102–109. [CrossRef]
41. Jemel, B.; Mottron, L.; Dawson, M. Impaired face processing in autism: Fact or artifact? *J. Autism Dev. Disord.* **2006**, *36*, 91–106. [CrossRef] [PubMed]
42. Adolphs, R.; Sears, L.; Piven, J. Abnormal processing of social information from faces in autism. *J. Cogn. Neuro Sci.* **2001**, *13*, 232–240. [CrossRef] [PubMed]
43. Harms, M.B.; Martin, A.; Wallace, G.L. Facial emotion recognition in autism spectrum disorders: A review of behavioral and neuroimaging studies. *Neuropsychol. Rev.* **2010**, *20*, 290–322. [CrossRef] [PubMed]
44. Nomi, J.S.; Uddin, L.Q. Face processing in autism spectrum disorders: From brain regions to brain networks. *Neuropsychologia* **2015**, *71*, 201–216. [CrossRef]
45. Constantino, J.N.; Gruber, C.P. *The Social Responsiveness Scale Manual*; Psychological Services: Los Angeles, CA, USA, 2005.
46. Happé, F. Autism: Cognitive deficit or cognitive style? *Trends Cogn. Sci.* **1999**, *3*, 216–222. [CrossRef]
47. Vivanti, G.; Hocking, D.R.; Fanning, P.; Dissanayake, C. Social affiliation motives modulate spontaneous learning in Williams syndrome but not in autism. *Mol. Autism* **2016**, *7*, 40. [CrossRef]
48. Bornstein, M.H.; Hahn, C.S.; Suwalsky, J.T. Physically developed and exploratory young infants contribute to their own long-term academic achievement. *Psychol. Sci.* **2013**, *24*, 1906–1917. [CrossRef]
49. Walker-Andrews, A.; Krogh-Jespersen, S.; Mayhew, E.; Coffield, C. The situated infant. In *Infant Mind: Origins of the Social Brain*; Legerstee, M., Haley, D., Bornstein, M., Eds.; Guilford Press: New York, NY, USA, 2013.
50. Fabbri-Destro, M.; Gizzonio, V.; Avanzini, P. Autism, motor dysfunctions and mirror mechanism. *Clin. Neuropsychiatry* **2013**, *10*, 177–187.

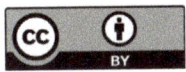

© 2020 by the authors. Licensee MDPI, Basel, Switzerland. This article is an open access article distributed under the terms and conditions of the Creative Commons Attribution (CC BY) license (http://creativecommons.org/licenses/by/4.0/).

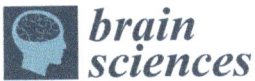
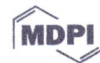

Article

Behavioral and Autonomic Responses in Treating Children with High-Functioning Autism Spectrum Disorder: Clinical and Phenomenological Insights from Two Case Reports

Lucia Billeci [1], Ettore Caterino [2], Alessandro Tonacci [1,*] and Maria Luisa Gava [3]

1. Institute of Clinical Physiology, National Research Council of Italy, 56124 Pisa, Italy; lucia.billeci@ifc.cnr.it
2. Azienda USL Sudest Toscana, Centro Autismo UFSMIA di Grosseto, Ospedale di Castel del Piano, 58033 Grosseto, Italy; ettore.caterino@uslsudest.toscana.it
3. Associazione Nazionale Famiglie di Persone con Disabilità Intellettiva e/o Relazionale (ANFFAS), 18100 Imperia, Italy; marialuisa.gava@gmail.com
* Correspondence: atonacci@ifc.cnr.it

Received: 9 June 2020; Accepted: 14 June 2020; Published: 17 June 2020

Abstract: In this study, we aimed to evaluate the process applied in subjects with Autism Spectrum Disorder (ASD) to elaborate and communicate their experiences of daily life activities, as well as to assess the autonomic nervous system response that subtend such a process. This procedure was evaluated for the first time in two eight-year-old girls with high-functioning ASDs. The subjects performed six months of training, based on the cognitive–motivational–individualized (c.m.i.®) approach, which mainly consisted in building domestic procedures and re-elaborating acquired experiences through drawing or the use of icons made by the children. Together with behavioral observations, the response of the autonomic nervous system during such re-elaboration was recorded. A change in communicative and interactive competences was observed, moving from a condition of spontaneity to one in which the girls were engaged in relating their experiences to a parent. Autonomic response highlighted how, in communicating their own experiences, they achieved a state of cognitive activation, which enabled a greater communicative and emotional connection with the interlocutor. This is a proof-of-concept study on the application of the c.m.i.®, which needs to be extensively validated in the clinical setting.

Keywords: high-functioning autism; language; experience; communication; autonomic nervous system; wearable technologies

1. Introduction

In the field of Autism Spectrum Disorders (ASD), several studies showed the importance of structuring a space, a time and a specific visual support as part of the related clinical intervention [1]. Many behavioral approaches provide a visual target to a child with ASD in order to implement the acquisition of a skill (i.e., washing the hands), assuming that the child would be more sensitized and would have a greater level of attention and orientation if induced to the object or action by an iconic structure.

However, according to our previous research study [2], our idea is that a child with ASD, somewhat similar to a typical developing child, should learn a procedure in a natural context (i.e., in their own environment) and then, eventually, use icons or visual references to recall the acquired skills. In this way, the child will be able to understand the real meaning of the visual reference used with respect to what the children have acquired during their own experience. In this way, the icons will only represent the starting point for recalling the actions the subject has previously learned (i.e., washing, dressing, cooking, etc.). Notably, this process requires the subject to be able to manipulate the experience acquired with a higher level of awareness and participation and then to verbalize and recall their own experiences. To recognize their experience, they should mentally manipulate the acquired contents (i.e., who, what, where and when) and the connections made among the motor actions performed. This is often difficult in children with high-functioning ASD due to the presence of deficits in executive functions [3,4], in social perception [5] and in narrative and pragmatic skills.

In this framework, the cognitive–motivational–individualized (c.m.i.®) approach is aimed at supporting an orientation and awareness process of personal reality and knowledge in subjects with verbal and/or cognitive and/or relational disabilities, so that they can organize and express their thoughts in a more understandable and orderly way. This approach, initially set up to facilitate work with augmentative and alternative communication (AAC) [6], represents a learning process since, through a specific reconstruction of daily life activities and work, the subject is helped to acquire these experiences in a more conscious and autonomous way. Specifically, to facilitate this process, a figurative reworking is proposed in order to make the experience concrete, visible and manually usable. From this perspective, the subject must retrace the practical process of the experience both on a symbolic plane and on a motor level, manipulating the components (i.e., what, where, who) and their connections or semantic constraints (i.e., what/where, who/what) in a praxis narrative form that refers to the experiential action. This would enable an understand of the process within which the subject retains the elements that are significant for them in reality (what he/she knows, what he/she does, what he/she likes, where the experiences take place and with whom they do these experiences) and how performing motor actions (acting on the images, the icons drawn from his/her everyday experience) re-elaborates his/her knowledge. The overall aim is to facilitate the integration between the experiential and phenomenal meaning performed with the body and language (lexical semantics) to avoid—as often happens in children with ASD—that, during the narration, the subject is only using the lexical meaning without the emotional content, which defines intentionality in the communication, the participation and, therefore, the intersubjective sense of language [7–9].

Together with behavioral observation, the assessment of physiological parameters during the task of reproducing the acquired experience in ASD subjects could help the clinician to understand the way the subjects are processing these experiences. In particular, several studies suggest that Autonomic Nervous System (ANS) activity is linked to social functioning in individuals with ASD [10–14]. Both the sympathetic (SNS) and parasympathetic (PNS) branches of the ANS contribute to social functioning and communication [15,16], with SNS activation reflecting a threat-oriented response, and PNS dominance easing adaptive social engagement [17]. More specifically, the PNS plays an important role in social functioning by innervating several organs in the face and in the neck and affecting various functions, including cardiac activity, which are related to social behavior and communication [18]. Thus, in a social setting, an increase in the PNS activity is related to an adaptive social behavior [13]. The SNS also plays an important role in social functioning, increasing heart rate (HR), sweating and alert state, mainly through acting on the so-called "fight or flight" mechanism [19,20].

Wearable technologies can be particularly relevant in the assessment of ANS in ASD due to their low obtrusiveness. In particular, the recording of the electrocardiogram (ECG) signal allows us to evaluate the activation of both the PNS and SNS by studying heart rate variability (HRV) [10]. On the other hand, the assessment of the galvanic skin response (GSR) is mainly related to the SNS, with a reduction in the signal associated with decreased SNS influence [21], whereas an increase in skin conductance during specific social tasks subtends higher SNS activation [22].

In this study, we aim to highlight how, in subjects with high-functioning ASD, it is a priority to enhance the mechanisms of self-awareness related to their experiences and knowledge rather than immediately using linguistic codes, icons or scripts or giving heuristic value to a phenomenological approach. More specifically, the objectives of the present study include: (i) to evaluate the behavior and communication of two subjects with ASD during the elaboration of an experiential content (procedural actions of shared daily life with the parent); (ii) to assess the ANS responses that underlie the subjects' behavior during such elaboration.

2. Materials and Methods

2.1. Participants

The subjects were two eight-year-old girls, with diagnoses of ASD, attending the "Autism service of the public health of the city of Grosseto". The protocol was approved by the Institutional Ethical Clearance board of the National Research Council (0087922/2019).

2.1.1. Subject 1—J

At the age of 3, J. received a clinical diagnosis of Autism Spectrum Disorder (ASD) confirmed with the Autism Diagnostic Observation Schedule-Generic (ADOS-G) [23]. Her non-verbal cognitive level, measured through Leiter-R [24] and Color Progressive Matrices [25] was average. In her clinical history, motor and language delays were reported. At the age of 3, J. showed a severe psychomotor and language regression. In this period, J. also partially lost sphincter control, showing sialorrhoea and feeding disturbance. She was severely apathetic. Before enrollment in this study, she started a psychoeducational intervention including speech and psychomotor therapies. At the age of the enrollment (6 y), J. presented a normostructured language with flat prosody and a socio-pragmatic disorder. Regarding her motor skills, she presented hypotonia and coarse-motor impairment, while she had adequate fine motor praxes and graph-pictorial skills.

2.1.2. Subject 2—B

At the age of 5, B. received a clinical diagnosis of Autism Spectrum Disorder (ASD) confirmed with ADOS-G. Her cognitive level, measured through Wechsler Preschool and Primary Scale of Intelligence (WPPSI-III) [26], was average (Full Scale Intelligence Quotient, FSIQ = 107). In her clinical history, language delay, marked issues in emotional dysregulation and Attention Deficit Hyperactivity Disorder (ADHD) were reported. Before enrollment in the study, she started a psychoeducational intervention. At the age of enrollment (6 y), B. was an hyperverbal child with high functioning ASD in comorbidity with ADHD and emotional dysregulation (i.e., meltdown). She used reinforcement strategies for performing school—and daily life—activities (i.e., planned and structured environments and activities, visual aids).

2.2. The c.m.i.® Approach

The c.m.i.® approach adopts a naturalistic and developmental approach (NBDI) [27]. It targets social, interactive and communication impairments in autism. The rationale is that children with autism would respond with enhanced communicative and social development to a style of parent communication adapted to their impairments [28]. The intervention is aimed to enhance the link between neuropsychological and relational skills. The rationale of c.m.i.® is the application of embodied cognition in the intervention for ASD. Inspired by Johnson-Glenberg and Megowan-Romanowicz [29], the three degrees of embodiment are considered: (a) sensorimotor experience; (b) link between body language and feelings; (c) emotional immersion experienced by the user.

The c.m.i.® methodology is aimed at supporting an orientation process and awareness of one's reality and knowledge in subjects with verbal, cognitive and relational disabilities so that they can organize and express their thoughts in a more comprehensible and orderly way. This experience is made explicit initially using the body—doing and perceiving also represent a form of non-verbal communication which subsequently and progressively evolves into language. The intervention allows a progressive maturation of orientation abilities in reality that affects the following dimensions: (i) spatial: where are things, people, objects; (ii) temporal: when events occur; (iii) instrumental: objects in the environment, their nature, their functions; (iv) relational: people around the subject.

2.3. Training According to the Cognitive Motivational Intervention (c.m.i.®)

The training of the two subjects according to the c.m.i.® approach was performed at home and involved the parents. It consisted of the following phases:

- Interview with the parents: During the interview, the parents were informed about the aims and modalities of the training approach and their involvement in the process. In addition, informed consent was obtained from the parents of the two girls enrolled, after receiving an exhaustive explanation of the study. Such explanation included: (a) the description of the theory of the cognitive motivational intervention; (b) the rationale of physiological signal acquisition and the procedures for data collection; (c) detailed description of home procedures; (d) the description of the re-elaboration of acquired experiences through drawing; (e) the modalities of using icons by the children.
- Observation of the two girls: This aimed at identifying the individual characteristics of the two girls. J. loves drawing and adds plenty of particulars in her drawings, although images look quite static. Conversely, B. is constantly in motion and uses continuous, redundant, sophisticated and dyspragmatic language. She does not like drawing, but rather prefers moving and talking. She has difficulties in maintaining task concentration. In order to manage individual differences among the subjects, meetings with parents were organized in order to explain to them the individual phenotypic profile of their child and how to manage the emotional experience of the child as well as their own. Specifically, therapists contacted the parents four times a month after the initial meeting.
- Training to realize the procedures: The parents were instructed how to guide the two girls in the acquisition of specific procedures, which consisted in cooking the girls' favorite foods (spaghetti for J. and biscuits for B.). Then, the girls were helped in acquiring information about the environments in which they were supposed to cook (which objects to use and where they are located). Once a week, the two girls were involved in making up their favorite food.

2.4. Evaluation of the Acquired Procedure

The evaluation of the acquired procedure was performed in a laboratory setting and was aimed at recalling the procedures acquired at home to allow the transition from praxis to a symbolic action when the girls reached a certain degree of autonomy. The session was guided by the experimenter who developed the c.m.i.® approach (M.L.G.).

The first phase of the evaluation (after six months) consisted in performing a graphical trace, which represented a symbolic reconstruction of the kitchen and objects used at home. Each girl was seated next to the experimenter at a table on which some papers and markers were positioned. First, the girl was guided in recovering the experience learned at home on the verbal level and subsequently in the drawing of the objects and the ingredients she used at home for cooking the selected food.

The second phase of the evaluation (after 10 months) consisted in the action on the represented, which dealt with the description of the experience acquired at home through the use of mobile icons to reproduce the motor action performed in the real scenario.

2.5. Physiological Signal Acquisition

During the evaluation procedure, the two subjects were equipped with two minimally obtrusive, wireless, wearable sensors for the monitoring of the electrocardiogram (ECG) and galvanic skin response (GSR). The ECG signal was acquired through the Shimmer ECG sensor (Shimmer Sensing, Dublin, Ireland) with a sampling frequency of 500 Hz, whereas the GSR signal was captured by the Shimmer3 GSR+ sensor (Shimmer Sensing, Dublin, Ireland) with a sampling frequency of 51.2 Hz. The Shimmer ECG acquired the relevant signal attached to a fitness-like chest strap manufactured by Polar Electro Oy (Kempele, Finland), whereas the Shimmer3 GSR+ captured the galvanic skin response by adhering to two nearby fingers of the subject's non-dominant hand through comfortable rings. The signals were acquired while the subject was seated on a chair at a table during the following phases:

- Baseline (3′): Basal measurement. Here, the subject was asked to stay as still as possible.
- Task (15′): Signal acquisition during the proposed tasks.
- Recovery (3′): Post-task basal measurement. The subject was required to stay as still as possible, similar to baseline.

2.6. Physiological Signal Analysis

The acquired physiological signals were processed using Matlab (Mathworks, Natick, MA, USA). In particular, the ECG signal was analyzed using home-made scripts for the calculation of the tachogram (RR series; i.e., the time elapsed between two successive R-waves) according to the Pan–Tompkins algorithm [30] and to extract both time and frequency domain features characterizing the ANS for each of the different phases.

The features extracted included:

- Heart rate (HR): the number of contractions of the heart occurring per time unit, expressed in bpm;
- Standard deviation of normal to normal RR intervals (SDNN): measure of heart rate variability (HRV), expressed in ms;
- Normalized component of the power spectral density of the ECG signal at low frequency (0.04–0.15 Hz) (nLF), which is related both to the sympathetic and parasympathetic response;
- Normalized component of the power spectral density of the ECG spectrum at high frequency (0.15–0.4 Hz) (nHF), which is mainly related to the parasympathetic response;
- Low versus high frequency components of the power spectral density of the ECG spectrum (LF/HF Ratio), which expresses the balance between the sympathetic and parasympathetic nervous system branches.

GSR signal was analyzed using Ledalab V3.4.9 (General Public License (GNU)), a Matlab-based tool enabling the user to extract typical features of the GSR signal, notably its tonic and phasic components [31]. Specifically—albeit both of the abovementioned components were extracted—for this work only the tonic phase was analyzed, since the rationale of the study aimed at comparing the signal in the different phases rather than evaluating the response to a given single stimulation.

Additional details about the analysis procedure can be found in previous studies [32,33].

3. Results

To assess the effects of treatment for every child and, keeping in line with the case series design, data were examined on an individual participant basis. Individual changes in social communication, adaptive behavior and neural response to social stimuli are discussed below.

3.1. Behavioral Observations

After a six month period (follow-up) of behavioral observations of the two subjects included in the present work, a critical evaluation was conducted concerning the experience carried out at home.

J. loved drawing. Compared to her previous drawings that were very static, she added an increasing number of dynamic characteristics in her storytelling and her drawings (i.e., climbing stairs, drying clothes). She was very precise and participated in the reconstruction of the objects, using language, eye contact and checking whether the therapist or the adult was able to listen to her and whether her work was being appreciated, as shown in Figure 1a.

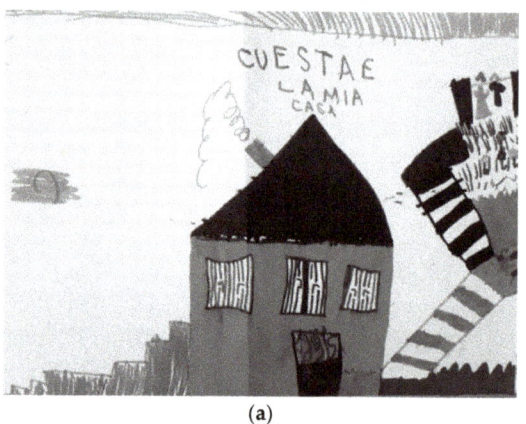 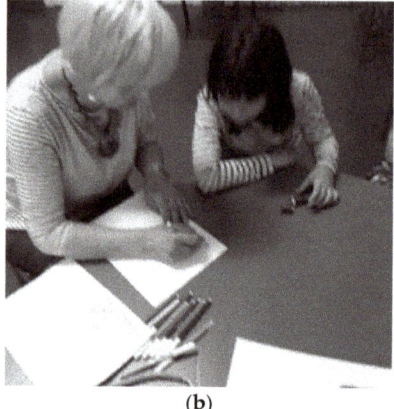

Figure 1. The first evaluation consisting in the graphical trace. (**a**) The drawing by J., (**b**) B. watches the experimenter drawing while she verbalizes.

B. reported difficulties in terms of the graphical realization of the tasks demanded. She preferred to use her voice to describe the steps of the recipe learned at home, while the experimenter realized the drawing, as shown in Figure 1b. She displayed quite rich and cogent language, albeit not always adherent to reality. The deposition of her mother was particularly interesting, as she reported significantly less automated language and an optimal self-care when physically engaged in actions.

After 10 months (second follow-up), the re-evaluation consisted in the action of the represented task, aimed at representing actions developed at home within the praxis procedure using mobile icons on a re-constructed background. The adult helped the child in re-constructing the kitchen on a paper sheet, positioning fixed objects (including furniture), whereas mobile ones were manipulated to narrate the procedure of cooked food.

J. verbalized the different phases, being very careful in adding elements related to the procedure, as shown in Figure 2a.

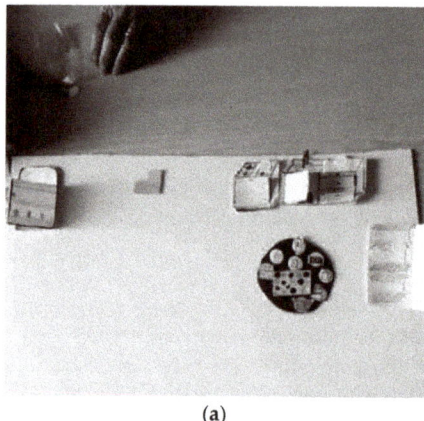 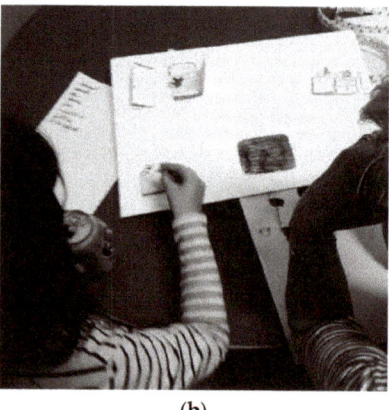

Figure 2. The second evaluation consisting in the action on the represented task. (**a**) The cooking of the biscuits realized with the icons by J., (**b**) B. reconstructing the procedure of cooking spaghetti.

B. often used mobile elements with good motor and language competence. Compared to the graphical trace evaluation, she expressed more self-control, as shown in Figure 2b.

Importantly, both girls' parents seemed to participate in their daughters' work. They highlighted with surprise and continuous discovery some characteristics of their daughters and they were more attentive about the movements of their children in the environment and about the way actions were followed (e.g., preparing "green" spaghetti and "white and black" biscuits, etc., spontaneously and with personal semantic links between objects and actions).

3.2. Autonomic Nervous System Response—Graphical Trace

With J., the task highlighted the presence of verbalization with and without ocular contact. When the drawing was similar to the experienced reality, the subject increased ocular contact with respect to the therapist, whereas a stereotyped drawing drove her to hypo-regulation and relational disinvestment.

According to behavioral observations, for J. the physiological signals were segmented in three different sub-phases during the execution of the task: verbalization with eye-contact, verbalization without eye-contact, and no response (during which she was concentrated on drawing and did not reply to the experimenter).

Concerning the ECG, an increased HR and a decreased HRV during verbalization with ocular contact was observed, as shown in Figure 3a,c. Conversely, during verbalization without eye contact, as well as during non-response phases and less cognitively-demanding tasks, the HRV was significantly increased, as shown in Figure 3c. Focusing on the SNS/PNS activation, it is worth noting that the SNS activity increased during the task, with somewhat of a SNS withdrawal during the verbalization with eye contact, probably due to a decrease in the stress level of the subject when interacting with the therapist, as shown in Figure 3b,d.

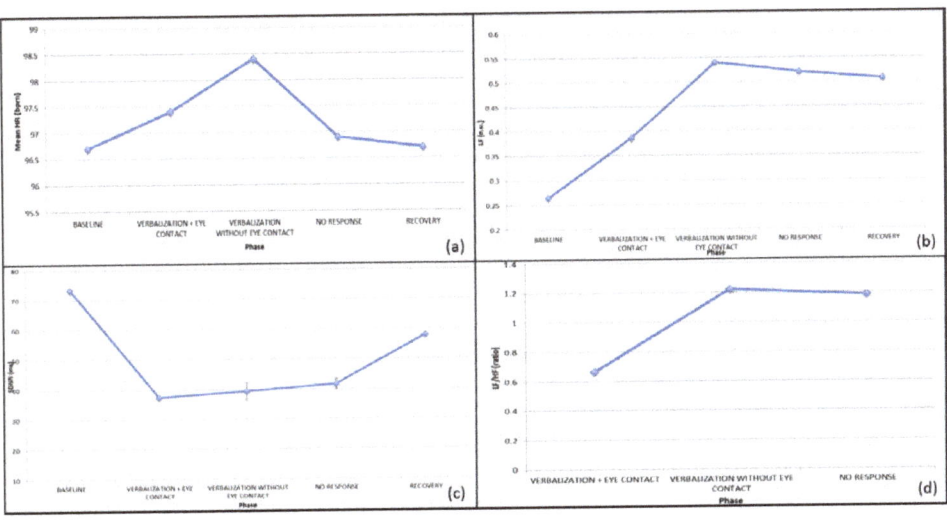

Figure 3. ECG features for J. during the various phases of the graphical trace: (**a**) HR, (**b**) LF, (**c**) SDNN, (**d**) LF/HF.

With J., the GSR signal displayed an increased phasic component, related to the response to a given stimulation during the task, whereas the tonic component mainly increased at recovery, indicating that the stress response, activated by the task performed, remained active after the completion of the task.

B. verbalized both during the execution of the graphical trace by the therapist and without the drawing. According to this behavioral observation, for B. the physiological signals were segmented in two different sub-phases during the execution of the task: verbalization with the graphical trace and verbalization without the graphical trace.

Concerning the ECG signal, the HR was increased from baseline to task during both phases, probably suggesting a higher arousal level while performing the tasks, followed by a similar decrease during recovery. Similar to the first subject, the HRV decreased here during the task, particularly while verbalizing and performing graphical trace (i.e., during a higher emotionally-demanding task), as shown in Figure 4a,c.

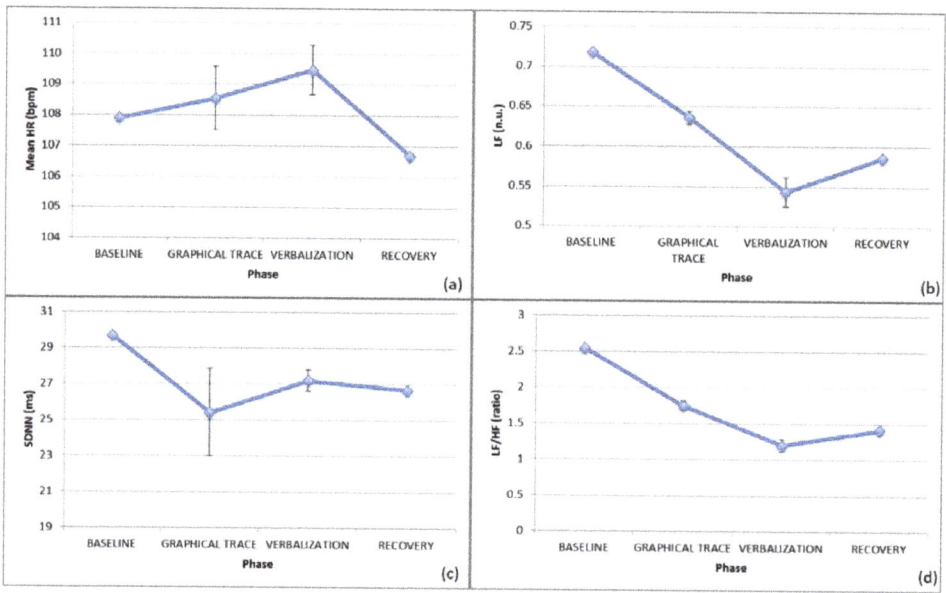

Figure 4. ECG features for B. during the various phases of the graphical trace: (**a**) HR, (**b**) LF, (**c**) SDNN, (**d**) LF/HF.

Focusing on the SNS/PNS activation, the second subject already displayed an over-activation of the SNS at baseline, with a PNS dominance during the task, ending with the return to a SNS prevalence at recovery, with the opposite trend with respect to the first individual analyzed, as shown in Figure 4b,d.

The GSR signal revealed an increased tonic and phasic component at task, with further stress evidence at recovery, possibly due to the environmental constraints necessarily applied to complete the experimental task (i.e., sitting on a given chair, staying in a given room, etc.).

3.3. Autonomic Nervous System Response—Action on the Represented

In the second task, the action on the represented task, no specific sub-phases could be defined, therefore the signals were not further segmented.

With J., an increased HR was observed with a contextual HRV decrease, probably suggesting significant cognitive involvement by the subject, as shown in Figure 5. Focusing on the SNS/PNS activation, the PNS component was dominating throughout the trial, with a slight increase in SNS activity at task.

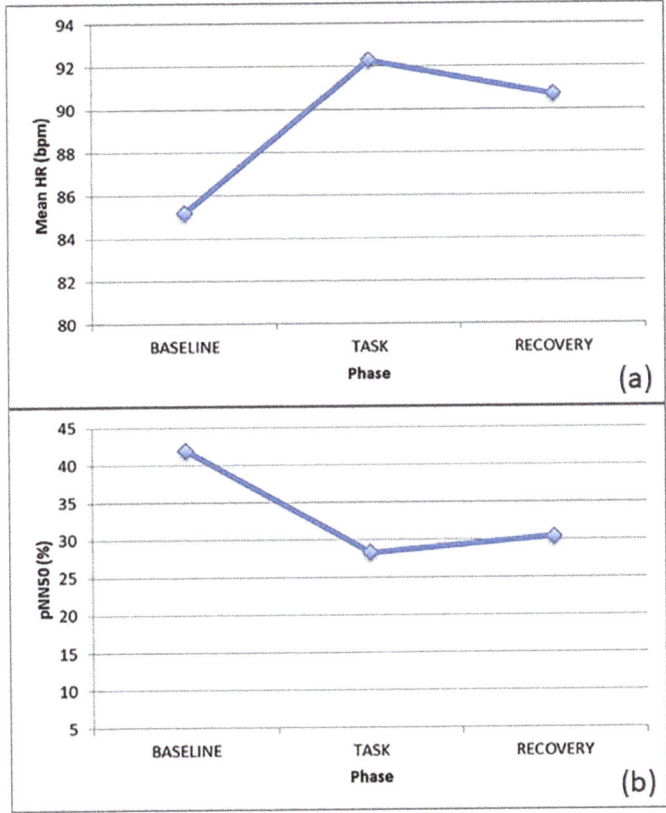

Figure 5. ECG features for J. during the various phases of the action on the represented: (a) HR, (b) pNN50.

The GSR signal showed an increased tonic component at task, probably suggesting an enhanced emotional involvement, whereas the phasic component appeared to be decreased, possibly because of the emotional involvement taking place for the engagement phase more than for the single tasks administered.

With B., a decreased HR and HRV at task was noticed, probably due to relaxation and enhanced task-demanded concentration, as shown in Figure 6.

The evaluation of SNS/PNS confirmed the tendency towards a SNS decrease at task, lasting up to the recovery phase, confirming the regulatory effect of the demanded task, considering the different basal involvement of the subject, who was more stressed at the beginning of the experimental protocol with respect to the previous individual.

Finally, as for the GSR signal, both the tonic and phasic components are higher as long as the test takes place, probably due to the abovementioned logistic constraints for the test administration for the previous subject tested.

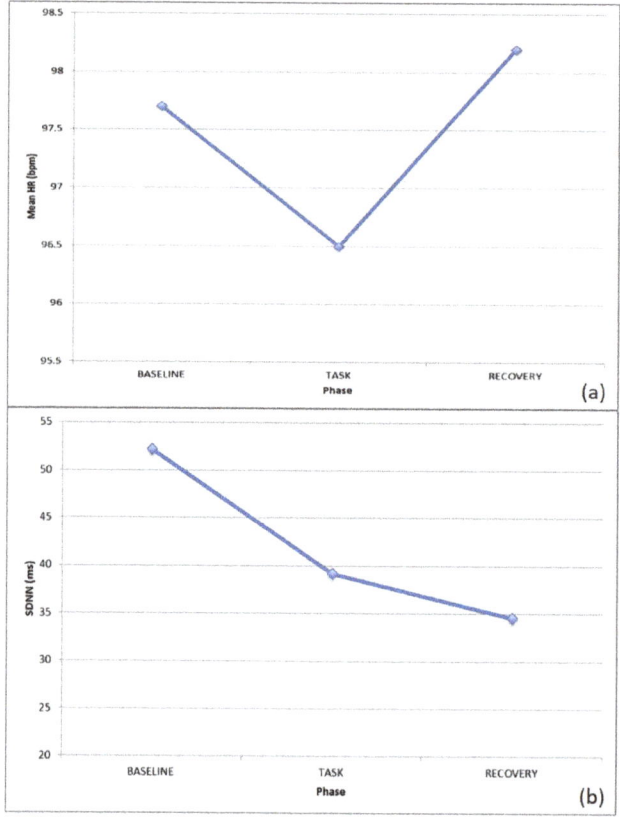

Figure 6. HR/HRV for B. during the various phases of the action on the represented: (**a**) HR, (**b**) SDNN.

4. Discussion

The most important lesson learned during the test administration and the discussion of the results of the present study protocol is the pivotal need for the personalization of the therapy that children with neurodevelopmental disorders should undergo. Indeed, despite the fact that the present study took into account just two subjects, with the same age and somewhat similar clinical characteristics, the personal attitudes, behaviors, and past histories surely played a significant role in their responses, with completely different neurophysiological adaptations to the tasks administered displayed by the two children. Indeed, different autonomic responses were seen between the two individuals, with different trends likely to be due to the personal attitudes of both subjects. With J., the clinical observation and the physiological parameters show how the girl, when left alone, tends towards a condition of hypo-regulation and relational closure. In this phase, she draws in a stereotyped way. When asked to design her own experiences, on the contrary, she expresses good communication skills, eye contact, and a greater adherence to the represented content. In this phase, the physiological parameters show that she is more engaged in the task and she has a good relationship with the examiner with the experiences she has learned in her own reality. With B.—who also has a hyper-regulated neurosensory profile at the baseline—progressive emotional regulation, emotional engagement and, therefore, good homeostasis, was obtained through cognitive reorganization (graphic trace, action on the represented task) and the narration of her experiences. Notably she remains regulated in the recovery phase after performing the drawing and the action on the represented task, as if, through this experience of reorganization, she could reach the regulation of her emotional components that usually tend to be dysregulated, impulsive and destabilizing.

These observations of individual characteristics and autonomic responses of the subjects, that happen quite often in presence of subjects with ASD, even with similar clinical characteristics, pave the way to a strongly personalized approach to the treatment.

To this extent, the proof of concept related to the importance of precision medicine in neurodevelopmental disorders has been already highlighted in past years, with interesting links postulated within the framework of genotype–phenotype relationships [34]. Indeed, treatment personalization might provide some benefit by addressing some of the deficits shown by children, even in the field of neurodevelopmental disorders [35].

The present work suggests that the cognitive–motivational–individualized (c.m.i.®) approach, the main focus of our investigation, sets its basis on this concept, completely relying on providing a complete overview of the individual aspects of a child and taking into account both cognitive and motivational dimensions to optimize the treatment outcome. In particular, the therapist administering the protocol should be able to empower the positive mindset of the individual treated. Indeed, ASD, even more than other neurodevelopmental disorders, presents individuals that are highly motivated to engage in their special interests, and are more motivated than non-ASD subjects (particularly typically developing controls) by intrinsic motivational factors, some of which are associated with positive effects [36]. Additionally, cognitive level should be taken into account in ASD, as demonstrated by the positive cognitive gains that behavioral and cognitive therapy has on individuals with ASD during adolescence (see [37] for an example) and even during adulthood [38].

Such positive preliminary impressions, albeit necessitating the confirmation on large-scale studies brought forward by the first results of this investigation, should be carefully considered, even in light of some acknowledged limitations. At first, the enrollment of just two subjects does not allow us to draw conclusions applicable to the general ASD population, or even to its subgroups (i.e., High-Functioning ASD); however, it gives us room for further investigation, applying c.m.i.® to larger cohorts likely to confirm an extreme heterogeneity of the treatment response. Notably, this study represents a proof-of-concept for the application of the c.m.i.® approach, which is based on a theoretical framework, and on the assessment of the physiological response of subjects with ASD during such treatment.

Second, the application, in this protocol, of c.m.i.® to only female subjects could reveal cognitive, behavioral and motivational characteristics that are specifically gender-biased, thus not reflecting the reality possibly observed among males, which represent the vast majority of ASD individuals (see [39] for some estimates).

Third, the fact that the two subjects enrolled belonged to an age group between 6 and 10 years, together with the absence of a control group, made it difficult to ascertain the likely positive effect due to c.m.i.® with respect to a general positive effect due to age. Therefore, future studies should include a control group to effectively discriminate further the contribution of c.m.i.® to the personal cognitive growth of ASD children.

Fourth, the use of wearables, even if recently more frequent in the scientific literature dealing with ASD (see, for example, [40,41]), should take advantage of a wider, better grounded amount of data, which will be possible step-by-step in next few years when such methodologies, still relatively new in the neurophysiological monitoring of ASD, will fully enter scientific society.

Under such premises, still taking into full consideration the abovementioned limitations, and if confirmed on large-scale studies, the proposed approach could flank traditional therapies, possibly improving the patients' outcomes based on their own specificities, paving the way for precision medicine in ASD and neurodevelopmental disorders. Further studies are needed to extensively apply and validate the proposed approach in a clinical setting.

5. Conclusions

The pilot study described here presented a novel approach for improving cognitive features of children and adolescents with ASD, leaning on personal motivations and own interests. Despite presenting some benefits for the patients included in the present study, the beneficial effects of this approach should be confirmed on larger cohorts, also taking advantage of the enrollment of control groups, lacking in our protocol. Eventual, likely positive results would further enable the large-scale application of the c.m.i. approach flanking traditional cognitive and behavioral therapies.

Author Contributions: Conceptualization, L.B., E.C. and M.L.G.; Data curation, L.B., A.T. and M.L.G.; Formal analysis, L.B. and A.T.; Funding acquisition, E.C. and M.L.G.; Investigation, L.B., E.C., A.T. and M.L.G.; Methodology, L.B., E.C. and M.L.G.; Project administration, L.B., E.C., A.T. and M.L.G.; Resources, E.C. and M.L.G.; Software, L.B. and A.T.; Supervision, E.C. and M.L.G.; Validation, L.B., E.C., A.T. and M.L.G.; Writing—original draft, L.B., E.C., A.T. and M.L.G.; Writing—review and editing, L.B., A.T. and M.L.G. All authors have read and agreed to the published version of the manuscript.

Funding: This research was funded by ANFFAS Onlus, Imperia.

Conflicts of Interest: The authors declare no conflict of interest.

References

1. Beadle-Brown, J.; Wilkinson, D.; Richardson, L.; Shaughnessy, N.; Trimingham, M.; Leigh, J.; Whelton, B.; Himmerich, J. Imagining Autism: Feasibility of a drama-based intervention on the social, communicative and imaginative behaviour of children with autism. *Autism* **2018**, *22*, 915–927. [CrossRef]
2. Gava, M.L.; Caterino, E. Autismo: Pensiero, azione, comunicazione. L'applicazione del metodo c.m.i.® (cognitivo-motivazionale-individualizzato) a soggetti con autismo a basso funzionamento. *Autismo Disturbi Dello Svilupp.* **2014**, *12*, 249–271.
3. Pennington, B.F.; Rogers, S.J.; Bennetto, L.; Griffith, E.M.; Reed, D.T.; Shyu, V. Validity tests of the executive dysfunction hypothesis of autism. In *Autism as an Executive Disorder*; Russell, J., Ed.; Oxford University Press (OUP): Oxford, UK, 1997; pp. 143–178.
4. Peristeri, E.; Baldimtsi, E.; Andreou, M.; Tsimpli, I.M. The impact of bilingualism on the narrative ability and the executive functions of children with autism spectrum disorders. *J. Commun. Disord.* **2020**, *85*, 105999. [CrossRef]
5. Narzisi, A.; Muratori, F.; Calderoni, S.; Fabbro, F.; Urgesi, C. Neuropsychological Profile in High Functioning Autism Spectrum Disorders. *J. Autism Dev. Disord.* **2012**, *43*, 1895–1909. [CrossRef]
6. Gava, M.L. *La Comunicazione Aumentativa Alternativa tra Pensiero e Parola*; Franco Angeli: Milan, Italy, 2013.
7. King, D.; Dockrell, J.E.; Stuart, M. Event narratives in 11-14 year olds with autistic spectrum disorder. *Int. J. Lang. Commun. Disord.* **2013**, *48*, 522–533. [CrossRef] [PubMed]
8. Losh, M.; Capps, L. Narrative ability in high-functioning children with autism or Asperger's syndrome. *J. Autism Dev. Disord.* **2003**, *33*, 239–251. [CrossRef] [PubMed]
9. Peristeri, E.; Andreou, M.; Tsimpli, I.M. Syntactic and Story Structure Complexity in the Narratives of High- and Low-Language Ability Children with Autism Spectrum Disorder. *Front. Psychol.* **2017**, *8*, 2027. [CrossRef]
10. Dawson, G.; Finley, C.; Phillips, S.; Lewy, A. A comparison of hemispheric asymmetries in speech-related brain potentials of autistic and dysphasic children. *Brain Lang.* **1989**, *37*, 26–41. [CrossRef]
11. Romanczyk, R.; Gillis, J.M.; Baron, M.G.; Groden, J.; Groden, G.; Lipsitt, L.P. Autism and the Physiology of Stress and Anxiety. In *Stress and Coping in Autism*; Baron, M.G., Groden, J., Groden, G., Lipsitt, L., Eds.; Oxford University Press (OUP): Oxford, UK, 2006; pp. 183–204.
12. Faja, S.; Murias, M.; Beauchaine, T.P.; Dawson, G. Reward-based decision making and electrodermal responding by young children with autism spectrum disorders during a gambling task. *Autism Res.* **2013**, *6*, 494–505. [CrossRef] [PubMed]
13. Sheinkopf, S.J.; Neal-Beevers, A.R.; Levine, T.P.; Miller-Loncar, C.; Lester, B. Parasympathetic Response Profiles Related to Social Functioning in Young Children with Autistic Disorder. *Autism Res. Treat.* **2013**, *2013*, 868396. [CrossRef] [PubMed]

14. Neuhaus, E.; Bernier, R.; Beauchaine, T.P. Brief Report: Social Skills, Internalizing and Externalizing Symptoms, and Respiratory Sinus Arrhythmia in Autism. *J. Autism Dev. Disord.* **2013**, *44*, 730–737. [CrossRef]
15. Porges, S.W. The polyvagal theory: Phylogenetic substrates of a social nervous system. *Int. J. Psychophysiol.* **2001**, *42*, 123–146. [CrossRef]
16. Porges, S.W. The Polyvagal Theory: Phylogenetic contributions to social behavior. *Physiol. Behav.* **2003**, *79*, 503–513. [CrossRef]
17. Bal, E.; Harden, E.; Lamb, D.; Van Hecke, A.V.; Denver, J.W.; Porges, S.W. Emotion Recognition in Children with Autism Spectrum Disorders: Relations to Eye Gaze and Autonomic State. *J. Autism Dev. Disord.* **2010**, *40*, 358–370. [CrossRef] [PubMed]
18. Neuhaus, E.; Bernier, R.A.; Beauchaine, T.P. Children with Autism Show Altered Autonomic Adaptation to Novel and Familiar Social Partners. *Autism Res.* **2016**, *9*, 579–591. [CrossRef] [PubMed]
19. Stifter, C.A.; Dollar, J.M.; Cipriano, E.A. Temperament and emotion regulation: The role of autonomic nervous system reactivity. *Dev. Psychobiol.* **2011**, *53*, 266–279. [CrossRef] [PubMed]
20. Diamond, L.M.; Cribbet, M.R. Links between adolescent sympathetic and parasympathetic nervous system functioning and interpersonal behavior over time. *Int. J. Psychophysiol.* **2013**, *88*, 339–348. [CrossRef] [PubMed]
21. Hubert, B.; Wicker, B.; Monfardini, E.; Deruelle, C. Electrodermal reactivity to emotion processing in adults with autistic spectrum disorders. *Autism* **2009**, *13*, 9–19. [CrossRef]
22. Mathersul, D.C.; McDonald, S.; Rushby, J. Autonomic arousal explains social cognitive abilities in high-functioning adults with autism spectrum disorder. *Int. J. Psychophysiol.* **2013**, *89*, 475–482. [CrossRef]
23. Lord, C.; Risi, S.; Lambrecht, L., Jr.; Cook, E.H.; Leventhal, B.L.; DiLavore, P.C.; Pickles, A.; Rutter, M. The Autism Diagnostic Observation Schedule—Generic: A Standard Measure of Social and Communication Deficits Associated with the Spectrum of Autism. *J. Autism Dev. Disord.* **2000**, *30*, 205–223. [CrossRef] [PubMed]
24. Lewis, M.; Norbury, C.; Luyster, R.; Schmitt, L.; McDuffie, A.; Haebig, E.; Murray, D.S.; Timler, G.; Frazier, T.; Holmes, D.L.; et al. Leiter International Performance Scale-Revised (Leiter-R). In *Encyclopedia of Autism Spectrum Disorders*; Volkmar, F.R., Ed.; Springer: New York, NY, USA, 2013.
25. Villardita, C. Raven's colored Progressive Matrices and intellectual impairment in patients with focal brain damage. *Cortex* **1985**, *21*, 627–634. [CrossRef]
26. Wechsler, D. *WPPSI-III: Technical and Interpretative Manual*; The Psychological Corporation: San Antonio, TX, USA, 2002.
27. Schreibman, L.; Dawson, G.; Stahmer, A.C.; Landa, R.J.; Rogers, S.J.; McGee, G.G.; Kasari, C.; Ingersoll, B.; Kaiser, A.; Bruinsma, Y.; et al. Naturalistic Developmental Behavioral Interventions: Empirically Validated Treatments for Autism Spectrum Disorder. *J. Autism Dev. Disord.* **2015**, *45*, 2411–2428. [CrossRef] [PubMed]
28. Green, J.; Charman, T.; McConachie, H.; Aldred, C.; Slonims, V.; Howlin, P.; Le Couteur, A.; Leadbitter, K.; Hudry, K.; Byford, S.; et al. Parent-mediated communication-focused treatment in children with autism (PACT): A randomised controlled trial. *Lancet* **2010**, *375*, 2152–2160. [CrossRef]
29. Johnson-Glenberg, M.C.; Megowan-Romanowicz, C. Embodied science and mixed reality: How gesture and motion capture affect physics education. *Cogn. Res. Princ. Implic.* **2017**, *2*, 27. [CrossRef]
30. Pan, J.; Tompkins, W.J. A real-time QRS detection algorithm. *IEEE Trans. Biomed. Eng.* **1985**, *32*, 230–236. [CrossRef]
31. Benedek, M.; Kaernbach, C. A continuous measure of phasic electrodermal activity. *J. Neurosci. Methods* **2010**, *190*, 80–91. [CrossRef]
32. Billeci, L.; Tonacci, A.; Narzisi, A.; Manigrasso, Z.; Varanini, M.; Fulceri, F.; Lattarulo, C.; Calderoni, S.; Muratori, F. Heart Rate Variability During a Joint Attention Task in Toddlers With Autism Spectrum Disorders. *Front. Physiol.* **2018**, *9*, 467. [CrossRef]
33. Tonacci, A.; Di Monte, J.; Meucci, M.B.; Sansone, F.; Pala, A.P.; Billeci, L.; Conte, R. Wearable Sensors to Characterize the Autonomic Nervous System Correlates of Food-Like Odors Perception: A Pilot Study. *Electronics* **2019**, *8*, 1481. [CrossRef]
34. Sahin, M.; Sur, M. Genes, circuits, and precision therapies for autism and related neurodevelopmental disorders. *Science* **2015**, *350*, aab3897. [CrossRef]

35. Waschbusch, D.A.; Willoughby, M.T.; Haas, S.M.; Ridenour, T.; Helseth, S.; Crum, K.I.; Altszuler, A.R.; Ross, J.M.; Coles, E.K.; Pelham, W.E. Effects of Behavioral Treatment Modified to Fit Children with Conduct Problems and Callous-Unemotional (CU) Traits. *J. Clin. Child Adolesc. Psychol.* **2019**, 1–12. [CrossRef]
36. Grove, R.; Roth, I.; Hoekstra, R.A. The motivation for special interests in individuals with autism and controls: Development and validation of the special interest motivation scale. *Autism Res.* **2016**, *9*, 677–688. [CrossRef] [PubMed]
37. White, S.W.; Schry, A.R.; Miyazaki, Y.; Ollendick, T.H.; Scahill, L. Effects of Verbal Ability and Severity of Autism on Anxiety in Adolescents With ASD: One-Year Follow-Up After Cognitive Behavioral Therapy. *J. Clin. Child Adolesc. Psychol.* **2015**, *44*, 839–845. [CrossRef] [PubMed]
38. Hesselmark, E.; Plenty, S.; Bejerot, S. Group cognitive behavioural therapy and group recreational activity for adults with autism spectrum disorders: A preliminary randomized controlled trial. *Autism* **2014**, *18*, 672–683. [CrossRef] [PubMed]
39. Kirkovski, M.; Enticott, P.; Fitzgerald, P.B. A Review of the Role of Female Gender in Autism Spectrum Disorders. *J. Autism Dev. Disord.* **2013**, *43*, 2584–2603. [CrossRef]
40. Di Palma, S.; Tonacci, A.; Narzisi, A.; Domenici, C.; Pioggia, G.; Muratori, F.; Billeci, L. Monitoring of autonomic response to sociocognitive tasks during treatment in children with Autism Spectrum Disorders by wearable technologies: A feasibility study. *Comput. Biol. Med.* **2017**, *85*, 143–152. [CrossRef] [PubMed]
41. Billeci, L.; Tonacci, A.; Tartarisco, G.; Narzisi, A.; Di Palma, S.; Corda, D.; Baldus, G.; Cruciani, F.; Anzalone, S.M.; Calderoni, S.; et al. An Integrated Approach for the Monitoring of Brain and Autonomic Response of Children with Autism Spectrum Disorders during Treatment by Wearable Technologies. *Front. Mol. Neurosci.* **2016**, *10*, 799. [CrossRef]

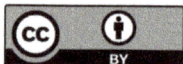

© 2020 by the authors. Licensee MDPI, Basel, Switzerland. This article is an open access article distributed under the terms and conditions of the Creative Commons Attribution (CC BY) license (http://creativecommons.org/licenses/by/4.0/).

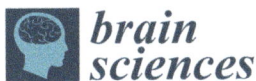

Article

Early Motor Development Predicts Clinical Outcomes of Siblings at High-Risk for Autism: Insight from an Innovative Motion-Tracking Technology

Angela Caruso [1], Letizia Gila [1], Francesca Fulceri [1], Tommaso Salvitti [1], Martina Micai [1], Walter Baccinelli [2], Maria Bulgheroni [2] and Maria Luisa Scattoni [1,*,†] on behalf of the NIDA Network Group

[1] Research Coordination and Support Service, Istituto Superiore di Sanità, Viale Regina Elena 299, 00161 Roma, Italy; angela.caruso@iss.it (A.C.); letizia.gila@iss.it (L.G.); francesca.fulceri@iss.it (F.F.); tommaso.salvitti@iss.it (T.S.); martina.micai@iss.it (M.M.)
[2] Ab.Acus srl, Milano, via F. Caracciolo 77, 20155 Milano, Italy; walterbaccinelli@ab-acus.eu (W.B.); mariabulgheroni@ab-acus.com (M.B.)
* Correspondence: marialuisa.scattoni@iss.it
† NIDA Network Group: Fabio Apicella, Andrea Guzzetta, Massimo Molteni, Giovanni Valeri, Stefano Vicari.

Received: 25 May 2020; Accepted: 12 June 2020; Published: 16 June 2020

Abstract: Atypical motor patterns are potential early markers and predictors of later diagnosis of Autism Spectrum Disorder (ASD). This study aimed to investigate the early motor trajectories of infants at high-risk (HR) of ASD through MOVIDEA, a semi-automatic software developed to analyze 2D and 3D videos and provide objective kinematic features of their movements. MOVIDEA was developed within the Italian Network for early detection of Autism Spectrum Disorder (NIDA Network), which is currently coordinating the most extensive surveillance program for infants at risk for neurodevelopmental disorders (NDDs). MOVIDEA was applied to video recordings of 53 low-risk (LR; siblings of typically developing children) and 50 HR infants' spontaneous movements collected at 10 days and 6, 12, 18, and 24 weeks. Participants were grouped based on their clinical outcome (18 HR received an NDD diagnosis, 32 HR and 53 LR were typically developing). Results revealed that early developmental trajectories of specific motor parameters were different in HR infants later diagnosed with NDDs from those of infants developing typically. Since MOVIDEA was useful in the association of quantitative measures with specific early motor patterns, it should be applied to the early detection of ASD/NDD markers.

Keywords: neurodevelopmental disorders; autism spectrum disorder; high-risk infants; motor development; screening; technology

---

1. Introduction

Neurodevelopmental disorders (NDDs) are a group of conditions with onset in the developmental period characterized by impairments of personal, social, and academic functioning (Diagnostic and statistical manual of mental disorders, DSM-5, APA 2013). The global rate of NDDs from 2009–2011 to 2015–2017 increased from 16.2% to 17.8% (e.g., Autism Spectrum Disorder (ASD): 1.1–2.5%; Attention-Deficit/Hyperactivity Disorder: 8.5–9.5%) [1]. Given the importance of early detection and intervention programs in improving infants' and parents' outcomes, previous research focused on the identification of early biomarkers and behavioral measures to determine risk status even before the emergence of clear behavioral symptoms [2,3]. In this scientific framework, the Italian National of Health hosts the Network for early detection of Autism Spectrum Disorders (NIDA Network), including pediatric hospitals and clinical research centers of Italian territory with high expertise in early detection and intervention programs in ASD. The NIDA Network delivered new tools and standards for research and clinical development across the nation and is currently coordinating the most extensive surveillance program of development in infants at risk for NDDs in Italy. The aim of the NIDA Network is the early detection of behavioral markers of NDDs to provide intervention programs in a timely manner.

Several studies revealed that some early behavioral measures might be effective in predicting abnormal developmental trajectories [4–7]. Moreover, a growing body of literature pointed toward nonsocial behavioral measures, such as motor skills, restricted and repetitive interests, sensory and visual processing, and attention disengagement [8–11]. Significant findings emerged from studies focusing on early motor development of children later diagnosed with NDDs [10,11]. Indeed, both fine and gross motor impairments are associated with NDD occurrence in the general population [8] and high-risk infants (i.e., siblings of children with a diagnosis of ASD, preterm and low birth weight infants) [9,10,12,13]. Overall, the most frequently reported early motor signs of NDDs are abnormalities in fluency, complexity, and variability of spontaneous general movements, and delays in early gross motor milestones [14,15], motor maturity [8,16], and motor functioning [17,18]. Findings reflect the heterogeneity of clinical symptomatology of NDDs, and instruments adopted to evaluate infants' motor patterns are extremely variable, ranging from analysis of General Movements (GMs) based on the Prechtl method assessment to parental reports and specific clinical motor batteries [19–25].

The study of motor development at an early age may be crucial in ASD research fields [26,27]. Indeed, several studies showed that the motor patterns of infants later diagnosed with ASD appeared consistently less developed than in neurotypical peers (see review [28,29]) and that spontaneous motor activity was impaired already in the first months of life [25,30]. Moreover, some studies addressing differences in motor milestones documented the presence of early repetitive behaviors in infants with ASD compared to ones with typical development or developmental disabilities, starting from six months of age [31–33].

Relevant findings emerged from studies regarding the early motor development of siblings of children with ASD (high-risk (HR) infants) who present an increased risk (~20%) of developing ASD compared to the general population [34]. Mounting research highlights that their motor developmental trajectories differ from those at low risk (LR; siblings of children without a diagnosis of ASD/NDD) at a mere six months of age [22,24,35–40]. A recent systematic review showed that fine motor competencies at six months predicted the clinical outcome [9] and language skills of siblings of children with ASD [22]. Moreover, very early repetitive/stereotypical behaviors and atypical body movements (6–12 months [41], 12 months [42], and from 18 months [43]) were reported to be associated with ASD outcome in HR infants, in line with the acknowledgement of restricted and repetitive behaviors as a core symptom of ASD.

Although the use of innovative technological instruments has increased over recent decades, limited impacts were observed on early screening and detection of ASD/NDDs [44]. Given the importance of further exploring early motor trajectories, more research should be promoted to implement technological tools to obtain objective measures of motor patterns and describe quantitative and qualitative features of infant movements. Over the last few decades, a set of innovative technologies, including computer vision and motion sensor-based approaches, as well as machine learning approaches, were implemented with the aim to emulate GM analysis and pinpoint objective measures of kinematic analysis [45–52], but none were transferred to clinical practice.

Recently, the NIDA Network developed a motion-tracking technology named MOVIDEA [46]. The technology was developed under the arising need to identify an easy, cost-effective instrument to investigate early motor markers of NDDs. MOVIDEA is a noninvasive technology measuring quantitative motor patterns in infants through two- and three-dimensional kinematic analyses [46]. The current study describes the application of MOVIDEA on a large library of video recordings of spontaneous movements of LR and HR infants. Our aim was to detect early quantitative differences in the motor trajectories of HR infants who received a diagnosis of NDDs or who did not receive a diagnosis compared to LR age-matched peers. Due to the small sample size of HR infants who developed ASD ($n = 3$), we included them in the group of infants who developed NDDs ($n = 15$), resulting in a total sample size of 18 infants with NDDs.

Evaluation of kinematic parameters permitted the investigation motor differences as a function of age and outcome, with the aim to improve early discrimination and screening of infants at higher risk of developing NDDs.

2. Materials and Methods

2.1. Participants

The current study was performed within the NIDA Network, enrolling LR and HR infants with the aim of detecting early signs of ASD/NDD through the recording and analysis of infant cry and motor patterns at 10 days and 6, 12, 18, and 24 weeks of age. At 6, 12, 18, 24, and 36 months, each infant/toddler underwent a comprehensive clinical/diagnostic assessment using standardized tools/tests and structured interviews, with parents for checking the presence/absence of an ASD or NDD diagnosis. Infant recruitment and data collection are still ongoing. The present study was carried out according to the standards for good ethical practice and the guidelines of the Declaration of Helsinki. The study protocol was approved by the Ethics Committee of the Italian Institute of Health (Approval Number: Pre 469/2016). A written informed consent from a parent/guardian of each participant was obtained.

For the purposes of the current study, the sample included data from 103 infants (54 females and 49 males), of which 53 were LR (infants with a sibling without any clinical diagnosis and no family history of ASD) and 50 were HR (infants with an older sibling with a clinical diagnosis of ASD). The inclusion criteria for infants were: (1) gestational age $\geq$ 36 weeks; (2) birth weight $\geq$ 2500 g; (3) Apgar index > 7 at the 5th minute; (4) absence of known medical, genetic, or neurological conditions associated with ASD; (5) absence of major complications in pregnancy and/or delivery likely to affect brain development.

HR infants were subdivided into two groups based on their clinical outcome at 24 or 36 months (using the Autism Diagnostic Observational Scale [53] and the DSM-5 criteria), as confirmed by expert clinicians of the NIDA team blinded to experimental data, resulting in 18 HR infants diagnosed with NDDs (HR-NDD) and 32 who did not receive any diagnosis (HR-no diagnosis). Infants in the LR group did not receive any clinical diagnosis at 24 or 36 months.

Video recordings of spontaneous movements were performed at 10 days and 6, 12, 18, and 24 weeks of age at home while the infant was lying on the bed (either naked or in a bodysuit not covering the limbs). To acquire images of spontaneous movement of the full infant body, the camera was placed 50 cm above the child and at chest height. See Table 1 for the description of the participants' characteristics and age during assessment.

Table 1. Video recordings available at various ages of assessment.

Age of Assessment	LR ($n = 53$)		HR-No Diagnosis ($n = 18$)		HR-NDD ($n = 32$)	
	Female	Male	Female	Male	Female	Male
	n	n	n	n	n	n
10 days	16	31	7	15	5	7
6 weeks	21	43	12	21	4	12
12 weeks	24	46	15	24	5	13
18 weeks	16	36	15	23	5	8
24 weeks	12	28	8	13	7	14

LR: Low-risk infants with a typical development; HR-NDD: High-risk infants diagnosed with NDDs; HR-No diagnosis: High-risk infants who did not receive any diagnosis.

2.2. Kinematic Analysis through MOVIDEA Software

Before applying MOVIDEA to the video library, each video was assessed for its eligibility for analysis. Then, one author cut each video to ensure the same properties, i.e., 3 min length, infant in supine position, in a condition of a quite awake state, well-being, and spontaneous motor activity, without crying or fussing episodes. Video frames containing interferences caused by the operator or parents or accidental movements of the camera were excluded from the analysis. Videos were analyzed by two coders blinded to the infant's risk status (LR or HR). Prior to starting coding, coders were trained and reached an excellent degree of agreement.

The MOVIDEA software computed the motor features using two different approaches. First, the trajectories covered by the infant's limbs during the free movement were extracted using a semi-automatic limb-tracking procedure. Second, movement quantification was performed through image processing techniques applied to the video frames. The software was developed using MATLAB ver. R2017a and its standard tools.

We analyzed the following set of kinematic features considered to eb meaningful for the identification of pathological motion patterns [46,54]:

- Quantity of motion (Qmean), i.e., the mean number of pixels where movement occurred divided by the total number of pixels in the image (percentage);
- Centroid of motion (C), i.e., the central point (2D coordinates measured in pixels) of the infant's movement computed for each motion image extracted from the video recording (Figure 1), with analysis of standard deviation in the X (Cxsd) and Y directions (Cysd), velocity (Vcmean), and acceleration (Acmean);
- Periodicity for the left and right hands (H-periodicity) and for the left and right feet (F-periodicity), which were nondimensional parameters aimed at measuring the presence of repetitive movements in the motion of the limbs.

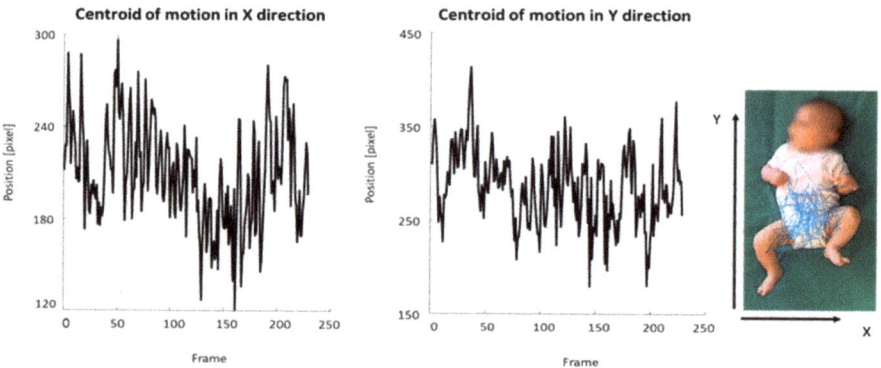

Figure 1. Graphic representation of the centroid of motion in the X and Y directions. The blue line depicts the trajectory of the centroid of motion of the infant's movement extracted from a video recording.

For details on the methods used to estimate measures as references and tracking methods, refer to Baccinelli and colleagues [46].

2.3. Statistical Analysis

An Analysis of Variance (ANOVA) with repeated measures was performed to analyze the kinematic parameters extracted by the MOVIDEA software (refer to Baccinelli and colleagues [46]), with the outcome (LR, HR-no diagnosis, and HR-NDD infants) as factor and age (10 days and 6, 12, 18, and 24 weeks) as the repeated measures. No significant sex differences were detected in the motor parameters analyzed. For this reason, data regarding sex were collapsed. Post-hoc comparisons were performed using Newman Keuls test. For all comparisons, significance was set at a *p*-value below 0.05. All statistical analyses were conducted using STATA 12.0 software (Stata Statistical Software: Release 12. College Station, TX, USA: StataCorp LP) [55,56].

3. Results

Using the MOVIDEA software, we evaluated specific kinematic parameters related to upper and lower limb movements in the space and using the head and the trunk as references (see Table 2).

Table 2. MOVIDEA kinematic parameters' means (SD) of the three groups of infants (LR, HR-no diagnosis, and HR-NDD).

Parameter	LR		HR-No Diagnosis		HR-NDD	
	n	Mean (SD)	n	Mean (SD)	n	Mean (SD)
Qmean						
10 days	31	0.008 (0.006)	15	0.008 (0.003)	7	0.006 (0.005)
6 weeks	43	0.012 (0.008)	21	0.014 (0.005)	12	0.016 (0.009)
12 weeks	46	0.011 (0.006)	24	0.015 (0.009)	13	0.019 (0.005)
18 weeks	36	0.010 (0.007)	23	0.018 (0.011)	8	0.012 (0.005)
24 weeks	28	0.011 (0.009)	13	0.016 (0.009)	14	0.017 (0.009)
Cxsd						
10 days	31	58.210 (21.422)	15	46.589 (13.116)	7	53.976 (13.967)
6 weeks	43	51.999 (13.722)	21	43.243 (10.278)	12	43.372 (9.371)
12 weeks	46	54.223 (14.314)	24	41.800 (10.001)	13	39.843 (9.384)
18 weeks	36	57.612 (16.725)	23	49.113 (23.310)	8	48.621 (15.325)
24 weeks	28	55.010 (15.419)	13	52.645 (19.299)	14	53.890 (16.267)
Cysd						
10 days	31	72.398 (31.810)	15	78.819 (34.812)	7	78.012 (23.567)
6 weeks	43	57.223 (19.110)	21	68.222 (23.111)	12	65.830 (21.765)
12 weeks	46	55.230 (20.111)	24	68.450 (20.701)	13	62.692 (18.991)
18 weeks	36	58.716 (25.416)	23	68.412 (24.411)	8	71.768 (26.802)
24 weeks	28	62.320 (18.799)	13	63.899 (23.789)	14	68.175 (16.267)
Acmean						
10 days	31	−0.015 (0.071)	15	0.017 (0.052)	7	0.161 (0.307)
6 weeks	43	−0.002 (0.024)	21	−0.002 (0.028)	12	−0.001 (0.043)
12 weeks	46	−0.004 (0.030)	24	0.001 (0.027)	13	−0.005 (0.015)
18 weeks	36	0.016 (0.052)	23	−0.005 (0.033)	8	−0.011 (0.034)
24 weeks	28	−0.017 (0.139)	13	−0.002 (0.041)	14	−0.023 (0.030)
Vcmean						
10 days	31	26.835 (7.432)	15	23.040 (5.128)	7	24.640 (5.665)
6 weeks	43	28.396 (6.225)	21	24.624 (5.356)	12	24.250 (4.036)
12 weeks	46	31.726 (7.301)	24	26.374 (5.170)	13	24.194 (4.570)
18 weeks	36	32.792 (8.828)	23	27.730 (9.116)	8	28.687 (6.638)
24 weeks	28	28.652 (7.402)	13	27.884 (10.032)	14	27.466 (8.335)
H-periodicity						
10 days	31	0.034 (0.012)	15	0.035 (0.006)	7	0.030 (0.004)
6 weeks	43	0.041 (0.011)	21	0.040 (0.013)	12	0.046 (0.014)
12 weeks	46	0.041 (0.010)	24	0.044 (0.018)	13	0.049 (0.013)
18 weeks	36	0.039 (0.010)	23	0.042 (0.018)	8	0.038 (0.010)
24 weeks	28	0.043 (0.013)	13	0.049 (0.023)	14	0.043 (0.011)
F-periodicity						
10 days	31	0.032 (0.007)	15	0.035 (0.007)	7	0.031 (0.003)
6 weeks	43	0.043 (0.011)	21	0.045 (0.014)	12	0.052 (0.018)
12 weeks	46	0.047 (0.015)	24	0.053 (0.022)	13	0.052 (0.017)
18 weeks	36	0.042 (0.015)	23	0.047 (0.016)	8	0.037 (0.010)
24 weeks	28	0.044 (0.014)	13	0.042 (0.012)	14	0.043 (0.010)

LR: Low-risk infants with typical development; HR-no diagnosis: High-risk infants who did not receive any diagnosis; HR-NDD: High-risk infants diagnosed with NDDs. Qmean: Quantity of motion; Cxsd: Standard deviation in the X direction of centroid of motion; Cysd: Standard deviation in the Y direction of centroid of motion; Acmean: Mean acceleration of centroid of motion; Vcmean: Mean velocity of centroid of motion; H-periodicity: Periodicity for the left and right hands; F-periodicity: Periodicity for the left and right feet.

3.1. Quantity of Motion

Analysis revealed a main effect of the outcome ($F(2,319) = 8.83$; $p = 0.0002$) with HR-NDD and HR-no diagnosis infants moving more than LR infants ($p = 0.001$ and $p < 0.0001$, respectively) and a main effect of the age ($F(4,319) = 7.16$; $p < 0.0001$) with differences at 10 days compared to 6, 12, 18, and 24 weeks ($p < 0.0001$ for all comparisons) (Figure 2).

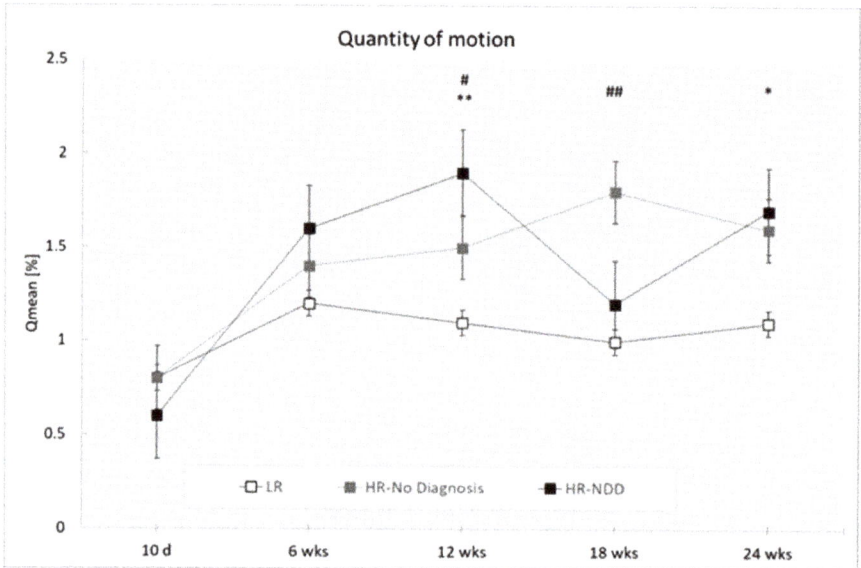

Figure 2. Quantity of motion in a 3-min session, measured at 10 days and 6, 12, 18, and 24 weeks in three groups of infants (LR, $n = 53$; HR-no diagnosis, $n = 32$; HR-NDD infants, $n = 18$). d = days; wks = weeks. Data are expressed as mean ± SEM. * $p < 0.05$ and ** $p < 0.01$ between HR-NDD and LR infants; # $p < 0.05$ and ## $p < 0.01$ between HR-no Diagnosis and LR infants.

Post-hoc comparisons performed on the two-way interaction outcome at x age ($F(8,319) = 1.69$; $p = 0.1003$) reported that HR-NDD and HR-no diagnosis infants moved more compared to LR infants at 12 weeks ($p = 0.001$ and $p = 0.023$, respectively). HR-no diagnosis infants moved more compared to LR infants at 18 weeks ($p < 0.0001$), and HR-NDD infants moved more compared to LR at 24 weeks ($p = 0.031$).

3.2. Centroid of Motion (Cxsd and Cysd)

Analysis revealed a main effect of the outcome (Cxsd: ($F(2,319) = 10.76$; $p < 0.0001$; Cysd ($F(2,319) = 4.81$; $p < 0.0088$. HR-NDD and HR-no diagnosis infants showed lower mean values of Cxsd compared to LR infants (respectively: $p = 0.001$; $p < 0.001$) (Figure 3) and a higher mean value of Cysd compared to LR infants (respectively: $p = 0.027$; $p = 0.003$) (Figure 4). Analysis revealed a main effect of age for Cxsd ($F(4,319) = 3.50$; $p = 0.0081$), with differences at 10 days compared to 6 weeks ($p = 0.025$) and 12 weeks ($p = 0.033$), at 6 weeks compared to 18 weeks ($p = 0.026$) and 24 weeks ($p = 0.026$), and at 12 weeks compared to 18 weeks ($p = 0.035$) and 24 weeks ($p = 0.034$). Analysis revealed a main effect of age for Cysd ($F(4,319) = 2.39$; $p = 0.0508$), with differences at 10 days compared to 6 weeks ($p = 0.002$), 12 weeks ($p < 0.0001$), 18 weeks ($p = 0.009$), and 24 weeks ($p = 0.013$).

Post-hoc comparisons performed on the two-way interaction outcome at x age (Cxsd: $F(8,319) = 0.67$; $p = 0.7198$; Cysd: $F(8,319) = 0.25$; $p = 0.9812$) revealed that HR-NDD infants showed a lower mean value of Cxsd in comparison to LR infants at 12 weeks ($p = 0.004$). HR-no diagnosis infants showed a lower mean value of Cxmean in comparison to LR infants at 10 days ($p = 0.019$), at 6 weeks ($p = 0.043$), at 12 weeks ($p = 0.002$), and at 18 weeks ($p = 0.046$). HR-No diagnosis infants showed a higher mean value of Cysd in comparison to LR infants at 18 weeks ($p = 0.027$).

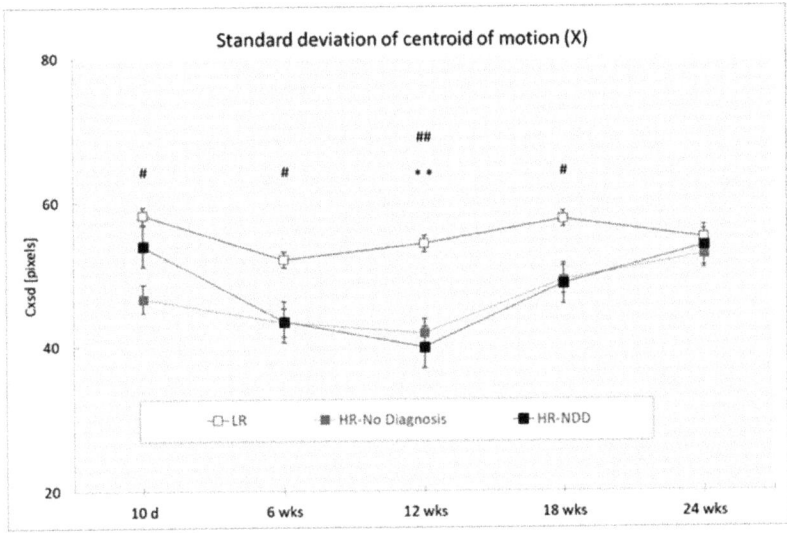

Figure 3. Standard deviation of centroid of motion in X direction (Cxsd) in a 3-min session, measured at 10 days and 6, 12, 18, and 24 weeks in three groups of infants (LR, $n = 53$; HR-no diagnosis, $n = 32$; HR-NDD infants, $n = 18$), d = days; wks = weeks. Data are expressed as mean ± SEM. ** $p < 0.01$ between HR-NDD and LR infants; # $p < 0.05$ and ## $p < 0.01$ between HR-no diagnosis and LR infants.

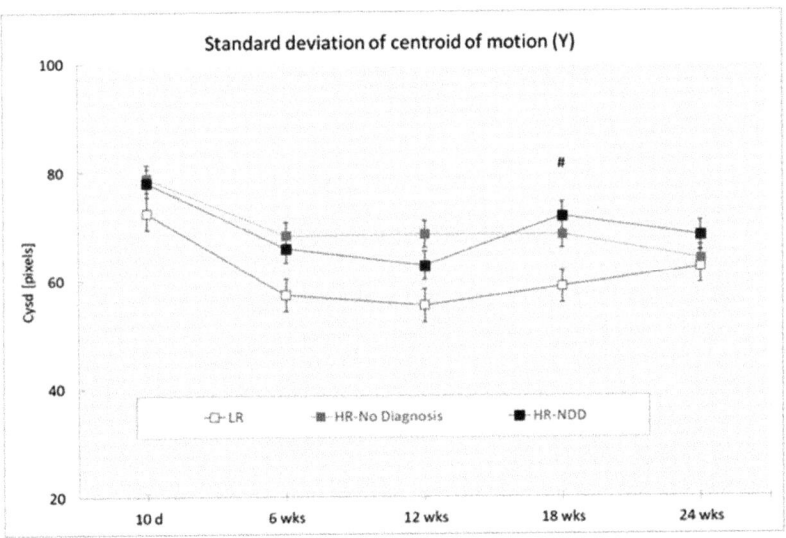

Figure 4. Standard deviation of centroid of motion in Y direction (Cxsd) in a 3-min session, measured at 10 days and 6, 12, 18, and 24 weeks in three groups of infants (LR, $n = 53$; HR-no diagnosis, $n = 32$; HR-NDD infants, $n = 18$). d = days; wks = weeks. Data are expressed as mean ± SEM. # $p < 0.05$ between HR-no diagnosis and LR infants.

3.3. Velocity of Centroid of Motion

Analysis revealed a main effect of the outcome (F(2,319) = 10.96; $p < 0.0001$), with HR-NDD and HR-no diagnosis infants showing reduced mean values of velocity of centroid of motion than LR infants ($p < 0.0001$ for both comparison groups) (Figure 5), and a main effect of age (F(4,319) = 3.22; $p = 0.0130$), with differences at 10 days compared to 12 weeks ($p = 0.005$), 18 weeks ($p < 0.0001$), and 24 weeks ($p = 0.041$), and at 6 weeks compared to 12 weeks ($p = 0.040$) and 18 weeks ($p = 0.001$).

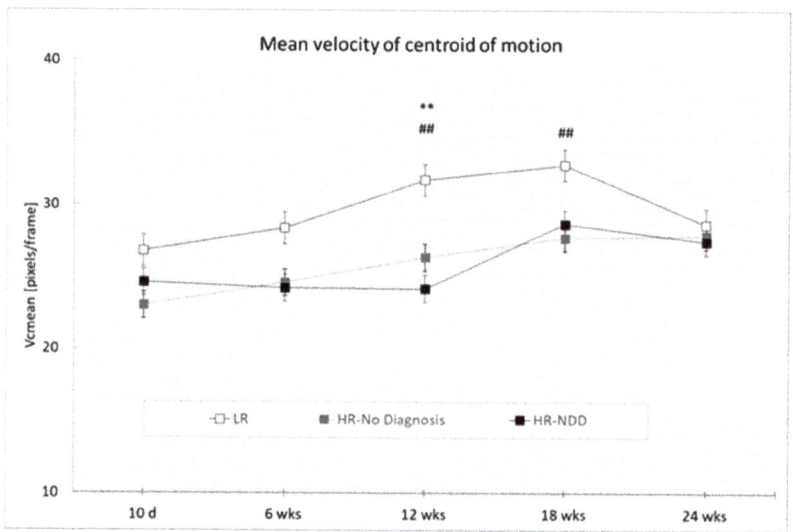

Figure 5. Mean velocity of centroid of motion in a 3-min session, measured at 10 days and 6, 12, 18, and 24 weeks in three groups of infants (LR, $n = 53$; HR-no diagnosis, $n = 32$; HR-NDD infants, $n = 18$). d = days; wks = weeks. Data are expressed as mean ± SEM. ** $p < 0.01$ between HR-NDD and LR infants; ## $p < 0.01$ between HR-no diagnosis and LR infants.

Post-hoc comparisons performed on the two-way interaction outcome at x age (F(8,319) = 0.72, $p = 0.6749$) revealed that HR-NDD and HR-no diagnosis infants showed reduced mean values of velocity of centroid of motion compared to LR infants at 12 weeks ($p = 0.001$ and $p = 0.003$, respectively) and HR-no diagnosis infants at 18 weeks compared to LR infants ($p = 0.008$).

3.4. Acceleration of Centroid of Motion

Analysis revealed a main effect of the outcome (F(2,319) = 3.25; $p = 0.0402$), with HR-NDD infants showing increased acceleration of centroid of motion than LR infants ($p = 0.050$), and a main effect of age (F(4,319) = 5.88; $p < 0.0001$), with differences at 10 days compared to 12 weeks ($p = 0.040$) and 24 weeks ($p = 0.009$).

Post-hoc comparisons performed on the two-way interaction outcome at x age (F(8,218) = 4.55; $p < 0.0001$) revealed that HR-NDD infants significantly differed from both LR and HR-no diagnosis infants at 10 days, showing a higher mean value of acceleration of centroid of motion ($p < 0.0001$ for both comparison groups) (Figure 6).

3.5. Periodicity

Analysis did not reveal a main effect of the outcome for either hand periodicity (F(2,319) = 1.28; $p = 0.2803$) or foot periodicity (F(2,319) = 1.22; $p = 0.2956$). Analysis revealed a main effect of age (hand periodicity: F(4,319) = 6.39; $p = 0.0001$; foot periodicity: F(4,319) = 10.66; $p < 0.0001$).

Hand periodicity was decreased at 10 days compared to 6, 12, 18, and 24 weeks ($p < 0.0001$) and at 18 compared to 24 weeks ($p = 0.041$) (Figure 7). Foot periodicity was decreased at 10 days compared to 6, 12, 18, and 24 weeks ($p < 0.0001$) and at 6 compared to 12 weeks ($p = 0.038$). By contrast, foot periodicity was increased at 12 weeks compared to 18 weeks ($p = 0.003$) and 24 weeks ($p = 0.011$) (Figure 8).

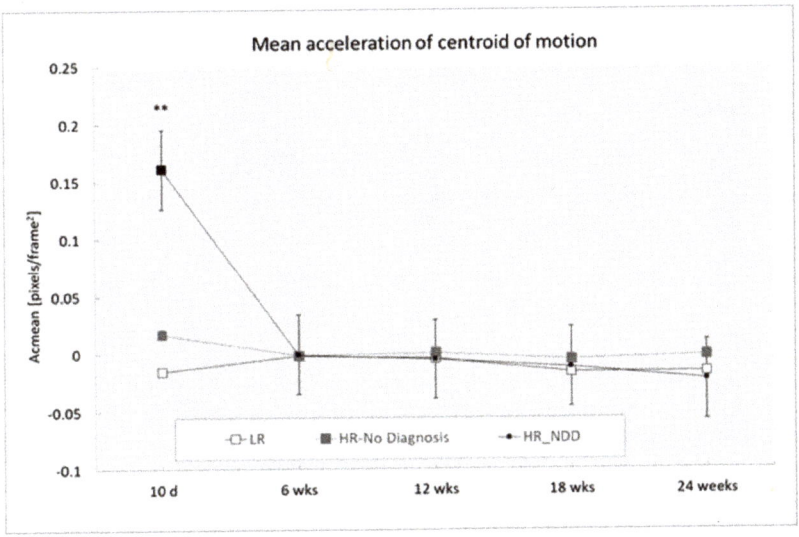

Figure 6. Mean acceleration of centroid of motion in a 3-min session, measured at 10 days and 6, 12, 18, and 24 weeks in three groups of infants (LR, $n = 53$; HR-no diagnosis, $n = 32$; HR-NDD infants, $n = 18$). d = days; wks = weeks. Data are expressed as mean ± SEM. ** $p < 0.01$ between HR-NDD and LR infants.

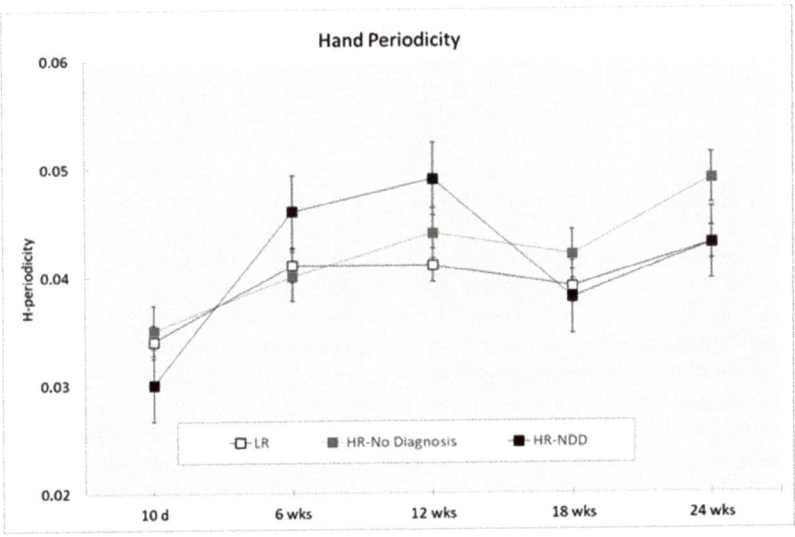

Figure 7. Hand periodicity in a 3-min session, measured at 10 days and 6, 12, 18, and 24 weeks in three groups of infants (LR, $n = 53$; HR-no diagnosis, $n = 32$; HR-NDD infants, $n = 18$). d = days; wks = weeks. Data are expressed as mean ± SEM. Periodicity is a nondimensional value.

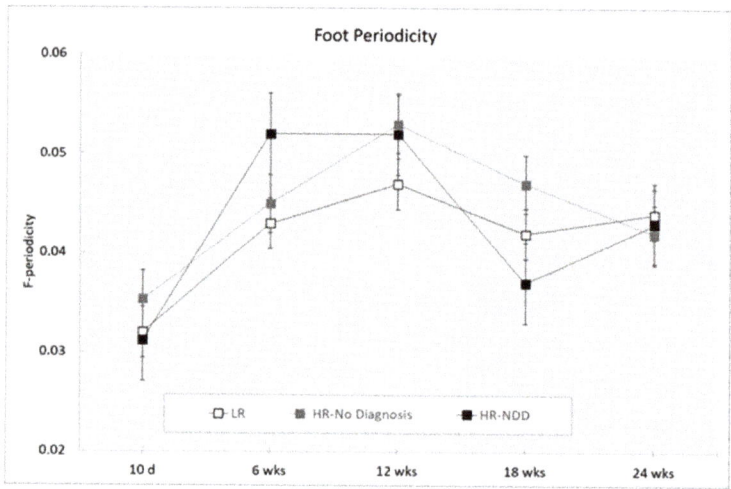

Figure 8. Foot periodicity in a 3-min session, measured at 10 days and 6, 12, 18, and 24 weeks in three groups of infants (LR, $n = 53$; HR-no diagnosis, $n = 32$; HR-NDD infants, $n = 18$). d = days; wks = weeks. Data are expressed as mean ± SEM. Periodicity is a nondimensional value.

4. Discussion

The study of early motor patterns might be effective in predicting abnormal developmental trajectories of infants at risk for developing ASD/NDD. Technological tools able to obtain objective measures of specific motor parameters might support the early detection of NDDs. To this aim, the Italian Network for early detection of Autism Spectrum Disorder (NIDA Network) developed a noninvasive motion-tracking technology, named MOVIDEA, to measure quantitative motor patterns in infants at risk for NDDs.

The main objective of this study was to investigate very early motor trajectories of infants at risk for developing ASD through MOVIDEA, a semi-automatic software able to analyze 2D and 3D videos and provide objective kinematic features of their movements. To our knowledge, this is the first research devoted to a detailed characterization of kinematic motor patterns in HR infants within the first six months of life. Overall, our findings revealed that early motor patterns of HR infants later diagnosed with NDDs (HR-NDD) differed from those of HR and LR infants who did not receive any diagnosis (HR-no diagnosis: high-risk infants who did not receive any diagnosis; LR: low-risk infants with typical development).

First, HR infants later diagnosed with NDDs moved more compared to typically developing LR infants and differences also emerged between HR infants who did not receive any diagnosis and LR infants at 12 and 18 weeks. Thus, HR infants seem to exhibit more active motor profiles during the first six months of life. One possible explanation may be their different abilities to perceive and respond to external stimuli and generate adequate motor responses to them. Abnormalities in the inhibition/excitation system in the cortical and subcortical motor regions could underlie general motor dysfunctions associated with NDDs [57]. Self-regulation behaviors (general irritability, range of states, state regulation, regulation capability) were described as predictors of psychomotor development at 4 and 12 months [58]. Self-regulation difficulties were reported to be present in children with ASD at only one year of age [59,60]. Moreover, neurobiological studies showed that self-regulation in ASD is related to dysfunction in certain brain circuits associated with social–emotional processing [59,61], suggesting the importance of assessing neonatal motor features during development [58].

Second, variability of the "centroid of motion" parameter was different between HR and LR infants. Since the centroid of motion is the central point of the infant's movement in a given motion image, its standard deviation in the X and Y directions throughout the video recording provide information regarding the variability of the location of the free movement's central point. On the other hand, the velocity and acceleration of the centroid of motion provide a measure regarding how fast the global movement changes over time and if significant jerks of movements are present. Our data reported that HR infants later diagnosed with NDDs moved in the X direction with reduced variability at 12 weeks of age at the same time point during which they expressed an increased quantity of motion compared to LR infants. Also, HR infants who did not receive any diagnosis moved in the X direction with reduced variability across several time points of development (from 10 days to 18 weeks of age), and increased variability of centroid of motion was measured in the vertical direction (Cysd) at 18 weeks of age. Differences also emerged in the acceleration and velocity of centroid of motion. HR infants later diagnosed with NDDs showed increased acceleration of centroid of motion at 10 days after birth, compared to HR and LR infants who did not receive any diagnosis. Also, HR infants later diagnosed with NDDs and HR who did not receive any diagnosis demonstrated decreased velocity of centroid of motion compared to LR infants at 12 weeks of age. Differences remained significant at 18 weeks for HR infants who did not receive any diagnosis. Even if MOVIDEA provided mixed findings, it seems that the movement of HR-NDD infants is characterized by reduced variability and velocity as well as increased acceleration. It is possible that abnormal patterns of centroid of motion in HR infants may reflect abnormal quality of movement, as already observed through the GM evaluation, and could be predictive of a later diagnosis of NDDs. Typical GMs are characterized by complexity and variation [62], supporting the hypothesis that motor variability and appropriate integration of sensorimotor information are expressions of typical motor development [63,64]. A lack of movement variability was mostly identified in infants who developed delays or disabilities [65–67] and abnormal GMs were reported in several infants with ASD and NDDs [25,30,68,69]. Moreover, a previous study measuring kinematic parameters using wearable sensors in 1–8-month-old infants detected different acceleration features between at-risk infants diagnosed with developmental delay or with no diagnosis and infants with typical development [70].

Finally, MOVIDEA detected changes across age of development in hand and foot periodic movements. Periodicity was described as the repetition of the same movement multiple times with high amplitude of the end effectors [54]. The presence of certain motor repetitive behaviors in early infancy is considered a necessary step for the development of voluntary purposeful movements and seems to have an adaptive role. Thus, these are considered to be indices of a typical psychomotor development [71]. However, increased frequency of repetitive movements was widely described in various NDDs [33,72], reflecting a continuum extending from typical to atypical development. We speculate that atypical periodicity, especially for the upper extremities, could interfere with later manual exploration or poor development of fine motor skills. During the fidgety period, the upper limb movement repertoire undergoes a maturational process, with the enrichment of motor patterns addressing the exploration of the body and environment, while the lower limb repertoire appears to be functionally limited [50].

In conclusion, our results revealed that HR infants who received a diagnosis of NDD showed an increased general motor activity associated with reduced variability and velocity, as well as increased acceleration of global movement in the space. Moreover, we reported patterns of increased periodicity of limbs, especially for the upper limbs, throughout the first 12 weeks of age. This developmental profile may reflect the motor difficulties of HR-NDD infants during the writhing and fidgety periods and provide a window into which it is possible to more deeply investigate the development of motor competences in high-risk infants.

The subtle motion analysis through MOVIDEA has several advantages and strengths. Nowadays, most movement assessment systems used for infants require external tracking equipment, i.e., special markers or wearable sensors to be located on the limbs, which are not easily adaptable to different recording settings [52]. Conversely, MOVIDEA gives the chance to obtain measurements via noninvasive assessment without any additional special devices that could interfere with spontaneous infant motor activity. It is important to consider that the use of noninvasive technology may well fit recordings in real-life settings and naturalistic neonatal environments (e.g., hospitals, pediatrician ambulatories, homes), thereby allowing detailed motion analysis. In particular, possible applications of the MOVIDEA tracking system may be on home-video segments, as well as on videos recorded in clinical settings to routinely monitor infants at neurodevelopmental risk. These videos may be recorded directly by parents/caregivers or professionals minimally trained to videotape infants, taking into account the experimental set-up described in the methodological section. Moreover, MOVIDEA collects measurable and quantifiable information not based on visual scoring of infant motor performances, completed by clinicians during well-child visits or trained operators. We believe that this computer-based analysis of infants' movements may support and integrate the analysis of motor patterns of infants at risk of NDDs in research settings [73,74]. Further studies could explore whether the features extracted by MOVIDEA software correlate with the qualitative and quantitative analysis performed by GM experts.

Some limitations of this study should be discussed. First, only a small sample size of HR-NDD infants was collected. Due to this limitation, it was not possible to carry out statistical analysis according to each separate NDD. Second, the accuracy of the extracted MOVIDEA features still need to be implemented and validated by experts in the field.

Overall, this experimental study identified potential early behavioral indexes that are related to later diagnosis of NDDs and may be precursors of altered movements during goal-directed behaviors. Moreover, the findings highlight the importance of a longitudinal assessment of motor development for LR and HR infants. Expanding knowledge regarding typical and atypical motor competencies is useful to detect a developmental motor trajectory as early as possible in the first weeks of life. Further video analyses should be carried out using the MOVIDEA software to increase the potential value of this objective, reliable, and quantifiable technology to identify early motor deficits in infants at risk for NDD.

Author Contributions: Conceptualization: M.L.S.; investigation: L.G., A.C., and NIDA Network group; formal analysis: T.S.; software: W.B. and M.B.; writing—original draft preparation: A.C., F.F., and M.M.; writing—review and editing: M.L.S and A.C.; funding acquisition: M.L.S. All authors have read and agreed to the published version of the manuscript.

Funding: This work was supported by the Italian Ministry of Health Grant "Italian Ministry of Health Network Project 'Italian Autism Spectrum Disorders Network: filling the gaps in the National Health System Care' (NET 2013- 02355263) and the MSCA-ITN-2018 - European Training Networks under Grant agreement ID: 814302 (SAPIENS) "Shaping the social brain through early interactions".

Conflicts of Interest: The authors declare no conflict of interest.

References

1. Zablotsky, B.; Black, L.I.; Maenner, M.J.; Schieve, L.A.; Danielson, M.L.; Bitsko, R.H.; Blumberg, S.J.; Kogan, M.D.; Boyle, C.A. Prevalence and Trends of Developmental Disabilities among Children in the United States: 2009–2017. *Pediatrics* **2019**, *144*, e20190811. [CrossRef] [PubMed]
2. Karmel, B.Z.; Gardner, J.M.; Meade, L.S.; Cohen, I.L.; London, E.; Flory, M.J.; Lennon, E.M.; Miroshnichenko, I.; Rabinowitz, S.; Parab, S.; et al. Early medical and behavioral characteristics of NICU infants later classified with ASD. *Pediatrics* **2010**, *126*, 457–467. [CrossRef] [PubMed]
3. McPartland, J.C. Considerations in biomarker development for neurodevelopmental disorders. *Curr. Opin. Neurol.* **2016**, *29*, 118–122. [CrossRef] [PubMed]
4. Licari, M.K.; Alvares, G.A.; Varcin, K.; Evans, K.L.; Cleary, D.; Reid, S.L.; Glasson, E.J.; Bebbington, K.; Reynolds, J.E.; Wray, J.; et al. Prevalence of Motor Difficulties in Autism Spectrum Disorder: Analysis of a Population-Based Cohort. *Autism Res.* **2020**, *13*, 298–306. [CrossRef]
5. Miller, M.; Iosif, A.M.; Young, G.S.; Hill, M.M.; Ozonoff, S. Early Detection of ADHD: Insights from Infant Siblings of Children With Autism. *J. Clin. Child Adolesc. Psychol.* **2018**, *47*, 737–744. [CrossRef]
6. Sacrey, L.A.; Bennett, J.A.; Zwaigenbaum, L. Early Infant Development and Intervention for Autism Spectrum Disorder. *J. Child Neurol.* **2015**, *30*, 1921–1929. [CrossRef]

7. Zwaigenbaum, L. Advances in the early detection of autism. *Curr. Opin. Neurol.* **2010**, *23*, 97–102. [CrossRef]
8. Athanasiadou, A.; Buitelaar, J.K.; Brovedani, P.; Chorna, O.; Fulceri, F.; Guzzetta, A.; Scattoni, M.L. Early motor signs of attention-deficit hyperactivity disorder: A systematic review. *Eur. Child Adolesc. Psychiatry* **2019**. [CrossRef]
9. Canu, D.; Van der Paelt, S.; Canal-Bedia, R.; Posada, M.; Vanvuchelen, M.; Roeyers, H. Early non-social behavioural indicators of autism spectrum disorder (ASD) in siblings at elevated likelihood for ASD: A systematic review. *Eur. Child Adolesc. Psychiatry* **2020**. [CrossRef]
10. Garrido, D.; Petrova, D.; Watson, L.R.; Garcia-Retamero, R.; Carballo, G. Language and motor skills in siblings of children with autism spectrum disorder: A meta-analytic review. *Autism Res.* **2017**, *10*, 1737–1750. [CrossRef]
11. Micai, M.; Fulceri, F.; Caruso, A.; Guzzetta, A.; Gila, L.; Scattoni, M.L. Early behavioral markers for neurodevelopmental disorders in the first 3 years of life: An overview of systematic reviews. manuscript submitted for publication.
12. Fuentefria, R.D.N.; Silveira, R.C.; Procianoy, R.S. Motor development of preterm infants assessed by the Alberta Infant Motor Scale: Systematic review article. *J. Pediatr.* **2017**, *93*, 328–342. [CrossRef] [PubMed]
13. Palomo, R.; Belinchon, M.; Ozonoff, S. Autism and family home movies: A comprehensive review. *J. Dev. Behav. Pediatr.* **2006**, *27*, S59–S68. [CrossRef] [PubMed]
14. Gurevitz, M.; Geva, R.; Varon, M.; Leitner, Y. Early markers in infants and toddlers for development of ADHD. *J. Atten. Disord.* **2014**, *18*, 14–22. [CrossRef] [PubMed]
15. Jaspers, M.; de Winter, A.F.; Buitelaar, J.K.; Verhulst, F.C.; Reijneveld, S.A.; Hartman, C.A. Early childhood assessments of community pediatric professionals predict autism spectrum and attention deficit hyperactivity problems. *J. Abnorm. Child Psychol.* **2013**, *41*, 71–80. [CrossRef] [PubMed]
16. Jacobvitz, D.; Sroufe, L.A. The early caregiver-child relationship and attention-deficit disorder with hyperactivity in kindergarten: A prospective study. *Child Dev.* **1987**, *58*, 1496–1504. [CrossRef]
17. Achermann, S.; Nystrom, P.; Bolte, S.; Falck-Ytter, T. Motor atypicalities in infancy are associated with general developmental level at 2 years, but not autistic symptoms. *Autism* **2020**. [CrossRef]
18. Focaroli, V.; Taffoni, F.; Parsons, S.M.; Keller, F.; Iverson, J.M. Performance of Motor Sequences in Children at Heightened vs. Low Risk for ASD: A Longitudinal Study from 18 to 36 Months of Age. *Front. Psychol.* **2016**, *7*, 724. [CrossRef]
19. Jasmin, E.; Couture, M.; McKinley, P.; Reid, G.; Fombonne, E.; Gisel, E. Sensori-motor and daily living skills of preschool children with autism spectrum disorders. *J. Autism Dev. Disord.* **2009**, *39*, 231–241. [CrossRef]
20. Landa, R.; Garrett-Mayer, E. Development in infants with autism spectrum disorders: A prospective study. *J. Child Psychol. Psychiatry* **2006**, *47*, 629–638. [CrossRef]
21. Landa, R.J.; Gross, A.L.; Stuart, E.A.; Faherty, A. Developmental trajectories in children with and without autism spectrum disorders: The first 3 years. *Child Dev.* **2013**, *84*, 429–442. [CrossRef]
22. LeBarton, E.S.; Landa, R.J. Infant motor skill predicts later expressive language and autism spectrum disorder diagnosis. *Infant Behav. Dev.* **2019**, *54*, 37–47. [CrossRef] [PubMed]
23. Libertus, K.; Landa, R.J. The Early Motor Questionnaire (EMQ): A parental report measure of early motor development. *Infant Behav. Dev.* **2013**, *36*, 833–842. [CrossRef] [PubMed]
24. Libertus, K.; Sheperd, K.A.; Ross, S.W.; Landa, R.J. Limited fine motor and grasping skills in 6-month-old infants at high risk for autism. *Child Dev.* **2014**, *85*, 2218–2231. [CrossRef] [PubMed]
25. Phagava, H.; Muratori, F.; Einspieler, C.; Maestro, S.; Apicella, F.; Guzzetta, A.; Prechtl, H.F.; Cioni, G. General movements in infants with autism spectrum disorders. *Georgian Med. News* **2008**, *156*, 100–105.
26. Harris, S.R. Early motor delays as diagnostic clues in autism spectrum disorder. *Eur. J. Pediatr.* **2017**, *176*, 1259–1262. [CrossRef]
27. Iverson, J.M. Early Motor and Communicative Development in Infants With an Older Sibling With Autism Spectrum Disorder. *J. Speech Lang Hear. Res.* **2018**, *61*, 2673–2684. [CrossRef]
28. Moseley, R.L.; Pulvermuller, F. What can autism teach us about the role of sensorimotor systems in higher cognition? New clues from studies on language, action semantics, and abstract emotional concept processing. *Cortex* **2018**, *100*, 149–190. [CrossRef]
29. West, K.L. Infant Motor Development in Autism Spectrum Disorder: A Synthesis and Meta-analysis. *Child Dev.* **2019**, *90*, 2053–2070. [CrossRef]

30. Einspieler, C.; Sigafoos, J.; Bolte, S.; Bratl-Pokorny, K.D.; Landa, R.; Marschik, P.B. Highlighting the first 5 months of life: General movements in infants later diagnosed with autism spectrum disorder or Rett Syndrome. *Res. Autism Spectr. Disord.* **2014**, *8*, 286–291. [CrossRef]
31. Kim, S.H.; Lord, C. Restricted and repetitive behaviors in toddlers and preschoolers with autism spectrum disorders based on the Autism Diagnostic Observation Schedule (ADOS). *Autism Res.* **2010**, *3*, 162–173. [CrossRef]
32. Morgan, L.; Wetherby, A.M.; Barber, A. Repetitive and stereotyped movements in children with autism spectrum disorders late in the second year of life. *J. Child Psychol. Psychiatry* **2008**, *49*, 826–837. [CrossRef] [PubMed]
33. Purpura, G.; Costanzo, V.; Chericoni, N.; Puopolo, M.; Scattoni, M.L.; Muratori, F.; Apicella, F. Bilateral Patterns of Repetitive Movements in 6- to 12-Month-Old Infants with Autism Spectrum Disorders. *Front. Psychol.* **2017**, *8*, 1168. [CrossRef]
34. Ozonoff, S.; Young, G.S.; Carter, A.; Messinger, D.; Yirmiya, N.; Zwaigenbaum, L.; Bryson, S.; Carver, L.J.; Constantino, J.N.; Dobkins, K.; et al. Recurrence risk for autism spectrum disorders: A Baby Siblings Research Consortium study. *Pediatrics* **2011**, *128*, e488–e495. [CrossRef] [PubMed]
35. Bryson, S.E.; Zwaigenbaum, L.; Brian, J.; Roberts, W.; Szatmari, P.; Rombough, V.; McDermott, C. A prospective case series of high-risk infants who developed autism. *J. Autism Dev. Disord.* **2007**, *37*, 12–24. [CrossRef] [PubMed]
36. Estes, A.; Zwaigenbaum, L.; Gu, H.; St John, T.; Paterson, S.; Elison, J.T.; Hazlett, H.; Botteron, K.; Dager, S.R.; Schultz, R.T.; et al. Behavioral, cognitive, and adaptive development in infants with autism spectrum disorder in the first 2 years of life. *J. Neurodev. Disord.* **2015**, *7*, 24. [CrossRef]
37. Flanagan, J.E.; Landa, R.; Bhat, A.; Bauman, M. Head lag in infants at risk for autism: A preliminary study. *Am. J. Occup. Ther.* **2012**, *66*, 577–585. [CrossRef]
38. Iverson, J.M.; Wozniak, R.H. Variation in vocal-motor development in infant siblings of children with autism. *J. Autism Dev. Disord.* **2007**, *37*, 158–170. [CrossRef]
39. Iverson, J.M.; Shic, F.; Wall, C.A.; Chawarska, K.; Curtin, S.; Estes, A.; Gardner, J.M.; Hutman, T.; Landa, R.J.; Levin, A.R.; et al. Early motor abilities in infants at heightened versus low risk for ASD: A Baby Siblings Research Consortium (BSRC) study. *J. Abnorm. Psychol.* **2019**, *128*, 69–80. [CrossRef]
40. Nickel, L.R.; Thatcher, A.R.; Keller, F.; Wozniak, R.H.; Iverson, J.M. Posture Development in Infants at Heightened vs. Low Risk for Autism Spectrum Disorders. *Infancy* **2013**, *18*, 639–661. [CrossRef]
41. Brian, J.; Bryson, S.E.; Garon, N.; Roberts, W.; Smith, I.M.; Szatmari, P.; Zwaigenbaum, L. Clinical assessment of autism in high-risk 18-month-olds. *Autism* **2008**, *12*, 433–456. [CrossRef]
42. Elison, J.T.; Wolff, J.J.; Reznick, J.S.; Botteron, K.N.; Estes, A.M.; Gu, H.; Hazlett, H.C.; Meadows, A.J.; Paterson, S.J.; Zwaigenbaum, L.; et al. Repetitive behavior in 12-month-olds later classified with autism spectrum disorder. *J. Am. Acad. Child Adolesc. Psychiatry* **2014**, *53*, 1216–1224. [CrossRef] [PubMed]
43. Chawarska, K.; Shic, F.; Macari, S.; Campbell, D.J.; Brian, J.; Landa, R.; Hutman, T.; Nelson, C.A.; Ozonoff, S.; Tager-Flusberg, H.; et al. 18-month predictors of later outcomes in younger siblings of children with autism spectrum disorder: A baby siblings research consortium study. *J. Am. Acad. Child Adolesc. Psychiatry* **2014**, *53*, 1317–1327. [CrossRef] [PubMed]
44. Bolte, S.; Bartl-Pokorny, K.D.; Jonsson, U.; Berggren, S.; Zhang, D.; Kostrzewa, E.; Falck-Ytter, T.; Einspieler, C.; Pokorny, F.B.; Jones, E.J.; et al. How can clinicians detect and treat autism early? Methodological trends of technology use in research. *Acta Paediatr.* **2016**, *105*, 137–144. [CrossRef] [PubMed]
45. Adde, L.; Helbostad, J.L.; Jensenius, A.R.; Taraldsen, G.; Stoen, R. Using computer-based video analysis in the study of fidgety movements. *Early Hum. Dev.* **2009**, *85*, 541–547. [CrossRef]
46. Baccinelli, W.; Bulgheroni, M.; Simonetti, V.; Fulceri, F.; Caruso, A.; Gila, L.; Scattoni, M.L. Movidea: A Software Package for Automatic Video Analysis of Movements in Infants at Risk for Neurodevelopmental Disorders. *Brain Sci.* **2020**, *10*, 203. [CrossRef]
47. Karch, D.; Wochner, K.; Kim, K.; Philippi, H.; Hadders-Algra, M.; Pietz, J.; Dickhaus, H. Quantitative score for the evaluation of kinematic recordings in neuropediatric diagnostics. Detection of complex patterns in spontaneous limb movements. *Methods Inf. Med.* **2010**, *49*, 526–530. [CrossRef]
48. Marchi, V.; Hakala, A.; Knight, A.; D'Acunto, F.; Scattoni, M.L.; Guzzetta, A.; Vanhatalo, S. Automated pose estimation captures key aspects of General Movements at eight to 17 weeks from conventional videos. *Acta Paediatr.* **2019**, *108*, 1817–1824. [CrossRef]
49. Marcroft, C.; Khan, A.; Embleton, N.D.; Trenell, M.; Plotz, T. Movement recognition technology as a method of assessing spontaneous general movements in high risk infants. *Front. Neurol.* **2014**, *5*, 284. [CrossRef]

50. Marchi, V.; Belmonti, V.; Cecchi, F.; Coluccini, M.; Ghirri, P.; Grassi, A.; Sabatini, A.M.; Guzzetta, A. Movement analysis in early infancy: Towards a motion biomarker of age. *Early Hum. Dev.* **2020**, *142*, 104942. [CrossRef]
51. Marschik, P.B.; Pokorny, F.B.; Peharz, R.; Zhang, D.; O'Muircheartaigh, J.; Roeyers, H.; Bolte, S.; Spittle, A.J.; Urlesberger, B.; Schuller, B.; et al. A Novel Way to Measure and Predict Development: A Heuristic Approach to Facilitate the Early Detection of Neurodevelopmental Disorders. *Curr. Neurol. Neurosci. Rep.* **2017**, *17*, 43. [CrossRef]
52. Tsuji, T.; Nakashima, S.; Hayashi, H.; Soh, Z.; Furui, A.; Shibanoki, T.; Shima, K.; Shimatani, K. Markerless Measurement and Evaluation of General Movements in Infants. *Sci. Rep.* **2020**, *10*, 1422. [CrossRef] [PubMed]
53. Lord, C.; Rutter, M.; DiLavore, P.C.; Risi, S.; Gotham, K.; Bishop, S.L. *Autism Diagnostic Observation Schedule*, 2nd ed.; Western Psychological Services: Torrance, CA, USA, 2012.
54. Meinecke, L.; Breitbach-Faller, N.; Bartz, C.; Damen, R.; Rau, G.; Disselhorst-Klug, C. Movement analysis in the early detection of newborns at risk for developing spasticity due to infantile cerebral palsy. *Hum. Mov. Sci.* **2006**, *25*, 125–144. [CrossRef]
55. Hsu, J.C. *Multiple Comparisons: Theory and Methods*; Hardback Published by Chapman & Hall in February 1996; The Ohio State University: Columbus, OH, USA, 1996.
56. Maxwell, S.E.; Delaney, H.D.; Kelley, K. *Designing Experiments and Analyzing Data: A Model Comparison Perspective*, 3rd ed.; Routledge: New York, NY, USA, 2018.
57. Sohal, V.S.; Rubenstein, J.L.R. Excitation-inhibition balance as a framework for investigating mechanisms in neuropsychiatric disorders. *Mol. Psychiatry* **2019**, *24*, 1248–1257. [CrossRef] [PubMed]
58. Canals, J.; Hernandez-Martinez, C.; Esparo, G.; Fernandez-Ballart, J. Neonatal Behavioral Assessment Scale as a predictor of cognitive development and IQ in full-term infants: A 6-year longitudinal study. *Acta Paediatr.* **2011**, *100*, 1331–1337. [CrossRef] [PubMed]
59. Christiansen, H.; Hirsch, O.; Albrecht, B.; Chavanon, M.L. Attention-Deficit/Hyperactivity Disorder (ADHD) and Emotion Regulation Over the Life Span. *Curr. Psychiatry Rep.* **2019**, *21*, 17. [CrossRef] [PubMed]
60. Gomez, C.R.; Baird, S. Identifying Early Indicators for Autism in Self-Regulation Difficulties. *Focus Autism Dev. Disabil. J.* **2005**, *20*, 106–116. [CrossRef]
61. Bachevalier, J.; Loveland, K.A. The orbitofrontal-amygdala circuit and self-regulation of social-emotional behavior in autism. *Neurosci. Biobehav. Rev.* **2006**, *30*, 97–117. [CrossRef]
62. Hadders-Algra, M. Neural substrate and clinical significance of general movements: An update. *Dev. Med. Child Neurol.* **2018**, *60*, 39–46. [CrossRef]
63. Dusing, S.C.; Brown, S.E.; Van Drew, C.M.; Thacker, L.R.; Hendricks-Munoz, K.D. Supporting Play Exploration and Early Development Intervention From NICU to Home: A Feasibility Study. *Pediatr. Phys. Ther.* **2015**, *27*, 267–274. [CrossRef]
64. Dusing, S.C.; Harbourne, R.T. Variability in postural control during infancy: Implications for development, assessment, and intervention. *Phys. Ther.* **2010**, *90*, 1838–1849. [CrossRef]
65. Adde, L.; Yang, H.; Saether, R.; Jensenius, A.R.; Ihlen, E.; Cao, J.Y.; Stoen, R. Characteristics of general movements in preterm infants assessed by computer-based video analysis. *Physiother. Theory Pract.* **2018**, *34*, 286–292. [CrossRef] [PubMed]
66. Hadders-Algra, M. Variation and variability: Key words in human motor development. *Phys. Ther.* **2010**, *90*, 1823–1837. [CrossRef] [PubMed]
67. Kyvelidou, A.; Harbourne, R.T.; Stergiou, N. Severity and characteristics of developmental delay can be assessed using variability measures of sitting posture. *Pediatr. Phys. Ther.* **2010**, *22*, 259–266. [CrossRef] [PubMed]
68. Hamer, E.G.; Bos, A.F.; Hadders-Algra, M. Specific characteristics of abnormal general movements are associated with functional outcome at school age. *Early Hum. Dev.* **2016**, *95*, 9–13. [CrossRef]
69. Zappella, M.; Einspieler, C.; Bartl-Pokorny, K.D.; Krieber, M.; Coleman, M.; Bolte, S.; Marschik, P.B. What do home videos tell us about early motor and socio-communicative behaviours in children with autistic features during the second year of life—An exploratory study. *Early Hum. Dev.* **2015**, *91*, 569–575. [CrossRef]
70. Abrishami, M.S.; Nocera, L.; Mert, M.; Trujillo-Priego, I.A.; Purushotham, S.; Shahabi, C.; Smith, B.A. Identification of Developmental Delay in Infants Using Wearable Sensors: Full-Day Leg Movement Statistical Feature Analysis. *IEEE J. Transl. Eng. Health Med.* **2019**, *7*, 2800207. [CrossRef]

71. Thelen, E. Rhythmical stereotypies in normal human infants. *Anim. Behav.* **1979**, *27*, 699–715. [CrossRef]
72. Leekam, S.; Tandos, J.; McConachie, H.; Meins, E.; Parkinson, K.; Wright, C.; Turner, M.; Arnott, B.; Vittorini, L.; Le Couteur, A. Repetitive behaviours in typically developing 2-year-olds. *J. Child Psychol. Psychiatry* **2007**, *48*, 1131–1138. [CrossRef]
73. Einspieler, C.; Prechtl, H.F. Prechtl's assessment of general movements: A diagnostic tool for the functional assessment of the young nervous system. *Ment. Retard. Dev. Disabil. Res. Rev.* **2005**, *11*, 61–67. [CrossRef]
74. Prechtl, H.F.; Einspieler, C.; Cioni, G.; Bos, A.F.; Ferrari, F.; Sontheimer, D. An early marker for neurological deficits after perinatal brain lesions. *Lancet* **1997**, *349*, 1361–1363. [CrossRef]

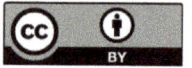

© 2020 by the authors. Licensee MDPI, Basel, Switzerland. This article is an open access article distributed under the terms and conditions of the Creative Commons Attribution (CC BY) license (http://creativecommons.org/licenses/by/4.0/).

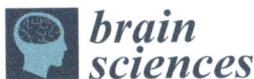 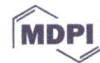

Article

Cerebrospinal Fluid Findings of 36 Adult Patients with Autism Spectrum Disorder

Kimon Runge [1,2], Ludger Tebartz van Elst [1,2,*], Simon Maier [1,2], Kathrin Nickel [1,2], Dominik Denzel [1,2], Miriam Matysik [1,2], Hanna Kuzior [1,2], Tilman Robinson [3], Thomas Blank [4], Rick Dersch [3], Katharina Domschke [2,5] and Dominique Endres [1,2]

1. Section for Experimental Neuropsychiatry, Department of Psychiatry and Psychotherapy, Medical Center, Faculty of Medicine, University of Freiburg, Freiburg im Breisgau, Germany; kimon.runge@uniklinik-freiburg.de (K.R.); simon.maier@uniklinik-freiburg.de (S.M.); kathrin.nickel@uniklinik-freiburg.de (K.N.); dominik.denzel@uniklinik-freiburg.de (D.D.); miriam.matysik@uniklinik-freiburg.de (M.M.); hanna.kuzior@uniklinik-freiburg.de (H.K.); dominique.endres@uniklinik-freiburg.de (D.E.)
2. Department of Psychiatry and Psychotherapy, Medical Center, Faculty of Medicine, University of Freiburg, Freiburg im Breisgau, Germany; katharina.domschke@uniklinik-freiburg.de
3. Department of Neurology, Medical Center, Faculty of Medicine, University of Freiburg, Freiburg im Breisgau, Germany; tilman.robinson@uniklinik-freiburg.de (T.R.); rick.dersch@uniklinik-freiburg.de (R.D.)
4. Institute of Neuropathology, Medical Center, Faculty of Medicine, University of Freiburg, Freiburg im Breisgau, Germany; thomas.blank@uniklinik-freiburg.de
5. Center for Basics in Neuromodulation, Faculty of Medicine, University of Freiburg, Freiburg im Breisgau, Germany
* Correspondence: tebartzvanelst@uniklinik-freiburg.de

Received: 12 April 2020; Accepted: 1 June 2020; Published: 8 June 2020

Abstract: Autism spectrum disorder (ASD) is a common neurodevelopmental disorder characterized by difficulties with social interaction, repetitive behavior, and additional features, such as special interests. Its precise etiology is unclear. Recently, immunological mechanisms, such as maternal autoantibodies/infections, have increasingly been the subject of discussion. Cerebrospinal fluid (CSF) investigations play a decisive role in the detection of immunological processes in the brain. This study therefore retrospectively analyzed the CSF findings of adult patients with ASD. CSF basic measures (white blood cell count, total protein, albumin quotient, immunoglobulin G (IgG) index, and oligoclonal bands) and various antineuronal antibody findings of 36 adult patients with ASD, who had received lumbar puncture, were compared with an earlier described mentally healthy control group of 39 patients with idiopathic intracranial hypertension. CSF protein concentrations and albumin quotients of patients with ASD were significantly higher as compared to controls (age corrected: $p = 0.003$ and $p = 0.004$, respectively); 17% of the patients with ASD showed increased albumin quotients. After correction for age and gender, the group effect for total protein remained significant ($p = 0.041$) and showed a tendency for albumin quotient ($p = 0.079$). In the CSF of two ASD patients, an intrathecal synthesis of anti-glutamate decarboxylase 65 (GAD65) antibodies was found. In total, more of the ASD patients (44%) presented abnormal findings in CSF basic diagnostics compared to controls (18%; $p = 0.013$). A subgroup of the patients with adult ASD showed indication of a blood–brain barrier dysfunction, and two patients displayed an intrathecal synthesis of anti-GAD65 antibodies; thus, the role of these antibodies in patients with ASD should be further investigated. The results of the study are limited by its retrospective and open design. The group differences in blood–brain barrier markers could be influenced by a different gender distribution between ASD patients and controls.

Keywords: Asperger syndrome; autism spectrum disorder; adults; cerebrospinal fluid; antibodies; blood–brain barrier; GAD65

1. Introduction

Autism spectrum disorder (ASD) is a common neurodevelopmental disorder characterized by deficits in social interaction and communication, unusually narrowed interests, and repetitive behavior in different situations [1]. Furthermore, the disorder involves specific alterations in social and sensory perception as well as in language [2]. The description of ASD in the Diagnostic and Statistical Manual of Mental Disorders, version 5 (DSM-5) demonstrates the clear tendency of the scientific community to subsume the various previous autism subtypes of the DSM-IV and of the International Statistical Classification of Diseases and Related Health Problems, version 10 (ICD-10) (childhood autism (ICD-10 F84.0, corresponding in the DSM-IV to autistic disorder 299.00), atypical autism (ICD-10 F84.1, not listed in the DSM-IV), and Asperger syndrome (ICD-10 F84.5, DSM-IV 299.80)) under a single diagnostic category [1,3,4]. ASD is a lifelong condition affecting predominantly males that is already present in early childhood, persists into adulthood, and is often accompanied by a variety of psychiatric comorbidities [1,2]. Despite the growing public and scientific interest in ASD over the past decades [5], which reflects increasing prevalence rates that are well above 1% and up to 2.7% depending on the populations studied [6,7], the disorder's precise etiology and pathophysiology remain elusive.

Genetic mechanisms certainly play an important role, and strong causal effects on ASD have long been known [8] for several rare genetic variants, such as tuberous sclerosis [9] and the fragile X syndrome [10]. Further genetic studies have shown the association of hundreds of distinct gene variants with autism, accounting, however, for only a fraction of ASD diagnoses [8,11]. Only recently, in the largest genome-wide association study (GWAS) for ASD to date, several single loci with genome-wide significance for association with ASD were reported for the first time [12]. Not only the phenotypic expression of ASD but also its etiology appear to be heterogeneous [13,14].

In recent studies, immunological mechanisms have increasingly been discussed as risk factors for altered neuronal development in ASD patients [15]. In particular, there is increasing evidence that maternal immune-dysfunction during gestation may lead to an ASD-like phenotype in susceptible offspring [11,16]. The first hints of the role of maternal prenatal infections were identified in the context of a significant increase in ASD after a rubella epidemic in the US in 1964 [17,18]. Furthermore, studies in large Danish registries found an elevated likelihood of ASD in children whose mothers were hospitalized during pregnancy due to a viral infection [19]. The possible importance of immune-dysfunction for an increased ASD risk is further supported by Scandinavian registry studies that reported a significant association between positive family history for autoimmune diseases and ASD [20,21]. Likewise, children of mothers with systemic lupus erythematosus have a doubled risk for ASD [22]. Potential mechanisms for an accentuated immune activation to affect neurological development are via cytokines, autoantibodies [11], or maternal anti-fetal brain antibodies [23,24]. In line with this, in post-mortem brains and the cerebrospinal fluid (CSF) of ASD patients, a proinflammatory cytokine profile has been found with activated microglia and astrocytes as signs of neuroinflammation [25].

In patients, CSF analysis is the most precise method for investigating subtle inflammation in the central nervous system (CNS) [26–28]. Furthermore, there is evidence that CSF circulation, which usually supplies growth hormones and signal molecules and cleanses the brain of harmful substances for proper brain development, is impaired in ASD [29]. Earlier CSF studies in ASD have analyzed children and infants as well as post-mortem material but not adult patients. This may be due to the fact that diagnostic procedures of potential brain disease are initiated at time of diagnosis (i.e., earlier in development and not in adulthood). Another reason might be that no CSF sampling is performed in adult ASD patients who are not characterized by mental retardation or further psychiatric/neurological symptoms. Therefore, this study's rationale is to retrospectively analyze the CSF findings of adult patients with ASD.

2. Participants and Methods

The study was part of a larger project of retrospective biomarker detection that was approved by the local ethics committee (Faculty of Medicine, Freiburg University, 396/18).

2.1. Study Sample

We included 36 patients with ASD who had received a lumbar puncture at our tertiary care hospital from 2010 to 2018. The patients were diagnosed by experienced senior physicians following German guidelines [30] as described in detail in earlier papers [31,32] and were classified following ICD-10. Patients with neurodegenerative disorders were excluded from the study; examples include mild cognitive impairment (ICD-10: F06.7) or dementia (ICD-10: F03), substance abuse (ICD-10: F1x.2), or severe neurological diseases other than epilepsy (because of its known association with ASD) [33,34]. The presence of other common comorbid conditions in patients with ASD was not defined as an exclusion criterion; examples include affective disorders (ICD-10: F30-F39), or neurodevelopmental disorders such as attention deficit hyperactivity disorder (ADHD; ICD-10: F90.x), or Tourette syndrome (ICD-10: F95.2).

The control group comprised 39 mentally healthy controls with idiopathic intracranial hypertension (IIH; ICD-10: G93.2), a non-inflammatory neurological disease characterized by increased intracranial pressure of unknown origin. All controls with clearly identifiable secondary forms of intracranial hypertension, those being treated with psychotropic drugs at the time of the lumbar puncture, and those with a history of psychiatric or neurological disorders (except headache) were excluded. This control group was collected in the context of a previous CSF study [35–37].

All the clinical and demographic data of the ASD patients were extracted from medical reports. Patients' psychometric data had been collected as part of routine clinical documentation, including the Clinical Global Impression (CGI) score [38], the Global Assessment of Functioning (GAF) score [4], and psychopathological scores based on the German Association for Methodology and Documentation in Psychiatry (AMDP) [39].

2.2. CSF and Instrument-Based Diagnostics

All of the included participants were informed about the lumbar puncture and gave their written informed consent. The CSF analyses were performed in the CSF laboratory at the Department of Neurology (https://www.uniklinik-freiburg.de/neurologie/klinik/diagnostische-einrichtungen/liquor-labor.html) as described in previous studies [40–42]. Routine CSF analysis included the determination of white blood cell (WBC) count, total protein concentration, albumin quotient (AQ), immunoglobulin G (IgG) index, and oligoclonal bands (OCBs). Antibodies against cell surface antigens (NMDA-receptor, LGI1, CASPR2, AMPA1/2-receptor, GABA-B-receptor) were identified in the CSF using fixed-cell assays (Euroimmun®). Antibodies in serum against paraneoplastic intracellular antigens (Yo, Hu, CV2/CRMP5, Ri, Ma1/2, SOX1, Tr, Zic4, glutamate decarboxylase 65 (GAD65), amphiphysin) were screened using immunoblots (Ravo line assay®). In individual cases, the anti-GAD65 antibody levels were measured in serum and CSF additionally using a radioimmunoassay (Medipan®, see [28] for comparison). All ASD patients received cerebral magnetic resonance imaging (MRI) assessed by experienced neuroradiologists as well as electroencephalograms (EEGs) assessed by the attending physicians.

2.3. Statistical Analyses

Data analysis was conducted with Statistical Package for the Social Sciences, version 25 (IBM Corp., Armonk, NY, USA). Group comparisons of categorical variables were conducted with Pearson's Chi-squared test. If the result in any of the cells of the contingency table was below 5, Fisher's exact test was used. One-way analyses of covariance (ANCOVAs) were conducted to determine whether there was a statistically significant difference between the patients and the controls in their CSF basis findings while controlling for the effect of age. Spearman's rank correlation coefficient was used for correlation analysis between CSF parameters (WBC count, protein concentration, AQ, and IgG index) of the ASD group and their psychometric scores, such as CGI, GAF, and AMDP as well as the number of inpatient stays, suicide attempts, and age. Further ANCOVAs were performed to detect significant influences of gender as well as the presence of abnormalities in EEGs or MRI on CSF parameters of ASD patients while controlling for the effect of age. To control the false discovery rate in multiple testing we calculated adjusted p-values with R (R Core Team, 2019) using the Benjamini–Hochberg procedure [43]. Thereby the p-values of the CSF basic diagnostics were adjusted together, then the p-values of the number of subjects with abnormal CSF diagnostics as a separate group and finally the p-values of each correlation of a CSF parameter with the psychometric data. A p-value of less than 0.05 was considered statistically significant.

3. Results

3.1. Clinical and Demographic Data

For clinical and demographic data of the patient and control samples see Table 1. The ASD and the control cohort differed significantly in gender ratio ($p < 0.001$) and age ($p = 0.03$). According to the ICD-10 subgroups of ASD, 34 patients were coded as diagnosed with Asperger syndrome (ICD-10: F84.5) and two with atypical autism (ICD-10: F84.1). All ASD patients had psychiatric comorbidities, of which depression was the most prevalent (75%).

Table 1. Clinical and demographic data of patients and controls.

	Patients with Autism ($n = 36$)	Controls ($n = 39$)	Statistics
Gender	13 F:23 M	33 F:6 M	$p < 0.001$
Average age at time of lumbar puncture (age range)	28.94 ± 9.9 (18–53 years)	34.6 ± 12.0 (18–61 years)	$p = 0.03$
Diagnosis			
F84.5	$n = 34$ (94.4%)	-	
F84.1	$n = 2$ (5.6%)	-	
G93.2	-	$n = 39$ (100%)	
Neuropsychiatric comorbidity			
Depression	$n = 27$ (86.1%)	-	
ADHD	$n = 6$ (16.7%)	-	
Schizophreniform disorders	$n = 5$ (13.9%)	-	
History of epilepsy	$n = 2$ (5.6%)	-	
Obsessive compulsive disorder	$n = 2$ (5.6%)	-	
Personality disorder	$n = 2$ (5.6%)	-	
Others	$n = 7$ * (19.4%)	-	
Civil status			
Single	$n = 31$ (86.1%)		
Married	$n = 3$ (8.3%)		
Unknown	$n = 2$ (5.6%)		
Educational level			
Low	$n = 5$ (13.9%)		
Intermediate	$n = 14$ (38.9%)		
High	$n = 14$ (38.9%)		
Unknown	$n = 3$ (8.3%)		
Employment			
Unemployed	$n = 7$ (19.4%)		
Working	$n = 11$ (30.6%)		
Education/training	$n = 11$ (30.6%)		
Occupational disability	$n = 4$ (11.1%)		
Others/unknown	$n = 3$ (8.3%)		
Living situation			
Alone	$n = 13$ (36.1%)		
With partner/family	$n = 2$ (5.6%)		
With parents/custodian	$n = 17$ (47.2%)		
Psychiatric transitional arrangement	$n = 1$ (2.8%)		
Others/unknown	$n = 3$ (8.3%)		

Table 1. *Cont.*

	Patients with Autism (*n* = 36)	Controls (*n* = 39)	Statistics
**Family history for any psychiatric disease **			
Positive	*n* = 23 (63.9%)		
Negative	*n* = 9 (25.0%)		
Unknown	*n* = 4 (11.1%)		
Number of previous inpatient stays			
None	*n* = 12 (33.3%)		
1	*n* = 4 (11.1%)		
2	*n* = 7 (19.4%)		
3	*n* = 3 (8.3%)		
More than 3	*n* = 7 (19.4%)		
Unknown	*n* = 3 (8.3%)		
Burden of acute events			
None	*n* = 6 (16.7%)		
Mild	*n* = 17 (47.2%)		
Intermediate	*n* = 5 (13.9%)		
Severe	*n* = 4 (11.1%)		
Extreme	*n* = 1 (2.8%)		
Unknown	*n* = 3 (8.3%)		
Burden of long-term life circumstances			
None	*n* = 2 (5.6%)		
Mild	*n* = 10 (27.8%)		
Intermediate	*n* = 9 (25.0%)		
Severe	*n* = 9 (25.0%)		
Extreme	*n* = 2 (5.6%)		
Unknown	*n* = 4 (11.1%)		
Number of suicide attempts			
None	*n* = 28 (77.8%)		
1	*n* = 6 (16.7%)		
2	*n* = 1 (2.8%)		
Unknown	*n* = 1 (2.8%)		

* Bipolar disorder, anorexia nervosa, narcolepsy, Tourette syndrome, insomnia, substance induced psychotic disorder, dissociative disorder. ** In first-degree relatives. Abbreviations: F = female, M = male, ADHD = attention deficit hyperactivity disorder, *n* = number.

Most of the ASD patients were single (86.1%), lived with their parents/guardians (47.2%) and were either working (30.6%) or in training (30.6%). The majority had achieved intermediate (38.9%) to high (38.9%) education. Most patients had a positive family history for some psychiatric disease in first-degree relatives (63.9%).

3.2. CSF Diagnostics

At the time of lumbar puncture, most of the ASD patients (75%) were treated with psychotropic medications, of which the most prevalent were atypical neuroleptics (52.8%) and antidepressants (55.6%). An exact listing of psychotropic medications used at the time of lumbar puncture is provided in Table 2.

Of the 36 ASD patients, three (8.3%) showed a slightly elevated WBC count, 12 (33.3%) an increased total protein, and six (16.7%) an increased age-dependent AQ. CSF-specific OCBs were found in one patient with ASD (2.8%) and in none of the control patients, and no patient showed an increased IgG index. In summary, 16 of the 36 patients (44.4%) presented abnormal CSF basic diagnostic findings, which differed significantly ($p = 0.013$) from respective findings in controls with abnormal CSF measures (7 of 39; 18%). The ANCOVAs conducted with age correction showed a significant difference between ASD patients and controls in total protein ($F_{(1,73)} = 6.450$, $p = 0.003$) and AQ ($F_{(1,73)} = 5.878$, $p = 0.004$), but not regarding WBC counts or IgG index. For this analysis, data from 36 ASD patients and 39 controls were evaluated except for the WBC count, for which data from only 35 controls were available. All results of the CSF basic diagnostic are summarized in Tables 3 and 4.

In a secondary analysis, we additionally investigated the effect of gender and the interaction between age and gender in these ANCOVAs. Here, the group effect for total protein remained significant ($F_{(1,70)} = 4.327$, $p = 0.041$) and for AQ a tendency could still be observed ($F_{(1,70)} = 3.167$, $p = 0.079$). We found a significant interaction between age and gender in the ANCOVAs for total protein ($F_{(1,70)}$ = 6.510, p = 0.013) as well as AQ ($F_{(1,70)}$ = 5.299, p = 0.024), but gender alone had no significant effect on the models for total protein ($F_{(1,70)}$ = 2.073, p = 0.154) and AQ ($F_{(1,70)}$ = 1.834, p = 0.180). For WBC count and IgG index no significant group effects or interactions were detected.

Most ASD patients additionally received screenings for antineuronal antibodies against cell surface antigens (n = 31) or intracellular antigens (n = 34) (Table 5). Two of the patients tested were positive for anti-GAD65 antibodies in serum and CSF, and one patient had a nonspecific reaction for anti-Yo antibodies in serum.

Table 2. Psychotropic medication at time of lumbar puncture.

	Patients with ASD (n = 36)
Class of Medication	
Selective serotonin reuptake inhibitor	n = 6 (16.7%)
Selective serotonin/noradrenaline reuptake inhibitor	n = 4 (11.1%)
Tricyclic antidepressants	n = 6 (16.7%)
Bupropion	n = 3 (8.3%)
Mirtazapine	n = 2 (5.6%)
Typical neuroleptics	n = 1 (2.8%)
Atypical neuroleptics	n = 19 (52.8%)
Lithium	n = 1 (2.8%)
Anticonvulsants	n = 7 (19.4%)
Benzodiazepine	n = 1 (2.8%)
Methylphenidate	n = 2 (5.6%)
Melatonin	n = 5 (13.9%)
Others	n = 4 * (11.1%)
Number of Different Medication Classes per Patient	
Same class/only one drug	n = 9 (25.0%)
Two drugs	n = 7 (19.4%)
Three drugs	n = 9 (25.0%)
More than three	n = 2 (5.6%)
Unmedicated	n = 9 (25.0%)

The number refers to different drug classes. If several drugs of the same class were taken, only one was included. * One patient with comorbid ADHD received atypical off-label treatment with levodopa + carbidopa (this was changed to bupropion after lumbar puncture); another patient took biperiden and clonidine. Abbreviations: ASD = Autism spectrum disorder; ADHD = attention deficit hyperactivity disorder; n = number.

Table 3. CSF basis diagnostics.

	Reference [44]	ASD Patients (n = 36)	Controls (n = 39)	Statistics (Unadjusted p-Value)
WBC count (Mean ± SD)	<5/µL	1.94 ± 1.37	2.60 ± 7.59 *	p = 0.698 (0.698)
Total protein (Mean ± SD)	≤450 mg/L	478.14 ± 391.1	309.33 ± 142.5	**p = 0.009 (0.003)**
Albumin quotient (Mean ± SD)	<40 years: 6.5 × 10^{-3}; 40–60 years: 8 × 10^{-3}; >60 years: 9.3 × 10^{-3}	5.84 ± 5.66	3.93 ± 1.81	**p = 0.009 (0.004)**
IgG index (Mean ± SD)	≤0.7 mg/L	0.50 ± 0.39	0.50 ± 0.038	p = 0.257 (0.193)

The control group was created for an earlier project and the results were published earlier [35–37]. Abbreviations: CSF = cerebrospinal fluid; WBC = white blood cell, SD = standard deviation, IgG = immunoglobulin G, n = number. * Data of only 35 controls are available. One of them suffered from pleocytosis (46 cells/µL), which normalized independently, and was interpreted as reactive pleocytosis. p-Values adjusted by Benjamini–Hochberg procedure. Bold = significant at p ≤ 0.05.

Table 4. Number of subjects with abnormal CSF diagnostics.

	ASD Patients (n = 36)	Controls (n = 39)	Statistics (Unadjusted p-Value)
Increased WBC count (≥5/μL)	n = 3 (8.3%) *	n = 1 (2.9%) **	p = 0.115 (0.086)
Increased total protein (>450 mg/L)	n = 12 (33.3%)	n = 6 (15.4%)	p = 0.115 (0.069)
Increased age-dependent albumin quotient (<40 years: 6.5×10^{-3}; 40–60 years: 8×10^{-3}; >60 years: 9.3×10^{-3})	n = 6 (16.7%)	n = 2 (5.1%)	p = 0.191 (0.143)
Increased IgG index (>0.7 mg/L)	n = 0	n = 0	-
CSF specific OCBs	n = 1 (2.8%) ***	n = 0 ****	p = 0.324 (0.324)
Patients with abnormal CSF basis diagnostics	16/36 (44.4%)	7/39 (18%)	p = 0.013

The control group was created for an earlier project and the results previously published (see [35–37]). The number of patients with abnormalities in CSF diagnostics, as a summary of previous tests, was not corrected for multiple testing. Abbreviations: WBC = white blood cell; SD = standard deviation; IgG = immunoglobulin G; OCBs = oligoclonal bands; n = number. * 5, 6 and 6 white blood cells without blood admixture. ** Only data of 35 controls are available. One of them suffered from reactive pleocytosis (46 cells/μL), which regressed independently to normal WBC counts and was interpreted as reactive pleocytosis. *** Two additional findings were not considered positive: one patient had an isolated OCB in the CSF, another patient had 1–2 very weak bands in the CSF. **** Only available from 38 (of 39) control patients. p-Values adjusted by Benjamini–Hochberg procedure. Bold = significant at $p \leq 0.05$.

Table 5. Antineuronal autoantibody findings.

Patients with ASD (n = 36)	Antibodies against Cell Surface Antigens in CSF	Antibodies against Paraneoplastic Intracellular Antigens in Serum
Not analyzed	n = 5 (13.9%)	n = 2 (5.6%)
Negative	n = 31 (86.1%)	n = 32 (88.2%)
Positive	n = 0	n = 2 * (5.6%)

* Two patients displayed anti-glutamate decarboxylase 65 (GAD65) antibodies, additionally one patient had a non-specific reaction for anti-Yo antibodies, which was not rated as a positive result. Abbreviations: ASD = Autism spectrum disorder, CSF = cerebrospinal fluid; n = number.

3.3. Instrument-Based Diagnostics

All patients received an EEG and an MRI scan of the brain. Sixteen ASD patients (44.4%) showed abnormalities in their MRI scans, the most frequent being white matter lesions/cerebral microangiopathy (25%). In the EEGs, generalized intermittent slow activity was found in five patients (13.9%) and focal slowing in three patients (8.3%). One patient (2.8%) had a history of epilepsy and showed corresponding epileptiform discharges with frontal spike wave complexes (Table 6).

Table 6. MRI and EEG pathologies in the ASD patient group.

MRI Abnormalities	Patients (n = 36)
White matter lesions/cerebral microangiopathy	n = 12 (33.3%)
Generalized cortical atrophy	n = 2 (5.6%)
Localized cortical atrophy	n = 1 (2.8%)
Pineal cyst	n = 4 (11.1%)
Other anatomical variants	n = 4 * (11.1%)
More than one abnormality	n = 7 (19.4%)
Normal findings	n = 20 (55.6%)
Total number of MRI abnormalities	16/36 patients (44.4%)
EEG pathologies	**Patients (n = 36)**
Continuous generalized/regional slow activity	-
Intermittent generalized slow activity	n = 5 (13.9%)
Intermittent focal slow activity	n = 3 (8.3%)
Epileptiform discharges	n = 1 (2.8%)
Absence of EEG pathologies	n = 28 (77.8%)
Total number of EEG pathologies	8/36 patients (22.2%)

* Arachnoidal cyst, asymmetric lateral ventricles, asymmetric vertebral artery, enlarged Virchow–Robin's space. Abbreviations: MRI = magnetic resonance imaging; EEG = electroencephalogram; n = number.

3.4. Clinical Characteristics of ASD Patients with Anti-GAD65 Antibodies

The two ASD patients who tested positive for anti-GAD65 antibodies in serum (patient (1): 14 U/mL; patient (2) 101 U/mL; reference <2.0 U/mL) displayed an increased antibody index (patient (1): 50.4, patient (2): 20.3; reference ≤1.5) indicating an intrathecal anti-GAD65 antibody synthesis. Both patients were relatively young, patient (1) was male and patient (2) was female. Both patients suffered from comorbid depression; patient (1) also suffered from tic disorder and patient (2) from anxious jitteriness and Hashimoto thyroiditis. Both patients had no diabetes mellitus (HbA1c levels were in the normal range) and no epilepsy. However, in patient (1), initially a slightly elevated WBC count in the CSF (6/µL; reference <5/µL; with normalization in the follow-up), increased streptolysin antibody levels, as well as anatomical alterations in the form of asymmetric lateral ventricles in the MRI and abnormal frontal slow waves in the EEG (which were partly generalized) were identified. A complementary [^{18}F] fluorodeoxyglucose positron emission tomography of the brain showed age-appropriate cerebral glucose utilization without patterns for an acute inflammatory CNS disease. In patient (2), the laboratory results, MRI, EEG, and CSF basis diagnostics were all essentially normal.

3.5. Correlation Analyses

For the ASD group we found significant negative correlations between WBC count and AMDP scores for formal thought disorders ($r = -0.336$, $p = 0.045$; $n = 36$) and delusion ($r = -0.457$, $p = 0.005$; $n = 36$) as well as number of suicide attempts ($r = -0.405$, $p = 0.014$; $n = 36$). This corresponds to moderate effect sizes of the correlation coefficients according to Cohen but were not significant after adjustments that control for the false discovery rate ($p = 0.27/0.09/0.126$). Furthermore, age correlated with total protein ($r = 0.338$, $p = 0.043$; $n = 36$) and AQ ($r = 0.474$, $p = 0.004$; $n = 36$). All other correlations between the CSF basic diagnostic parameters and the psychometric data were not significant. No significant influence of gender or the presence of EEG or MRI abnormalities on CSF parameters of ASD patients was detected.

4. Discussion

The main findings of this study are higher CSF levels of AQs in patients with ASD indicate potential blood–brain barrier (BBB) dysfunction and an intrathecal synthesis of anti-GAD65 antibodies in two patients with ASD. Overall, we found abnormal CSF basic findings in almost half of the ASD patients—significantly more than in the control group.

4.1. Significance of Increased CSF Protein Levels

Altogether the ASD group presented significantly higher CSF levels of total protein (478.1 vs. 309.3 mg/dL) and AQs (5.84 vs. 3.93) compared to the control group. Accordingly, 33.3% of ASD patients had an increased total protein and 16.7% an increased albumin ratio, which compares well to figures in similarly aged patients with schizophreniform psychosis (total protein increase in psychosis in 42.4%, increased AQs in 21.8%) [40] and to the previously reported proportion of neurological patients with a non-inflammatory disease of the CNS with isolated BBB dysfunction (17.5%) [45]. The serum/CSF AQ is clinically considered the "gold standard" for the assessment of BBB function [46]. Since albumin is only produced in the liver, it can reach the CSF only via the BBB. Nevertheless, it is still a matter of debate whether BBB dysfunction as measured with elevated AQs is the sequel of "leakage" at the site of small vessels and capillaries or a reduced CSF drainage in the context of disturbances of CSF flow [47,48]. For ASD, an altered CSF flow was suggested by Shen et al. [29]. In their study of the MRIs of infants who later developed autism, the authors observed an increased extra-axial CSF volume as a possible sign of reduced CSF circulation [49]. Interestingly, the protein concentration in the extra-axial CSF was also significantly elevated compared to healthy children [29]. Thus, it has been suggested that an impaired CSF circulation may lead to an altered distribution of growth factors

4.2. EEG and MRI Findings

The link between epilepsy and autism is well known, and thus an EEG is an important diagnostic procedure in patients with ASD. However, in addition to the detection of epileptiform discharges in a subgroup of patients, increased nonspecific EEG abnormalities in the form of, for example, slowing or asymmetries [50], as well as hints of long-range underconnectivity [51] in ASD patients have been described. The current study included one patient with comorbid epilepsy and epileptiform discharges, and 19% of the patients presented only focal or generalized slow activity. A previous study with a small sample size discerned a statistically significant difference between ASD patients and healthy controls in the rate of slow activity after hyperventilation [52]. One quarter of ASD patients in the current study showed nonspecific white matter alterations in their MRI. Other mental illnesses, such as depression, present similar rates [41]. It is assumed that these are caused by micro- or macroangiopathic diseases resulting from a dysfunction of the neurovascular unit, which can also lead to a BBB dysfunction [53]. Neuroinflammation can lead to defects in the neovascular unit and, reciprocally, defects in the neurovascular unit can also promote neuroinflammatory processes in the brain. However, the significance and clinical relevance of these white matter alterations remain unclear. Further studies in larger and more homogeneous subgroups of ASD patients are needed to develop a better understanding.

4.3. Antibody Findings

The presence of brain-reactive antibodies in patients with ASD has been reported in numerous studies [54]. Accordingly, Singer et al. [55] observed a greater prevalence of autoantibodies in the serum of autistic children than in their non-autistic siblings or healthy controls (in human brain slices of the caudate nucleus, putamen, prefrontal cortex, cerebellum, and cingulate gyrus). Moreover, the presence of brain-reactive antibodies in either the patient or the mother is associated with a more severe degree of autism [56] and has been reported to lead to markedly greater brain enlargement in preschool children who later develop ASD [57]. In the current study, the authors identified two patients (5.6%) who presented an intrathecal synthesis of anti-GAD65 antibodies. GAD65 is an enzyme that catalyzes the intracellular synthesis of the inhibitory neurotransmitter γ-amino butyric acid (GABA) through the decarboxylation of glutamate in brain cells and the pancreatic islet β-cells of the pancreas. Autoantibodies against GAD65 are common at the onset of type I diabetes but have also been reported in various neurological disorders, such as stiff person syndrome, cerebral ataxia, and, in some cases, in epilepsy and limbic encephalitis [58,59]. Interestingly, type I diabetes is a common co-morbidity not only of patients with ASD but also of their mothers and first-degree relatives [54,60,61]. In the healthy population, the prevalence of anti-GAD65 antibodies ranged from 0.5% to 1.1% [62,63]. Small studies in patients with ASD have described a higher incidence in ASD patients, ranging from 5% (three of 60 patients) [64] to 15% (three of 20 patients) [65]. There are, however, contradictory findings that may be related to diverse subgroups of ASD patients or to measurement techniques for anti-GAD65 antibodies [66]. It is important to note that most studies only tested antibodies in serum and did not comment on BBB integrity or the presence of antibodies in the CSF. Presumably, the antibodies are relevant for brain alteration only when they can reach the brain tissue from the serum through a "leaky" BBB due, for instance, to injury or inflammation or when they are synthesized intrathecally [67]. Although why are anti-GAD65 antibodies associated with diabetes mellitus in one patient, stiff person syndrome in another, and with autism in a third? The time at which antibodies reach specific organs as well as genetic predispositions (HLA haplotype) seem to play important roles [68], and environmental factors may be important. The pathophysiology of neuropsychiatric disease in association with anti-GAD65 antibodies is poorly understood to date. The gene expression of GAD65 appears to be reduced in ASD patients in certain brain regions, such as the cerebellar dentate nuclei [69,70], and also in the cortex of mice whose mothers during pregnancy received the anti-epileptic drug valproate, which is associated with a high risk of autism [71]. Moreover, hypermethylation of the *GAD1* promoter has been observed in the offspring of mice that received a nonspecific immune response by means of a poly (I:C) injection during pregnancy [72]. One possible pathomechanism is the direct intracellular binding of anti-GAD65 antibodies to the cytoplasmic GAD65 through unknown mechanisms leading to a change in GABAergic transmission. While a strong binding has been demonstrated in vitro [73], the application of anti-GAD65 antibodies in the CSF of mice in vivo did not lead to a change in hippocampal GABAergic transmission [74]. Thus, the pathophysiological functioning of anti-GAD65 antibodies seems to be more complex than, for example, in the case of the immunoglobulin G antibodies against the surface N-methyl D-aspartate receptor. In this context, we need to consider that GAD65 antibodies themselves may not be pathophysiologically active, but rather an immunological epiphenomenon of an unknown underlying pathomechanism [75]. Thus, the formation of anti-GAD65 antibodies could be secondary to the destruction of GABAergic neurons by, for instance, hitherto unidentified antibodies and the release of intracellular GAD into CSF [75,76]. This would also explain the clinical heterogeneity of diseases associated with anti-GAD65 antibodies and their different responsiveness to immunosuppressive therapies. In all cases, anti-GAD65 antibodies function at least as a disease marker of an unknown but most likely immune mediated process [76].

Case reports have described severe neurological diseases in association with anti-GAD65 antibodies, such as limbic encephalitis and epilepsy, that barely responded to classical immunotherapy, such as steroids or intravenous immunoglobulins (IVIGs), and required more aggressive treatment with monoclonal antibodies, such as basiliximab or rituximab [77,78]. Nevertheless, it has been reported at least in one patient with ASD with clinically relevant high anti-GAD65 antibodies and comorbid type I diabetes, that there was a relevant benefit from therapy with IVIGs [64].

4.4. Limitations

This study was performed openly and retrospectively. The decision to conduct lumbar punctures followed clinical criteria to exclude a secondary organic pathology and was not a routine procedure; therefore, the patient group is not representative of all patients with ASD. In addition, the control group's unclear IIH pathophysiology may have introduced a confounder to data in this group. In patients with IIH, larger amounts of CSF were removed due to therapy. Given that a clear reduction of the AQ between the first 4 mL and the last 4 mL of a total of 24 mL of CSF of a lumbar puncture has been described [79,80], false low values in the control group are possible. Moreover, the AQ may vary due to body weight, smoking, degenerative disc disease, hypothyroidism, or gender [80,81]. Particularly noteworthy is the gender difference between our patient and control groups. However, we did not find a gender effect in our secondary analysis of the CSF parameters but in the gender corrected ANOVA, however, only the group difference in the protein concentrations was still significant, whereas the AQ showed only a tendential increase in the ASD patients. Our findings could therefore be partly caused by a gender difference. Furthermore, the measured values for total protein and sometimes additionally AQ of one third of the ASD patients were also increased compared to established reference values. Differences on other CSF parameters like WBC and IgG due to gender have not been observed.

Psychotropic medication may also have had an influence on the total protein in the CSF and AQs. While three quarters of the ASD patients were medicated, the control group did not receive psychiatric medication. It has been indicated that, for example, antipsychotic drugs in bipolar patients may lead to an increased AQ [82]. However, other studies found no influence of antipsychotic [83–85] or antidepressant [86] medication on CSF properties. Finally, depression and other comorbidities may have confounded our results.

5. Conclusions

The present retrospective study on CSF measures provides no clear-cut positive evidence for relevant inflammatory alterations in adult ASD, however, it does suggest a trend toward a BBB dysfunction in some adult patients with ASD. The identification of anti-GAD65 antibodies in some patients with ASD may be relevant for future research in an effort to define etiological and clinical sub-phenotypes of ASD informing more personalized treatment approaches.

Author Contributions: K.R., L.T.v.E., and D.E. designed the study. K.R. and D.E. performed the data research and created the structure of the paper. H.K. and M.M. supported data search. K.R. wrote the first manuscript, and D.E. critically revised it. T.R. and R.D. helped in interpreting the CSF basic analyses. T.B. supported the neuroanatomical interpretation. S.M. supported statistical analyses. L.T.v.E., K.N., D.D., M.M., H.K., and K.D. critically revised the clinical interpretation of our findings. All authors were critically involved in the theoretical discussion and composition of the manuscript. All authors have read and approved the final version of the manuscript.

Funding: The article processing charge was funded by the German Research Foundation (DFG) and the University of Freiburg in the funding programme Open Access Publishing.

Acknowledgments: D.E. was supported by the Berta-Ottenstein-Programme for Advanced Clinician Scientists, Faculty of Medicine, University of Freiburg.

Conflicts of Interest: K.R., S.M., K.N., D.D., M.M., H.K., T.B., and D.E. declare no conflicts of interest; L.T.v.E.: Advisory boards, lectures, or travel grants within the last three years: Roche, Eli Lilly, Janssen-Cilag, Novartis, Shire, UCB, GSK, Servier, Janssen and Cyberonics; T.R.: Travel grants from Biogen and Novartis; R.D.: Lecture fees from Roche and travel grants from Biogen; K.D.: Steering Committee Neurosciences, Janssen; The funders had no role in the design of the study; in the collection, analyses, or interpretation of data; in the writing of the manuscript, or in the decision to publish the results.

Abbreviations

ADHD	Attention deficit hyperactivity disorder
AMDP	Association for Methodology and Documentation in Psychiatry (in German: Arbeitsgemeinschaft für Methodik und Dokumentation in der Psychiatrie)
ANCOVA	One-way analysis of covariance
AQ	Albumin quotient
ASD	Autism spectrum disorder
BBB	Blood–brain barrier
CGI	Clinical Global Impression
CNS	Central nervous system
CSF	Cerebrospinal fluid
EEG	Electroencephalography
F	Female
GABA	γ-amino butyric acid
GAD65	Glutamate decarboxylase 65
GAF	Global Assessment of Functioning
GWAS	Genome-wide association study
IgG	Immunoglobulin G
IIH	Idiopathic intracranial hypertension
IVIG	Intravenous immunoglobulins
M	Male
MRI	Magnetic resonance imaging
n	Number
OCB	Oligoclonal band
SD	Standard deviation
WBC	White blood count
y	Years

References

1. World Health Organization. *ICD-10 International Statistical Classification of Diseases and Related Health Problems: 10th Revision ICD-10*, 5th ed.; World Health Organization: Geneva, Switzerland, 2016.
2. Van Elst, L.T.; Pick, M.; Biscaldi, M.; Fangmeier, T.; Riedel, A. High-functioning autism spectrum disorder as a basic disorder in adult psychiatry and psychotherapy: Psychopathological presentation, clinical relevance and therapeutic concepts. *Eur. Arch. Psychiatry Clin. Neurosci.* **2013**, *263*, 189–196. [CrossRef] [PubMed]

3. American Psychiatric Association. *Diagnostic and Statistical Manual of Mental Disorders: DSM-5*, 5th ed.; American Psychiatric Publishing: Washington, DC, USA, 2013.
4. American Psychiatric Association. *Diagnostic and Statistical Manual of Mental Disorders: DSM-IV-TR*, 4th ed.; American Psychiatric Association: Arlington, VA, USA, 2009.
5. Lai, M.-C.; Lombardo, M.V.; Baron-Cohen, S. Autism. *Lancet* **2014**, *383*, 896–910. [CrossRef]
6. Baio, J.; Wiggins, L.; Christensen, D.L.; Maenner, M.J.; Daniels, J.; Warren, Z.; Kurzius-Spencer, M.; Zahorodny, W.; Robinson, C.; Rosenberg, C.R.; et al. Prevalence of Autism Spectrum Disorder Among Children Aged 8 Years—Autism and Developmental Disabilities Monitoring Network, 11 Sites, United States, 2014. *MMWR. Surveill. Summ.* **2018**, *67*, 1–23. [CrossRef] [PubMed]
7. Kim, Y.S.; Leventhal, B.L.; Koh, Y.-J.; Fombonne, E.; Laska, E.; Lim, E.-C.; Cheon, K.-A.; Kim, S.-J.; Kim, Y.-K.; Lee, H.; et al. Prevalence of Autism Spectrum Disorders in a Total Population Sample. *Am. J. Psychiatry* **2011**, *168*, 904–912. [CrossRef]
8. Vorstman, J.A.S.; Parr, J.R.; Moreno-De-Luca, D.; Anney, R.J.L.; Nurnberger, J.I., Jr.; Hallmayer, J.F. Autism genetics: Opportunities and challenges for clinical translation. *Nat. Rev. Genet.* **2017**, *18*, 362–376. [CrossRef]
9. Crino, P.B.; Nathanson, K.L.; Henske, E.P. The Tuberous Sclerosis Complex. *N. Engl. J. Med.* **2006**, *355*, 1345–1356. [CrossRef]
10. Kidd, S.A.; Lachiewicz, A.; Barbouth, D.; Blitz, R.K.; Delahunty, C.; McBrien, D.M.; Visootsak, J.; Berry-Kravis, E. Fragile X Syndrome: A Review of Associated Medical Problems. *Pediatrics* **2014**, *134*, 995–1005. [CrossRef]
11. Meltzer, A.; Van De Water, J. The Role of the Immune System in Autism Spectrum Disorder. *Neuropsychopharmacology* **2016**, *42*, 284–298. [CrossRef]
12. Grove, J.; Ripke, S.; Als, T.D.; Mattheisen, M.; Walters, R.K.; Won, H.; Pallesen, J.; Agerbo, E.; Andreassen, O.A.; Autism Spectrum Disorder Working Group of the Psychiatric Genomics Consortium; et al. Identification of common genetic risk variants for autism spectrum disorder. *Nat. Genet.* **2019**, *51*, 431–444. [CrossRef]
13. Happé, F.; Ronald, A.; Plomin, R. Time to give up on a single explanation for autism. *Nat. Neurosci.* **2006**, *9*, 1218–1220. [CrossRef]
14. Levy, S.E.; Mandell, D.S.; Schultz, R.T. Autism. *Lancet* **2009**, *374*, 1627–1638. [CrossRef]
15. Edmiston, E.; Ashwood, P.; Van De Water, J. Autoimmunity, Autoantibodies, and Autism Spectrum Disorder. *Boil. Psychiatry* **2016**, *81*, 383–390. [CrossRef] [PubMed]
16. Onore, C.; Careaga, M.; Ashwood, P. The role of immune dysfunction in the pathophysiology of autism. *Brain Behav. Immun.* **2011**, *26*, 383–392. [CrossRef] [PubMed]
17. Chess, S.; Fernandez, P.; Korn, S. Behavioral consequences of congenital rubella. *J. Pediatr.* **1978**, *93*, 699–703. [CrossRef]
18. Chess, S. Autism in children with congenital rubella. *J. Autism Dev. Disord.* **1971**, *1*, 33–47. [CrossRef] [PubMed]
19. Atladóttir, H.Ó.; Thorsen, P.; Østergaard, L.; Schendel, D.E.; Lemcke, S.; Abdallah, M.; Parner, E. Maternal Infection Requiring Hospitalization During Pregnancy and Autism Spectrum Disorders. *J. Autism Dev. Disord.* **2010**, *40*, 1423–1430. [CrossRef]
20. Atladóttir, H.Ó.; Pedersen, M.G.; Thorsen, P.; Mortensen, P.B.; Deleuran, B.; Eaton, W.W.; Parner, E.; Sutton, R.M.; Niles, D.E.; Nysaether, J.; et al. Association of Family History of Autoimmune Diseases and Autism Spectrum Disorders. *Pediatrics* **2009**, *124*, 687–694. [CrossRef]
21. Keil, A.P.; Daniels, J.L.; Forssén, U.; Hultman, C.; Cnattingius, S.; Söderberg, K.C.; Feychting, M.; Sparén, P. Parental Autoimmune Diseases Associated With Autism Spectrum Disorders in Offspring. *Epidemiology* **2010**, *21*, 805–808. [CrossRef]
22. Vinet, E.; Pineau, C.A.; Clarke, A.; Scott, S.; Fombonne, E.; Joseph, L.; Platt, R.; Bernatsky, S. Increased Risk of Autism Spectrum Disorders in Children Born to Women With Systemic Lupus Erythematosus: Results From a Large Population-Based Cohort. *Arthritis Rheumatol.* **2015**, *67*, 3201–3208. [CrossRef]
23. Braunschweig, D.; Ashwood, P.; Krakowiak, P.; Hertz-Picciotto, I.; Hansen, R.; Croen, L.A.; Pessah, I.N.; Van De Water, J. Autism: Maternally derived antibodies specific for fetal brain proteins. *NeuroToxicology* **2007**, *29*, 226–231. [CrossRef]
24. Braunschweig, D.; Krakowiak, P.; Duncanson, P.; Boyce, R.; Hansen, R.L.; Ashwood, P.; Hertz-Picciotto, I.; Pessah, I.N.; Van De Water, J. Autism-specific maternal autoantibodies recognize critical proteins in developing brain. *Transl. Psychiatry* **2013**, *3*, e277. [CrossRef]

25. Vargas, D.L.; Nascimbene, C.; Krishnan, C.; Zimmerman, A.W.; Pardo, C.A. Neuroglial activation and neuroinflammation in the brain of patients with autism. *Ann. Neurol.* **2004**, *57*, 67–81. [CrossRef]
26. Bechter, K. CSF diagnostics in psychiatry—Present status—Future projects. *Neurol. Psychiatry Brain Res.* **2016**, *22*, 69–74. [CrossRef]
27. Endres, D.; Bechter, K.; Prüss, H.; Hasan, A.; Steiner, J.; Leypoldt, F.; Van Elst, L.T. Autoantikörper-assoziierte schizophreniforme Psychosen: Klinische Symptomatik. *Der Nervenarzt* **2019**, *90*, 547–563. [CrossRef]
28. Van Elst, L.T.; Bechter, K.; Prüss, H.; Hasan, A.; Steiner, J.; Leypoldt, F.; Endres, D. [Autoantibody-associated schizophreniform psychoses: Pathophysiology, diagnostics, and treatment]. *Der Nervenarzt* **2019**, *90*, 745–761. [CrossRef]
29. Shen, M.D. Cerebrospinal fluid and the early brain development of autism. *J. Neurodev. Disord.* **2018**, *10*, 39. [CrossRef]
30. Arbeitsgemeinschaft der Wissenschaftlichen Medizinischen Fachgesellschaften (AWMF). Autismus-Spektrum-Störungen im Kindes-, Jugend- und Erwachsenenalter. 2016. Available online: https://www.awmf.org/uploads/tx_szleitlinien/028-018l_S3_Autismus-Spektrum-Stoerungen_ASS-Diagnostik_2016-05.pdf (accessed on 15 December 2019).
31. Van Elst, L.T.; Maier, S.; Fangmeier, T.; Endres, D.; Mueller, G.T.; Nickel, K.; Ebert, D.; Lange, T.; Hennig, J.; Biscaldi, M.; et al. Disturbed cingulate glutamate metabolism in adults with high-functioning autism spectrum disorder: Evidence in support of the excitatory/inhibitory imbalance hypothesis. *Mol. Psychiatry* **2014**, *19*, 1314–1325. [CrossRef]
32. Endres, D.; Van Elst, L.T.; Meyer, S.A.; Feige, B.; Nickel, K.; Bubl, A.; Riedel, A.; Ebert, D.; Lange, T.; Glauche, V.; et al. Glutathione metabolism in the prefrontal brain of adults with high-functioning autism spectrum disorder: An MRS study. *Mol. Autism* **2017**, *8*, 10. [CrossRef]
33. Patterson, P.H. Maternal infection and immune involvement in autism. *Trends Mol. Med.* **2011**, *17*, 389–394. [CrossRef]
34. van Tebartz Elst, L.; Perlov, E. *Epilepsie und Psyche: Psychische Störungen bei Epilepsie—Epileptische Phänomene in der Psychiatrie*, 1st ed.; Kohlhammer: Stuttgart, Germany, 2013.
35. Kuzior, H.; Fiebich, B.; Yousif, N.M.; Saliba, S.W.; Ziegler, C.; Nickel, K.; Maier, S.; Süß, P.; Runge, K.; Matysik, M.; et al. Increased IL-8 Concentrations in the Cerebrospinal Fluid of Patients with Unipolar Depression. **2020**, under review.
36. Balla, A.; Endres, D.; Fiebich, B.; Stich, O.; Dersch, R.; van Tebartz Elst, L. The role of intrathecal-specific antibody synthesis against neurotropic infectious agents in patients with schizophreniform disorders. Poster-Session P-02. Poster 009. In Proceedings of the WPA XVII World Congress of Psychiatry Berlin 2017, Berlin, Germany, 8–12 October 2017.
37. Kuzior, H.; Fiebich, B.; Saliba, S.W.; Yousif, N.; Gargouri, B.; Blank, T.; Ziegler, C.; van Tebartz Elst, L.; Endres, D. Erhöhte Interleukin-8 Levels im Liquor von Patienten mit unipolaren Depressionen. In Proceedings of the Poster 012, DGPPN Congress Berlin 2018, Berlin, Germany, 28 November–1 December 2018.
38. Rush, A.J. *Handbook of Psychiatric Measures*, 1st ed.; American Psychiatric Association: Washington, DC, USA, 2000.
39. *Das AMDP-System: Manual zur Dokumentation Psychiatrischer Befunde*, 10th ed.; Hogrefe: Göttingen, Germany, 2018.
40. Endres, D.; Perlov, E.; Baumgartner, A.; Hottenrott, T.; Dersch, R.; Stich, O.; Van Elst, L.T. Immunological findings in psychotic syndromes: A tertiary care hospital's CSF sample of 180 patients. *Front. Hum. Neurosci.* **2015**, *9*, 897. [CrossRef]
41. Endres, D.; Perlov, E.; Dersch, R.; Baumgärtner, A.; Hottenrott, T.; Berger, B.; Stich, O.; Van Elst, L.T. Evidence of cerebrospinal fluid abnormalities in patients with depressive syndromes. *J. Affect. Disord.* **2016**, *198*, 178–184. [CrossRef]
42. Endres, D.; Dersch, R.; Hottenrott, T.; Perlov, E.; Maier, S.; Van Calker, D.; Hochstuhl, B.; Venhoff, N.; Stich, O.; Van Elst, L.T. Alterations in Cerebrospinal Fluid in Patients with Bipolar Syndromes. *Front. Psychol.* **2016**, *7*, 1689. [CrossRef]
43. Benjamini, Y.; Hochberg, Y. Controlling the False Discovery Rate: A Practical and Powerful Approach to Multiple Testing. *J. R. Stat. Soc. Ser. B* **1995**, *57*, 289–300. [CrossRef]

44. Hufschmidt, A.; Lücking, C.H.; Rauer, S.; Glocker, F.X. (Eds.) *Neurologie Compact: Für Klinik und Praxis*, 7th ed.; Georg Thieme Verlag: Stuttgart, Germany; New York, NY, USA, 2017.
45. Brettschneider, J.; Claus, A.; Kassubek, J.; Tumani, H. Isolated blood–cerebrospinal fluid barrier dysfunction: Prevalence and associated diseases. *J. Neurol.* 2005, *252*, 1067–1073. [CrossRef]
46. Reiber, H.; Peter, J.B. Cerebrospinal fluid analysis: Disease-related data patterns and evaluation programs. *J. Neurol. Sci.* 2001, *184*, 101–122. [CrossRef]
47. Asgari, M.; De Zélicourt, D.; Kurtcuoglu, V. Barrier dysfunction or drainage reduction: Differentiating causes of CSF protein increase. *Fluids Barriers CNS* 2017, *14*, 14. [CrossRef]
48. Reiber, H. Flow rate of cerebrospinal fluid (CSF)—A concept common to normal blood-CSF barrier function and to dysfunction in neurological diseases. *J. Neurol. Sci.* 1994, *122*, 189–203. [CrossRef]
49. Shen, M.D.; Kim, S.H.; McKinstry, R.C.; Gu, H.; Hazlett, H.C.; Nordahl, C.W.; Emerson, R.W.; Shaw, D.; Elison, J.T.; Swanson, M.R.; et al. Increased Extra-axial Cerebrospinal Fluid in High-Risk Infants Who Later Develop Autism. *Boil. Psychiatry* 2017, *82*, 186–193. [CrossRef]
50. Keller, R.; Basta, R.; Salerno, L.; Elia, M. Autism, epilepsy, and synaptopathies: A not rare association. *Neurol. Sci.* 2017, *38*, 1353–1361. [CrossRef]
51. O'Reilly, C.; Lewis, J.D.; Elsabbagh, M. Is functional brain connectivity atypical in autism? A systematic review of EEG and MEG studies. *PLoS ONE* 2017, *12*, e0175870. [CrossRef]
52. Endres, D.; Maier, S.; Feige, B.; Posielski, N.A.; Nickel, K.; Ebert, D.; Riedel, A.; Philipsen, A.; Perlov, E.; Van Elst, L.T. Altered Intermittent Rhythmic Delta and Theta Activity in the Electroencephalographies of High Functioning Adult Patients with Autism Spectrum Disorder. *Front. Hum. Neurosci.* 2017, *11*, 27. [CrossRef]
53. Najjar, S.; Pearlman, D.; Devinsky, O.; Najjar, A.; Zagzag, D. Neurovascular unit dysfunction with blood-brain barrier hyperpermeability contributes to major depressive disorder: A review of clinical and experimental evidence. *J. Neuroinflamm.* 2013, *10*, 142. [CrossRef]
54. Hughes, H.K.; Ko, E.M.; Rose, D.; Ashwood, P. Immune Dysfunction and Autoimmunity as Pathological Mechanisms in Autism Spectrum Disorders. *Front. Cell. Neurosci.* 2018, *12*, 405. [CrossRef]
55. Singer, H.S.; Morris, C.M.; Williams, P.N.; Yoon, D.Y.; Hong, J.J.; Zimmerman, A.W. Antibrain antibodies in children with autism and their unaffected siblings. *J. Neuroimmunol.* 2006, *178*, 149–155. [CrossRef]
56. Piras, I.S.; Haapanen, L.; Napolioni, V.; Sacco, R.; Van De Water, J.; Persico, A.M. Anti-brain antibodies are associated with more severe cognitive and behavioral profiles in Italian children with Autism Spectrum Disorder. *Brain Behav. Immun.* 2014, *38*, 91–99. [CrossRef]
57. Nordahl, C.W.; Braunschweig, D.; Iosif, A.-M.; Lee, A.; Rogers, S.; Ashwood, P.; Amaral, D.G.; Van De Water, J. Maternal autoantibodies are associated with abnormal brain enlargement in a subgroup of children with autism spectrum disorder. *Brain Behav. Immun.* 2013, *30*, 61–65. [CrossRef]
58. Kaufman, D.L.; Erlander, M.G.; Clare-Salzler, M.; Atkinson, M.A.; MacLaren, N.K.; Tobin, A.J. Autoimmunity to two forms of glutamate decarboxylase in insulin-dependent diabetes mellitus. *J. Clin. Investig.* 1992, *89*, 283–292. [CrossRef]
59. Lancaster, E.; Dalmau, J. Neuronal autoantigens–pathogenesis, associated disorders and antibody testing. *Nat. Rev. Neurol.* 2012, *8*, 380–390. [CrossRef]
60. Chen, M.-H.; Su, T.-P.; Chen, Y.-S.; Hsu, J.-W.; Huang, K.-L.; Chang, W.-H.; Chen, T.-J.; Bai, Y.-M. Comorbidity of allergic and autoimmune diseases in patients with autism spectrum disorder: A nationwide population-based study. *Res. Autism Spectr. Disord.* 2013, *7*, 205–212. [CrossRef]
61. Comi, A.M.; Zimmerman, A.W.; Frye, V.H.; Law, P.A.; Peeden, J.N. Familial clustering of autoimmune disorders and evaluation of medical risk factors in autism. *J. Child Neurol.* 1999, *14*, 388–394. [CrossRef]
62. Dahm, L.; Ott, C.; Steiner, J.; Stepniak, B.; Teegen, B.; Saschenbrecker, S.; Hammer, C.; Borowski, K.; Begemann, M.; Lemke, S.; et al. Seroprevalence of autoantibodies against brain antigens in health and disease. *Ann. Neurol.* 2014, *76*, 82–94. [CrossRef]
63. Rolandsson, O.; Hägg, E.; Hampe, C.; Sullivan, E.P., Jr.; Nilsson, M.; Jansson, G.; Hallmans, G.; Lernmark, Å. Glutamate decarboxylase (GAD65) and tyrosine phosphatase-like protein (IA-2) autoantibodies index in a regional population is related to glucose intolerance and body mass index. *Diabetologia* 1999, *42*, 555–559. [CrossRef]
64. Connery, K.; Tippett, M.; Delhey, L.M.; Rose, S.; Slattery, J.C.; Kahler, S.G.; Hahn, J.; Kruger, U.; Cunningham, M.W.; Shimasaki, C.; et al. Intravenous immunoglobulin for the treatment of autoimmune encephalopathy in children with autism. *Transl. Psychiatry* 2018, *8*, 148. [CrossRef]

65. Rout, U.K.; Mungan, N.K.; Dhossche, D.M. Presence of GAD65 autoantibodies in the serum of children with autism or ADHD. *Eur. Child Adolesc. Psychiatry* **2012**, *21*, 141–147. [CrossRef]
66. Kalra, S.; Burbelo, P.D.; Bayat, A.; Ching, K.H.; Thurm, A.; Iadarola, M.J.; Swedo, S.E. No evidence of antibodies against GAD65 and other specific antigens in children with autism. *BBA Clin.* **2015**, *4*, 81–84. [CrossRef]
67. Ehrenreich, H. Autoantibodies against N-methyl-d-aspartate receptor 1 in health and disease. *Curr. Opin. Neurol.* **2018**, *31*, 306–312. [CrossRef]
68. Belbezier, A.; Joubert, B.; Montero-Martin, G.; Fernandez-Vina, M.; Fabien, N.; Rogemond, V.; Mignot, E.; Honnorat, J. Multiplex family with GAD65-Abs neurologic syndromes. *Neurol. Neuroimmunol. Neuroinflamm.* **2017**, *5*, e416. [CrossRef]
69. Yip, J.; Soghomonian, J.-J.; Blatt, G.J. Decreased GAD65 mRNA levels in select subpopulations of neurons in the cerebellar dentate nuclei in autism: An in situ hybridization study. *Autism Res.* **2009**, *2*, 50–59. [CrossRef]
70. Blatt, G.J.; Fatemi, S. Alterations in GABAergic Biomarkers in the Autism Brain: Research Findings and Clinical Implications. *Anat. Rec. Adv. Integr. Anat. Evol. Boil.* **2011**, *294*, 1646–1652. [CrossRef]
71. Chau, D.K.-F.; Choi, A.Y.-T.; Yang, W.; Leung, W.N.; Chan, C.W. Downregulation of glutamatergic and GABAergic proteins in valproric acid associated social impairment during adolescence in mice. *Behav. Brain Res.* **2017**, *316*, 255–260. [CrossRef]
72. Labouesse, M.A.; Dong, E.; Grayson, D.R.; Guidotti, A.; Meyer, U. Maternal immune activation induces GAD1 and GAD2 promoter remodeling in the offspring prefrontal cortex. *Epigenetics* **2015**, *10*, 1143–1155. [CrossRef]
73. Dalakas, M.C.; Li, M.; Fujii, M.; Jacobowitz, D.M. Stiff person syndrome: Quantification, specificity, and intrathecal synthesis of GAD65 antibodies. *Neurology* **2001**, *57*, 780–784. [CrossRef]
74. Hackert, J.K.; Müller, L.; Rohde, M.; Bien, C.G.; Bien, C.G.; Kirschstein, T. Anti-GAD65 Containing Cerebrospinal Fluid Does not Alter GABAergic Transmission. *Front. Cell. Neurosci.* **2016**, *10*, 923. [CrossRef]
75. Dalakas, M.C. Advances in the pathogenesis and treatment of patients with stiff person syndrome. *Curr. Neurol. Neurosci. Rep.* **2008**, *8*, 48–55. [CrossRef]
76. Stagg, C.J.; Lang, B.; Best, J.G.; McKnight, K.; Cavey, A.; Johansen-Berg, H.; Vincent, A.; Palace, J. Autoantibodies to glutamic acid decarboxylase in patients with epilepsy are associated with low cortical GABA levels. *Epilepsia* **2010**, *51*, 1898–1901. [CrossRef]
77. Widman, G.; Golombeck, K.; Hautzel, H.; Gross, C.C.; Quesada, C.M.; Witt, J.-A.; Rota-Kops, E.; Ermert, J.; Greschus, S.; Surges, R.; et al. Treating a GAD65 Antibody-Associated Limbic Encephalitis with Basiliximab: A Case Study. *Front. Neurol.* **2015**, *6*, 167. [CrossRef]
78. Daif, A.; Lukas, R.V.; Issa, N.P.; Javed, A.; VanHaerents, S.; Reder, A.T.; Tao, J.X.; Warnke, P.; Rose, S.; Towle, V.L.; et al. Antiglutamic acid decarboxylase 65 (GAD65) antibody-associated epilepsy. *Epilepsy Behav.* **2018**, *80*, 331–336. [CrossRef]
79. Blennow, K.; Fredman, P.; Wallin, A.; Gottfries, C.-G.; Långström, G.; Svennerholm, L. Protein Analyses in Cerebrospinal Fluid. *Eur. Neurol.* **1993**, *33*, 126–128. [CrossRef]
80. Brainin, M.; Barnes, M.P.; Gilhus, N.E. (Eds.) *European Handbook of Neurological Management: Volume 1*, 2nd ed.; Wiley-Blackwell: Chichester, West Sussex, UK, 2010.
81. Castellazzi, M.; Morotti, A.; Tamborino, C.; Alessi, F.; Pilotto, S.; Baldi, E.; Caniatti, L.M.; Trentini, A.; Casetta, I.; Granieri, E.; et al. Increased age and male sex are independently associated with higher frequency of blood–cerebrospinal fluid barrier dysfunction using the albumin quotient. *Fluids Barriers CNS* **2020**, *17*, 1–9. [CrossRef]
82. Zetterberg, H.; Jakobsson, J.; Redsäter, M.; Andreasson, U.; Pålsson, E.; Ekman, C.J.; Sellgren, C.M.; Johansson, A.G.; Blennow, K.; Landen, M. Blood–cerebrospinal fluid barrier dysfunction in patients with bipolar disorder in relation to antipsychotic treatment. *Psychiatry Res.* **2014**, *217*, 143–146. [CrossRef]
83. Kirch, D.G.; Kaufmann, C.A.; Papadopoulos, N.M.; Martin, B.; Weinberger, D.R. Abnormal cerebrospinal fluid protein indices in schizophrenia. *Boil. Psychiatry* **1985**, *20*, 1039–1046. [CrossRef]
84. Axelsson, R.; Martensson, E.; Alling, C. Impairment of the Blood-Brain Barrier as an Aetiological Factor in Paranoid Psychosis. *Br. J. Psychiatry* **1982**, *141*, 273–281. [CrossRef]

85. Bauer, K.; Kornhuber, J. Blood-cerebrospinal fluid barrier in schizophrenic patients. *Eur. Arch. Psychiatry Clin. Neurosci.* **1987**, *236*, 257–259. [CrossRef]
86. Pitts, A.F.; Carroll, B.T.; Gehris, T.L.; Kathol, R.G.; Samuelson, S.D. Elevated CSF protein in male patients with depression. *Boil. Psychiatry* **1990**, *28*, 629–637. [CrossRef]

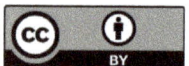

© 2020 by the authors. Licensee MDPI, Basel, Switzerland. This article is an open access article distributed under the terms and conditions of the Creative Commons Attribution (CC BY) license (http://creativecommons.org/licenses/by/4.0/).

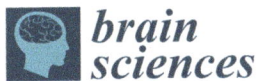 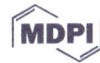

Article

Psychosocial and Behavioral Impact of COVID-19 in Autism Spectrum Disorder: An Online Parent Survey

Marco Colizzi [1,2,3,*], Elena Sironi [3], Federico Antonini [3], Marco Luigi Ciceri [3], Chiara Bovo [4] and Leonardo Zoccante [3]

1. Section of Psychiatry, Department of Neurosciences, Biomedicine and Movement Sciences, University of Verona, 37134 Verona, Italy
2. Department of Psychosis Studies, Institute of Psychiatry, Psychology and Neuroscience, King's College London, London SE5 8AF, UK
3. Child and Adolescent Neuropsychiatry Unit, Maternal-Child Integrated Care Department, Integrated University Hospital of Verona, 37126 Verona, Italy; sironi.elena@yahoo.it (E.S.); fede187ant@gmail.com (F.A.); marcoluigi.ciceri@aovr.veneto.it (M.L.C.); leonardo.zoccante@aovr.veneto.it (L.Z.)
4. Medical Direction, Integrated University Hospital of Verona, 37126 Verona, Italy; direzione.sanitaria@aovr.veneto.it
* Correspondence: marco.colizzi@univr.it; Tel.: +39-045-812-6832

Received: 17 May 2020; Accepted: 1 June 2020; Published: 3 June 2020

Abstract: The 2019 coronavirus disease (COVID-19) outbreak could result in higher levels of psychological distress, especially among people suffering from pre-existing mental health conditions. Young individuals with autism spectrum disorders (ASD) are particularly at risk due to their vulnerability to unpredictable and complex changes. This study aimed to investigate the impact of the COVID-19 pandemic on ASD individuals, whether any pre-pandemic sociodemographic or clinical characteristics would predict a negative outcome, and to narratively characterize their needs. Parents and guardians of ASD individuals filled out an online survey consisting of 40 questions investigating socio-demographic and clinical characteristics of their children, impact of the COVID-19 outbreak on their wellbeing and needs to deal with the emergency. Data were available on 527 survey participants. The COVID-19 emergency resulted in a challenging period for 93.9% of families, increased difficulties in managing daily activities, especially free time (78.1%) and structured activities (75.7%), and, respectively, 35.5% and 41.5% of children presenting with more intense and more frequent behavior problems. Behavior problems predating the COVID-19 outbreak predicted a higher risk of more intense (odds ratio (OR) = 2.16, 95% confidence interval (CI) 1.42–3.29) and more frequent (OR = 1.67, 95% CI 1.13–2.48) disruptive behavior. Even though ASD children were receiving different types of support, also requiring specialist (19.1%) or emergency (1.5%) interventions in a relatively low proportion of cases, a number of needs emerged, including receiving more healthcare support (47.4%), especially in-home support (29.9%), as well as interventions to tackle a potentially disruptive quarantine (16.8%). The COVID-19 outbreak has undoubtedly resulted in increased difficulties among ASD individuals.

Keywords: coronavirus; 2019-nCoV; neurodevelopment; child and adolescent psychiatry; mental health prevention

---

1. Introduction

After the Severe Acute Respiratory Syndrome (SARS) Coronavirus outbreak of 2002–2003, the International Health Regulations (IHR) of the World Health Organization (WHO), which had been first adopted in 1969, were revised in 2005 to extend their scope to any public health risk that might affect human health, irrespective of the source. Emphasis was put on the risk that the increasing international travel and trade could facilitate the international spread of disease, requiring a coordinated international response. Since the 2005 IHR adoption, the WHO has formally declared six Public Health Emergencies of International Concern (PHEIC), the latter of which, the 2019 coronavirus disease (COVID-19), is still ongoing [1]. COVID-19 is caused by a newly identified coronavirus which can induce SARS in man (SARS-CoV-2), as a consequence of a probable zoonotic spillover [2], firstly reported in Central China in December 2019 [3]. Due to person-to-person transmission, it has rapidly spread in Europe [4], with northern Italy becoming Europe's epicenter [5], and USA [6]. As of 1 May 2020, over 3 million cases have been reported worldwide, affecting more than 200 countries.

Since the beginning of the pandemic, most clinical and research efforts have been allocated to advance our understanding of the virus properties and pathogenic armory in order to treat the infection and protect from it [7]. However, according to some research evidence, the COVID-19 pandemic is also unraveling a potential gap in mental health services during emergencies [8]. In particular, the COVID-19 outbreak would result in higher levels of psychological distress among the general population [8] as well as a higher risk or symptom exacerbation among people suffering from a pre-existing mental health condition [9], possibly triggered by concerns about its rapid escalation and global spread [1] as a deadly threat [10]. Furthermore, alarming media reports may unintendedly amplify fear reactions [11], with potential detrimental consequences for people susceptible to negative emotional states. Importantly, the pandemic has required unprecedented measures by national governments including imposing quarantine to citizens [12]. The experience of being quarantined may be negative, as evidence suggests a wide range of long-lasting mental health problems in a substantial proportion of individuals [13]. While there is no strong evidence that any particular demographic factors carry a higher risk of poor psychological outcome following the obligation of home quarantine [13], a pre-existing psychiatric history seems to predict a worse outcome [14] and a higher need for support during quarantine [13].

Among vulnerable populations, young individuals with autism spectrum disorders (ASD) are of particular concern for the impact that the COVID-19 outbreak may have on their wellbeing as well as the specific support they may need to preserve their mental health through the pandemic [15]. ASD are a group of conditions characterized by social communication problems, difficulties with reciprocal social interactions, and unusual patterns of repetitive behavior [16]. Such features are associated with a preference for highly predictable environments, whereas ASD individuals may feel stressed, anxious or confused if unpredictable or complex changes occur [17]. The COVID-19 outbreak has undoubtedly led to a quick-paced and rapidly shifting social situation which may increase ASD individuals' difficulties.

The purpose of this study was threefold. The main aim was to rapidly investigate the impact of the COVID-19 outbreak on ASD individuals through an online parent survey carried in Northern Italy, one of the European regions mostly affected [5]. Due to the ASD individuals' difficulty to deal with the unexpected, a mainly unfavorable psychosocial and behavioral outcome was hypothesized. A further aim was to investigate whether any pre-pandemic sociodemographic or clinical characteristics would predict a negative impact of the pandemic on ASD individuals' wellbeing. Based on previous evidence [13,14], psychological problems predating the emergency were hypothesized to predict a poor outcome. Finally, the survey served to characterize the needs of ASD individuals and their families from a narrative perspective, by collecting the parents' perceptions, as a first step to improving their quality of health care.

2. Materials and Methods

2.1. Research Design

Google Forms was used to create an online parent survey to be shared through the dissemination of a hyperlink. The survey was available online from the 6 April to the 20 April 2020. All participants provided electronic informed consent that contained information about the purpose of the study, procedures, benefits of participating, voluntary participation, and contact information of the researchers.

The survey was part of a larger study which was approved by the research ethics committee at the Integrated University Hospital of Verona (CESC 2242 and CESC 2243).

2.2. Participants

Parents and guardians of individuals with an ASD diagnosis were asked by healthcare professionals affiliated with the Veneto Autism Spectrum Disorder Regional Centre at the Integrated University Hospital of Verona to fill out the online survey. Autism advocacy and family support networks were additionally used to distribute and directly encourage survey participation. Children' ASD diagnosis was self-reported.

2.3. Instrument

The parent survey was developed by a focus group of physicians, psychologists, and child life specialists, also taking the advice from parents of children with ASD. The survey consisted of 40 questions (18 multiple choice questions, 20 yes/no questions, and 2 open-response questions) in 3 categories: (i) ASD individuals' socio-demographic and clinical characteristics, (ii) impact of the COVID-19 outbreak on their wellbeing, and (iii) needs to deal with the emergency. Participants were allowed to select only 1 item for each multiple-choice question.

2.4. Analyses

The final raw data were downloaded from Google Forms into a Microsoft Excel file for analysis using SPSS software (Version 26.0; IBM Corp, Armonk, NY, USA). Descriptive statistics were used to provide baseline information concerning survey participants' ASD children. Then, multiple logistic regressions were performed to investigate whether any ASD individuals' socio-demographic or clinical characteristics would predict a greater frequency and intensity of behavior problems following the COVID-19 outbreak.

The open-response questions did not have a scoring system. The needs identified by the survey responses were gathered with the intent of informing healthcare professionals in their assessment and management of individuals with an ASD diagnosis during the ongoing COVID-19 emergency. Two authors independently evaluated such answers and pooled them into categories (e.g., healthcare, social, financial needs, etc.). In the rare instances of discrepant category attribution, consensus was reached through discussion with a third senior clinical researcher.

The survey was not intended to formally assess severity of ASD among participants' children.

3. Results

A total of 529 respondents participated in the survey. As 2 participants did not answer any questions at all, a total of 527 participants were included in the study. Across the 38 closed questions, survey participants provided 18,738 answers, while 373 answers were missing (<2%). Further, 34 answers and 1 missing item were deemed inconsistent (<0.2%) and excluded from the final analyses.

3.1. Socio-Demographic and Clinical Characteristics

The mean age of participants' children was 13 years (SD = 8.1). Almost all of them were from the Veneto region (99.4%) and the large majority were living in married or cohabiting couple families (88.2%). Most children had at least 1 sibling (71.6%), and one out every 10 siblings had a neurodevelopmental disorder (NDD) diagnosis (10.2%). Most children were receiving private therapy (66.2%) and most parents were members of autism advocacy and family support networks (67.1%) (Table 1).

Table 1. Socio-demographic and clinical characteristics.

	M	(SD)
Age (years)	13	8.1
	N	(%)
Veneto Region Province		
Belluno	41	7.8
Padova	88	16.8
Rovigo	26	5
Treviso	40	7.6
Venezia	73	13.9
Verona	149	28.4
Vicenza	105	20
Other Region	3	0.6
Missing	2	
Parenting couple situation		
Married/Cohabiting	463	88.2
Separated	31	5.9
Single parent	31	5.9
Missing	2	
Only child		
No	374	71.6
Yes	148	28.4
Missing	2	
Number of siblings *		
1	290	77.5
2	65	17.4
3	15	4
4	3	0.8
5	1	0,3
Missing	0	
Siblings diagnosed with NDD (ASD, ADHD, etc.) *		
No	336	89.8
Yes	38	10.2
Missing	0	
Child receiving private therapy		
No	175	33.8
Yes	342	66.2
Missing	4	
Membership in Autism advocacy/family support networks		
No	172	32.9
Yes	351	67.1
Missing	4	

Table 1. Cont.

	M	(SD)
Child's language level		
Fluent speech	174	33.1
Phrase speech	146	27.8
No phrase speech	205	39
Missing	2	
The child was presenting with behavior problems from before COVID-19		
No	251	48.5
Yes	266	51.5
Missing	6	
Pharmacological treatment for behavior problems **		
No	152	57.8
Yes	111	42.2
Missing	3	
Comorbid medical conditions		
No	377	72.2
Yes	145	27.8
Missing	5	

* Of those reporting siblings; ** Of those reporting behavior problems from before COVID-19; NDD, Neurodevelopment disorder; ASD, Autism spectrum disorder; ADHD, Attention Deficit Hyperactivity Disorder.

Only one every three children had a fluent language (33.1%). About half of the entire sample was presenting with behavior problems from before the outbreak of COVID-19 (51.5%); among those, 42.2% were receiving pharmacological treatment. At least 1 comorbid medical condition was reported in 27.8% of ASD individuals, with neuromotor and gastrointestinal conditions and allergies and food sensitivity being the conditions most frequently reported (Table 1 and Supplementary Table S1).

3.2. Psychosocial and Behavioral Impact of the Emergency Outbreak

COVID-19 positivity was reported among 1.3% of nuclear family members and 4.4% of extended family members, with bereavement occurring in 2.3% of cases. Approximately one out of four parents stopped working due the emergency outbreak (26.1% of mothers and 27.5% of fathers). The large majority of them evaluated the current period of change and restrictions as challenging or very challenging (93.9%) and more challenging than before the emergency outbreak (77%) (Table 2).

Following the emergency outbreak, a proportion of parents reported support from the Local Healthcare Services (27.7%), with the large majority of them reporting both direct (70.1%; e.g., calls, videocalls) and indirect (84%; e.g., text messages, homework assignments) school support as well as support from the private therapist (73.3%). For each type of support, an only slightly lower proportion of parents considered it from sufficiently useful to very useful during the ongoing emergency (Table 2).

A proportion of parents reported difficulties in managing their child's meals (23%), autonomies (31%), free time (78.1%), and structured activities (75.7%). For each activity, an almost overlapping proportion of parents reported such activity as more difficult than before the emergency outbreak. Overall, compared to before the emergency outbreak, behavior problems were reported being more intense (35.5%) and more frequent (41.5%) in a substantial proportion of ASD individuals. Due to the onset of behavior problems, an emergency contact with the child's Neuropsychiatrist was required in 19.1% of cases, while an access to the Accident and Emergency (A&E) happened in 1.5% of cases (Table 2).

Table 2. Psychosocial and behavioral impact of the emergency outbreak.

	N	(%)
COVID-19 positivity among nuclear family members		
No	519	98.7
Yes	7	1.3
Missing	1	
COVID-19 positivity among extended family members		
No	500	95.6
Yes	23	4.4
Missing	4	
Bereavement due to COVID-19		
No	514	97.7
Yes	12	2.3
Missing	1	
Mother's current working situation		
Regularly commuting to work	92	17.6
Smart working	98	18.7
Not working because of COVID-19	137	26.1
Not working since before COVID-19	197	37.6
Missing	3	
Father's current working situation		
Regularly commuting to work	212	42
Smart working	104	20.6
Not working because of COVID-19	139	27.5
Not working since before COVID-19	50	9.9
Missing	22	
Judgement on this period of change and restrictions		
Very challenging	284	54
Challenging	210	39.9
Not challenging	32	6.1
Missing	1	
Judgement on this period of change and restrictions as compared to before COVID-19		
More challenging	405	77
Equally challenging	86	16.3
Less challenging	35	6.7
Missing	1	
Support by Local Healthcare Services since COVID-19		
Daily contacts	7	1.4
Weekly contacts	98	19.4
Twice weekly contacts	35	6.9
No contact	366	72.3

Table 2. *Cont.*

	N	(%)
Missing	21	
Usefulness of support by Local Healthcare Services during COVID-19		
Very useful	10	2.2
Useful	28	6.1
Sufficiently useful	65	14.1
Not very useful	93	20.1
Not useful	266	57.6
Missing	65	
Direct school support since COVID-19		
Daily contacts	110	22.5
Weekly contacts	157	32.2
Twice weekly contacts	75	15.4
No contact	146	29.9
Missing	39	
Indirect school support since COVID-19		
Daily contacts	138	28.7
Weekly contacts	159	33.1
Twice weekly contacts	106	22.1
No contact	77	16
Missing	47	
Usefulness of school support during COVID-19		
Very useful	60	12.9
Useful	113	24.4
Sufficiently useful	116	25
Not very useful	93	20
Not useful	82	17.7
Missing	63	
Private therapist support since COVID-19		
Daily contacts	43	12.6
Weekly contacts	148	43.4
Twice weekly contacts	59	17.3
No contact	91	26.7
Missing	1	
Usefulness of private therapist during COVID-19		
Very useful	65	19.6
Useful	80	24.1
Sufficiently useful	64	19.3
Not very useful	50	15.1
Not useful	73	22

Table 2. Cont.

	N	(%)
Missing	10	
Difficulties in managing the child's meals since COVID-19		
No	404	77
Yes	121	23
Missing	2	
Greater difficulties in managing the child's meals as compared to before COVID-19		
No	378	71.9
Yes	148	28.1
Missing	1	
Difficulties in managing the child's autonomies since COVID-19		
No	361	69
Yes	162	31
Missing	4	
Greater difficulties in managing the child's autonomies as compared to before COVID-19		
No	372	71
Yes	152	29
Missing	3	
Difficulties in managing the child's free time since COVID-19		
No	115	21.9
Yes	411	78.1
Missing	1	
Greater difficulties in managing the child's free time as compared to before COVID-19		
No	97	18.4
Yes	429	81.6
Missing	1	
Difficulties in managing the child's structured activities since COVID-19		
No	126	24.3
Yes	393	75.7
Missing	8	
Greater difficulties in managing the child's structured activities as compared to before COVID-19		
No	123	23.8
Yes	394	76.2
Missing	10	
Intensity of the child's behavior problems as compared to before COVID-19		
More intense	183	35.5
Equally intense	264	51.3

Table 2. Cont.

	N	(%)
Less intense	68	13.2
Missing	12	
Frequency of the child's behavior problems as compared to before COVID-19		
More frequent	216	41.5
Equally frequent	229	44
Less frequent	76	14.6
Missing	6	
Contacts with the child's Neuropsychiatrist due to behavioral problems since COVID-19		
No	424	80.9
Yes	100	19.1
Missing	3	
Access to A&E for child's behavioral problems since COVID-19		
No	514	98.5
Yes	8	1.5
Missing	5	

3.3. Predictors of Emergency Outbreak Negative Impact on Wellbeing

A multiple logistic regression tested for an effect of (i) behavior problems predating the emergency (yes/no), (ii) age, (iii) language (fluent/non-fluent), (iv) being an only child (yes/no) as a proxy of greater social isolation in quarantine, (v) medical comorbidity (yes/no), (vi) parenting couple situation (married or cohabiting/separated or single parent), (vii) support by Local Healthcare Services since COVID-19 (yes/no), (viii) direct school support since COVID-19 (yes/no), (ix) indirect school support since COVID-19 (yes/no), (x) private therapist support since COVID-19 (yes/no or no private therapist from before COVID-19) on the intensity of the behavior problems following the emergency outbreak (more intense/equally or less intense). The logistic regression model was statistically significant, χ^2 (10, N = 440) = 32.338, $p < 0.001$. ASD individuals with preexisting behavior problems were 2.16 times more likely to exhibit more intense behavior problems that those without preexisting behavior problems. Increasing age and living with a separated or single parent were associated with a reduction in the likelihood of exhibiting more intense behavior problems, while not receiving indirect school support during the emergency tended to be associated with an increased likelihood of exhibiting more intense behavior problems (Table 3).

A further multiple logistic regression tested for the effect of (i) behavior problems predating the emergency (yes/no), (ii) age, (iii) language (fluent/non-fluent), (iv) being an only child (yes/no), (v) medical comorbidity (yes/no), (vi) parenting couple situation (married or cohabiting/separated or single parent), (vii) support by Local Healthcare Services since COVID-19 (yes/no), (viii) direct school support since COVID-19 (yes/no), (ix) indirect school support since COVID-19 (yes/no), (x) private therapist support since COVID-19 (yes/no or no private therapist from before COVID-19) on the frequency of the behavior problems following the emergency outbreak (more frequent/equally or less frequent). The logistic regression model was statistically significant, χ^2 (10, N = 444) = 18.502, $p = 0.047$. ASD individuals with preexisting behavior problems were 1.67 times more likely to exhibit more frequent behavior problems that those without preexisting behavior problems (Table 4).

Table 3. Predictors of emergency outbreak negative impact on intensity of behavior problems.

	B	S.E.	Wald Chi-Square	p-Value	OR	95% CI
Age	−0.037	0.019	3.981	0.046	0.963	0.929–0.999
Behavior problems predating COVID-19	0.770	0.215	12.869	<0.001	2.160	1.418–3.291
Non-fluent language	0.352	0.243	2.100	0.147	1.422	0.883–2.290
Medical comorbidity	0.317	0.241	1.726	0.189	1.372	0.856–2.201
Only child	0.286	0.233	1.507	0.220	1.331	0.843–2.102
Separated/single parent	−0.778	0.383	4.127	0.042	0.459	0.217–0.973
No support from Local Health Service	0.050	0.241	0.043	0.836	1.051	0.656–1.685
No direct support from school	−0.127	0.255	0.247	0.619	0.881	0.534–1.453
No indirect support from school	0.605	0.322	3.540	0.060	1.831	0.975–3.439
No support from private therapist	−0.073	0.214	0.118	0.732	0.929	0.610–1.414

Note: OR, odds ratio; CI, confidence interval.

Table 4. Predictors of emergency outbreak negative impact on frequency of behavior problems.

	B	S.E.	Wald Chi-Square	p-Value	OR	95% CI
Age	−0.024	0.018	1.841	0.175	0.976	0.943–1.011
Behavior problems predating COVID-19	0.513	0.201	6.509	0.011	1.670	1.126–2.477
Non-fluent language	0.304	0.226	1.800	0.180	1.355	0.869–2.111
Medical comorbidity	0.221	0.229	0.933	0.334	1.248	0.796–1.954
Only child	−0.004	0.224	0.000	0.984	0.996	0.642–1.544
Separated/ single parent	−0.229	0.329	0.486	0.486	0.795	0.417–1.515
No support from Local Health Service	−0.312	0.227	1.888	0.169	0.732	0.469–1.142
No direct support from school	−0.334	0.246	1.849	0.174	0.716	0.442–1.159
No indirect support from school	0.406	0.312	1.694	0.193	1.501	0.814–2.769
No support from private therapist	−0.137	0.203	0.455	0.500	0.872	0.586–1.298

Note: OR, odds ratio; CI, confidence interval.

3.4. Needs to Deal with the Emergency: A Narrative Perspective

Out of 527 survey participants, 406 parents (77%) reported at least one need to the open-response question about what could be of help do deal with the ongoing emergency. Ten of them reported more than one need (4 participants reported 2 needs, 6 participants reported 3 needs), for a total of 422 responses. The most commonly reported need was for in-home healthcare support (29.9%), followed by center-based healthcare support (10.4%), loosening quarantine restrictions (9.7%), ending lockdown (7.1%), and in-hospital healthcare support (7.1%; Table 5).

Table 5. Responses to the open-response question about what could be of help do deal with the ongoing emergency.

	N	%
In-home healthcare support	126	29.9
Center-based healthcare support	44	10.4
Loosening quarantine restrictions	41	9.7
Ending lockdown	30	7.1
In-hospital healthcare support	30	7.1

Table 5. Cont.

	N	%
Increase school support	29	6.9
Help setting a daily schedule	21	5
"Nothing"	20	4.7
"Don't know"	14	3.3
Parent support	13	3.1
Peer relationship	12	2.8
Structured physical activity	9	2.1
Community support	9	2.1
Financial family support	8	1.9
Work support	6	1.4
Spiritual and religious reflections	4	0.9
Information technology support	3	0.7
Pharmacological support	3	0.7

4. Discussion

To our knowledge, this is the first study which systematically explored the impact of the COVID-19 outbreak in a population of individuals suffering from an autism spectrum disorder (ASD). Results from this parent survey indicate that the large majority of parents of ASD individuals consider the period of change and restrictions that has followed the onset of the emergency as challenging and requiring more commitment than before. Most support was delivered by school services, followed by private therapists and local healthcare services. Consistent with previous reports of executive functioning deficits making ASD individuals more vulnerable to routine disruption [18], an elevated number of parents reported difficulties in managing their children's daily activities, especially in terms of free time and structured activities. Despite requiring specialist intervention in a relatively small proportion of cases, and almost never ending in hospital emergency assessments, behavior problems worsened in more than one third of ASD individuals.

In line with previous evidence that pre-existing psychological difficulties seem to be the only clear predictor of poorer mental health outcomes following respiratory syndromes [14] and quarantine [13], the most relevant finding of this survey is that ASD individuals with behavior problems predating the COVID-19 outbreak are twice as likely to experience more intense and more frequent behavior problems since the beginning of the emergency. As independent evidence supports decreasing symptom levels from childhood to young adulthood in ASD, especially in verbally fluent individuals [19], we also tested whether the age and language level of survey participants' children with ASD would predict a worsening of the behavior problems. Results suggest that older age may play a protective role with regards to the emergency-induced intensification of behavior problems, while the effect of language failed to reach statistical significance. Furthermore, despite social isolation and mental health problems may co-occur in childhood [20], as well as medical conditions and ASD [21], being an only child, as a proxy of greater social isolation, and comorbid medical conditions did not predict a poorer outcome in terms of more intense or more frequent behavior problems following the COVID-19 outbreak and the implementation of restrictive measures and quarantine. Interestingly, living with a separated or single parent was associated with a better outcome in terms of intensity of behavior problems. Despite being counterintuitive, such a finding may reflect a more simplified parent–child interaction which could be effective in preventing the deterioration of the child's wellbeing during quarantine and restrictions. Future studies would need to clarify this issue. Furthermore, it is important to highlight that such evidence does not necessarily apply to other social contexts. Finally, ASD individuals not receiving school support since the COVID-19 outbreak tended to express more intense behavior problems, suggesting the importance of maintaining contact with the school during the emergency.

The last scope of this study was to narratively collect the parents' perceived needs through the emergency by offering an open-response question at the end of the survey. About half of the participants reported needing support from healthcare services, especially in-home services. Interestingly, almost one every five parents reported that loosening restrictions or ending the lockdown would be of help.

Outbreaks of emerging infections such as COVID-19 can elicit strong fear reactions and preoccupations with downstream effects on physical and mental health, especially in vulnerable individuals [22]. Moreover, such negative impacts on health could be worsened by the experience of being quarantined [13]. Autism is no exception. Even though it is a complex genetic disorder, the effect of the environment in shaping the behavioral phenotype should not be underestimated. In fact, a high emotional climate, such as that resulting from the COVID-19 emergency outbreak, has been associated with increased levels of maladaptive behavior in ASD over time [23]. Furthermore, families of individuals with ASD have been reported to experience greater stress than families whose children suffer from other disabilities [24,25], making a compelling case for the implementation of youth-oriented mental health prevention and early intervention strategies [26,27]. Evidence supports the effectiveness of such interventions in mitigating disabilities and even improving skills among young individuals with ASD [28].

Surveys performed during previous Public Health Emergencies of International Concern (PHEIC) have provided timely data to inform best practices in responding to the emergency [29]. Similarly, the online survey presented here has proved to be a powerful data collection tool, benefiting from the strengths that have been associated to this type of instrument such as having a large sample size, fast response times, timely data processing, and low costs [30]. Moreover, thanks to the solid infrastructure of autism advocacy and family support networks, we were able to mitigate the risk of poor response rates and improve sample representativeness, collecting data from over five hundred ASD individuals and their families in a catchment area (the Veneto Region) of about 5 million people. However, the findings of this study have to be seen in light of some limitations. In particular, in spite of the aforementioned advantages, the survey suffered from the lack of a standardized assessment of clinical features such as language and behavior problems. Such aspects may limit the comparability of outcomes among different studies as well as internal comparisons in any follow-up assessments. Furthermore, despite collecting information on children's language and behavior problems predating the emergency as a proxy of their baseline cognitive and adaptive functioning, due to its nature, the online survey did not allow investigating such aspects through a standard method such as psychometric tests. Furthermore, information on the gender of ASD children was not available through the online survey. Even though the main aim of the study was not to investigate gender differences in response to the COVID-19 outbreak in ASD, we acknowledge the limitation.

In conclusion, the present survey indicates that the ongoing COVID-19 emergency has resulted in a challenging period for most ASD individuals and their families, with increased difficulties in managing daily activities and at least one in every three children presenting with more frequent or more intense behavior problems. Children with behavior problems predating the COVID-19 outbreak were found to be particularly at risk to present with more intense and more frequent disruptive behavior. Even though ASD children were receiving different types of support, also requiring specialist or emergency interventions in a relatively low proportion of cases, a number of needs emerged, including receiving more healthcare support, especially from in-home services, as well as interventions to tackle a potentially disruptive quarantine.

Supplementary Materials: The following are available online at http://www.mdpi.com/2076-3425/10/6/341/s1. Table S1: Responses to the open-response question about what medical comorbidity was present in children with ASD.

Author Contributions: Conceptualization, M.C., E.S., F.A., M.L.C., C.B., and L.Z.; methodology, M.C., E.S., F.A., M.L.C., and L.Z.; validation, M.C., C.B. and L.Z.; formal analysis, M.C., E.S., and L.Z.; investigation, M.C., E.S., F.A., M.L.C., and L.Z.; resources, M.C., E.S., F.A., M.L.C., C.B., and L.Z.; data curation, M.C., E.S., and L.Z.; writing—original draft preparation, M.C.; writing—review and editing, M.C., E.S., F.A., M.L.C., C.B., and L.Z.; visualization, M.C., E.S., F.A., M.L.C., C.B., and L.Z.; supervision, L.Z.; project administration, C.B. and L.Z. All authors have read and agreed to the published version of the manuscript.

Funding: This research did not receive any specific grant from funding agencies in the public, commercial, or not-for-profit sectors.

Acknowledgments: The authors would like to thank the survey participants and their families for their cooperation and commitment as well as acknowledge infrastructure from the Integrated University Hospital of Verona and the University of Verona.

Conflicts of Interest: The authors declare no conflict of interest.

References

1. Cucinotta, D.; Vanelli, M. WHO Declares COVID-19 a Pandemic. *Acta Biomed.* **2020**, *91*, 157–160. [CrossRef]
2. Lu, R.; Zhao, X.; Li, J.; Niu, P.; Yang, B.; Wu, H.; Wang, W.; Song, H.; Huang, B.; Zhu, N.; et al. Genomic characterisation and epidemiology of 2019 novel coronavirus: Implications for virus origins and receptor binding. *Lancet* **2020**, *395*, 565–574. [CrossRef]
3. Li, Q.; Guan, X.; Wu, P.; Wang, X.; Zhou, L.; Tong, Y.; Ren, R.; Leung, K.S.M.; Lau, E.H.Y.; Wong, J.Y.; et al. Early Transmission Dynamics in Wuhan, China, of Novel Coronavirus-Infected Pneumonia. *N. Engl. J. Med.* **2020**, *382*, 1199–1207. [CrossRef] [PubMed]
4. Rothe, C.; Schunk, M.; Sothmann, P.; Bretzel, G.; Froeschl, G.; Wallrauch, C.; Zimmer, T.; Thiel, V.; Janke, C.; Guggemos, W.; et al. Transmission of 2019-nCoV Infection from an Asymptomatic Contact in Germany. *N. Engl. J. Med.* **2020**, *382*, 970–971. [CrossRef] [PubMed]
5. Gagliano, A.; Villani, P.G.; Cò, F.M.; Paglia, S.; Bisagni, P.A.G.; Perotti, G.M.; Storti, E.; Lombardo, M. 2019-ncov's epidemic in middle province of northern Italy: Impact, logistic & strategy in the first line hospital. *Disaster Med. Public Health Prep.* **2020**, 1–15. [CrossRef]
6. Ghinai, I.; McPherson, T.; Hunter, J.; Kirking, H.; Christiansen, D.; Joshi, K.; Rubin, R.; Morales-Estrada, S.; Black, S.; Pacilli, M.; et al. First known person-to-person transmission of severe acute respiratory syndrome coronavirus 2 (SARS-CoV-2) in the USA. *Lancet* **2020**, *395*, 1137–1144. [CrossRef]
7. Berger, Z.D.; Evans, N.G.; Phelan, A.L.; Silverman, R.D. Covid-19: Control measures must be equitable and inclusive. *BMJ* **2020**, *368*, m1141. [CrossRef]
8. Lima, C.K.T.; Carvalho, P.M.M.; Lima, I.A.A.S.; Nunes, J.V.A.O.; Saraiva, J.S.; de Souza, R.I.; da Silva, C.G.L.; Neto, M.L.R. The emotional impact of Coronavirus 2019-nCoV (new Coronavirus disease). *Psychiatry Res.* **2020**, *287*, 112915. [CrossRef]
9. Yao, H.; Chen, J.H.; Xu, Y.F. Patients with mental health disorders in the COVID-19 epidemic. *Lancet Psychiatry* **2020**, *7*, e21. [CrossRef]
10. Onder, G.; Rezza, G.; Brusaferro, S. Case-Fatality Rate and Characteristics of Patients Dying in Relation to COVID-19 in Italy. *JAMA* **2020**. [CrossRef]
11. Garfin, D.R.; Silver, R.C.; Holman, E.A. The novel coronavirus (COVID-2019) outbreak: Amplification of public health consequences by media exposure. *Health Psychol.* **2020**. [CrossRef] [PubMed]
12. Wilder-Smith, A.; Freedman, D.O. Isolation, quarantine, social distancing and community containment: Pivotal role for old-style public health measures in the novel coronavirus (2019-nCoV) outbreak. *J. Travel Med.* **2020**, *27*. [CrossRef] [PubMed]
13. Brooks, S.K.; Webster, R.K.; Smith, L.E.; Woodland, L.; Wessely, S.; Greenberg, N.; Rubin, G.J. The psychological impact of quarantine and how to reduce it: Rapid review of the evidence. *Lancet* **2020**, *395*, 912–920. [CrossRef]
14. Jeong, H.; Yim, H.W.; Song, Y.J.; Ki, M.; Min, J.A.; Cho, J.; Chae, J.H. Mental health status of people isolated due to Middle East Respiratory Syndrome. *Epidemiol. Health* **2016**, *38*, e2016048. [CrossRef] [PubMed]
15. Narzisi, A. Handle the Autism Spectrum Condition During Coronavirus (COVID-19). *Brain Sci.* **2020**, *10*, 207. [CrossRef] [PubMed]
16. American Psychiatric Publishing. *Diagnostic and Statistical Manual of Mental Disorders*; APA: Arlington, VA, USA, 2013.

17. Baron-Cohen, S. The hyper-systemizing, assortative mating theory of autism. *Prog. Neuropsychopharmacol. Biol. Psychiatry* **2006**, *30*, 865–872. [CrossRef]
18. Narzisi, A.; Muratori, F.; Calderoni, S.; Fabbro, F.; Urgesi, C. Neuropsychological Profile in High Functioning Autism Spectrum Disorders. *J. Autism Dev. Disord.* **2013**, *43*, 1895–1909. [CrossRef]
19. Bal, V.H.; Kim, S.H.; Fok, M.; Lord, C. Autism spectrum disorder symptoms from ages 2 to 19 years: Implications for diagnosing adolescents and young adults. *Autism Res.* **2019**, *12*, 89–99. [CrossRef]
20. Matthews, T.; Danese, A.; Wertz, J.; Ambler, A.; Kelly, M.; Diver, A.; Caspi, A.; Moffitt, T.E.; Arseneault, L. Social isolation and mental health at primary and secondary school entry: A longitudinal cohort study. *J. Am. Acad. Child Adolesc. Psychiatry* **2015**, *54*, 225–232. [CrossRef]
21. Tye, C.; Runicles, A.; Whitehouse, A.; Alvares, G. Characterizing the Interplay Between Autism Spectrum Disorder and Comorbid Medical Conditions: An Integrative Review. *Front. Psychiatry* **2019**, *9*. [CrossRef]
22. Colizzi, M.; Bortoletto, R.; Silvestri, M.; Mondini, F.; Puttini, E.; Cainelli, C.; Gaudino, R.; Ruggeri, M.; Zoccante, L. Medically unexplained symptoms in the times of Covid-19 pandemic: A case-report. *Brain Behav. Immun. Health* **2020**, 100073. [CrossRef] [PubMed]
23. Greenberg, J.; Seltzer, M.; Hong, J.; Orsmond, G. Bidirectional effects of expressed emotion and behavior problems and symptoms in adolescents and adults with autism. *Am. J. Ment. Retard.* **2006**, *111*, 229–249. [CrossRef]
24. Seltzer, M.; Krauss, M. Quality of life of adults with mental retardation/developmental disabilities who live with family. *Ment. Retard. Dev. Disabil. Res. Rev.* **2001**, *7*, 105–114. [CrossRef] [PubMed]
25. Drogomyretska, K.; Fox, R.; Colbert, D. Brief Report: Stress and Perceived Social Support in Parents of Children with ASD. *J. Autism Dev. Disord.* **2020**. [CrossRef]
26. Colizzi, M.; Lasalvia, A.; Ruggeri, M. Prevention and early intervention in youth mental health: Is it time for a multidisciplinary and trans-diagnostic model for care? *Int. J. Ment. Health Syst.* **2020**, *14*. [CrossRef]
27. Vivanti, G.; Kasari, C.; Green, J.; Mandell, D.; Maye, M.; Hudry, K. Implementing and evaluating early intervention for children with autism: Where are the gaps and what should we do? *Autism Res.* **2018**, *11*, 16–23. [CrossRef]
28. French, L.; Kennedy, E. Annual Research Review: Early intervention for infants and young children with, or at-risk of, autism spectrum disorder: A systematic review. *J. Child Psychol. Psychiatry* **2018**, *59*, 444–456. [CrossRef]
29. Abir, M.; Moore, M.; Chamberlin, M.; Koenig, K.; Hirshon, J.; Singh, C.; Schneider, S.; Cantrill, S. Using Timely Survey-Based Information Networks to Collect Data on Best Practices for Public Health Emergency Preparedness and Response: Illustrative Case From the American College of Emergency Physicians' Ebola Surveys. *Disaster Med. Public Health Prep.* **2016**, *10*, 681–690. [CrossRef]
30. Evans, J.; Mathur, A. The value of online surveys: A look back and a look ahead. *Internet Res.* **2018**, *28*, 854–887. [CrossRef]

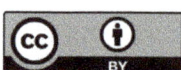

© 2020 by the authors. Licensee MDPI, Basel, Switzerland. This article is an open access article distributed under the terms and conditions of the Creative Commons Attribution (CC BY) license (http://creativecommons.org/licenses/by/4.0/).

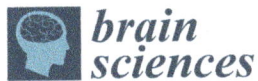 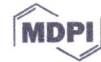

Article

Sensory Profiles of Children with Autism Spectrum Disorder with and without Feeding Problems: A Comparative Study in Sicilian Subjects

Simonetta Panerai [1,*], Raffaele Ferri [1], Valentina Catania [1], Marinella Zingale [1], Daniela Ruccella [2], Donatella Gelardi [1], Daniela Fasciana [3] and Maurizio Elia [1]

1. Oasi Research Institute-IRCCS, 94018 Troina, Italy; rferri@oasi.en.it (R.F.); vacatania@oasi.en.it (V.C.); mzingale@oasi.en.it (M.Z.); dgelardi@oasi.en.it (D.G.); melia@oasi.en.it (M.E.)
2. Psychoeducational Service for Children with Autism and Intellectual Disability, Società Cooperativa Sociale "I Corrieri dell'Oasi" (CdO), 94100 Enna, Italy; danielaruccella82@gmail.com
3. Center for Diagnosis and Early Intensive Treatment of Autism Spectrum Disorder, 93100 ASP Caltanissetta, Italy; danifasciana@gmail.com
* Correspondence: spanerai@oasi.en.it; Tel.: +39-38-9432-0329

Received: 27 April 2020; Accepted: 28 May 2020; Published: 31 May 2020

Abstract: The aim of this study is to better understand the relationship between sensory and feeding problems in Autism Spectrum Disorder (ASD) by comparing sensory responsiveness of ASD children with (ASD-W) and without (ASD-WO) feeding problems. The feeding and sensory characteristics of 111 children with ASD (37 ASD-W and 74 ASD-WO) were assessed by using two questionnaires tapping on feeding problems and two on sensory problems. A comparative study was carried out with between-group as well as intra-group comparisons design; a correlation analysis was also added. A statistically significant correlation was found between sensory and feeding problems. ASD-W children showed more severe and extensively impaired sensory responses than ASD-WO, with lower sensory adaptation and more generalized and severe deficits in all subdomains. Taste/Smell sensitivity was strongly impaired only in ASD-W, whereas in ASD-WO it was found to be a point of strength. Both groups showed a Hyporesponsive profile, though it was more marked in ASD-W. Both groups showed strengths in Visual/Auditory sensitivity, Low-Energy/Weak, and Movement sensitivity, again more marked in ASD-WO. These results might prove to be particularly useful for sensory training and psychoeducational treatment.

Keywords: autism spectrum disorder (ASD); sensory profile; sensory responsiveness; feeding problems; short sensory profile (SSP); sensory experience questionnaire (SEQ)

1. Introduction

Sensory impairments are frequent in children with Autism Spectrum Disorder (ASD) [1–7], with over 90% of cases presenting severe sensory symptoms in multiple sensory domains, as reported in some studies [2,4]. They form a group of disorders that involve challenges in modulation, integration, organization, and discrimination of sensory inputs, leading to either inappropriately responding to those inputs or experiencing disruptions in daily activities and emotional-behavioral patterns. In particular, sensory modulation disorders are classified into three subtypes: (1) over-responsivity (or hyperresponsiveness), characterized by exaggerated, rapid onset and/or prolonged reactions to sensory stimulation; (2) under-responsivity (or hyporesponsiveness), with unawareness or slow response to sensory input; and (3) seeking for, involving craving of, and interest in sensory experiences that are prolonged or intense [8]. Some patterns, such as hypo- and hyperresponsiveness, are also known to co-occur in children with ASD [9–12], especially in children showing a generalized sensory impairment [13]. Results of a meta-analysis by Ben Sasson et al. [14] showed a significantly high difference between ASD and Typically Developing (TD) groups in sensory modulation, with the greatest difference in under-responsivity, followed by over-responsivity and sensation seeking. Although the three sensory modulation disorder subtypes are hypothetical, some physiological research supports these distinctions. A review by Suarez [4] reported some results of these physiological studies: in over-responsivity a low threshold for one or multiple sensation channels has been hypothesized, resulting, for example, in exaggerated reactions to textures or noises. On the contrary, in under-responsivity, a high threshold has been hypothesized, so that only intense and sustained stimuli can obtain attention by children, resulting in diminished or no response, for example, to name or pain. Studies using physiological tools, such as electrodermal sensors or cardiac vagal tone index, found a decreased or increased activation of the electrodermal responses (in under-responsive and in over-responsive children respectively) and an impaired less effective parasympathetic system.

The most affected sensory modalities in children with ASD seem to be auditory filtering and tactile sensitivity [3,15–18]. Sensory dysfunctions also seem to be related to the severity of ASD [5,14,19] and to stereotyped interests and behaviors [16,20]. Limited and stereotyped behaviors, interests and activities can be observed also in the feeding domain [21,22] and a strong sensitivity to sensory information has been associated with feeding problems, especially food fussiness, in both children with typical and atypical development [23]. However, in children with atypical development, feeding concerns still persist beyond childhood. With age, children with typical development change their appetite, food preferences, and eating habits, but the social and emotional dimensions of food remain stable and expand over time. Furthermore, in children with ASD, feeding involves both the nutritional and the emotional-relational dimensions. The term "eating problems" typically refers to oral consumption of nutrients that deviates from the norm, enough to lead to negative emotional, social or health consequences. The prevalence of feeding problems in children with ASD is estimated to be approximately 90%, with 70% of children showing food selectivity [24–26]. It has been suggested that feeding problems might be related to sensory modulation disorders as well [4,27–30]. The study by Zobel-Lachiusa et al. [28] investigated differences in feeding behaviors and sensory characteristics of children with ASD compared to TD children. Statistically significant differences between the two groups were found in all the measures administered, as well as a moderate to strong positive correlation between feeding problems and sensory impairments in children with ASD. Nadon et al. [29] found a definite and probable difference in sensory processing (as measured by using the Short Sensory Profile—SSP) [31] in 65% of children (N = 95) with ASD, aged 3 to 10 years; these results were also related to increased feeding problems in the sample. Chistol et al. [30] found higher levels of food refusal in ASD children with atypical oral sensitivity compared to those showing a typical oral sensitivity. McCormick et al. [7] showed no significant differences between ASD and Developmentally Delayed children, except for the Taste/Smell and Visual/Auditory sensitivity (SSP subsections).

Children with ASD present with higher sensory problems than TD, with a prevalence ranging from 65.3% to 84.8% [3,28,32]; moreover, sensory and feeding problems seem to be correlated. Objective of our study was to investigate whether ASD children with feeding problems (ASD-W) show the same sensorimotor features as the ASD without feeding problems (ASD-WO): which sensory modalities are impaired and to what extent? Our study is not directed to feeding per se, as a purely physiological process, but to the behavioral components accompanying the feeding act.

Our hypothesis is that sensory profiles might present different characteristics in specific subgroups of children with autism (with and without feeding problems), and that ASD-W children might show higher sensory impairments than ASD-WO, with Taste/Smell sensitivity mostly affected. In order to carry out this assessment, we used four measures: two questionnaires for the detection of feeding problems, and two for the detection of sensorimotor features. We are not aware of previous studies in the literature on such a topic. A better understanding of the association between feeding problems and sensory factors in children with autism, might bring benefits for the physical health of ASD children, since it might provide some ideas and guide for treatment: for example, feeding training might include behavioral techniques to gradually decrease the negative sensory experiences related to food consumption, and encourage familiarity and acceptance of foods.

2. Materials and Methods

2.1. Study Design

A comparative study was carried out. The four questionnaires were administered by clinical psychologists, working in the diagnostic services of three Sicilian specialized centers, throughout interviews to parents, as part of the psychological and psychoeducational assessment. Recruitment and organization of the sample are described in the following paragraph.

2.2. Participants

A total of 111 children with ASD, aged 2 to 12 years (86 males and 25 females; median chronological age 62 months, interquartile range 44–75 months), were consecutively recruited from specialized services of diagnosis and treatment of autism during the year 2019, in three specialized centers of Eastern Sicily provinces (Enna, Caltanissetta and Catania). All participants were diagnosed by a multidisciplinary team, following the DSM-5 criteria [21]. The severity of their disorders was classified into three levels (1 to 3) accordingly. Approximately 65% ($N = 72$) of children showed a severity level of 3, about 27% ($N = 30$) a severity level of 2, and about 8% ($N = 9$) a severity level of 1; moreover, the majority of them (91%, $N = 101$) presented with comorbid Intellectual Disability (ID). Diagnoses were further confirmed using at least one of the most common diagnostic scales (the Autism Diagnostic Interview-Revised, the Autism Diagnostic Observation Schedules or the Childhood Autism Rating Scale-Second edition). Based on the results obtained at the Brief Autism Mealtime Behaviors Inventory (BAMBI-18) [33], the sample was divided into two subgroups, which included ASD-W ($N = 37$, 33%; scores at BAMBI ≥ 34) and ASD-WO ($N = 74$, 67%; scores at BAMBI < 34) children. The characteristics of the two subgroups are shown in Table 1 (N of males and females, level of severity, chronological ages, total and sub-domain scores obtained at mealtime behavior measures).

Table 1. Characteristics of the sample and scores obtained at BAMBI 18 and CEBQ, expressed as medians and interquartile ranges.

TitleSample Features	ASD-W	ASD-WO	z =	p ≤	Effect Size [3] r
N =	37	74			
Males/Females	30/7	56/18		NS [1]	
Severity level 3/2/1	27/8/2	45/22/7		NS [1]	
Chronological age, months	60 (44–76)	63.5 (45.2–74.0)		NS [2]	
BAMBI 18 total scores	41 (38–46)	26.5 (22.25–29.75)	−8.44	0.00001 [2]	0.8
BAMBI 18 subdomains					
Food Selectivity	14 (12–16)	9 (7–11)	−7.1	0.00001 [2]	0.67
Disruptive Behaviors	13 (10–16)	7.5 (6–9)	−6.48	0.00001 [2]	0.61
Food Refusal	7 (5–9)	4 (3–4.75)	−7.02	0.00001 [2]	0.67
Mealtime Rigidity	8 (6–11)	4 (3–7)	−5.69	0.00001 [2]	0.54
CEBQ	93 (84–105)	10 (7–16)	−8.54	0.00001 [2]	0.81
CEBQ subdomains					
Food Responsiveness	12 (7–16)	10 (7–16)	−0.424	NS [2]	
Emotional Over-eating	5 (4–8)	6 (4–7)	0.237	NS [2]	
Enjoyment of food	13 (10–16)	16 (13–17)	2.939	0.038 [2]	0.28
Desire to Drink	7 (5–9)	6 (5–8)	−0.88	NS [2]	
Satiety responsiveness	12 (10–15)	11 (8–13)	−2.36	0.018 [2]	0.22
Slowness in Eating	12 (10–15)	9 (8–12)	−2.13	0.033 [2]	0.2
Emotional Under-eating	10 (6–12)	8 (6–12)	−1.84	NS [2]	
Food Fussiness	21 (18–26)	16 (12–19)	−4.58	0.00001 [2]	0.435

ASD = Autism Spectrum Disorder; ASD-W = ASD With feeding problems; ASD-WO = ASD WithOut feeding problems; Severity level: 3 = requiring very substantial support, 2 = requiring substantial support, 1 = requiring support; BAMBI = Brief Autism Mealtime Behaviour Inventory; CEBQ = Child Eating Behaviour Questionnaire; NS = Not Significant; [1] Chi-square test; [2] Mann-Whitney's U Test; [3] Effect size calculated by using $r = z/\sqrt{N}$ formula.

2.3. Measures

BAMBI 18 [33,34] is an 18-item interview for assessing mealtime behavior problems. A 5-point Likert scale is used, ranging from 1 = never/rarely to 5 = always, including a neutral midpoint; a total frequency score is derived from the sum of the items; higher scores indicate more problematic mealtime behaviors. Undesirable behaviors can be analyzed also on the basis of four main factors, and namely: limited variety/food selectivity, disruptive mealtime behaviors, food refusal and mealtime rigidity [34]. Original test-retest reliability was reported at 0.87 (TD children $N = 40$ and ASD children $N = 68$, aged 3 to 11 years), and interrater reliability at 0.78 [31]. The scale internal consistency was 0.88 (Cronbach's alpha). A cut-off total score of 34 was found by DeMand et al. [34].

CEBQ [35] is a tool for assessing children's eating styles. It is an interview including 35 items; a 5-point Likert scale is used, ranging from 1 = never to 5 = always. It includes eight scales: Food responsiveness, Emotional over-eating, Enjoyment of food, Desire to drink, Satiety responsiveness, Slowness in eating, Emotional under-eating, and Food fussiness. Internal reliability, derived from two samples ($N = 177$ and $N = 222$, respectively) for the eight factors, ranged from 0.72 to 0.91 (Cronbach's alpha). Test-retest reliability ($N = 160$) ranged from 0.52 to 0.87.

SSP [31] is a 38-item caregiver questionnaire, scored on a 5-point Likert scale (ranging from 1 = always to 5 = never). The lower the score, the more atypical sensory responses. The SSP consists of a total score and 7 subsection scores: Tactile sensitivity (7 items, mostly focusing on tactile avoiding and expression of distress: for example, fights or cries during hair cutting, fingernail cutting or face washing; emotional or aggressive reactions to touch; difficulty in standing in line or close to other people; avoids going barefoot, especially over sand or grass); Taste/Smell sensitivity (4 items, focusing on food avoiding and selectivity: for example, avoiding certain tastes or food smells that are typically part of children's diet; eating only certain foods or limiting to particular food textures/temperatures; picky eating); Movement sensitivity (3 items, focusing on anxiety due to specific postures: for example, becoming anxious or distressed when feet leave the ground, disliking activities where head is upside down); Under-responsive/Seeks sensation (7 items, focusing on actions adding more intense sensations and inattention during social interactions: for example, seeking to make noises, or enjoying strange noises; fidgeting, and not seating still; seeking all kinds of movement, touching people and objects, jumping from one activity to another, not noticing messy face or hands); Auditory Filtering (6 items, focusing on distraction and inattention caused by auditory stimuli in the environment: for example, being distracted by noises, and impossibility to work with background noises; not hearing what he/she is told, not responding to his/her name, ignoring persons interacting with him/her); Low Energy/Weak (6 items, focusing on weakness and easy fatigue: for example, getting easily tired, especially when standing or holding particular body positions; weak grasping; not lifting heavy objects in comparison to children with the same age); Visual/Auditory sensitivity (5 items, focusing on negative responses to unexpected or loud stimuli: for example, negative responses to unexpected or loud noises, protecting ears from sound or eyes from light, being bothered by bright light). The SSP total score and the subsection scores can be used to classify children's sensory impairments into three categories: Typical Performance, Probable Difference, and Definite Difference. Cut-off points to define these categories are available for the total and the subsection scores. A discriminant validity > 95% in differentiating children with and without sensory impairments was found [36]. The internal reliability was reported as ranging between 0.70 to 0.90. Internal validity correlations for the subsections ranged from 0.25 to 0.76 and were all significant at $p < 0.01$ [31].

The Sensory Experience Questionnaire (SEQ Version 1) [10,37] is a brief caregiver interview designed to assess sensory problems in young children with ASD and related Developmental Disorders. A 5-point Likert scale is used, ranging from 1 = almost never to 5 = almost always. Higher scores indicate higher sensory problems. The SEQ measures the Hyper- and Hyporesponsive patterns across social and nonsocial contexts. Hypo- is considered as a lack of or delayed response to sensory stimuli [14,38]). Hyper- is defined as an exaggerated or avoidant response to sensory stimuli [39,40]. SEQ yields both a total score as well as four-dimensional subscale scores. The psychometric properties of SEQ were evaluated by Little et al. [35] by means of 358 caregiver questionnaires; internal consistency and test–retest reliability were 0.80 (Cronbach's coefficient alpha); intraclass correlation coefficients was 0.92.

2.4. Statistical Analysis

Non-parametric statistics were used because most of the variables did not show a normal distribution, based on asymmetry and kurtosis. The between-group comparisons were carried out by means of the Mann-Whitney's U test; the significance level was set at $p < 0.05$. Effect sizes were calculated by means of the $r = z/\sqrt{N}$ formula, where N is the total number of the sample participants. The r value of 0.1, 0.3 and 0.5 indicated a small, a medium, and a large effect size respectively; the absolute value of r has been reported. The Chi-square test was used for frequency data, including the intra-group comparisons; effect size was calculated by means of the Cramer's V test, where scores ≤0.2 indicate a small effect size, while scores between 0.2 and ≤ 0.6 a moderate effect size, and >0.6 a strong effect size. For intra-group comparisons, the Friedman and the Wilcoxon matched pair tests were used. Effect sizes were calculated by means of $r = z/\sqrt{N}$ formula. A correlation analysis between sensory and feeding problems was carried out for the whole sample, by using the Spearman's test.

2.5. Ethics Committee Approval

Approval was obtained from the Local Ethics Committee "Comitato Etico IRCCS Sicilia–Oasi Maria SS.", approval date 7 July 2018, approval code: 2018/07/18/CE-IRCCS-OASI/14. All parents provided written informed consent prior to the administration of the questionnaires.

3. Results

No significant differences were found between ASD-W and ASD-WO subgroups, neither in the chronological ages, nor in the number of male and female participants, or in the levels of disorder severity (Table 1); therefore, the two subgroups were comparable.

Table 1 shows statistically significant differences at BAMBI and CEBQ questionnaires, both investigating feeding problems. In all the BAMBI subdomains (selectivity, disruptive behaviors, refusal, and mealtime rigidity), statistically significant differences were obtained with medium to large effect sizes. In the CEBQ, the statistically significant differences were found only in some subdomains, namely enjoyment of food, satiety responsiveness, slowness in eating, and, above all, food fussiness, including food selectivity items. Therefore, the two subgroups turned out to be clearly distinguished from each another as for feeding behaviors.

3.1. Comparisons Between ASD-W and ASD-WO Subgroups

Statistically significant differences were found in the comparisons between ASD-W and ASD-WO subgroups (Mann Whitney's U test; Table 2).

Table 2. Scores obtained from ASD-W and ASD-WO subgroups at the SSP and SEQ, expressed as medians and interquartile ranges.

MeasuresTitle	ASD-W break//N = 37	ASD-WO N = 74	z =	$p \le$ [1]	Effect Size $r =$ [2]
SEQ Total scores	51 (41–62)	46.5 (39–57)	−1.94	0.026	0.18
SEQ subsections					
HY	21 (18–28)	19 (16–23)	−2.49	0.006	0.24
HY-S	11 (8–15)	10 (7–12)	−1.75	0.04	0.17
HY-NS	11 (10–13)	10 (7.25–12)	−2.52	0.006	0.24
HO	29 (23–34)	29 (22–34)	−1.03	NS	
HO-S	8 (5–9)	7 (5–9)	−1.13	NS	
HO-NS	22 (18–24)	20 (17–25.75)	−0.89	NS	

Table 2. Cont.

MeasuresTitle	ASD-W break//N = 37	ASD-WO N = 74	z =	$p \leq$ [1]	Effect Size $r =$ [2]
SSP Total scores	132 (113–149)	156 (140.25–165.5)	4.5	0.00001	0.43
SSP subsections					
Tactile sensitivity	27 (23–31)	30.5 (28–33)	2.99	0.0014	0.28
Taste/Smell sensitivity	9 (7–13)	18 (14–20)	5.42	0.00001	0.515
Movement sensitivity	13 (10–15)	15 (11.25–15)	1.87	0.03	0.18
Under-responsive/Seeks sensation	21 (17–22)	24.5 (19.25–27.75)	3.43	0.0003	0.33
Auditory filtering	16 (14–22)	22 (20–24)	3.79	0.00008	0.36
Low energy/Weak	26 (20–28)	28 (25.25–30)	2.77	0.028	0.26
Visual/Auditory sensitivity	20 (17–22)	21 (18–23)	1.004	NS	

ASD = Autism Spectrum Disorder; ASD-W = ASD With feeding problems; ASD-WO = ASD WithOut feeding problems; SEQ = Sensory Experience Questionnaire; HY = Hyperresponsiveness; HY-S = HY social items; HY-NS = HY non-social items; HO = Hyporesponsiveness; HO-S = HO social items; HO-NS = HO non-social items; SSP = Short Sensory Profile; NS = Not significant; [1] Mann Whitney's U Test; [2] Effect size calculated by using the formula: $r = z/\sqrt{N}$.

As far as the SSP results are concerned, differences were found in the total score, with a medium effect size, and in almost all the subsections, with a large effect size in Taste/Smell sensitivity, a medium effect size in Auditory Filtering and Under-responsive/Seeks sensation, and a small effect size in Tactile sensitivity, Low Energy/Weak, and Movement sensitivity. Higher sensory impairments turned out to characterize the ASD-W subgroup. No differences were found in the Visual/Auditory sensitivity.

Statistically significant differences emerged from SEQ, both in the total score, with a small effect size, and in the Hyperresponsiveness subsection (in total score and responsiveness toward social and non-social stimuli), with most impairments in the ASD-W subgroup. No statistically significant differences were found in Hyporesponsiveness subsection, impaired in both subgroups (see median scores). Table 3 shows the SSP performance categories (Definite Difference, Probable Difference, and Typical Performance in both total and subsection scores), expressed in percentages of children, and the results from the comparisons between the two subgroups (Chi Square test).

Table 3. SSP performances from the whole ASD sample and from each of the ASD-W and ASD-WO subgroups (expressed as percentages of children); statistically significant differences between ASD-W and ASD-WO subgroups; percentages of children as reported in other studies.

SSP Performance Categories Title	All ASD (N = 111)	ASD-W (N = 37)	ASD-WO (N = 74)	ASD-W vs. ASD-WO $p \le 1$	Cramer's V Effect Size	Tomchek and Dunn, 2007 [3]	Nadon et al., 2011 [29]	Al-Heizan et al., 2015 [32]
SSP Total scores								
Definite Difference	43.2	73	28.4	0.00001 [3]	0.46	83.6	65.3 [2]	84.8
Probable Difference	15.3	10.8	17.6			11.4	21.1	8.7
Typical Performance	41.4	16.2	54			5	13.7	6.5
SSP subsections:								
Tactile sensitivity								
Definite Difference	28.8	48.6	19	0.000015 [4]	0.33	60.9	36.8	60.9
Probable Difference	22.5	21.6	23			18.5	24.2	21.7
Typical Performance	48.7	29.7	58			20.6	37.9	17.4
Taste/Smell sensitivity								
Definite Difference	28.8	62.2	12.2	0.00001 [5]	0.54	54.1	48.4	52.2
Probable Difference	18.9	16.2	20.2			13.9	15.8	19.6
Typical Performance	52.3	21.6	67.6			32	34.7	28.26
Movement sensitivity								
Definite Difference	14.4	24.3	9.5	0.0013 [6]	0.26	23.1	28.4	50
Probable Difference	17.1	8.1	21.6			21	20	15.2
Typical Derformance	68.5	67.6	68.9			55.9	51.6	34.8
Under-responsive/Seeks sensation								
Definite Difference	54.1	78.4	41.9	0.00001 [7]	0.38	86.1	67.4	89.1
Probable Difference	22.5	13.5	27			7.5	16.8	2.2
Typical Derformance	23.4	8	31.1			6.4	15.8	8.7
Auditory Filtering								
Definite Difference	39.6	70.3	24.3	0.00001 [8]	0.47	77.6	55.8	73.9
Probable Difference	23.5	8.1	31.1			14.6	24.2	8.7
Typical Derformance	36.9	21.6	44.6			7.8	20	17.4
Low Energy/Weak								
Definite difference	26.1	37.8	20.2	0.0035 [9]	0.24	23.1	43.2	58.7
Probable difference	7.2	10.8	5.4			18.9	12.6	10.9
Typical performance	66.7	51.3	74.3			58	44.2	30.4
Visual/Auditory sensitivity								
Definite difference	10.8	13.5	9.5	NS		43.8	22.1	34.8
Probable difference	23.4	27	21.6			25.3	31.6	19.6
Typical performance	65.8	59.4	68.9			31	46.3	45.7

ASD = Autism Spectrum Disorder; ASD-W = ASD With feeding problems; ASD-WO = ASD WithOut feeding problems; SSP = Short Sensory Profile; NS = Not significant; [1] Chi-square test; [2] In this group a mean of 15.5 ± 6 presented with feeding problems; Definite difference vs. Typical performance: [3] $p < 0.00001$, Cramer's V = 0.49; [4] $p < 0.00001$, Cramer's V = 0.38; [5] $p < 0.00001$, Cramer's V = 0.59; [6] $p < 0.00001$, Cramer's V = 0.18; [7] $p < 0.00001$, Cramer's V = 0.38; [8] $p < 0.0018$, Cramer's V = 0.415; [9] $p < 0.0017$, Cramer's V = 0.23.

The percentage of Definite Difference in ASD-W subgroup was higher than ASD-WO in both the SSP total score and the subsections; on the contrary, higher percentages of ASD-WO children fell into the Typical Performance of SSP total and subsection scores. Statistically significant differences were found in the comparisons between the two subgroups, with moderate effect sizes in the total score and in all the subsections, except for Visual/Auditory sensitivity performance, in which no statistically significant difference was found. When comparing Definite Differences vs. Typical performance, statistically significant differences and moderate effect sizes were found.

3.2. ASD-WO Intra-Group Analysis

In the ASD-WO subgroup, a statistically significant difference ($p < 0.00001$; Friedman's test) was found between the SSP subsection scores, expressed as medians of the ratios between the scores obtained and the maximum possible scores; the medians of the ratios ranged from 0.8 to 1, (the highest SSP score, the lowest impairment) in the following subdomains: Tactile, Taste/Smell, Movement, Visual/Auditory sensitivity and Low Energy/Weak; and from 0.7 to 0.75 in Under-responsive/Seeks sensation and Auditory Filtering (Figure 1A).

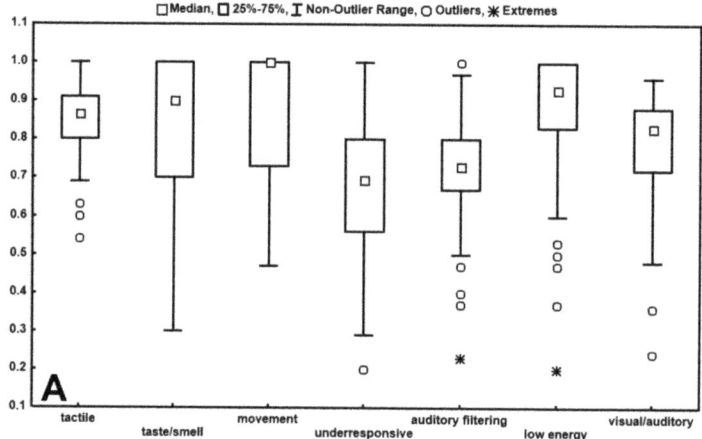

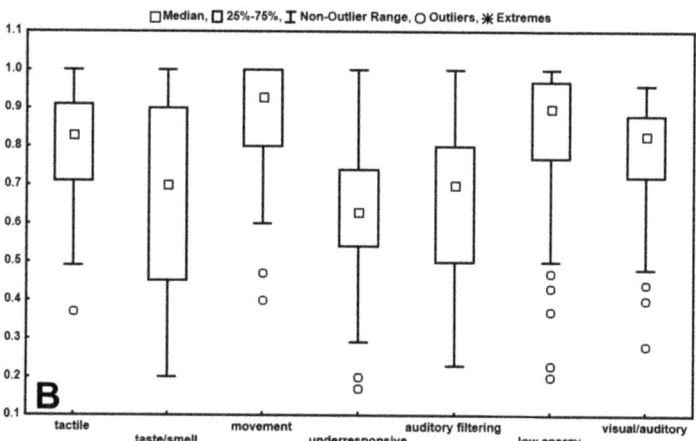

Figure 1. Scores obtained from ASD-WO (**A**) and ASD-W (**B**) in the SSP subdomains (expressed as medians of the ratios between obtained scores and maximum possible scores).

Both Under-responsive/Seeks sensation (US) and Auditory Filtering (AF) showed statistically significant differences (Wilcoxon matched pairs test) when compared to the other SSP subdomains, and namely: US vs. Tactile, Movement, and Low Energy $p < 0.000001$, with large effect sizes ($z = 6.78$, 6.45, 5.98 respectively; $r = 0.79, 0.75, 0.69$ respectively); US vs. Visual/Auditory $p < 0.000002$, with large effect size ($z = 4.73$; $r = 0.55$); US vs. Taste/Smell $p = 0.000014$, with large effect size ($z = 4.35$; $r = 0.506$); US vs. AF $p = 0.012$, with small effect size ($z = 2.51$; $r = 0.29$); AF vs. Tactile, Movement, Low Energy $p < 0.000001$, with large effect sizes ($z = 5.76, 5.53, 5.98$ respectively; $r = 0.67, 0.64, 0.69$ respectively); AF vs. Taste/Smell $p = 0.001$, with medium effect size ($z = 3.27$; $r = 0.38$), AF vs. Visual/Auditory $p = 0.002$, with medium effect size ($z = 3.1$; $r = 0.36$).

As far as the SEQ is concerned, a statistically significant difference with large effect size between the Hyperresponsiveness and Hyporesponsiveness subdomains (Wilcoxon matched pairs test, $p < 0.00001$, $z = -5.22$, $r = 0.07$) was found, with higher scores in Hyporesponsiveness. Within the Hyporesponsiveness subdomain, a statistically significant difference with medium effect size was found between responses to social and non-social stimuli (Wilcoxon matched pairs test, $p = 0.006$, $z = 2.73$, $r = 0.036$), with response to non-social stimuli being more impaired. Within the Hyperresponsiveness subdomain, no significant difference was found between responses to social and non-social stimuli.

3.3. ASD-W Intra-Group Analysis

In the ASD-W subgroup, a statistically significant difference ($p < 0.00001$, Friedman's test) was found between the SSP subsection scores, expressed as medians of the ratios between the scores obtained and the maximum possible scores. The medians of the ratios ranged from 0.75 to 0.9 in the following subdomains: Tactile, Movement, Visual/Auditory and Low Energy/Weak; from 0.53 and 0.45 in Auditory Filtering, Under-responsive/Seeks sensation, and Taste/Smell sensitivity (Figure 1 B). No statistically significant differences were found either between Taste/Smell and both Under-responsive and Auditory Filtering, or between Under-responsive and Auditory filtering (Wilcoxon matched pairs test). Taste/Smell, Under-responsive and Auditory Filtering subsections showed statistically significant differences and large effect sizes in comparison with the others SSP subdomains, and namely: Taste/Smell (TS) vs. Tactile $p = 0.000004$, $z = 4.62$, $r = 0.76$; TS vs. Movement $p = 0.000003$, $z = 4.71$, $r = 0.77$; TS vs. Low Energy $p = 0.000016$, $z = 4.32$, $r = 0.71$; TS vs. Visual/Auditory $p = 0.000017$, $z = 4.31$, $r = 0.71$; US vs. Tactile $p = 0.000002$, $z = 4.8$, $r = 0.79$; US vs. Movement and Visual/Auditory $p = 0.000001$, $z = 5.1$ and 4.82 respectively; $r = 0.84$ and 0.79 respectively; US vs. Low Energy $p = 0.000007$, $z = 4.51$, $r = 0.74$ (Wilcoxon matched pairs test).

As far as the SEQ is concerned, a statistically significant difference between the Hyperresponsiveness and Hyporesponsiveness subdomains and a large effect size (Wilcoxon matched pairs test $p < 0.015$, $z = -3.39$, $r = 0.09$) were found, with sensory Hyporesponsiveness being prevalent; no statistically significant differences were found either in Hyperresponsiveness or Hyporesponsiveness subdomains (responses to social and non-social stimuli).

3.4. Correlation Analysis

Statistically significant correlations (Spearman's test; $p < 0.05$) between the total scores of sensory and mealtime behaviors questionnaires were found (BAMBI vs. CEBQ = 0.61; SSP vs. SEQ = −0.59; SSP vs. BAMBI = −0.46; SSP vs. CEBQ = −0.61; SEQ vs. BAMBI = 0.3; SEQ vs. CEBQ = 0.33). A positive correlation was found between the two questionnaires on feeding problems (increased scores in one questionnaire corresponded to increased scores in the other), and between SEQ and each of the mealtime measures (increasing scores in feeding problems corresponded to increasing scores in sensory impairments, investigated by SEQ). A negative correlation was found between each mealtime measure and SSP: increasing scores in BAMBI or CEBQ corresponded to decreasing scores in SSP, that is, decreased typical sensory performances.

4. Discussion

Children with ASD seem to show more sensory problems than children with TD, and a relationship between sensory and feeding problems was hypothesized by some authors [4,26–29]. To the best of our knowledge, no studies on ASD sensory processing have so far reported any comparisons between sensory characteristics of ASD children with and without feeding problems. The aim of our study was to shed light on this aspect, starting from the hypothesis that ASD-W children presented with higher sensory impairments than ASD-WO, with Taste/Smell sensitivity particularly affected.

In our ASD sample, the percentage of feeding problems turned out to be lower than those reported in other studies [24,25,41,42], probably due to the specific cut-off used in our study for classifying children with feeding problems. This result should be further investigated in future studies with larger samples.

The Spearman's test showed a statistically significant correlation between feeding behaviors and responses to sensory stimuli, especially between SSP and the two mealtime behaviors measures, thus confirming the findings of the studies above mentioned [4,27–30].

Results obtained from the between-group comparisons seem to confirm our hypothesis. Statistically significant differences in the total scores of both SSP and SEQ were found, with higher impairments in the ASD-W subgroup. As stated by O'Donnell et al. [43], the SSP total score is considered as the most sensitive indicator of sensory dysfunction. As for the SSP subsections, differences turned out to be particularly marked in the Taste/Smell sensitivity, and this is certainly consistent with our expectations, since the Taste/Smell sensitivity is a factor that strongly influences feeding behaviors. The presence of olfactory and gustatory dysfunctions in children with ASD have already been reported in the literature [44,45], even if they remain still understudied. The olfactory system is mainly implicated in detection, identification, memory and recognition of odors. The principal function of taste is to analyze chemosensory, somesthetic and hedonic features of gustatory stimuli. Results from the few studies in which physiological measures were used, found significant differences in odor and taste identification in children with ASD compared with TD, but not in detection thresholds, thus suggesting cortical rather than brainstem dysfunction [45]. A recent study by Koehler et al. [46] on odor threshold and odor identification in children with ASD, using structural magnetic resonance imaging, found decreased threshold and identification functions, and a decreased activation of the pyriform cortex, suggesting that olfactory impairments in people with ASD has its correspondence in the primary olfactory cortex. A study by Avery et al. [47] on taste reactivity in ASD found an aberrant function of the primary gustatory cortex (anterior insula and frontal operculum) and other brain regions associated with social functioning. Taste and smell cerebral pathways present some similarities, since they both involve regions such as the orbitofrontal cortex, the insula, the limbic system and the hypothalamus. However, studies have so far found no clear link between impaired responses to sensory stimuli and the underlying brain sensory processing; therefore, the unusual sensory responses in children with autism still need a reliable explanation. We know that these cortex areas are connected not only to the olfactory and gustatory systems, but also to emotions and social behaviors; therefore, it is possible to hypothesize that the altered perception of taste/smell stimuli in children with autism can contribute to their social and emotional deficits.

As far as the other results of our study are concerned, statistically significant differences were found in all the other SSP subsections, especially in Auditory Filtering and Under-responsive/Seeks sensation (Tables 2 and 3), and also in Tactile sensitivity, Movement sensitivity and Low Energy/Weak (Table 3). These results indicate that feeding behaviors of children with autism seem to be affected not only by Taste/Smell sensitivity, but also by multiple sensory experiences, and that a generalized impairment of all sensory modalities occurs more in children with ASD-W than in children with ASD-WO. This generalized sensory impairment, especially in children with ASD-W, might find an explanation in the theory of imbalance in excitatory and inhibitory processes in the brain, resulting in increased excitation (greater glutamatergic signaling) and reduced inhibition (reduced GABA inhibitory neurotransmitters) [48,49]. Increased activation was found in children with ASD in primary sensory cortices, amygdala, hippocampus and orbitofrontal cortex, also related to cognitive, emotional, and social processing; reduced GABA levels were found in auditory, motor and frontal cortex. However, a link between changes in neurotransmitters and the anomalous behavioral responses to sensory stimuli has not been established yet.

The presence and severity of sensory dysfunctions in our sample seemed to be related to feeding problems, rather than to the autism severity (as stated by some authors) [7,15,18]; in fact, the two subgroups did not differ from each other as for the severity of autistic symptoms (see Table 1). Visual/Auditory sensitivity did not seem to affect feeding behaviors: a high percentage of children (about 60% of ASD-W and 70% of ASD-WO) showed a Typical Performance in this sensory modality, therefore it was not widely impaired in our whole sample.

In a study by Lane et al. [50], using the SSP, four distinct sensory subtypes were identified: sensory adaptive, consisting in typical functioning in five of the seven SSP subsections; taste smell sensitive, consisting in extreme Taste/Smell sensitivity and clinically significant concerns in Auditory Filtering and Under-responsive/Seeks sensation; postural inattentive, consisting in extreme score in Low Energy/Weak and clinically significant concerns in Auditory Filtering and Under-responsive/Seeks sensation; and generalized sensory difference, in which all sensory domains were affected. We applied these subtypes to both ASD-W and ASD-WO children, thus confirming our results as described above: ASD-W children fell into the Taste/Smell sensitive subtype, and showed a more generalized sensory difference than the ASD-WO subgroup; on the contrary, ASD-WO children were sensory adaptive in about half of the cases.

The SSP performance classifications in our study appeared to be different from those obtained in previous studies [3,29,32] (Table 3), either in the whole ASD sample, or in the ASD-WO subgroup. In fact, the percentages of Definite Differences were lower, while those of Typical Performance higher; our percentages were close to those of the studies mentioned above only in the case of the ASD-W subgroup. This might be due to the fact that these studies included ASD children with and without feeding problems, but their percentages were not specified. Nadon et al. [29], however, suggested that the presence of feeding problems might have affected the results of their study.

As far as the SEQ is concerned, Hyporesponsiveness turned out to be impaired in both ASD-W and ASD-WO children. This is consistent with previous studies [14] and confirms data obtained in the SSP Under-responsive/Seeks sensation subsection. Statistically significant differences were found by comparing the two subgroups, both in the SEQ total score and Hyperresponsive subsection, and ASD-W appeared to be more affected than ASD-WO children; however, the effect sizes were small, therefore these results need to be confirmed by further studies. In the ASD-W subgroup the dysfunctioning seemed to be more generalized, because no differences were found in the responses to social and non-social stimuli in Hyporesponsiveness.

Results from the intra-group SSP analysis (Figure 1) are also consistent with those described above: in the ASD-WO children, the Under-responsive/Seeks sensations and Auditory Filtering subsections appeared to be the most impaired, unlike Tactile, Taste/Smell, Movement, Low Energy/Weak, and Visual-Auditory subsections, which turned out to be points of strength. The strengths of the ASD-W subgroup seem to be Movement, Low Energy/Weak, and Visual/Auditory sensitivity, unlike Under-responsive/Seeks sensation, Auditory Filtering, and Taste/Smell subsections, which turned out to be strongly impaired.

Results from our study might offer some suggestions about the opportunity to include individualized sensory training within the psychoeducational treatments. Whereas these trainings seem to be useful for ASD-WO children with no typical performance, they become essential for children with ASD-W, because of their generalized sensory dysfunctioning that requires a multisensory stimulation treatment. The multisensory stimulation treatment should be individually designed to decrease the functional limitations due to the impaired sensory modulation and should involve active participation of children to produce adaptive responses. A play context might encourage children participation. Individualized sensory trainings might provide multiple benefits: (1) normalizing the deficient responses to tactile, olfactory and tasting stimuli, so as to provide the opportunity for learning adequate mealtime behaviors and other functional self-care skills; (2) providing the appropriate required level of sensory stimulation—through Applied Behavior Analysis procedures—that would replace sensations typically experienced from repetitive behaviors or stereotypies; (3) capturing and maintaining attention on the provided stimuli (especially auditory stimuli); (4) using visual/auditory and kinesthetic stimulation (in which the ASD-W children appear to be more adapted) as a bridge to more easily accept sensory stimuli generally avoided.

Our study has some limitations: first of all, the absence of a TD control group. The comparison with TD peers would highlight any statistically significant differences with ASD sensory profiles, especially for the ASD-WO subjects, who showed more adaptive sensory responsiveness. Second, the absence of other clinical control groups, for example peers with ID, with and without feeding problems, that might allow us to better understand whether different clinical populations would show different sensory profiles. To this regard, for example, McCormick et al. [7] did not find any differences between ASD and Developmentally Delayed children in the SSP total scores, except for Taste/Smell and Visual/Auditory sensitivities. Third, the relatively small sample size, especially the ASD-W subgroup: a future study with larger samples might confirm the similarities and differences found here between ASD-W and ASD-WO sensory profiles; moreover, larger samples might be useful to establish whether changes in the sensory processing occur across different age ranges. Finally, our sample mainly included children with moderate to severe disorder (predominantly showing severity levels 2 and 3), therefore our results might be not generalizable to ASD children with a severity level 1. Fourth, to investigate children's response to sensory stimuli we used only questionnaires to parents, that present a certain degree of subjectivity. More psychophysical investigations are needed in order to decrease the subjectivity of data, although the biological mechanisms underlying sensory processing are not easy to determine due to the heterogeneity of the disorder and the difficulty in applying physiological measures to low functioning and little collaborating subjects.

5. Conclusions

We were able to confirm our original hypothesis of the existence of a significant correlation between sensory and feeding problems in ASD. We may suggest that ASD-W children show a more severe and more extensive impaired sensory processing than ASD-WO children, and that feeding behaviors of children with autism are affected not only by Taste/Smell, but also by multiple sensory experiences. ASD-W and ASD-WO subgroups showed a Hyporesponsive profile. Both subgroups showed impairments in Under-responsive/Seeks sensation and Auditory Filtering, more marked in ASD-W than in ASD-WO children. Taste/Smell sensitivity was strongly impaired only in ASD-W, whereas in ASD-WO subgroup it turned out to be a strength. ASD-W showed a more severe impairment also in Tactile sensitivity. Both subgroups showed strengths in Visual/Auditory sensitivity, Low-Energy/Weak, and Movement sensitivity, though more marked in ASD-WO. Based on our results, some useful suggestions on sensory trainings and psychoeducational treatments might be provided. However, a deeper knowledge of sensory dysfunctions in larger samples of ASD-W and ASD-WO children would be desirable for better orienting psychoeducational treatments by providing pointly suggestions about specific and individualized sensory trainings.

Author Contributions: Conceptualization, S.P. and M.E.; Data curation, V.C., M.Z., D.R., D.G. and D.F.; Formal analysis, S.P. and R.F.; Methodology, S.P.; Supervision, R.F.; Writing—original draft, S.P.; Writing—review & editing, S.P., R.F. and M.E. All authors have read and agreed to the published version of the manuscript.

Funding: This study was funded by the Italian Ministry of Health (Ricerca Corrente 2018–2020, Project No. 2757322).

Acknowledgments: We acknowledge the valuable contribution of all families who joined the study. We are grateful to Rosa Di Giorgio for her contribution to the final version of this paper. We are also grateful to the "I Corrieri dell'Oasi" Professional Team–Enna and Adrano (Psychologists, Pedagogues, Professional Educators, Speech-therapists, Psychomotor Therapists, Rehabilitation Therapists, Occupational Therapists, Art Teachers, and Health Care Assistants), to Danila Polizzi (Pedagogue), and Michele Lipani (Coordinator of the Center for Diagnosis and EIT for children with ASD-Caltanissetta).

Conflicts of Interest: The authors have no conflict of interest to declare.

References

1. Watling, R.; Deitz, J.; White, O. Comparison of sensory profile scores of young children with and without autism spectrum disorders. *Am. J. Occup. Ther.* **2001**, *55*, 416–423. [CrossRef] [PubMed]
2. Leekam, S.R.; Nieto, C.; Libby, S.J.; Wing, L.; Gould, J. Describing the sensory abnormalities of children and adults with autism. *J. Autism Dev. Disord.* **2007**, *37*, 894–910. [CrossRef] [PubMed]
3. Tomchek, S.D.; Dunn, W. Sensory processing in children with and without autism: A comparative study using the short sensory profile. *Am. J. Occup. Ther.* **2007**, *61*, 190–200. [CrossRef] [PubMed]
4. Suarez, M.A. Sensory processing in children with autism spectrum disorders and impact on functioning. *Pediatr. Clin. N. Am.* **2012**, *59*, 203–214. [CrossRef]
5. Brockevelt, B.L.; Nissen, R.; Schweinle, W.E.; Kurtz, E.; Larson, K.J. A comparison of the Sensory Profile scores of children with autism and an age- and gender-matched sample. *S. D. J. Med.* **2013**, *66*, 463–465.
6. Green, D.; Chandler, S.; Charman, T.; Simonoff, E.; Baird, G. Brief Report: DSM-5 Sensory behaviours in children with and without an Autism Spectrum Disorder. *J. Autism Dev. Disord.* **2016**, *46*, 3597–3606. [CrossRef]
7. McCormick, C.; Hepburn, S.; Young, G.S.; Rogers, S.J. Sensory symptoms in children with autism spectrum disorder, other developmental disorders and typical development: A longitudinal study. *Autism* **2016**, *20*, 572–579. [CrossRef]
8. Miller, L.J.; Anzalone, M.E.; Lane, S.; Cermak, S.A.; Osten, E. Concept evolution in sensory integration: A proposed nosology for diagnosis. *Am. J. Occup. Ther.* **2007**, *61*, 135–140. [CrossRef]
9. Ausderau, K.; Sideris, J.; Furlong, M.; Little, L.; Bulluck, J.C.; Baranek, G.T. National survey of sensory features in children with ASD: Factor structure of the sensory experience questionnaire (3.0). *J. Autism Dev. Disord.* **2014**, *44*, 915–925. [CrossRef]
10. Baranek, G.T.; David, F.J.; Poe, M.D.; Stone, W.L.; Watson, L.R. Sensory Experiences Questionnaire: Discriminating sensory features in young children with autism, developmental delays, and typical development. *J. Child Psychol. Psychiatry* **2006**, *47*, 591–601. [CrossRef]
11. Lane, A.E.; Young, R.L.; Baker, A.E.; Angley, M.T. Sensory processing subtypes in autism: Association with adaptive behavior. *J. Autism Dev. Disord.* **2010**, *40*, 112–122. [CrossRef] [PubMed]
12. Liss, M.; Saulnier, C.; Fein, D.; Kinsbourne, M. Sensory and attention abnormalities in autistic spectrum disorders. *Autism* **2006**, *10*, 155–172. [CrossRef] [PubMed]
13. Ausderau, K.K.; Furlong, M.; Sideris, J.; Bulluk, J.; Little, L.M.; Watson, L.R.; Boyd, B.A.; Belger, A.; Dickie, V.A.; Baranek, G.T. Sensory subtypes in children with autism spectrum disorder: Latent profile transition analysis using a national survey of sensory features. *J. Child Psychol. Psychiatry* **2014**, *55*, 935–944. [CrossRef] [PubMed]
14. Ben-Sasson, A.; Hen, L.; Fluss, R.; Cermak, S.A.; Engel-Yeger, B.; Gal, E. A meta-analysis of sensory modulation symptoms in individuals with autism spectrum disorders. *J. Autism Dev. Disord.* **2009**, *39*, 1–11. [CrossRef]
15. Ashburner, J.; Ziviani, J.; Rodger, S. Sensory processing and classroom emotional, behavioral, and educational outcomes in children with autism spectrum disorder. *Am. J. Occup. Ther.* **2008**, *62*, 564–573. [CrossRef]
16. Wiggins, L.D.; Robins, D.L.; Bakeman, R.; Adamson, L.B. Brief report: Sensory abnormalities as distinguishing symptoms of autism spectrum disorders in young children. *J. Autism Dev. Disord.* **2009**, *39*, 1087–1091. [CrossRef]
17. Fernández-Andrés, M.I.; Pastor-Cerezuela, G.; Sanz-Cervera, P.; Tárraga-Mínguez, R. A comparative study of sensory processing in children with and without autism spectrum disorder in the home and classroom environments. *Res. Dev. Disabil.* **2015**, *38*, 202–212. [CrossRef]
18. Sanz-Cervera, P.; Pastor-Cerezuela, G.; González-Sala, F.; Tárraga-Mínguez, R.; Fernández-Andrés, M.I. Sensory processing in children with autism spectrum disorder and/or attention deficit/hyperactivity disorder in the home and classroom context. *Front. Psychol.* **2017**, *8*, 1772. [CrossRef]
19. Sanz-Cervera, P.; Pastor-Cerezuela, G.; Fernández-Andrés, M.I.; Tárraga-Mínguez, R. Sensory processing in children with autism spectrum disorder: Relationship with non-verbal IQ, autism severity and attention deficit/hyperactivity disorder symptomatology. *Res. Dev. Disabil.* **2015**, *45*, 188–201. [CrossRef]

20. Kargas, N.; López, B.; Reddy, V.; Morris, P. The relationship between auditory processing and restricted, repetitive behaviors in adults with autism spectrum disorders. *J. Autism Dev. Disord.* **2015**, *45*, 658–668. [CrossRef]
21. American Psychiatric Association. *Diagnostic and Statistical Manual of Mental Disorders*, 5th ed.; American Psychiatric Publishing: Arlington, VA, USA, 2013.
22. Balıkçi, Ö.S.; Çiyiltepe, M. Feeding problems of children with autism. *Int. J. Soc. Sci.* **2017**, *3*, 870–880. [CrossRef]
23. Smith, B.; Rogers, S.L.; Blisset, J.; Ludlow, A.K. The relationship between sensory sensitivity, food fussiness and food preferences in children with neurodevelopmental disorders. *Appetite* **2020**, *150*, 104643. [CrossRef] [PubMed]
24. Kodak, T.; Piazza, C.C. Assessment and behavioral treatment of feeding and sleeping disorders in children with autism spectrum disorders. *Child Adolesc. Psychiatr. Clin. N. Am.* **2008**, *17*, 887–905. [CrossRef] [PubMed]
25. Twachtman-Reilly, J.; Amaral, S.C.; Zebrowsk, P.P. Addressing feeding disorders in children on the autism spectrum in school- based settings: Physiological and behavioral issues. *Lang. Speech Hear. Serv.* **2008**, *39*, 261–272. [CrossRef]
26. Panerai, S.; Suraniti, G.S.; Catania, V.; Carmeci, R.; Elia, M.; Ferri, R. Improvements in mealtime behaviors of children with special needs following a day-center-based behavioral intervention for feeding problems. *Riv. Psichiatr.* **2018**, *53*, 299–308. [CrossRef]
27. Cermak, S.A.; Curtin, C.; Bandini, L.G. Food selectivity and sensory sensitivity in children with autism spectrum disorders. *J. Am. Diet. Assoc.* **2010**, *110*, 238–246. [CrossRef]
28. Zobel-Lachiusa, J.; Andrianopoulos, M.V.; Mailloux, Z.; Cermak, S.A. Sensory differences and mealtime behavior in children with Autism. *Am. J. Occup. Ther.* **2015**, *69*, 6905185050p1–6905185050p8. [CrossRef]
29. Nadon, G.; Feldman, D.E.; Dunn, W.; Gisel, E. Association of sensory processing and eating problems in children with autism spectrum disorders. *Autism Res. Treat.* **2011**, *2011*, 541926. [CrossRef]
30. Chistol, L.T.; Bandini, L.G.; Must, A.; Phillips, S.; Cermak, S.A.; Curtin, C. Sensory sensitivity and food selectivity in children with autism spectrum disorder. *J. Autism Dev. Disord.* **2018**, *48*, 583–591. [CrossRef]
31. Dunn, W. *The Sensory Profile: User's Manual*; Psychological Corporation: San Antonio, TX, USA, 1999.
32. Al-Heizan, M.O.; AlAbdulwahab, S.S.; Kachanathu, S.J.; Natho, M. Sensory processing dysfunction among Saudi children with and without autism. *J. Phys. Ther. Sci.* **2015**, *27*, 1313–1316. [CrossRef]
33. Lukens, C.T.; Linscheid, T.R. Development and validation of an inventory to assess mealtime behavior problems in children with autism. *J. Autism Dev. Disord.* **2008**, *38*, 342–352. [CrossRef] [PubMed]
34. DeMand, A.; Johnson, C.; Foldes, E. Psychometric Properties of the Brief Autism Mealtime Behaviors Inventory. *J. Autism Dev. Disord.* **2015**, *45*, 2667–2673. [CrossRef] [PubMed]
35. Wardle, J.; Guthrie, C.A.; Sanderson, S.; Rapoport, L. Development of the children's eating behaviour questionnaire. *J. Child Psychol. Psychiatry* **2001**, *42*, 963–970. [CrossRef] [PubMed]
36. McIntosh, D.N.; Miller, L.J.; Shyu, V. Development and validation of the short sensory profile (SSP). In *The Sensory Profile: Examiner's Manual*; Dunn, W., Ed.; The Psychological Corporation: San Antonio, TX, USA, 1999; pp. 59–73.
37. Little, L.M.; Freuler, A.C.; Houser, M.B.; Guckian, L.; Carbine, K.; David, F.J.; Baranek, G.T. Psychometric validation of the sensory experiences questionnaire. *Am. J. Occup. Ther.* **2011**, *65*, 207–210. [CrossRef] [PubMed]
38. Baranek, G.T.; Watson, L.R.; Boyd, B.A.; Poe, M.D.; David, F.J.; McGuire, L. Hyporesponsiveness to social and nonsocial sensory stimuli in children with autism, children with developmental delays, and typically developing children. *Dev. Psychopathol.* **2013**, *25*, 307–320. [CrossRef]
39. Baranek, G.T.; Boyd, B.A.; Poe, M.D.; David, F.J.; Watson, L.R. Hyperresponsive sensory patterns in young children with autism, developmental delay, and typical development. *Am. J. Ment. Retard.* **2007**, *112*, 233–245. [CrossRef]
40. Schoen, S.A.; Miller, L.J.; Green, K.E. Pilot study of the sensory over-responsivity scales: Assessment and inventory. *Am. J. Occup. Ther.* **2008**, *62*, 393–406. [CrossRef]
41. Ledford, J.R.; Gast, D.L. Feeding problems in children with autism spectrum disorders: A review. *Focus Autism Dev. Disabil.* **2006**, *21*, 153–166. [CrossRef]

42. Sharp, W.G.; Berry, R.C.; McCracken, C.; Nuhu, N.; Marvel, E.; Saulnier, C.A.; Klin, A.; Jones, W.; Jaquess, D.L. Feeding problems and nutrient intake in children with autism spectrum disorders: A meta-analysis and comprehensive review of the literature. *J. Autism Dev. Disord.* **2013**, *43*, 2159–2173. [CrossRef]
43. O'Donnell, S.; Deitz, J.; Kartin, D.; Nalty, T.; Dawson, G. Sensory processing, problem behavior, adaptive behavior, and cognition in preschool children with autism spectrum disorders. *Am. J. Occup. Ther.* **2012**, *66*, 586–594. [CrossRef]
44. Boudjarane, M.A.; Grandgeorge, M.; Marianowski, R.; Misery, L.; Lemonnier, E. Perception of odors and tastes in autism spectrum disorders: A systematic review of assessments. *Autism Res.* **2017**, *10*, 1045–1057. [CrossRef] [PubMed]
45. Bennetto, L.; Kuschner, E.S.; Hyman, S.L. Olfaction and taste processing in autism. *Biol. Psychiatry* **2007**, *62*, 1015–1021. [CrossRef] [PubMed]
46. Baum, S.H.; Stevenson, R.A.; Wallace, M.T. Behavioral, perceptual, and neural alterations in sensory and multisensory function in autism spectrum disorder. *Prog. Neurobiol.* **2015**, *134*, 140–160. [CrossRef] [PubMed]
47. Avery, J.A.; Ingeholm, J.E.; Wohltjen, S.; Collins, M.; Riddell, C.D.; Gotts, S.J.; Kenworthy, L.; Wallace, G.L.; Simmons, W.K.; Martin, A. Neural correlates of taste reactivity in autism spectrum disorder. *NeuroImage Clin.* **2018**, *19*, 38–46. [CrossRef] [PubMed]
48. Mikkelsen, M.; Wodka, E.L.; Mostofsky, S.H.; Puts, N.A.J. Autism spectrum disorder in the scope of tactile processing. *Dev. Cogn. Neurosci.* **2018**, *29*, 140–150. [CrossRef] [PubMed]
49. Koehler, L.; Fournel, A.; Albertowski, K.; Roessner, V.; Gerber, J.; Hummel, C.; Hummel, T.; Bensafi, M. Impaired odor perception in autism spectrum disorder is associated with decreased activity in olfactory cortex. *Chem. Senses* **2018**, *43*, 627–634. [CrossRef]
50. Lane, A.E.; Molloy, C.A.; Bishop, S.L. Classification of children with autism spectrum disorder by sensory subtype: A case for sensory-based phenotypes. *Autism Res.* **2014**, *7*, 322–333. [CrossRef]

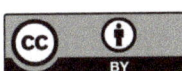

© 2020 by the authors. Licensee MDPI, Basel, Switzerland. This article is an open access article distributed under the terms and conditions of the Creative Commons Attribution (CC BY) license (http://creativecommons.org/licenses/by/4.0/).

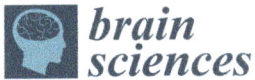 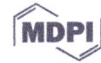

Article

Disentangling Restrictive and Repetitive Behaviors and Social Impairments in Children and Adolescents with Gilles de la Tourette Syndrome and Autism Spectrum Disorder

Mariangela Gulisano [1,*], Rita Barone [1], Salvatore Alaimo [2], Alfredo Ferro [2], Alfredo Pulvirenti [2], Lara Cirnigliaro [1], Selena Di Silvestre [1], Serena Martellino [1], Nicoletta Maugeri [1], Maria Chiara Milana [1], Miriam Scerbo [1] and Renata Rizzo [1]

[1] Child and Adolescent Psychiatric Section, Department of Clinical and Experimental Medicine, Catania University, Via Santa Sofia 78, 95123 Catania, Italy; rbarone@unict.it (R.B.); laracirnigliaro92@gmail.com (L.C.); selena_disilvestre@yahoo.it (S.D.S.); serena.martellino@live.it (S.M.); nico_maugeri@hotmail.it (N.M.); mariachiara.milana@gmail.com (M.C.M.); mimiscerbo@gmail.com (M.S.); rerizzo@unict.it (R.R.)
[2] Bioinformatics Unit, Department of Clinical and Experimental Medicine, Catania University, Viale Andrea Doria 6, 95125 Catania, Italy; alaimos@gmail.com (S.A.); ferro@dmi.unict.it (A.F.); apulvirenti@dmi.unict.it (A.P.)
* Correspondence: mariangelagulisano@gmail.com; Tel.: +39-328-7380-316; Fax: +39-095-3782-779

Received: 1 May 2020; Accepted: 15 May 2020; Published: 18 May 2020

Abstract: Gilles de la Tourette syndrome (GTS) and autism spectrum disorder (ASD) are two neurodevelopmental disorders with male predominance, frequently comorbid, that share clinical and behavioral features. The incidence of ASD in patients affected by GTS was reported to be between 2.9% and 22.8%. We hypothesized that higher ASD rates among children affected by GTS previously reported may be due to difficulty in discriminating GTS sub-phenotypes from ASD, and the higher scores in the restrictive and repetitive behaviors in particular may represent at least a "false comorbidity". We studied a large population of 720 children and adolescents affected by GTS ($n = 400$) and ASD ($n = 320$), recruited from a single center. Patients were all assessed with The Yale Global Tic Severity Rating Scale (YGTSS), The Autism Diagnostic Observation Schedule (ADOS), The Autism Diagnostic Interview Revised (ADI-R), The Children's Yale–Brown Obsessive–Compulsive Scale (CY-BOCS), and The Children's Yale–Brown Obsessive–Compulsive Scale for autism spectrum disorder (CY-BOCS ASD). Our results showed statistically significant differences in ADOS scores for social aspects between GTS with comorbid attention deficit hyperactivity disorder (ADHD) and obsessive–compulsive disorder (OCD) sub-phenotypes and ASD. No differences were present when we compared GTS with comorbid ASD sub-phenotype to ASD, while repetitive and restrictive behavior scores in ASD did not present statistical differences in the comparison with GTS and comorbid OCD and ASD sub-phenotypes. We also showed that CY-BOCS ASD could be a useful instrument to correctly identify OCD from ASD symptoms.

Keywords: autism spectrum disorder; Gilles de la Tourette; obsession; compulsion; social behavior; social impairment

1. Introduction

Autism spectrum disorder (ASD) is a neurodevelopmental disorder with an onset in early childhood characterized by persistent deficits in social communication and social interaction across multiple contexts alongside restricted and repetitive patterns of behavior and interests or activities [1].

Social problems are the most characteristic and persistent components of the behavioral phenotype. Autism is 4.5 times more common in males than in females. The prevalence of ASD is approximately 1% in the general population [2].

Gilles de la Tourette syndrome (GTS) is a neurodevelopmental disorder characterized by motor tics and at least one vocal tic that occurs for more than 1 year, with an age of onset before 18 years [1]. It is also characterized by male predominance. In addition to sharing some symptomatology and sexual dysmorphism, these disorders are commonly comorbid [3].

This comorbidity might partly reflect common etiological mechanisms in children and adolescents affected by GTS, and the strong heritability of both ASD and GTS implies genetic etiology [4]; the Brainstorm consortium (2018) reported shared heritability in both disorders [5]. However, another study examining the shared genetic etiology through analysis of heritability among brain phenotypes found common genetic variation across a number of neuropsychological disorders and proposed a specific relationship between GTS and ASD [6]. A large body of literature has convincingly shown that many similarities are present in genetic factors, functional and structural brain characteristics, and cognitive profiles. In particular, recent studies have found similar overlapping alterations of functional connectivity in ASD and GTS patients [7]. Compulsive attachment to routines and stereotypical behaviors in ASD are associated with changes in the corticostriatal circuitry especially involving the caudate [8]. Likewise, compulsions observed in obsessive–compulsive disorder (OCD) were shown to be associated with alteration of the orbitofrontal circuitry and caudate nucleus dysfunction [9].

The incidence of ASD in patients affected by GTS was reported to be between 2.9% and 4.9% in two clinical populations, using DSM-5 criteria for the diagnoses of both GTS and ASD [10,11]. The first study [10] analyzed the data of 3500 patients from the Tourette Syndrome International Database Consortium Registry that comprised 83 active sites, while the second reported a small group (35 patients) of Iranian children and adolescents aged 6–18 years [11].

More recently Huisman-van Dijk et al. and Darrow et al. [12,13] studied two large clinical cohorts of GTS patients and their family members using two screening instruments, the Autism Quotient and the Social Responsiveness Scale (SRS), to characterize ASD symptoms and reported a higher incidence of "probable" ASD between 20% and 22.8%.

Social communication and interaction challenges as well as the presence of functionally disabling restricted repetitive behaviors are characteristic of ASD. Symptoms such as obsessions, compulsive behaviors, echolalia and palilalia are common in both conditions [14].

Repetitive behaviors are observed in as many as 65% of patients with GTS and can be classified as "tic-like" or OCD-like symptoms according to clinical phenomenology [15]. Repetitive behaviors in ASD typically overlap with phenomena in GTS. It may be challenging to distinguish phenomenological characteristics of ASD from GTS. In clinical practice, medical professionals often struggle to define which disorder best describes the child's symptoms.

Our hypothesis is that higher ASD rates among children affected by GTS reported by Darrow et al. [13] and Huiss Van Dick et al. [12] may be due to the difficulty in discriminating complex tics and OCD symptoms from ASD symptoms, and the higher scores in the repetitive behaviors in particular may represent at least a "false comorbidity".

The primary aim of this study was to disentangle repetitive behavior features and social impairment in two large populations from a single center, GTS patients compared to ASD patients. Specifically, we aimed to determine whether features related to autism as measured by ADOS subscales and CY-BOCS differ for GTS sub-phenotype patients in relation to ASD.

2. Materials and Methods

2.1. Patient Selection

Participants were recruited from a larger database on clinical and molecular features of GTS and ASD that was assembled over a twenty-year period and is still being updated.

Participants in the present study were 720 children and adolescents with a primary diagnosis of GTS or ASD, according to DSM-5 criteria (APA 2013), recruited from January 2016 to February 2019 at the outpatient clinic of the Child and Adolescent Neuropsychiatry Unit at Catania University Hospital. We excluded patients who showed 1) evidence of primary psychiatric disorders different from GTS or ASD and 2) severe neurological or physical impairments or who were minimally verbal.

2.2. Procedures

The study was approved by the local Ethics Committee. Investigations were carried out as part of the routine clinical care of the patients in accordance with the ethical standards laid down in the 1964 Declaration of Helsinki and its later amendments (Helsinki Declaration 1975, revision 2013). All parents gave written informed consent, and the subjects assented when possible. All patients underwent physical examination and blood and urine analyses to rule out systemic diseases (e.g., inherited metabolic disorders). Diagnoses of GTS and comorbid disorders and ASD were performed according to DSM5 criteria, and neuropsychological evaluation was carried out by an expert team of child and adolescent neurologists, supervised by R.R., M.G., and R.B.

2.3. Measures

All parents participated in a medical history interview to determine prenatal, perinatal, and psychosocial risk factors as well as socio-economic status. Before inclusion in the study, all patients were screened with the Schedule for affective disorders and Schizophrenia for School age children—present and lifetime (Kiddie-SADS-PL) to rule out primary psychiatric disorders considered as criteria of exclusion. The Kiddie-SADS-PL is a semi-structured interview tool developed by Kauffman et al. (1997) that can be used in children and adolescents aged between 6–18 years [16]. This evaluation includes fundamental diagnosis of various psychiatric disorders. All patients underwent neuropsychological evaluation for GTS and related comorbidities.

2.3.1. Tics

To assess tic disorders, the National Hospital Interview Schedule for GTS (NHIS) [17], a semi-structured interview was used to diagnose GTS and its associated conditions, behaviors, and relevant family history. The Yale Global Tic Severity Rating Scale (YGTSS) [18] is an 11-item clinician rated interview that is able to evaluate motor and phonic tic severity considering the number, frequency, and impairments that tics are able to provoke in the patient. The score of the YGTSS ranges from 0 to 100, including the impairment section. Higher scores indicate greater severity of symptoms and impairment.

2.3.2. Obsessive–Compulsive Disorder

To evaluate OCD, the Children's Yale–Brown Obsessive–Compulsive Scale (CY-BOCS) [19] and the ASD CY-BOCS [20] were used. The CY-BOCS is a semi-structured interview conducted principally with parents, even if patients are encouraged to participate. This interview is able to assess the severity of obsessive–compulsive symptoms in children. The total score of CY-BOCS ranges between 0 and 40. It is possible to evaluate an obsession and a compulsion score separately. Higher scores indicate greater severity of symptoms and impairment.

2.3.3. Autism Spectrum Disorder

The Autism Diagnostic Observation Schedule (ADOS) [21] was used for ASD diagnosis. The ADOS is a standardized evaluation scale that is considered the gold standard for the diagnosis of ASD. It is structured in four domains of exploration (A), social interaction (B), imagination (C), and repetitive and stereotyped behaviors (D). Items are scored from 0 to 3 on the basis of severity (3: more severe).

The ADOS provides a total score and partial scores related to Social Affect (SA) and Restricted, Repetitive Behavior (RRB).

The Autism Diagnostic Interview Revised (ADI-R) [22] is a structured interview conducted with the parents/guardians. Its purpose is to investigate the same areas of ADOS based on the judgment of parents/guardians with respect to their children's symptoms. Items are scored from 0 to 3 on the basis of severity (3: more severe).

The Children Yale Brown Obsessive–Compulsive Scale for Autism Spectrum Disorder is a semi-structured interview conducted with patients and parents that was developed after CY-BOCS by Schahill et al. (2014) to detect the differences between obsession and compulsion in OCD and repetitive and restrictive behaviors, interests, and stereotypes in ASD [20]. For this purpose, the scale is structured with a Symptom Checklist (behavior present or absent) and five sub-schedules (Time Spent, Interference, Distress, Resistance, and Control). Each item ranges from 0 (not present) to 4 (severe), and the total score is between 0 and 20. The interview includes a symptom checklist of possible repetitive behaviors grouped into eight categories (e.g., washing rituals, checking behaviors). Each category allows the interviewer to describe "other" behaviors presumed relevant to that overall category. The severity of each item is anchored to the past week and scored from 0 (not present) to 4 (severe) for a total score of 0 to 20 [20].

2.4. Statistical Analysis

Clinical covariates were identified within each psycho-diagnostic class that might be able to detect affected subjects and their comorbidities from healthy individuals. Analyzed psycho-diagnostic classes included ADI-R, ADOS, YGTSS, CY-BOCS, and CY-BOCS ASD.

The identification of class-specific clinical covariates, which have statistically different values, is a fundamental process to identify common elements among different conditions and to stratify affected subjects according to comorbidities. For this purpose, we employed the R software suite to perform statistical analyses using a two-sided t-test or ANOVA and to build a risk classification model based on C-Tree Induction [23].

Risk models were developed with the use of decision-tree induction from class-labeled training records, i.e., the training set was composed of records in which one attribute was the class label (or dependent variable), and the remaining attributes were the predictor variables; the individual records were the tuples for which the class label was known.

The aim of this analysis was the objective identification of the classification power of evaluation metrics used in the context of Gilles de la Tourette syndrome and the assessment of a joint model to distinguish between pure GTS, GTS plus comorbidities, and ASD. For this purpose, the usage of a classification model is crucial to study the predictive power of a set of diagnostic metrics. The classification, starting from the characteristics (in our case the independent variables are those reported in Table 1), named predictor variables, of the examined subjects, aims to infer a set of rules allowing the prediction of covariate values, named class labels (or dependent variables). Each node of the tree analyzes a covariate by computing an optimal binary split. The goodness of the split is supported by a two-sample statistical test based on a permutation analysis.

In our study the objective was to distinguish six different classes: GTS, GTS + OCD, GTS + attention deficit hyperactivity disorder (ADHD), GTS + OCD + ADHD, GTS + ASD, and ASD.

The performance of the classification model was analyzed, randomly splitting the data in the training set (2/3 of the records) and the testing Set (1/3 of the records); this partition was repeated 100 times, and the classification accuracy was taken as the average of each accuracy measurement. All differences were considered statistically significant at a 5% probability level.

Table 1. Demographic and clinical features.

	GTS (pt 400)	ASD (pt 320)
M/F	274/62	196/37
Mean age	11.4 (± 3.1)	11.1 (± 3.5)
IQ		
TIQ	91.7 (± 17.9)	77.2 (± 24.4)
PIQ	91.61 (± 18.0)	79.1 (± 24)
VIQ	92.87 (± 18.5)	77.7 (± 25.1)
YGTSS	19.54 (± 9.4)	1.4 (± 2.6)
CY-BOCS	15.61 (± 10.9)	13,9 (± 11,3)
CY-BOCS ASD	6.2 (± 4.4)	17 (± 3.2)

GTS: Gilles de la Tourette Syndrome; ASD: Autism Spectrum Disorder; CY-BOCS: Children Yale Brown Obsessive–Compulsive Scale; CY-BOCS ASD: Children Yale Brown Obsessive–Compulsive Scale for Autism Spectrum Disorder; YGTSS: Yale Global Tic Severity Scale; TIQ: Total Intelligence Quotient; PIQ: Performance Intelligence Quotient; VIQ: Verbal Intelligence Quotient.

3. Results

We recruited a clinical cohort of 720 patients aged 6–18 years, mean age 11.3 (±3.3) years. Of this cohort, 400 subjects were affected by GTS. They were 274 males and 62 females, with a mean age of 11.4 (±3.1) years. Patients with ASD (n = 320) included 196 males and 37 females, with a mean age of 11.1 (±3.5). Demographic and clinical characteristics of the study samples are reported in Table 1. The GTS clinical cohort had a significantly higher mean IQ (91.7 ± 17.9) than that of the ASD patients (77.2 ± 24.4) (Table 1).

Nearly all subjects with GTS presented at least one comorbidity. The results of the neuropsychological evaluation enabled assessment of GTS clinical sub-phenotypes distributed as follows: GTS only (15.5%), GTS + ADHD (32%), GTS + OCD (33.5%), GTS + ADHD + OCD (10.25%), and GTS + ASD (8.9%). GTS sub-phenotypes were compared to the ASD clinical group.

3.1. Yale Global Tic Severity Rating Scale

GTS patients presented a mean YGTSS total score of 19.5 (±9.4). The YGTSS score in the GTS clinical sub-phenotypes was as follows: pure GTS, 16.1 (±7); GTS+ADHD, 19.1 (±1); GTS+OCD, 22.2 (±9.7); GTS + ADHD + OCD, 25.9 (±9); and GTS + ASD, 11.7 (±3.2). The ASD group presented a mean YGTSS of 2.3 (±1.8). Statistically significant differences were observed in the comparisons of YGTSS scores between the GTS sub-phenotypes and ASD clinical cohort ($p < 0.001$) (see Figure 1 and Table 2).

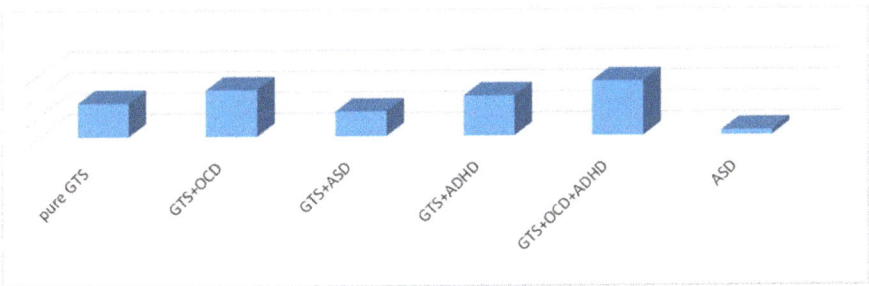

Figure 1. YGTSS score between clinical groups. GTS: Gilles de la Tourette Syndrome; ASD: Autism Spectrum Disorder; OCD: Obsessive–Compulsive Disorder; ADHD: Attention Deficit Hyperactivity Disorder; YGTSS: Yale Global Tic Severity Scale.

Table 2. Comparison between mean YGTSS values in each sub-phenotype and statistical significance.

	GTS Only	GTS + OCD	GTS + ASD	GTS + ADHD	GTS + OCD + ADHD	ASD	*p*-Value
YGTSS	16.1 (±7)	22.2 (±9.7)	11.7 (3.2)	19.1 (±1)	25.9 (±9.6)	2.3 (±108)	0.0005

GTS: Gilles de la Tourette Syndrome; ASD: Autism Spectrum Disorder; OCD: Obsessive–Compulsive Disorder; ADHD: Attention Deficit Hyperactivity Disorder; YGTSS: Yale Global Tic Severity Scale.

3.2. Children's Yale–Brown Obsessive–Compulsive Scale

GTS patients presented a mean CY-BOCS of 15.6 (±1). With regard to GTS clinical sub-phenotypes, the following mean CY-BOCS scores were computed: pure GTS, 7.6 (±6); GTS + ADHD, 9.9 (±7.8); GTS + OCD, 23.5 (±8.3); GTS + ADHD + OCD, 27.1 (±1); and GTS + ASD, 12.1 (±6.1). ASD patients presented a mean CY-BOCS score of 17.9 (±3.1) (Figure 2, Table 3).

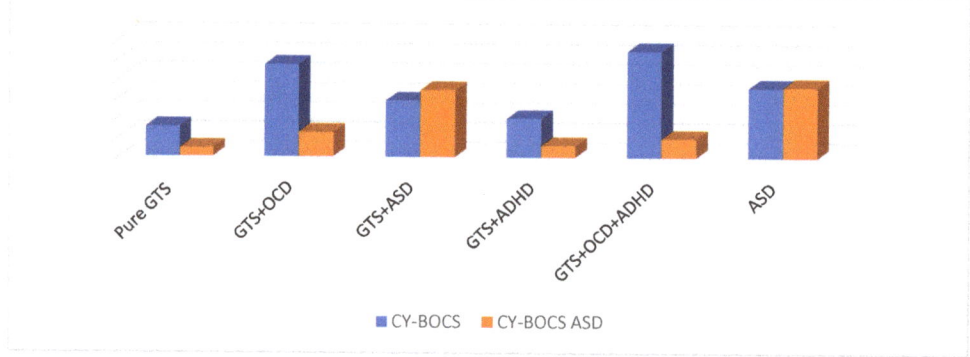

Figure 2. Comparison between CY-BOCS and CY-BOCS ASD scores between clinical groups. GTS: Gilles de la Tourette Syndrome; ASD: Autism Spectrum Disorder; OCD: Obsessive–Compulsive Disorder; ADHD: Attention Deficit Hyperactivity Disorder; CY-BOCS: Children Yale Brown Obsessive–Compulsive Scale; CY-BOCS ASD: Children Yale Brown Obsessive–Compulsive Scale for Autism Spectrum Disorder.

Table 3. Comparison between mean values of measures in each sub-phenotype and statistical significance.

	Pure GTS	GTS + OCD	GTS + ASD	GTS + ADHD	GTS + OCD + ADHD	ASD	*p*-Value
CY-BOCS	7.6 (±6)	23.5 (±8.3)	14.4 (9.3)	9.9 (±7.8)	27.1 (±1)	17.9 ± 3.1	0.0005
CY-BOCS ASD	2.2 (±1.9)	6.2 (±4.4)	17.1 (4.1)	3 (±1.9)	4.8 (±2.1)	18.1 ± 3.2	0.0005

GTS: Gilles de la Tourette Syndrome; ASD: Autism Spectrum Disorder; OCD: Obsessive–Compulsive Disorder; ADHD: Attention Deficit Hyperactivity Disorder; CY-BOCS: Children Yale Brown Obsessive–Compulsive Scale; CY-BOCS ASD: Children Yale Brown Obsessive–Compulsive Scale for Autism Spectrum Disorder.

3.3. Children's Yale–Brown Obsessive–Compulsive Scale: Autism Spectrum Disorder

GTS patients presented a mean CY-BOCS ASD of 6.2 (±4.4). In detail, GTS clinical sub-phenotypes presented the following mean scores: pure GTS, 2.2 (±1.9); GTS + ADHD, 2.9 (±1.9); GTS + OCD, 6.2 (±4.4); GTS + ADHD + OCD, 3.1 (±2.1); and GTS + ASD, 17.9 (±2.9). ASD patients presented a mean CY-BOCS ASD score of 18.1 (±3.2) (Figure 2, Table 3).

Figure 3 shows a decision tree. Among all the inferred models, we showed the one built as a function of the CY-BOCS ASD variable. Each internal node of the tree represents a statistical test (on such a variable, the two departing branches split the data according to the most discriminant threshold). These analyses revealed that when the score of CY-BOCS ASD was lower than 1, the analyses were able to detect GTS only, whereas when the CY-BOCS ASD score was higher than 14, the more represented clinical group was that with pure ASD, followed by GTS+ASD. However, the overall accuracy of the model is 46,35%, which means that this variable is not reliable for detection of GTS + comorbidities when its value is between 1 and 14.

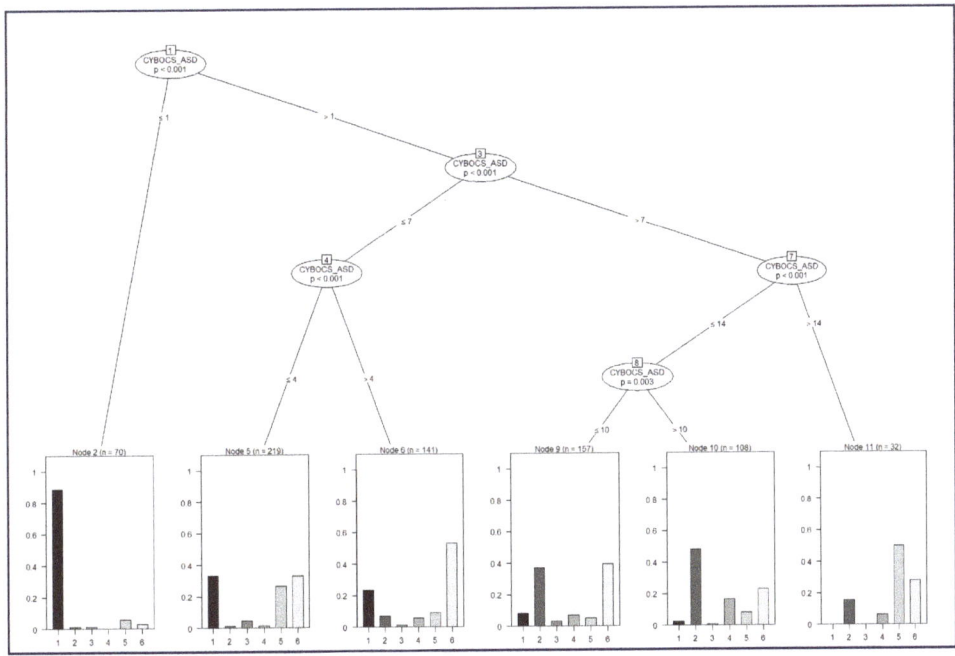

Figure 3. Decision tree. Clinical groups: 1: pure GTS; 2: GTS+ OCD; 3: GTS + ADHD; 4: GTS + ADHD + OCD + OCD; 5: GTS + ASD; 6 ASD.

3.4. Autism Diagnostic Observation Schedule

For all ADOS scales, ASD and GTS + ASD presented scores that fulfilled the diagnosis of ASD. No significant differences in scores were observed between these groups. In contrast, GTS presented significantly lower mean scores in ADOS scales compared to those of ASD and GTS + ASD.

With regard to ADOS-SA "Social Interaction", "Imagination", and "Communication, Language, and Behavior", the GTS sub-phenotypes always presented significantly lower scores than ASD and GTS + ASD sub-phenotypes. When ADOS-RR subscale scores of "restricted and repetitive behaviors" from the GTS sub-phenotype were analyzed in detail, different results related to the compared groups in each ADOS subscale were computed. In particular, no significant differences were detected when comparing GTS sub-phenotypes and ASD as follows: GTS + ASD vs. GTS + OCD in D3 (repetitive and stereotyped behavior) and D4 (compulsions); GTS + ASD vs. GTS + OCD + ADHD in D4 (compulsion); ASD vs. GTS + OCD in D1 (unusual interests), D3 (repetitive and stereotyped behavior), and D4 (compulsions) (Figure 4 and Table 4).

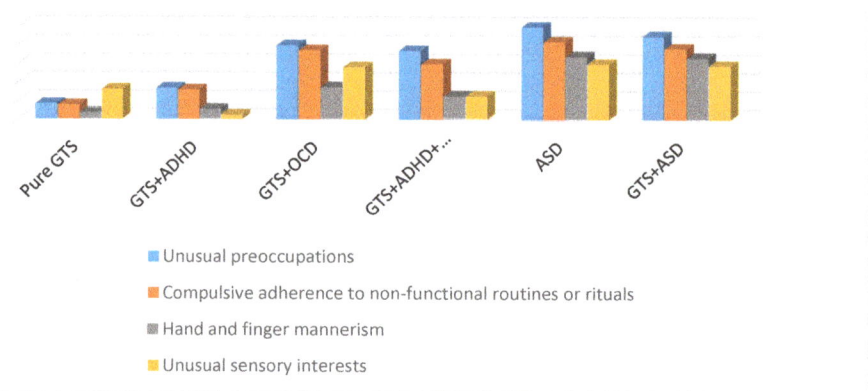

Figure 4. ADOS (D scale) restricted and repetitive behaviors: comparison between clinical sub-phenotypes. GTS: Gilles de la Tourette Syndrome; ASD: Autism Spectrum Disorder; OCD: Obsessive–Compulsive Disorder; ADHD: Attention Deficit Hyperactivity Disorder.

Table 4. ADOS Restricted and repetitive behaviors (D Scale): statistical significance in comparison with clinical sub-phenotypes.

	D. Total	D1	D2	D3	D4
"GTS + ASD" vs. "Pure GTS"	0.0005	0.0005	0.0005	0.0005	0.0005
"GTS + ASD" vs. "GTS + OCD"	0.0045	0.0205	0.0005	0.3828	0.9716
"GTS + ASD" vs. "GTS + ADHD"	0.0051	0.0095	0.0061	0.0065	0.0051
"GTS + ASD" vs. "GTS + OCD + ADHD"	0.0002	0.0071	0.0005	0.0005	0.7991
"ASD" vs. "Pure GTS"	0.0005	0.0005	0.0005	0.0005	0.0061
"ASD" vs. "GTS + OCD"	0.0065	0.1287	0.0005	0.6742	0.7789
"ASD" vs. "GTS + ADHD"	0.0005	0.0005	0.0054	0.0067	0.0065
"ASD" vs. "GTS + OCD + ADHD"	0.0005	0.0005	0.0005	0.0005	0.0005

GTS: Gilles de la Tourette Syndrome; ASD: Autism Spectrum Disorder; OCD: Obsessive–Compulsive Disorder; ADHD: Attention Deficit Hyperactivity Disorder. D1: unusual interests; D2: hand mannerisms and complex mannerisms; D3: repetitive and stereotyped behavior items; D4: compulsions. * represents a statistically significant p-value <0.05.

3.5. Autism Diagnostic Interview Revised

For all ADI-R scales, ASD and GTS + ASD presented scores that fulfilled the diagnosis of ASD. No significant differences in ADI-R scores were found between these groups. Pure GTS ADI-R scores did not fulfill the diagnosis of ASD and were significantly lower compared to those of ASD and GTS + ASD. Regarding the ADI-R scale "Restricted and Repetitive Behaviors" (C scale), no significant differences were detected when comparing GTS sub-groups and ASD as follows: GTS + ASD vs. GTS + OCD in C1 (unusual preoccupations), C2 (rituals), C3 (mannerism), and C4 (unusual interests); GTS + OCD vs. ASD in C2 (rituals) (Figure 5 and Table 5).

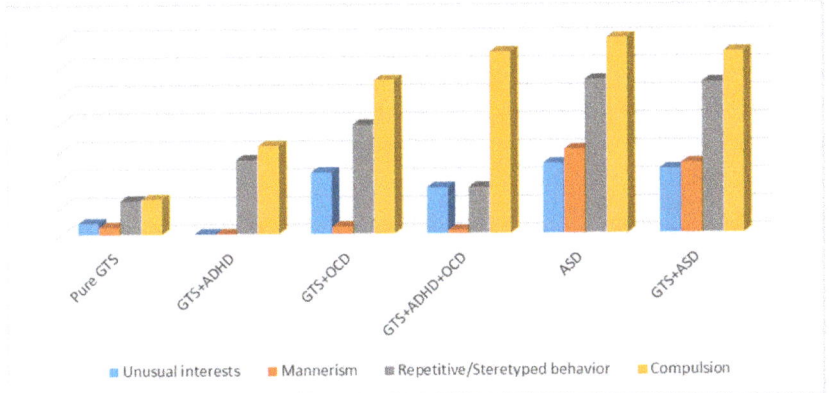

Figure 5. ADI-R, Restricted and Repetitive Behaviors (C Scale): comparison between clinical sub-phenotypes.

Table 5. ADI Restricted and repetitive behaviors (C): comparison between GTS clinical sub-phenotypes.

	C Total	C1	C2	C3	C4
"GTS + ASD" vs. "Pure GTS"	0.0005	0.0005	0.0005	0.0005	0.0005
"GTS + ASD" vs. "GTS + OCD"	0.0155	0.7586	0.4183	0.1235	0.0956
"GTS + ASD" vs. "GTS + ADHD"	0.0005	0.0005	0.0335	0.0005	0.0005
"GTS + ASD" vs. "GTS + OCD + ADHD"	0.0335	0.1924	0.1639	0.001	0.0205
"ASD" vs. "Pure GTS"	0.0005	0.0005	0.0005	0.0005	0.0005
"ASD" vs. "GTS + OCD"	0.0032	0.0038	0.2365	0.0042	0.0005
"ASD" vs. "GTS + ADHD"	0.0005	0.0005	0.0005	0.0005	0.0005
"ASD" vs. "GTS + OCD + ADHD"	0.0005	0.0005	0.0005	0.0005	0.0005

C1: unusual preoccupations; C2: compulsive adherence to non-functional routines or rituals; C3: hand and finger mannerisms; C4: unusual sensory interests; GTS: Gilles de la Tourette Syndrome; ASD: Autism Spectrum Disorder; OCD: Obsessive–Compulsive Disorder; ADHD: Attention Deficit Hyperactivity Disorder. * represents a statistically significant $p < 0.05$.

4. Discussion

Along with a deficit in social communication and interaction, restricted and repetitive behaviors constitute the defining core features of ASD; however, GTS also shares RRB and social communication and interaction problems with ASD.

In this study, we explored the prevalence and pattern of ASD symptoms in relation to GTS and other comorbid disorders, comparing the two distinct cohorts of individuals affected by GTS and ASD. We systematically assessed a large sample of children and adolescents affected by GTS and compared them to an ASD group of children and adolescents with verbal capacity.

As our primary hypothesis was that the higher percentage of ASD in GTS recently reported by other authors [12,13] showed a false comorbidity due to overlap between symptoms that were in common in both conditions, the study examined the degree to which the gold standard instruments for autism diagnosis, the ADI-R and ADOS, disentangle restrictive and repetitive behaviors and social impairment in children and adolescents affected by GTS and ASD and verify the hypothesis that, in particular, the presence of GTS + OCD and related symptoms could mimic ASD symptoms. The patients were also assessed by CY-BOCS and CY-BOCS ASD to investigate the overlap between ASD symptoms and GTS in affected individuals.

The results supported these hypotheses by indicating that higher ASD rates reported in other samples may be due to the confounding of tic or OCD symptoms for ASD or vice versa. In our samples of children and adolescents, 8.9% of patients affected by GTS presented comorbid ASD, in contrast with the incidences of 20% and 28% reported by Darrow et al. and Huisman-van Dijk et al., respectively [12,13].

In particular, when we compared ADOS and ADI-R with GTS and ASD, for ADOS scores, we did not observe any significant differences between GTS + ASD and GTS + OCD in D3 (repetitive and stereotyped behavior) and D4 (compulsions); GTS + ASD and GTS + OCD + ADHD in D4 (compulsion); or ASD and GTS + OCD in D1 (unusual interests), D3 (repetitive and stereotyped behavior), and D4 (compulsions). When examining ADI-R, no significant differences were detected between GTS + ASD and GTS + OCD in C1 (unusual preoccupations), C2 (rituals), C3 (mannerism), and C4 (unusual interests); GTS + ASD and GTS + OCD + ADHD in C1 (unusual preoccupations); and GTS + OCD and ASD in C2 (rituals).

Darrow et al. (2017) studied 535 GTS patients and used the Social Responsiveness Scale Second Edition (SRS) as a measure of ASD symptoms. The SRS contains five treatment subscales including the following domains: social awareness, social cognition, social communication (SC), social interaction (SCI), and restricted interests and repetitive behaviors (RRB).

When they examined the relationship between SRS total score and GTS sub-phenotypes, there were significant differences in SRS scores among the different classes. The highest SRS scores were found in the two classes that endorsed OCD symptoms (GTS + OCD + ADHD, OCD symmetry). These two classes had significantly higher SC and RRB scores than the other classes.

Our findings show that GTS + OCD and GTS + ASD sub-phenotypes were in line with this work; however, they reported a higher percentage (23%) of GTS-affected participants that met the cut-off criteria for probable ASD (83% of whom also met criteria for OCD). In our opinion this is because, as stated in previous studies, children [24] with mood and anxiety disorders have elevated rates of ASD based on SRS cut-off criteria, suggesting that some of the elevation in SRS scores may reflect underlying psychiatric impairment rather than being specific to ASD.

The fact that scores for the RRB subscales were higher for individuals who had OCD symptoms suggests that these SRS subscales may in fact be tapping into common repetitive behaviors in individuals with GTS and/or OCD that could be confused with stereotypies seen in ASD [13]

This is also supported by Huisman-van Dijk et al. (2016) in their significant paper, where items measuring repetitive behaviors in autism were loaded into a factor with OCD related items rather than into a factor with social communication items. Interestingly, the autism factor including lack of social skills as well as non-functional child routines, attention switching problems, and lack of investigation was not related to any of the tic or OCD symptom factors. This autism dimension might be etiologically distinct from the second factor characterized by repetitive behaviors [12].

In our study, the differences between GTS + OCD, GTS + ASD, and ASD samples were significant except in the ADOS and ADI-R domains of restrictive and repetitive behaviors.

More recently, Eapen et al. [25] in a sample of 203 participants, 44 with GTS and 26 with ASD compared to the general sample of 133 with a mean age of 18.17 years, examined the occurrence of autism related features measured by the Social Communication Questionnaire (SCQ) focusing on areas of overlap and differences.

They found that the GTS sample had significantly higher mean SCQ scores than the general population but generally lower scores than the ASD sample. The group differences in mean SCQ scores between GTS and ASD samples were significant except in the domain of RRB.

Eapen et al. suggested that symptom overlap may represent a true overlap through a shared phenotype or that the overlap may be a phenocopy where the clinical symptoms, for example, complex tics and related obsessive–compulsive symptoms of GTS, may mimic ASD symptoms and vice versa where stereotypic and repetitive behaviors characteristic of ASD may mimic GTS. In their study on the domain level, they found a close concordance between the two disorders on restricted and repetitive behaviors and less on social communication.

These results are in line with our study. ADOS differences between GTS clinical sub-phenotypes and ASD were significant in social interaction, imagination, and communication language and behavior; when RRB was analyzed, there were no significant differences.

However, restricted and repetitive behaviors are some of the major impairments shown in ASD and GTS. Having a measure that disentangles these two domains easily in a clinical setting is important for the clinicians who may use it as a basis for their treatment recommendations. We also assessed our clinical sample with CY-BOCS and CY-BOCS ASD.

CY-BOCS had the unique ability to detect symptomatology that differed from ASD characteristics, whereas other measures assessing obsessive–compulsive symptoms did not [26].

Several original CY-BOCS checklist items are nevertheless irrelevant for children with ASD. However, the results of this study provide an incremental refinement for measuring repetitive behavior in children and adolescents with GTS and ASD. Nonetheless, certain repetitive behaviors in children with ASD may have been overlooked due to sample characteristics of children with verbal capacity and normal or mild intellectual disability. Lower-functioning or non-verbal children were more likely to engage in hand and finger stereotypy and object manipulation. With regard to obsession and compulsion measured with CY-BOCS, no significant differences were detected in the comparison of scores in ASD, GTS + OCD, and GTS + ASD patients in our sample.

CY-BOCS ASD results provided a reliable and valid measure of repetitive behavior in youths with ASD and underscored differences in repetitive behavior in ASD compared to GTS [20]. With CY-BOCS ASD, no significant differences were found between GTS + ASD and ASD groups. The score obtained in the GTS + OCD, compared to the ASD group and GTS +ASD, was significantly lower. The clinical implications of these findings are important for clinicians who may use the CY-BOCS ASD as a diagnostic tool. The CY-BOCS ASD yields a total score based on the impact of the symptoms present rather than subscale scores. The results suggest that the CY-BOCS ASD is a valid and reliable measure of repetitive behavior in youths with ASD [27]. It is easy to use in a clinical setting, and clinicians may use it as a basis for their treatment recommendations.

Limitations

The principal limitation of our study is that our Tourette Clinic is a tertiary level center. For this reason, we assessed and followed complicated cases that may have not been representative of the general population affected. The different sex distribution is a limitation of this sample because we analyzed two disorders with a high prevalence in males. Finally, another limitation was related to GTS sub-phenotype analysis and the comparison of GTS sub-phenotypes with ASD without comorbidities.

5. Conclusions

To conclude, the similarities largely contained within the RRS domain rather than across the RRS and social communication domains support our hypothesis that higher ASD rates among children affected by GTS may make it difficult to discriminate between specific features of GTS and ASD, contributing to the representation of a false comorbidity.

However, another possibility exists that certain symptoms may be duplicated due to environmental or other factors rather than due to a common genetic basis. The similarities could be due to a phenocopy rather than phenotypic overlap as suggested by Eapen et al. [25].

Genetic studies together with clinical task-based RMN functional studies could contribute to a better understanding of the underlying mechanism involved in the etiology of ASD and GTS and could be critical in obtaining better treatments.

Compared to their peers with GTS but not ASD, children with GTS and ASD have greater treatment needs (that are either unmet needs or treatment usage). This finding aligns with previous literature focused on children with ASD, which found high rates of service needs, particularly among children diagnosed with co-occurring conditions [28].

When symptoms are not correctly managed, more severe psychopathology may develop, alongside poorer interpersonal, school, family, and cognitive functioning and life outcomes among this population relative to that of controls. The possibility of individualizing symptoms to treat (e.g., compulsions, rituals, and repetitive behaviors) could improve the children's quality of life and, consequently, other social aspects of their life. To our knowledge, this is the first study on a large unique cohort that analyzed symptoms that could mimic diagnosis. ADOS and ADI-R are the gold standard scales for diagnosis, and they are always able to individualize diagnosis. However, it might be helpful to define differences that could individualize treatment and help clinicians in the management of specific patients with GTS and comorbid OCD. In line with previous research [20], we suggest refining ASD diagnosis by using CY-BOSC ASD to better distinguish repetitive behaviors from compulsion and rituals.

Author Contributions: Conceptualization, M.G. and R.R.; Data curation, M.G., R.B., L.C., S.D.S., S.M. and N.M.; Formal analysis, A.F. and A.P.; Investigation, M.C.M. and M.S.; Project administration, R.R.; Software, S.A., A.F. and A.P.; Writing—original draft, R.R.; Writing—review and editing, R.R., M.G. and R.B. All authors have read and agreed to the published version of the manuscript.

Funding: This research received no external funding.

Acknowledgments: This study was funded by the 2016/2018 Research Plan of the University of Catania, Department of Clinical and Experimental Medicine.

Conflicts of Interest: The authors declare that the research was conducted in the absence of any commercial or financial relationships that could be construed as potential conflicts of interest.

References

1. American-Psychiatric-Association. *Diagnostic and Statistical Manual of Mental Disorders*; American Psychiatric Publishing: Washington, DC, USA, 2013.
2. Lord, C.; Elsabbagh, M.; Baird, G.; Veenstra-Vanderweele, J. Autism spectrum disorder. *Lancet* **2018**, *392*, 508–520. [CrossRef]
3. Rapanelli, M.; Frick, L.M.; Pittenger, C. The role of interneurons in autism and Tourette syndrome. *Trends Neurosci.* **2017**, *40*, 397–407. [CrossRef] [PubMed]
4. State, M.W. The genetics of child psychiatric disorders: Focus on autism and Tourette syndrome. *Neuron* **2010**, *68*, 254–269. [CrossRef]
5. Benedicto, C.F. Analysis of shared heritability in common disorder of the brain in The Brainstorm Consortium. *Science* **2018**, *22*, 360.
6. Antilla, V.; Bullik-Sullivan, B.; Finucane, H.K. Analysys of shared heritability in common disorders of the brain. *BioRxiv* **2016**. [CrossRef]
7. Worbe, Y.; Marrakchi-Kacem, L.; Lecomte, S.; Valabregue, R.; Poupon, F.; Guevara, P.; Tucholka, A.; Mangin, J.F.; Vidailhet, M.; Lehericy, S.; et al. Altered structural connectivity of cortico-striato-pallido-thalamic networks in Gilles de la Tourette syndrome. *Brain* **2015**, *138*, 472–482. [CrossRef]
8. Langen, M.; Durston, S.; Kas, M.J.; Van Engeland, H.; Staal, W.G. The neurobiology of repetitive behavior: ... and men. *Neurosci. Biobehav. Rev.* **2011**, *35*, 356–365. [CrossRef]
9. Markarian, Y.; Larson, M.J.; Aldea, M.A.; Baldwin, S.A.; Good, D.; Berkeljon, A.; Murphy, T.K.; Storch, E.A.; McKay, D. Multiple pathways to functional impairment in obsessive-compulsive disorder. *Clin. Psychol. Rev.* **2010**, *30*, 78–88. [CrossRef]
10. Burd, L.; Li, Q.; Kerbeshian, J.; Klug, M.G.; Freeman, R.D. Tourette syndrome and comorbid pervasive developmental disorders. *J. Child Neurol.* **2009**, *24*, 170–175. [CrossRef]
11. Ghanizadeh, A.; Mosallaei, S. Psychiatric disorder and behavioral problems in children and adolescents with Tourette syndrome. *Brain Develop.* **2009**, *31*, 15–19. [CrossRef]
12. Huisman-van Dijk, H.M.; Schoot, R.V.; Rijkeboer, M.M.; Mathews, C.A.; Cath, D.C. The relationship between tics, OC, ADHD and autism symptoms: A cross-disorder symptom analysis in Gilles de la Tourette syndrome patients and family-members. *Psych. Res.* **2016**, *237*, 138–146. [CrossRef]

13. Darrow, S.M.; Grados, M.; Sandor, P.; Hirschtritt, M.E.; Illmann, C.; Osiecki, L.; Dion, Y.; King, R.; Pauls, D.; Budman, C.L.; et al. Autism spectrum symptoms in a Tourette syndrome sample. *J. Am. Acad. Child Adolesc. Psychiatry* **2017**, *56*, 610–617. [CrossRef] [PubMed]
14. Rizzo, R.; Gulisano, M.; Domini, C.N.; Ferro, M.C.; Curatolo, P. The relationship between autism spectrum disorder and tourette syndrome in childhood: An overview of shared characteristics. *J. Pediatr. Neurol.* **2017**, *15*, 115–122.
15. Worbe, Y.; Gerardin, E.; Hartmann, A.; Valabrégue, R.; Chupin, M.; Tremblay, L.; Vidailhet, M.; Colliot, O.; Lehéricy, S. Distinct structural changes underpin clinical phenotypes in patients with Gilles de la Tourette syndrome. *Brain* **2010**, *133*, 3649–3660. [CrossRef] [PubMed]
16. Kaufman, J.; Birmaher, B.; Brent, D.; Rao, U.; Flynn, C.; Moreci, P.; Williamson, D.; Ryan, N. Schedule for affective disorders and schizophrenia for school-age children-present and lifetime version (K-SADS-PL): Initial reliability and validity data. *J. Am. Acad. Child Adolesc. Psychiatry* **1997**, *36*, 980–988. [CrossRef]
17. Robertson, M.; Eapen, V. The National Hospital Interview Schedule for the assessment of Gilles de la Tourette syndrome. *Int. J. Methods Psychiatr. Res.* **1996**, *6*, 203–226. [CrossRef]
18. Leckman, J.F.; Riddle, M.A.; Hardin, M.T.; Ort, S.I.; Swartz, K.L.; Stevenson, J.; Cohen, D.J. The yale global tic severity scale: Initial testing of a clinician-rated scale of tic severity. *J. Am. Acad. Child Adolesc. Psychiatry* **1989**, *28*, 566–573. [CrossRef]
19. Scahill, L.; Riddle, M.A.; McSwiggin-Hardin, M.; Ort, S.I.; King, R.A.; Goodman, W.K.; Cicchetti, D.; Leckman, J.F. Children's Yale-Brown Obsessive Compulsive Scale: Reliability and validity. *J. Am. Acad. Child Adolesc. Psychiatry* **1997**, *36*, 844–852. [CrossRef]
20. Scahill, L.; Specht, M.; Page, C. The prevalence of tic disorders and clinical characteristics in children. *J. Obs. Compuls. Relat. Disord.* **2014**, *3*, 394–400. [CrossRef]
21. Lord, C.; Risi, S.; Lambrecht, L.; Cook, E.H., Jr.; Leventhal, B.L.; DiLavore, P.C.; Pickles, A.; Rutter, M. The autism diagnostic observation schedule-generic: A standard measure of social and communication deficits associated with the spectrum of autism. *J. Autism Dev. Disord.* **2000**, *30*, 205–223. [CrossRef]
22. Kim, S.H.; Lord, C. New autism diagnostic interview-revised algorithms for toddlers and young preschoolers from 12 to 47 months of age. *J. Autism Dev. Disord.* **2012**, *42*, 82–93. [CrossRef] [PubMed]
23. Hothorn, T.; Hornik, K.; Zeileis, A. Unbiased recursive partitioning: A conditional inference framework. *J. Comput. Graph. Stat.* **2006**, *15*, 651–674. [CrossRef]
24. Pine, D.S.; Guyer, A.E.; Goldwin, M.; Towbin, K.A. Autism spectrum disorder scale scores in pediatric mood and anxiety disorders. *Child Adolesc Psychiatry* **2008**, *47*, 652–661. [CrossRef] [PubMed]
25. Eapen, V.; McPherson, S.; Karlov, L.; Nicholls, L.; Črnčec, R.; Mulligan, A. Social communication deficits and restricted repetitive behavior symptoms in Tourette syndrome. *Neuropsychiatr. Dis. Treat.* **2019**, *15*, 2151–2160. [CrossRef]
26. Wu, M.S.; McGuire, J.F.; Arnold, E.B.; Lewin, A.B.; Murphy, T.K.; Storch, E.A. Psychometric properties of the Children's Yale-Brown Obsessive Compulsive Scale in youth with autism spectrum disorders and obsessive-compulsive symptoms. *Child Psychiatry Hum. Dev.* **2014**, *45*, 201–211. [CrossRef] [PubMed]
27. Scahill, L.; McDougle, C.J.; Williams, S.K.; Dimitropoulos, A.; Aman, M.G.; McCracken, J.T.; TIERNEY, E.; Arnold, L.E.; Cronin, P.; Grados, P.; et al. Children's Yale-Brown Obsessive Compulsive Scale modified for pervasive developmental disorders. *J. Am. Acad. Child Adolesc. Psychiatry* **2006**, *45*, 1114–1123. [CrossRef] [PubMed]
28. Zablotsky, B.; Black, L.I.; Maenner, M.J.; Schieve, L.A.; Blumberg, S.J. Estimated prevalence of autism and other developmental disabilities following questionnaire changes in the 2014 National Health Interview Survey. *Natl. Health Stat. Rep.* **2015**, *13*, 1–20.

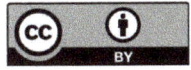

© 2020 by the authors. Licensee MDPI, Basel, Switzerland. This article is an open access article distributed under the terms and conditions of the Creative Commons Attribution (CC BY) license (http://creativecommons.org/licenses/by/4.0/).

MDPI
St. Alban-Anlage 66
4052 Basel
Switzerland
Tel. +41 61 683 77 34
Fax +41 61 302 89 18
www.mdpi.com

Actuators Editorial Office
E-mail: actuators@mdpi.com
www.mdpi.com/journal/actuators

www.ingramcontent.com/pod-product-compliance
Lightning Source LLC
LaVergne TN
LVHW070248100526
838202LV00015B/2191